SIXTH EDITION

Introduction to
PUBLIC HEALTH

Mary-Jane Schneider, PhD
Clinic Associate Professor and Assistant Dean Emerita
Department of Health Policy, Management and Behavior
School of Public Health
State University of New York at Albany
Rensselaer, New York

with

Henry S. Schneider, PhD
Associate Professor
Department of Public Health Sciences
School of Medicine
and
Stephen J.R. Smith School of Business
Queen's University
Kingston, Ontario

Drawings by Henry S. Schneider

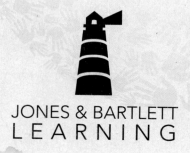

JONES & BARTLETT
LEARNING

World Headquarters
Jones & Bartlett Learning
5 Wall Street
Burlington, MA 01803
978-443-5000
info@jblearning.com
www.jblearning.com

Jones & Bartlett Learning books and products are available through most bookstores and online booksellers. To contact Jones & Bartlett Learning directly, call 800-832-0034, fax 978-443-8000, or visit our website, www.jblearning.com.

Substantial discounts on bulk quantities of Jones & Bartlett Learning publications are available to corporations, professional associations, and other qualified organizations. For details and specific discount information, contact the special sales department at Jones & Bartlett Learning via the above contact information or send an email to specialsales@jblearning.com.

19770-9

Production Credits
VP, Product Management: Amanda Martin
Director of Product Management: Laura Pagluica
Product Manager: Sophie Fleck Teague
Product Specialist: Sara Bempkins
Senior Project Specialist: Dan Stone
Senior Digital Project Specialist: Angela Dooley
Senior Marketing Manager: Susanne Walker
Product Fulfillment Manager: Wendy Kilborn

Composition: Exela Technologies
Cover Design: Michael O'Donnell
Cover Image/Part Opener Image: © Vectomart/Shutterstock
Text Design: Michael O'Donnell
Senior Media Development Editor: Troy Liston
Rights Specialist: Maria Leon Maimone
Printing and Binding: LSC Communications

Library of Congress Cataloging-in-Publication Data
Library of Congress Control Number: 2020930218

6048

Printed in the United States of America
25 24 23 22 21   10 9 8 7 6 5 4 3

To Allan S. Schneider

We will miss you

Brief Contents

Contents

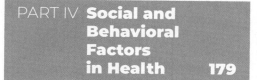

**PART IV Social and
Behavioral
Factors
in Health   179**

**PART VII The Future of
Public Health 445**

**Bonus Material in the eBook:
Learning from the COVID-19
Pandemic**

Preface

In the Preface to the *First Edition*, I wrote about the public's general ignorance of the field of public health and my own uncertainty about what public health was when, in 1986, I first went to work for the newly established School of Public Health, a collaboration between the University at Albany and the New York State Department of Health. After working with public health professionals from the Department of Health to design curricula for the programs at the school, and after teaching an introductory course in public health for more than 10 years in collaboration with many of the same health department faculty, I feel much more confident about what the term means. After the bioterrorism scare of 2001 and the public health disasters of Hurricane Katrina in 2005 and Hurricane Sandy in 2012, I believe that the public has a better sense of the field as well.

As I wrote in the Preface to the *First Edition*, I believe that every citizen should know something about public health, just as they should know something about democracy, law, and other functions of government. Public health issues are inherently interesting and important to almost everyone. They are featured almost every day on the front pages of newspapers and in the headlines of television news programs, although often they are not labeled as public health issues. One of my goals is to help people put these news stories into context when they occur.

The *Sixth Edition* of this text follows the plan of the first five editions, bringing it up-to-date and including new developments in infectious disease, injury control, environmental health controversies, the reform of the American healthcare system, and many other issues. I have illustrated public health principles by presenting stories that have been in the news; some of these stories have been ongoing sagas that have been supplemented with each edition. The *Second* and *Third Editions* focused on political interference with science, but as discussed in the *Fourth Edition*, the Obama administration vowed to restore honest science as a basis of policy decisions. Issues new to the *Fifth Edition* included the Ebola epidemic, the risks of traumatic brain injury to retired professional athletes, and the implementation of President Obama's healthcare reform law, the Patient Protection and Affordable Care Act. The *Sixth Edition* takes up the disaster of the opioid crisis, the arrival of the Zika virus and the resurgence of measles; the risks of driving while drugged, which the United States must now face with changing marijuana laws; and the rapid spread of vaping among America's youth. It also describes the reemergence of political interference with science during the Trump administration.

I have tried to make this text easily comprehensible to the general reader. One of the things that makes public health fascinating to me is the fact that it is often controversial, depending on political decisions as well as scientific evidence. The politics are frustrating to many practitioners, but it is often the politics that puts public health in the headlines. I hope that by describing both the science and the politics, I will contribute to making public health as fascinating to the readers as it is to me.

Mary-Jane Schneider

Public Health in the News

What is public health? It is an abstract concept, hard to pin down. Reports about public health appear in the news every day, but they are not labeled as public health stories, and most people do not recognize them as such. Here in the prologue are four major public health stories of the modern era that bring the abstraction to life. The ongoing AIDS epidemic, perhaps the greatest challenge that the public health community has faced in the past 50 years, illustrates the multidisciplinary nature of the field and the complex ethical and political issues that are often an inherent component of public health. The outbreak of waterborne disease that sickened more than 400,000 people in Milwaukee, Wisconsin, in 1993 was the consequence of a breakdown in a routine public health measure that has protected the populations of developed countries for most of the past century. Lest we forget that maintaining the health of the population requires constant vigilance, it has become apparent that white non-Hispanic American men and women in midlife, especially those with a high-school education or less, have been experiencing increases in mortality and morbidity since the turn of the century. The face of this decline is the opioid crisis, but the problems are rooted in more basic social and economic trends. Finally, the terrorist attacks in the fall of 2001 made it clear that the national security of the United States depends not only on the U.S. Department of Defense, but also on the American public health system.

AIDS Epidemic

On July 3, 1981, *The New York Times* ran a story with the headline: "Rare Cancer Seen in 41 Homosexuals."[1] The cancer was Kaposi's sarcoma, a form of skin cancer that is rare in the United States but more common in equatorial Africa. The victims were young gay men living in New York City or San Francisco, and 8 of the 41 had died within 24 months of being diagnosed. The report noted that several of the victims had been found to have severe defects in their immune systems, but it was not known whether the immune defects were the underlying problem or had developed later. Most of the victims had engaged in multiple and frequent sexual encounters with different partners, the article said, but there was no evidence that the disease was contagious, since none of the patients knew each other.

On August 29 of that same year, there was another story: "2 Fatal Diseases Focus of Inquiry."[2] A rare kind of pneumonia called pneumocystis had been striking gay men with a 60% fatality rate. According to *The New York Times*, 53 cases of pneumocystis had been diagnosed. Also, the number of cases of Kaposi's sarcoma had grown to 47, and 7 patients had both diseases. No one knew why gay men were affected, but speculation suggested that there might be a link to their sexual lifestyle, drug use, or some other environmental cause. The article noted without comment that one woman had also been reported to have pneumocystis pneumonia. A scientific task force had been formed at the Centers for Disease Control and Prevention (CDC) to investigate what was going on. There was no further news in *The New York Times* about what would become known as AIDS until May 1982.[3] In that article, the underlying commonality of the immune defect was recognized, and the condition was called gay-related immune deficiency syndrome (GRID). While immune deficiencies had been known and studied previously, most were genetic conditions that afflicted children from birth or were caused by immunosuppressive drugs used to prevent rejection of transplanted organs. The total suppression of the immune system by whatever means leads to many infections, one of which eventually kills the victim. Speculation about the cause of GRID generally focused on a sexually transmitted infectious agent, although there was a suspicion that multiple factors might be involved, perhaps including drugs or an immune response to the introduction of sperm into the blood through sexual contact.

As the number of reported cases grew, CDC scientists interviewed people with GRID, questioning them about their sexual behavior and partners. The sexual activities of gay men became the focus of scientists and the news media alike—reports of promiscuous and anonymous sex in public baths and use of drugs to enhance sexual pleasure emerged—which tended to worsen many people's already negative view of gay men. Linkages were found that began to confirm that a sexually transmitted infectious agent was responsible. But the investigations were hampered by lack of funding. President Ronald Reagan had been inaugurated

in January 1981 on a conservative platform, and his administration was not interested in a disease that affected people who behaved in ways so unappealing to the general population. Nor was there much concern on the part of the general public. Most people felt no threat to themselves, although people who lived in New York, San Francisco, Los Angeles, and Miami, where most of the cases had been reported, might have felt more cause for concern.

Since early in the epidemic, occasional reports had noted the presence of the immune deficiency in women and heterosexual men, many of them intravenous drug users. By the summer of 1982, cases of the syndrome had also been reported in people with hemophilia who were exposed to blood products used to make a clotting factor and in patients who had received blood transfusions. A study of female sexual partners of men with the syndrome suggested that the disease might also be transmitted by heterosexual relations. A number of babies turned up with a syndrome that resembled GRID, possibly transmitted from their mothers before or at birth. It was clear that the condition was not limited to gay men, and its name was changed to acquired immunodeficiency syndrome (AIDS). The public began to take notice.

By mid-1983, the public began to panic. A report by a pediatrician in New Jersey suggested that AIDS had spread within a family by routine household contact. That scared a lot of people: AIDS was a fatal disease, and people did not want to take any chances of catching it. Inmates in a New York State prison refused to eat meals in a mess hall used by a fellow inmate who had died of AIDS. A New York City sanitation worker with no known risk factors contracted AIDS, perhaps from a syringe protruding from a trash bag. In San Francisco, with its large gay population, the police officers demanded special masks and gloves for handling people suspected of being infected with AIDS. Blood banks reported that blood supplies were critically low because people wrongly feared that they could contract AIDS through donating blood. In New York City, tenants of a cooperative apartment building tried to evict a doctor known for treating people with AIDS. In a few well-publicized incidents, schools refused to allow children with AIDS—usually children with hemophilia—into the classroom. A special telephone information number on AIDS, set up by the federal government, was swamped with 8000 to 10,000 calls per day. Fundamentalist preachers and conservative legislators fulminated that AIDS was God's punishment for abominable behavior and that people with AIDS deserved their fate.

Meanwhile, although controversy still restricted federal funding for AIDS research, biomedical scientists were competing to identify the infectious agent, which most scientists believed would turn out to be a virus. Despite the ill repute of many AIDS patients, the disease was of great scientific interest, and the growing public concern promised to reward with acclaim and financial benefits the scientist who isolated the virus. On April 23, 1984, the U.S. Secretary of Health and Human Services convened a press conference to announce that Dr. Robert Gallo of the National Cancer Institute had discovered the virus—now known as the human immunodeficiency virus (HIV)—and that a vaccine would be available within five years.[4] While both of those statements proved to be less than accurate—Gallo's priority claim was disputed and eventually disproved, and after more than 35 years an effective vaccine has still not been developed—the discovery did promise to allow testing of blood for exposure to the virus. Just a year later, blood banks in the United States began screening donated blood, greatly reducing the risk to transfusion recipients and people with hemophilia.

Now, nearly four decades after the first reports on AIDS were publicized, most of the hysteria has faded, while many of the direst predictions have been realized. By the end of 2015, more than 1.2 million people in the United States had been diagnosed with AIDS, and approximately 700,000 had died, while an estimated 1,122,900 people were living in the United States with HIV.[5,6] The proportion of women diagnosed with HIV infection increased steadily over the first two decades and has remained stable since then at approximately 20%.[7] A great deal more is known about the disease. New drugs have "miraculously" restored health to some dying patients and offer hope that HIV is becoming a chronic, manageable condition rather than a progressively fatal disease. However, there is still no cure, and the only prevention is the avoidance of risky behaviors.

The question of how the government should respond to the AIDS epidemic raised some of the most difficult ethical and political issues imaginable in public health. Every new scientific discovery stimulated new dilemmas. Most of the controversies pitted two opposing principles against each other: the protection of the privacy and freedom of the individual suspected of being ill, and the protection of the health of potential victims at risk of being exposed. This conflict is common to many public health problems. Historically, the protection of the public has taken precedence over the rights of the individual. Thus, the principle of quarantining patients with dangerous infectious diseases such as plague, smallpox, or tuberculosis has been generally accepted and upheld by the courts. However, in the case of AIDS, the issues were more complicated.

Because people with AIDS belonged to stigmatized groups who may have been exposed to the virus through illegal behavior (intravenous drug use or homosexual acts that were still illegal in many states), they bitterly opposed being publicly identified. Gay men, who had only recently achieved a degree of liberation from public oppression, were very well organized politically; they effectively opposed some measures that would have normally been considered standard public health practice, such as reporting the names of diagnosed patients to the health department. They had well-founded fears of being discriminated against for jobs, housing, access to health insurance, and so on. Major political battles erupted over issues such as whether gay bathhouses should be closed and whether AIDS should be declared a communicable disease, which would legally require names of patients to be reported to the local health department. As HIV infection has become more controllable, much of the controversy surrounding it has subsided.

AIDS is particularly difficult for government to deal with because the only effective way to prevent its spread is to change people's behavior. There are precedents for governmental efforts aimed at promoting behavior change—campaigns to promote smoking cessation, use of bicycle helmets, and healthy diet and exercise—but their success has been mixed. Generally, the weight of a law adds significantly to the government's success in promoting healthy behavior, as in the case of seat belt laws and laws against drunk driving. However, the behavior that spreads HIV is very difficult to control by law; intravenous drug use is already illegal under federal law everywhere in the United States, and homosexual acts were also illegal in many states until the U.S. Supreme Court declared these laws unconstitutional in 2003. From the beginning, public health officials recognized that AIDS could be prevented only by persuading people to reduce their risk by limiting their exposure, which requires convincing them to control powerful biological and social urges.

Beginning with the earliest attempts at AIDS education, conflict arose between the attempt to communicate effectively with people most likely to be at risk and the likelihood of offending the general public by seeming to condone obscene or illegal acts. Conservatives argued—and still argue—that the only appropriate AIDS education message is abstinence from sex and drugs. C. Everett Koop, the Surgeon General of the United States when the AIDS epidemic emerged, was originally known for his right-to-life views. Later he became an unexpected hero to public health advocates by taking a strong stand in favor of frank AIDS education. While stressing the importance of mutually faithful monogamous sexual relationships and avoiding injected drugs, he nevertheless advocated education about the advantages of condoms and clean needles, and he urged schools to teach children about safe sex. In response, Senator Jesse Helms, a powerful conservative from North Carolina, denounced safe sex materials aimed at gay men as "promotion of sodomy" by the government and sponsored an amendment banning the use of federal funds "to provide AIDS education, information, or prevention materials and activities that promote or encourage, directly or indirectly, homosexual activities."[8(p.218)] Today, sexual education and condom availability programs, while not as strictly limited as they were in past decades, still face barriers. In New York City, for example, many public-school building are leased by the New York City Department of Education from the Catholic Church, which allows only abstinence-based sexual education and forbids condom availability programs on their premises.[9]

Drug regimens introduced in the mid-1990s that are capable of controlling the damage the virus wreaks on the immune system stimulated new medical, ethical, and economic challenges. These drugs have side effects that may prove fatal for some patients and have long-term adverse effects in others. Complicated regimens for taking many pills per day have been simplified, but new problems of viral strains resistant to the drugs have arisen. These strains may be transmitted to others. Moreover, the drugs are expensive, representing 60% of the projected $326,500 lifetime cost of HIV treatment per infected individual in the United States,[10] well beyond the budget of most patients, although government programs pay for the treatment of many patients. The federal government allocated $21.5 billion for HIV-related medical care in the United States in 2019.[11]

The history of the AIDS epidemic vividly illustrates that public health involves both science and politics. It took the science of epidemiology—the study of disease in human populations—to determine the basic nature of the disease and how it is transmitted. The biomedical sciences, especially virology and immunology, were crucial in identifying the infectious agent, determining how it causes its dire effects on the human organism, developing methods to identify virus-infected blood, and devising drugs that can hold the virus at bay. Biostatisticians help design the trials that test the effectiveness of new drugs and, eventually it is hoped, vaccines—believed to be the greatest hope for controlling the virus. In the meantime, behavioral scientists must find ways to convince people to avoid actions that spread the virus.

The politics of the AIDS epidemic shows the tension between individual freedom and the health of the community. There is a strong tradition of the use of police powers to protect the health of the public in all civilized societies. But the United States also has a strong tradition of individual liberty and civil rights. Politics determines the path the government will take in balancing these traditions. Public health is not based on scientific facts alone, but rather depends on politics to choose the values and ethics that determine how science will be applied to preserve people's health while protecting their fundamental rights.

Cryptosporidium in Milwaukee Water

In early April 1993, an outbreak of "intestinal flu" struck Milwaukee, causing widespread absenteeism among hospital employees, students, and schoolteachers. The symptoms included watery diarrhea that lasted for several days. The Milwaukee Department of Health, concerned about the burgeoning number of cases, contacted the Wisconsin State Health Department, and an investigation began.[12]

Stool samples from the most severely ill patients had been sent to clinical laboratories for testing, and these tests yielded the first clues about the cause of the illness. Two laboratories reported to the city health department that they had identified Cryptosporidium in samples

from seven adults. This organism was not one that most laboratories routinely tested for, but starting April 7, all 14 clinical laboratories began looking for it in all stool samples submitted to them—and they began finding it. Ultimately, 739 stool samples tested between March 1 and May 30 were found positive for Cryptosporidium.

Cryptosporidium is an intestinal parasite that is most commonly spread through contaminated water. In people who are basically healthy, the severe symptoms last a week or so. In addition to the watery diarrhea, the symptoms of infection with this pathogen include varying degrees of cramps, nausea, vomiting, and fever. The infection can be fatal in people with a compromised immune system, such as AIDS patients or people taking immunosuppressive drugs for organ transplants or cancer treatment.

In Milwaukee, public health officials immediately suspected the municipal water supply, which comes from Lake Michigan. They inspected records from the two water treatment plants that supplied the city, and suspicion immediately fell on the southern plant. The inspectors noted that the water's turbidity, or cloudiness, which was monitored once every 8 hours, had increased enormously beginning on March 21, an ominous sign. On April 7, city officials issued a warning, advising customers of the Milwaukee Water Works to boil their water before drinking it. On April 9, they temporarily closed the plant. Looking for evidence that the water was indeed contaminated with Cryptosporidium, they discovered that a southern Milwaukee company had produced and stored blocks of ice on March 25 and April 9. Testing confirmed that the organism was present in the ice.

Meanwhile, public health investigators were trying to determine how many people had been made sick by the contaminated water. Reasoning that only the most severely affected patients would go to a doctor and have their stools tested, they began a telephone survey of Milwaukee residents. On April 9, 10, and 12, they called randomly selected phone numbers and asked the first adult who answered whether anyone in the household had been sick since March 1. Of 482 respondents, 42% reported having had watery diarrhea, which was considered to be the defining symptom of the illness. In a more extensive telephone survey conducted on 1663 people in the greater Milwaukee area between April 28 and May 2, 30% of the respondents reported having had diarrhea. Half of the respondents whose water came from the southern plant reported the symptoms, while only 15% of those whose homes did not get water from the Milwaukee Water Works had been ill. These individuals had probably been exposed at work or from visiting the affected region.[12]

The investigators, who reported the results of their study in the *New England Journal of Medicine*, estimated that at least 403,000 people were made ill by the *Cryptosporidium* contamination of the Milwaukee water supply.[12] The number of deaths has been estimated to be 54; 85% of them were AIDS patients, whose compromised immune systems made them especially vulnerable.[13] In discussing how the contamination had occurred, the investigators speculated that unusually large amounts of the organism may have come from cattle farms, slaughterhouses, or human sewage swept into Lake Michigan by heavy spring rains and snow runoff. Flaws in the water treatment process of the southern plant led to inadequate removal of the parasites. After the problem was diagnosed, the southern water treatment plant was thoroughly cleaned, and a continuous turbidity monitor was installed that automatically sounds an alarm and shuts down the system if the turbidity rises above a certain level.

Cryptosporidium contamination is probably much more common than is generally recognized. It is difficult to control because the organisms are both widespread in the environment and resistant to chlorination and other commonly used water disinfection methods. *Cryptosporidium* was first recognized as a waterborne pathogen during an outbreak in Texas in 1984 that sickened more than 2000 people.[14] Many other pathogens may potentially surprise us with waterborne outbreaks; according to a report by the Institute of Medicine, only 1% of the organisms associated with disease that might be found in water have been identified.[15]

The United States has one of the safest public water supplies in the world. Nonetheless, according to the CDC, an estimated 4 million to 33 million cases of gastrointestinal illness associated with public drinking water systems occur annually.[16] Many communities are still using water treatment technology dating to World War I, while population growth, modern agricultural technology, toxic industrial wastes, and shifts in weather patterns due to climate change are challenging the limits of the aging infrastructure. Updating the infrastructure is expensive—but waterborne disease outbreaks are also expensive. An analysis of the Milwaukee outbreak in terms of medical and productivity costs done by scientists from the CDC, the City of Milwaukee Department of Health, the Wisconsin State Division of Public Health, and Emory University yielded an estimate of $96.2 million.[17] These authors estimated that, based on the approximately 7.7 million cases of waterborne disease annually, waterborne disease outbreaks cost $21.9 billion each year in the United States. They recommended that the cost of the outbreaks should be considered when costs of maintaining safe water supplies are calculated. Safe drinking water—one of the most fundamental public health measures—is by no means assured in the United States.

Deaths of Despair: The Declining Life Expectancy of White Americans

In 2012, the life expectancy of Americans at birth was 78.8 years. In 2017, it was 78.6 years.[18] This small downtick may at first glance seem innocuous, but it was the first time in nearly 80 years that life expectancy in the United States fell over a five-year period. Moreover, there were no contemporaneous high-casualty wars or disease outbreaks during this period, a major expansion of health insurance coverage had occurred, and the economy was increasingly thriving. The steady march forward in longevity in the United States, an apparent triumph of public health and modern medicine, had stopped. What was happening to the health of Americans?

A closer look at the data shows that the worrisome trend began in the late 1990s, and was driven by a sharp increase in mortality among less-educated middle-aged white Americans. The left panel of **Figure 1** shows this trend for 45- to 49-year-olds, along with the near mirror image for less-educated middle-aged black Americans. The deteriorating health of white Americans appears even more striking when juxtaposed to the continuing improvements among middle-aged residents of other rich countries, shown in the right panel of Figure 1. The gap in mortality rates between black and white Americans is shrinking, but perversely this is because white Americans are dying at increasing rates.

One immediate cause is what researchers Anne Case and Angus Deaton have famously called "deaths of despair"—suicide, alcohol-associated deaths, and drug overdoses, especially from opioids. **Figure 2** shows these alarming trends and how they center on the less educated.[19]

In 2017, there were 72,284 fatal drug overdoses in the United States (provisional data show a slight downtick since then, to 69,029 deaths over the 12 months ending February 2019).[20] This exceeds the peak annual number of U.S. deaths attributable to car crashes, 54,589 (in 1972); HIV, 50,628 (in 1995); and guns, 39,773 (in 2017).[21–23] The rate of fatal drug overdoses among whites ages 45 to 54 reached 40 per 100,000 in 2017, and overdose is now the leading cause of death of Americans younger than the age of 50.[23]

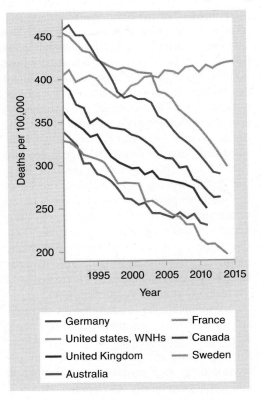

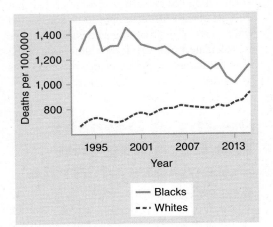

Figure 1 All-Cause Mortality Rates
Left panel: Black and white non-Hispanic Americans, ages 50 to 54, with a high school degree or less education, 1992–2015. Right panel: White non-Hispanic Americans (WNHs) and residents of other countries, ages 45 to 54, 1990–2015.

Reproduced from A. Case and A. Deaton, "Mortality and Morbidity in the 21st Century," *Brookings Papers on Economic Activity* 2017, no. 1 (2017), Figures 1.2 and 1.3.

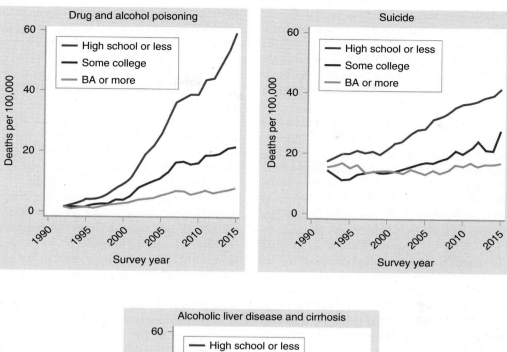

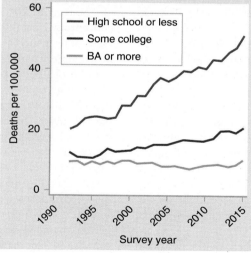

Figure 2 White Non-Hispanic Mortality of Americans Ages 50 to 54 by Education Class, 1992–2015

Reproduced from A. Case and A. Deaton, "Mortality and Morbidity in the 21st Century: Appendix," *Brookings Papers on Economic Activity* 2017, no. 1 (2017), Figure 7.

Nevertheless, deaths of despair do not wholly explain the increasing mortality. The other major contributor is a slowing in the decrease in heart disease mortality rate among whites. This rate had been falling by about 2% per year in the decades prior to 1999, but thereafter slowed to approximately 1% per year, with no decline at all occurring over the period 2009 to 2015. For blacks and Hispanics, heart disease mortality rates have continued to decline, falling 2.7% and 2.5% per year from 1999 to 2015, respectively. The reason for the slowing improvement in heart disease among whites is not entirely clear, but some experts believe the obesity epidemic in the United States, long expected to affect long-term health outcomes, is starting to appear. This explanation alone is not entirely satisfactory, however, as obesity rates for black and Hispanic Americans have also been increasing but without a slowing of heart disease improvements.[19]

Two factors in particular triggered the opioid crisis. First, in the 1990s, medical groups began arguing that untreated pain was pervasive and should be treated more aggressively. Previously, the medical profession had focused on treating acute pain, such as that experienced after surgery, but not chronic pain, such as that from a back injury.[24] Second, the pharmaceutical company Purdue Pharma introduced the painkiller OxyContin and undertook an intense marketing effort for this medication. The company's CEO stated that "the launch of OxyContin tablets will be followed by a blizzard of prescriptions that will bury the competition. The prescription blizzard will be so deep, dense, and white." The company's sales representatives advised doctors to push the highest doses possible because they were the most profitable, telling doctors that fewer than 1% of patients were susceptible to the risk of addiction—a wildly inaccurate claim with no scientific basis. The apparent logic was that the long-acting nature of OxyContin, compared to shorter-acting competitors like Percocet and Vicodin, would appeal less to drug abusers. The U.S. Food and Drug Administration (FDA) accepted this claim despite the lack of evidence, and it became the company's chief marketing message.[25]

Reports soon emerged that OxyContin was finding its way onto the black market, where users discovered they could crush the pills into white powder to create a pure high-grade heroin-like narcotic.[26] Despite the mounting human toll, the company continued to claim its drug was less addictive than alternatives and hired former New York City mayor and September 11 hero Rudolph (Rudy) Giuliani in 2002 to fend off governmental action.[27] These efforts generally worked until 2007, at which point the company was forced to settle claims that it had misrepresented the dangers of the drug. The company payed $635 million in fines and its top three executives pled guilty to misbranding the drug.[25] As researcher Angus Deaton noted in his 2018 testimony before the Joint Economic Committee of the U.S. Congress, "Selling heroin is profitable and illegal. Selling prescription drugs is profitable and legal. . . . Our health care system has sometimes been better at generating wealth than at generating health."[28]

In response to the alarming trends, Purdue eventually did replace OxyContin, in August 2010, with an abuse-deterrent reformulation, which when crushed turned into a gummy substance that was not easily snorted or injected. The street quickly adapted by moving from OxyContin to heroin, which had become readily available and was less expensive, and the rates of addiction and overdoses only accelerated.[24]

Starting in 2013, fentanyl, an even more concentrated painkiller, which had legitimate medical uses such as treating pain from open-heart surgery, emerged on the black market. Because of its low price and high potency, it was being cut into the formulation of illicit opioids. But the unregulated nature of this market meant that users often did not know what they were taking, leading many to consume far higher doses than they expected. This, in turn, has pushed the rate of overdoses even higher. **Figure 3** shows the trends in fatal opioid overdoses over the last two decades, including the three waves—prescription pills, heroin, fentanyl—that have killed so many Americans, among them musicians Prince, Tom Petty, Lil Peep, and Mac Miller, and actors Philip Seymour Hoffman and Heath Ledger.

While the drug epidemic has played a central role in the deteriorating health of less-educated white Americans, opioids are less the root cause than, in the words of Case and Deaton, "an accelerant . . . that added fuel to the fire, and made an already bad situation much worse."[28] The root cause is more complex and must also explain the

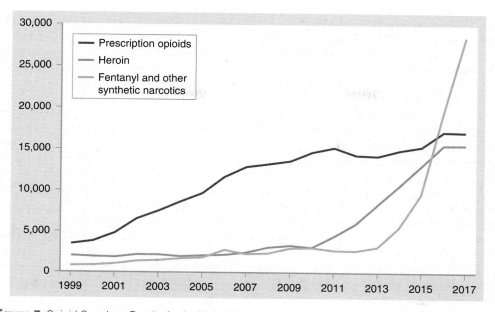

Figure 3 Opioid Overdose Deaths in the United States, 1999–2017

Data from National Center on Health Statistics, "Number of National Drug Overdose Deaths Involving Select Prescription and Illicit Drugs," CDC WONDER, National Institute on Drug Abuse, https://wonder.cdc.gov/mcd.html, accessed September 16, 2019.

continuing improvements in the health of more-educated white Americans, black and Hispanic Americans of all educational levels and ages, and residents of other rich countries. (Canada is perhaps most similar to the United States in having had 4460 opioid overdose fatalities—73% involving fentanyl—in 2018, in a country with about one-tenth of the U.S. population.[29]) The root cause must additionally account for the dramatic rise in suicide and alcohol deaths, both of which were well-known causes of death long before these recent trends emerged.

The increase in deaths of despair seems rooted in the sea change in American society that occurred in the 1980s and 1990s. Less-educated whites born in the 1960s and 1970s were hard hit by globalization and technological advances that shipped much of the manufacturing sector overseas, including its well-paying and previously stable careers that allowed people with limited formal education to enter the middle class. The deterioration of unions, due in part to conservative political

trends of the 1980s, facilitated this transition. Women became increasingly independent and had less practical need for men without stable earnings. The influence of religion and other social institutions that connected communities was waning. Collectively, these factors meant that the social fabric of society had weakened significantly for some Americans.[19]

To illustrate the point, among white Americans with a high school degree or less, only 7% of the cohort born in 1960 were out of the workforce by age 35 (in 1995). For the cohort born in 1980, 18% were out of the workforce by age 35 (in 2015). Similarly, for the 1960 cohort, 13% had never been married by age 35, while for the 1980 cohort, 20% had never been married at age 35. In contrast, more-educated white Americans showed no change in these life determinants over time.[19] Moreover, survey evidence shows that half of men out of the workforce are taking pain medication, and two-thirds of these are taking prescription painkillers such as opioids.[30] In the words of Case and Deaton, "These slow acting and cumulative social forces . . . work through their effects on family, on spiritual fulfillment, and on how people perceive meaning and satisfaction in their lives in a way that goes beyond material success. At the same time, cumulative distress, and the failure of life to turn out as expected is consistent with people compensating through other risky behavior such as abuse of alcohol, overeating, or drug use."[19]

It now appears that Purdue Pharma, the maker of OxyContin, will settle lawsuits filed against the company on behalf of the roughly 200,000 Americans who have died, and for the additional damage that has been caused, from its products. The company and the family that owns it are expected to pay approximately $15 billion to more than 2000 state and local governments in an outcome reminiscent of the Tobacco Master Settlement Agreement of 1998 (discussed in Chapter 15, Public Health Enemy Number One: Tobacco). The company will also be dissolved and a new one will be formed that will continue to sell pharmaceuticals, but with its profits going to the plaintiffs. Meanwhile, Purdue Pharma will develop and provide drugs for addiction and overdose treatment.[31] Unfortunately, the problems facing less-educated middle-aged white Americans may get worse before they get better: As they reach old age, their health problems are likely to compound.

The declining health of less-educated white Americans illustrates the complex interaction between class, race, societal institutions, and availability of vices such as opioids in determining the health of the public. Some of these factors fall squarely within the domain of public health to address, whereas others are more entrenched and require broader efforts to rectify.

Public Health and Terrorism

On September 11, 2001, the United States was attacked by foreign terrorists, and Americans entered a new phase of civic life. Four passenger airliners were simultaneously hijacked;

three were crashed into buildings filled with people going about their work, and one crashed in an empty field in Pennsylvania, apparently headed for another target but stopped by passengers.

The immediate public reaction to these disasters was the activation of emergency response plans in the regions where the crashes occurred. Police, firefighters, and ambulances rushed to the scenes; hospital emergency rooms were alerted; extra doctors and nurses were called in. In the New York City area, healthcare facilities in the whole region readied themselves to receive the expected large numbers of people wounded at the World Trade Center. Unfortunately, much of this preparation was not utilized because there were so few injured people who survived.

Although the disaster of September 11 was unprecedented in its magnitude, it was similar in kind to other emergencies and disasters for which communities plan: plane and train crashes, factory explosions, earthquakes, hurricanes, and so on. In New York, public health agencies were concerned not only with coordinating emergency medical care, but also with ensuring the safety of cleanup workers and area residents. Problems with polluted water, contaminated air, spoiled food, infestation of vermin, and so on, had to be dealt with in lower Manhattan just as they must be dealt with after any natural disaster. The longer-term response to September 11 has focused on law enforcement and national defense, with the goal of preventing future hostile acts by terrorists. The federal government has tightened security at airports and borders; it has attacked or warned foreign countries thought to harbor terrorists; and national intelligence agencies have increased their surveillance of persons and groups suspected of being a threat to the United States, to the extent that there are concerns that civil liberties are being eroded.

In contrast to the dramatic events of September 11, the second terrorist attack occurring in autumn 2001 became apparent only gradually. On October 2, Robert Stevens, an editor for a supermarket tabloid, was admitted to a Florida hospital emergency room suffering from a high fever and disorientation. An infectious disease specialist made a diagnosis of anthrax, in part because of heightened suspicions of bioterrorism provoked by the September 11 attacks. The doctor notified the county health department, which notified the state and the CDC. After further tests, the health agencies announced on October 4 that a case of inhalational anthrax had been confirmed. An intensive investigation into the source of exposure began at once. Stevens died on October 5.[32,33]

On that same day, another case was diagnosed in a worker at the same tabloid office where Stevens worked. Tests done throughout the building detected a few anthrax spores on Stevens's computer keyboard and more in the mailroom. The building was closed, and all employees were offered antibiotics to protect them against the development of disease.

On October 9, the New York City Department of Health announced that a newsroom worker at NBC in New York City had developed cutaneous anthrax. She had handled a suspicious letter containing a powder, later identified as anthrax spores.[34] Shortly after, a 7-month-old infant, who had visited his mother's workplace at ABC-TV 2 weeks earlier, was diagnosed with cutaneous anthrax. The child had developed a severe, intractable skin lesion that progressed to severe anemia and kidney failure, but anthrax had not been suspected as a cause of these symptoms. After two weeks in the hospital, the infant was correctly diagnosed with anthrax and given antibiotics; he gradually recovered, as did the NBC worker.[35] By this time, it was clear that the outbreak was intentionally caused and that a bioterror attack was under way.

On October 15, a staff member working in Senator Tom Daschle's office in Washington, D.C., opened a letter and noticed a small burst of powder from it. Alert to the threat of anthrax, the aide notified the police and the Federal Bureau of Investigation (FBI), and the area was vacated. The letter tested positive for anthrax. Staff and visitors who were potentially exposed were offered antibiotics, as were workers in the Capitol's mailrooms.[36]

The bad news continued. At about the same time that workers in the media and in Congress were being exposed to anthrax, the disease was breaking out in postal workers in New Jersey, Maryland, and Virginia, although it took days to weeks to recognize what was happening. While it was known by mid-October that anthrax spores were being sent through the mail, they were not believed to escape from sealed envelopes. As it turned out, postal workers were among the most affected by the outbreak. The Brentwood Mail Processing and Distribution Center in the District of Columbia was closed on October 21 after four postal workers were hospitalized with inhalational anthrax; two of these workers died.[37]

All told, a total of 22 cases of anthrax were diagnosed over a 2-month period, of which 11 were the inhalational form. Five of the latter group died, one of whom was a 94-year-old woman in Connecticut whose source of exposure was never verified. It was surmised that a piece of mail received at her home had been cross-contaminated by another piece of mail at a postal facility.[38] The CDC estimated that 32,000 potentially exposed people received prophylactic antibiotic therapy, which may have prevented many more cases.[39] Contaminated buildings, including five U.S. Postal Service facilities, had to be closed and laboriously decontaminated; some of these buildings could not be reopened for more than a year.[40,41]

Investigation of postal service records determined that letters to the media were mailed in Trenton, New Jersey, in mid-September. The letter to Senator Daschle and one to Senator Patrick Leahy, which was not opened until it was irradiated to kill the bacteria, were mailed in Trenton on October 9. A number of hoax letters—similar to the anthrax letters, and some containing innocuous white powder—were also mailed to media and government offices from St. Petersburg, Florida. Since they were sent before the news broke about the anthrax letters, they were presumably sent by the same person.

The perpetrator of the anthrax mailings was finally identified in 2008 as a scientist working on drugs and vaccines against anthrax at the U.S. Army Medical Research Institute of Infectious Diseases. As the FBI began to close in on him as a suspect, Bruce Ivins committed suicide. Many of his colleagues doubt that he was responsible, and the case will never be proven in court. The U.S. Department of Justice released its evidence against Ivins and requested that the National Academy of Sciences conduct a review of the evidence.[42] The Academy's report concluded that the evidence was consistent with Dr. Ivins's lab being the source of the anthrax spores but did not prove it.[43] Meanwhile, the anthrax letters that were sent to Senators Daschle and Leahy, and the New Jersey mail collection box from which the letter was mailed, were decontaminated and in 2014 were put on display at the Smithsonian Institution's National Postal Museum in Washington, D.C.[44]

The anthrax attacks terrorized the population far beyond the actual damage done. They also disrupted the public health and emergency response systems out of proportion to the actual threat. Any encounter with white powder evoked panic, causing people to send samples to public health laboratories for testing. At New York State's Wadsworth Center in Albany, scientists worked around the clock throughout the fall, testing more than 900 samples. Some of the unlikely specimens sent for testing were a pair of jeans, a box of grape tomatoes, a box of Tic Tac breath fresheners, and several packets of cash from automatic teller machines. The largest amount of cash submitted at one time was $8000, carefully guarded and picked up by police immediately after the anthrax tests proved to be negative (L. Sturman, personal communication).

The events that occurred in the autumn of 2001 disturbed Americans' sense of security within their borders. The 9/11 terrorists' hijacking of four airplanes prompted major efforts to strengthen homeland security through more rigorous screening of airline passengers and of international travelers at the borders—precautions that are now routine and are expected to be maintained. The anthrax attacks called attention to the fact that the public health system is America's best protection from bioterrorism. Increased funding for disease surveillance, public health laboratories, and emergency response systems has strengthened the ability of the public health system to respond to bioterrorist attacks as well as to natural disasters and epidemics. These precautions are just as important as other homeland security measures for Americans to be safe in their homeland.

References

1. L. Altman, "Rare Cancer Seen in 41 Homosexuals," *The New York Times*, July 3, 1981.
2. Associated Press, "2 Fatal Diseases Focus of Inquiry," *The New York Times*, August 29, 1981.
3. L. Altman, "New Homosexual Disorder Worries Health Officials," *The New York Times*, May 11, 1982.
4. L. Garrett, *The Coming Plague: Newly Emerging Diseases in a World Out of Balance* (New York, NY: Farrar, Straus, and Giroux, 1994).
5. Centers for Disease Control and Prevention, "HIV in the United States: At a Glance," https//www.cdc.gov/hiv/statistics/basics/ataglance.html, accessed September 4, 2015 and July 24, 2019.
6. Centers for Disease Control and Prevention, "CDC Fact Sheet: Today's HIV/AIDS Epidemic," https://www.cdc.gov/nchhstp/newsroom/docs/factsheets/todaysepidemic-508.pdf, accessed July 24, 2019.
7. Centers for Disease Control and Prevention, "HIV Surveillance Report, 2016," 2017, https://www.cdc.gov/hiv/library/reports/hiv-surveillance.html, accessed July 24, 2019.

8. R. Bayer, *Private Acts, Social Consequences: AIDS and the Politics of Public Health* (New York, NY: Free Press, 1989), p. 218.

9. Office of the New York City Comptroller Scott M. Stringer, "Healthy Relationships: A Plan for Improving Health and Sexual Education in New York City Schools," September 2017, https://comptroller.nyc.gov/wp-content/uploads/documents/Comprehensive_Sex-Ed_Final.pdf, accessed July 24, 2019.

10. E. G. Martin and B. R. Schackman. "Treating and Preventing HIV with Generic Drugs: Barriers in the United States," *New England Journal of Medicine* 378 (2018): 316–319.

11. Kaiser Family Foundation, "Fact Sheet: U.S. Federal Funding for HIV/AIDS: Trends Over Time," March 2019, https://www.kff.org/hivaids/fact-sheet/u-s-federal-funding-for-hivaids-trends-over-time/, accessed July 24, 2019.

12. W. R. MacKenzie, N. J. Hoxie, M. E. Proctor, M. S. Gradus, K. A. Blair, D. E. Peterson, et al., "A Massive Outbreak in Milwaukee of Cryptosporidium Infection Transmitted Through the Public Water Supply," *New England Journal of Medicine* 331 (1994): 161–167.

13. N. J. Hoxie, J. P. Davis, J. M. Vergeront, R. D. Nashold, and K. A. Blair, "Cryptosporidiosis-Associated Mortality Following a Massive Waterborne Outbreak in Milwaukee, Wisconsin," *American Journal of Public Health* 87 (1997): 2032–2035.

14. U.S. Environmental Protection Agency, "Cryptosporidium: Drinking Water Health Advisory," EPA-822-R-01-009, March 2001, https://www.epa.gov/sites/production/files/2015-10/documents/cryptosporidium-report.pdf, accessed September 23, 2019.

15. L. Reiter et al., eds., *From Source Water to Drinking Water: Workshop Summary* (Washington, DC: National Academies Press, 2004).

16. Centers for Disease Control and Prevention, "Notice to Readers: National Drinking Water Week—May 4–10, 2008," *Morbidity and Mortality Weekly Report* 57 (2008): 465–466.

17. P. S. Corso, M. H. Kramer, K. A. Blair, D. G. Addiss, J. P. Davis, and A. C. Haddix, "Cost of Illness in the 1993 Waterborne *Cryptosporidium* Outbreak, Milwaukee, Wisconsin," *Emerging Infectious Diseases* 9 (2003): 426–431.

18. Centers for Disease Control and Prevention, "United States Life Tables, 2017," *National Statistics Vital Reports* 68, no. 7 (2019), https://www.cdc.gov/nchs/data/nvsr/nvsr68/nvsr68_07-508.pdf, accessed September 14, 2019.

19. A. Case and A. Deaton, "Mortality and Morbidity in the 21st Century." *Brookings Papers on Economic Activity 2017*, no. 1 (2017).

20. Centers for Disease Control and Prevention, "Provisional Drug Overdose Death Counts," Vital Statistics Rapid Release, https://www.cdc.gov/nchs/nvss/vsrr/drug-overdose-data.htm, accessed September 16, 2019.

21. J. Katz, "Drug Deaths in America Are Rising Faster Than Ever," *The New York Times*, June 5, 2017.

22. Centers for Disease Control and Prevention, "HIV Surveillance—United States, 1981–2008," *Morbidity and Mortality Weekly Report* 60, no. 21 (2011).

23. Centers for Disease Control and Prevention, "Deaths: Final Data for 2017," *National Vital Statistics Report* 68, no. 9 (June 24, 2019): Table 6, https://www.cdc.gov/nchs/data/nvsr/nvsr68/nvsr68_09-508.pdf, accessed September 16, 2019.

24. W. N. Evans, E. M. J. Lieber, and P. Power, "How the Reformulation of OxyContin Ignited the Heroin Epidemic," *Review of Economics and Statistics* 101, no. 1 (2019).

25. B. Meier, "Origins of an Epidemic: Purdue Pharma Knew Its Opioids Were Widely Abused," *The New York Times*, May 29, 2018.

26. B. Meier, "Sacklers Directed Efforts to Mislead Public About OxyContin, Court Filing Claims," *The New York Times*, January 15, 2019.

27. B. Meier and E. Lipton, "Under Attack, Drug Maker Turned to Giuliani for Help," *The New York Times*, December 28, 2007.

28. A. Deaton, "Economic Aspects of the Opioid Crisis," Testimony Before the Joint Economic Committee of the United States Congress, June 8, 2017.

29. Government of Canada, "National Report: Apparent Opioid-related Deaths in Canada," June 2019, https://health-infobase.canada.ca/datalab/national-surveillance-opioid-mortality.html, accessed September 17, 2019.

30. A. B. Krueger, "Where Have All the Workers Gone? An Inquiry into the Decline of the US Labor Force Participation Rate," *Brookings Papers on Economic Activity 2017*, no. 2 (2017).

31. J. Hoffman, "Sacklers Would Give up Ownership of Purdue Pharma Under Settlement Proposal, *The New York Times*, August 27, 2019.

32. Centers for Disease Control and Prevention, "Update: Investigation of Anthrax Associated with Intentional Exposure and Interim Public Health Guidelines," *Morbidity and Mortality Weekly Report* 50 (October 2001): 889–891.

33. S. G. Stolberg, "Anthrax Threat Points to Limits in Health System," *The New York Times*, October 14, 2001.

34. L. K. Altman, "A Nation Challenged: NBC; Doctor in City Reported Anthrax Case Before Florida," *The New York Times*, October 18, 2001.

35. D. Grady, "Report Notes Swift Course of Inhalational Anthrax," *The New York Times*, February 20, 2002.

36. Centers for Disease Control and Prevention, "Update: Investigation of Bioterrorism-Related Anthrax and Interim Guidelines for Exposure Management and Antimicrobial Therapy, October 2001," *Morbidity and Mortality Weekly Report* 50 (2001): 909–919.

37. Centers for Disease Control and Prevention, "Evaluation of *Bacillus anthracis* Contamination Inside the

Brentwood Mail Processing and Distribution Center—District of Columbia, October 2001," *Morbidity and Mortality Weekly Report* 50 (2001): 1129–1133.

38. Centers for Disease Control and Prevention, "Update: Investigation of Bioterrorism-Related Anthrax—Connecticut, 2001," *Morbidity and Mortality Weekly Report* 50 (2001): 1077–1079.

39. Centers for Disease Control and Prevention, "Update: Investigation of Bioterrorism-Related Anthrax and Adverse Events from Antimicrobial Prophylaxis, 2001," *Morbidity and Mortality Weekly Report* 50 (2001): 973–976.

40. Centers for Disease Control and Prevention, "Follow-up of Deaths Among U.S. Postal Service Workers Potentially Exposed to *Bacillus anthracis*—District of Columbia, 2001–2002," *Morbidity and Mortality Weekly Report* 52 (2003): 937–938.

41. I. Peterson, "Postal Center Hit by Anthrax Is Now Clean, Officials Say," *The New York Times*, February 10, 2004.

42. S. Shane, "Portrait Emerges of Anthrax Suspect's Troubled Life," *The New York Times*, January 3, 2009.

43. National Research Council, Review of the Scientific Approaches Used During the FBI's Investigation of the 2001 Anthrax Letters (Washington, DC: National Academies Press, 2011); https://www.nap.edu/catalog/13098/review-of-the-scientific-approaches-used-during-the-fbis-investigation-of-the-20010anthrax-letters, accessed September 23, 2019.

44. J. Landers, "The Anthrax Letters That Terrorized a Nation Are Now Contaminated and on Public View," *Smithsonian.com*, September 12, 2016, https://www.smithsonianmag.com/smithsonian-institution/anthrax-letters-terrorized-nation-now-decontaminated-public-view-180960407/, accessed July 24, 2019.

About the Authors

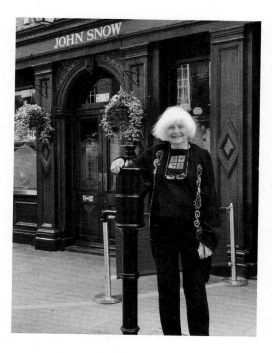

Mary-Jane Schneider earned a B.S. in chemistry at the University of Rochester and a Ph.D. in biophysics in 1967 at the University of California, Berkeley, where she met her husband, Allan, also a Ph.D. student. They spent two years as postdoctoral fellows at the Weizmann Institute of Science in Israel. On returning to the United States, Mary-Jane worked as a science writer at the National Cancer Institute in Bethesda, Maryland. She and Allan then moved to New York City where their sons Henry and Joseph were born, and Mary-Jane continued writing about science at the New York Academy of Sciences and then at the Albert Einstein College of Medicine.

In 1986, the family moved to Albany, New York, where Mary-Jane accepted a position at the newly formed School of Public Health, a collaboration between the University at Albany of the State University of New York and the New York State Department of Health. She worked with faculty committees to design academic programs for the School, including Master of Public Health and Doctor of Public Health programs. She later became the director of those programs. Once the School was firmly established, administrators at the University pressed the School to teach an undergraduate course, so as to introduce undergraduate students to the field. Mary-Jane volunteered to coordinate that course, which was team taught by faculty from the Department of Health and the University, beginning in 1994. She searched for a textbook and, finding none, decided to write one herself. That first edition was dated 2000. Much of what she initially learned about public health and included in the book came from attending those lectures by practitioners of the field.

A fortunate result of his mom's career path was that **Henry Schneider** has been immersed in public health from a young age, discussing the issues of the day at the dinner table with his mother Mary-Jane. Henry went on to study physics at Wesleyan University, where he received a B.S. in 1996, and economics at Yale University, where he received a Ph.D. in 2006. Following graduate work, Henry was a professor at Cornell University for a decade. In 2016, he moved across the border to Canada, where he is now a professor in both the Department of Public Health Sciences and the Stephen J.R. Smith School of Business at Queen's University, one of the leading research schools in Canada. Inspired by pathbreaking work in medicine, his recent research examines how checklists affect worker behavior, including why checklists seem to improve the quality of medical care in some settings but not in others. His other recent work examines how small psychologically based interventions – so-called "nudges" – can influence people to make healthier and more fulfilling decisions. Henry's background and knowledge has been an invaluable contribution and support in the development of this text.

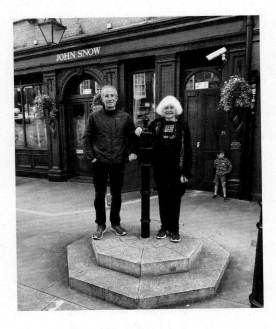

Mary-Jane and **Henry** in London at the Broad Street pump, the birthplace of modern epidemiology, in October 2019. Henry's son Gus is in the background, leaning against the John Snow Pub, which is named after the famous first epidemiologist, Dr. John Snow, who identified the Broad Street pump as the source of the 1854 cholera epidemic that killed 616 local residents. (See Chapter 4, *Epidemiology: The Basic Science of Public Health*, for more on John Snow and his work.)

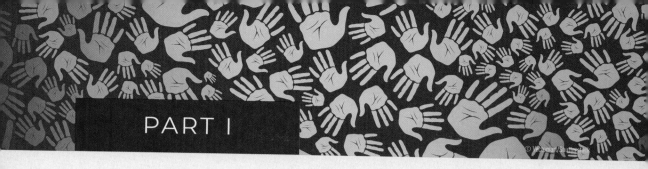

PART I

What Is Public Health?

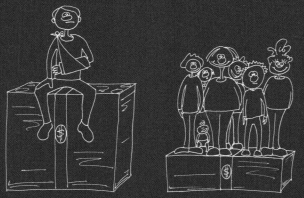

CHAPTER 1

Medical Care Versus Public Health

Public Health: Science, Politics, and Prevention

KEY TERMS

Assessment
Assurance
Biomedical sciences
Bioterrorism
Community

Epidemiology
Infectious disease
Interventions
Life expectancy
Policy development

Primary prevention
Public health
Secondary prevention
Statistics
Tertiary prevention

One expectation about living in a civilized society is that the living conditions will be basically healthy. Unless something unusual happens, like the outbreak of *Cryptosporidium* that affected the Milwaukee, Wisconsin, water supply, people assume that they are basically safe: Their water is safe to drink; the hamburger they buy at the fast-food restaurant is safe to eat; the aspirin they take for a headache is what the label says it is; and they are not likely to be hit by a car—or a bullet—if they use reasonable caution in walking down the street.

In historical terms, this expectation is a relatively recent development. In the mid-19th century, when record-keeping began in England and Wales, death rates were very high, especially among children. Of every 10 newborn infants, two or three never reached their first birthday. Five or six died before they were six years old, and only about

three of the 10 lived beyond the age of 25.[1] Tuberculosis was the single largest cause of death in the mid-19th century. Epidemics of cholera, typhoid, and smallpox swept through communities, killing people of all ages and making them afraid to leave their homes. Injuries—often fatal—to workers in mines and factories were common due to unsafe equipment, long working hours, poor lighting and ventilation, and child labor.

There are a number of reasons why people's lives are generally healthier today than they were 150 years ago: cleaner water, air, and food; safe disposal of sewage; better nutrition; more knowledge concerning healthy and unhealthy behaviors; and many others. Most of these factors fall within the domain of **public health**. In fact, the term "public health" refers to two different but related concepts. First, we can say that public health has improved since the 19th century, meaning that the general state of people's health is now much better than it was. Second, the measures that people take as a society to bring about and maintain that improvement are also known as public health.

Although many sectors of the **community** may be involved in promoting public health, people most often look to government—at the local, state, or national level—to take the primary responsibility for this realm. Governments provide pure water and efficient sewage disposal. Governmental regulations ensure the safety of the food supply. They also ensure the quality of medical services provided through hospitals, nursing homes, and other institutions. Laws regulating people's behavior prevent them from injuring each other. Laws requiring immunization of school-aged children prevent the spread of **infectious diseases**. Governments also sponsor research and education programs on causes and prevention of disease.

What Is Public Health?

Public health is not easy to define or to comprehend. A telephone survey of registered voters conducted in 1999 by a charitable foundation found that more than half of the 1234 respondents misunderstood the term.[2] Leaders in the field have themselves struggled to understand the mission of public health, to explain what it is, why it is important, and what it should do. Charles-Edward A. Winslow, a theoretician and leader of American public health during the first half of the 20th century, defined public health in 1920 this way:

> The science and the art of preventing disease, prolonging life, and promoting physical health and efficiency through organized community efforts for the sanitation of the environment, the control of community infections, the education of the individual in principles of personal hygiene, the

organization of medical and nursing services for the early diagnosis and preventive treatment of disease, and the development of the social machinery which will ensure to every individual in the community a standard of living adequate for the maintenance of health.[3(p.1)]

Winslow's definition is still considered valid today.

Over the following decades, public health had many successes, carrying out many of the tasks described in Winslow's definition. It was highly effective in reducing the threat of infectious diseases, thereby increasing the average lifespan of Americans by several decades. By the 1980s, public health was taken for granted, and most people were unaware of its activities. Yet some signs indicated that the system was not functioning well. Government expenditures on health were alarmingly high, but most of the spending was directed toward medical care. No one was talking about public health. At the same time, new health problems began appearing: The acquired immunodeficiency syndrome (AIDS) epidemic broke out, concern about environmental pollution was growing, the aging population was demanding increased health services, and social problems such as teenage pregnancy, violence, and substance abuse were becoming more common. There was a sense that public health was not prepared to deal with these problems, in part because people were not thinking of them as public health problems.

A study conducted by the Institute of Medicine (now the National Academy of Medicine) and published in 1988 called *The Future of Public Health* refocused attention on the importance of public health and did a great deal to revitalize the field. One of the first tasks the study committee set for itself was to reexamine the definition of public health, reasoning that for it to be effective, public health had to be broadly defined.[4] The committee's report gives a four-part definition describing public

---

Table 1-1 **The Ten Essential Public Health Services**

Assessment

1. Monitor health status to identify community health problems

2. Diagnose and investigate health problems and health hazards in the community

Policy Development

3. Inform, educate, and empower people about health issues

4. Mobilize community partnerships to identify and solve health problems

5. Develop policies and plans that support individual and community health efforts

Assurance

6. Enforce laws and regulations that protect health and ensure safety

7. Link people to needed personal health services and assure the provision of health care when otherwise unavailable

8. Assure a competent public health and personal healthcare workforce

9. Evaluate effectiveness, accessibility, and quality of personal and population-based health services

Serving All Functions

10. Research for new insights and innovative solutions to health problems

---

health's mission, substance, organizational framework, and core functions.

The Future of Public Health defines the mission of public health as "the fulfillment of society's interest in assuring the conditions in which people can be healthy."[4(p.40)] The substance of public health is "organized community efforts aimed at the prevention of disease and the promotion of health."[4(p.41)] The organizational framework of public health encompasses "both activities undertaken within the formal structure of government and the associated efforts of private and voluntary organizations and individuals."[4(p.42)] Public health has the following three core functions:

1. Assessment
2. Policy development
3. Assurance[4(p.43)]

Another committee later translated these core functions into a more concrete set of activities called the Ten Essential Public Health Services (**Table 1-1**).

Public Health Versus Medical Care

One way to better understand public health and its functions is to compare and contrast them with medical practice. Whereas medicine is concerned with individual patients, public health regards the community as its patient, trying to improve the health of the population. Medicine focuses on healing patients who are ill; public health focuses on preventing illness.

In carrying out its core functions, public health—like a doctor working with a patient—assesses the health of a population, diagnoses its problems, seeks the causes of those problems, and devises strategies to cure them. **Assessment** constitutes the diagnostic function, in which a public health agency collects, assembles, analyzes, and makes available information on the health of the population. **Policy development**, like a doctor's development of a treatment plan for a sick patient, involves the use of scientific knowledge to develop a strategic approach to improving the community's health. **Assurance** is equivalent to the doctor's actual treatment of the patient. Public health has the responsibility of assuring that the services needed for the protection of public health in the community are available and accessible to everyone. These include environmental, educational, and basic medical services. If public health agencies do not provide these services themselves, they must encourage others to do so or require such actions through regulation.

Public health's focus on prevention makes it more abstract than medicine, and its achievements are therefore more difficult to recognize. The doctor who cures a sick person has achieved a real, recognizable benefit, and the patient is grateful. Public health cannot point to the people who have been spared illness by its efforts. As Winslow wrote in 1923, "If we had but the gift of second sight to transmute abstract figures into flesh and blood, so that as we walk along the street we could say, 'That man would be dead of typhoid fever,' 'That woman would have succumbed to tuberculosis,' 'That rosy infant would be in its coffin,'— then only should we have a faint conception of the meaning of the silent victories of public health."[3(p.65)]

This "silence" accounts in large part for the relative lack of attention paid to public health by politicians and the general public in comparison with medical care. It is estimated that less than 3% of the United States' total health spending is devoted to public health.[5]

During the presidential campaigns leading up to the 2016 and 2020 elections, virtually all of the discussion related to health focused on how to pay for medical care, ranging from a Medicare-for-all–style single-payer system at one extreme to a privatized Medicare at the other extreme, yet very little attention was paid to funding for public health. In contrast, President Barack Obama's health reform law, passed in 2010, did include significant provisions and funding for prevention, wellness, and public health.[6]

Effective public health programs clearly save money on medical costs in addition to saving lives. Moreover, public health contributes a great deal more to the health of a population than medicine does. While the **life expectancy** of Americans increased from 47 to 77 years over the course of the 20th century, only 5 of those 30 additional years can be attributed to the work of the medical care system.[7,8] The majority of the gain has come from improvements in public health, broadly defined as including better nutrition, housing, sanitation, and occupational safety. The striking benefits of public health continue apace. According to recent analyses, the introduction of the pneumococcal conjugate vaccine into the routine infant immunization program in the United States in 2000 prevented 13,000 deaths between 2000 and 2008, while an improvement in this vaccine in 2010 averted an additional 1000 deaths per year.[9,10] One responsibility of public health, therefore, as noted in the Institute of Medicine report, is to educate the public and politicians about "the crucial role that a strong public health capacity must play in maintaining and improving the health of the public . . . By its very nature, public health requires support by members of the public—its beneficiaries."[4(p.32)]

Public health, like medical practice, is based on science. However, even when public health scientists are certain they know all about the causes of a problem and what should be done about it, a political decision is generally necessary before action can be taken to solve it. When a doctor diagnoses a patient's illness and recommends a treatment, the patient has the prerogative to accept or reject the doctor's recommendation. When the "patient" is a community or a whole country, usually a government—federal, state, or local—must make the decision to accept or reject the recommendations of public health experts. Sometimes the process starts within the community when, like a patient going to a doctor with a complaint, the people recognize a problem and demand that the government take action. This has occurred in many communities when victims of drunk drivers form organizations such as Mothers Against Drunk Driving (MADD) to lobby for stricter laws, or when neighbors of pollution-generating factories demand that the government force the industry to clean up the environment.

Politics enters the public health process as part of the policy development function and especially as part of the assurance function. Since the community will have to pay for the "treatments," usually through taxes, they must decide how much "health" they are willing to fund. They also must decide whether they are willing to accept the possible limitations on their freedom that may be required to improve the community's health. Among the assurance functions of public health is the provision of basic medical services: How this should be done has been a matter of great political controversy. Public health professionals are often impatient with politics, as the Institute of Medicine report notes, seeming to "regard politics as a contaminant of an ideally rational decision-making process rather than as an essential element of democratic governance."[4(p.5)]

The Sciences of Public Health

The scientific knowledge on which public health is based spans a broad range of professional disciplines. The Institute of Medicine report notes that "public health is a coalition of professions united by their shared mission" as well as by "their focus on disease prevention and health promotion; their prospective approach in contrast to the reactive focus of therapeutic medicine, and their common science, epidemiology."[4(p.40)] The disciplines of public health can be divided somewhat arbitrarily into six areas. Epidemiology and statistics are the basis for the assessment functions of public health, including the collection and analysis of information. Both assessment and policy development need an understanding of the causes of health problems in the community—an understanding that depends on biomedical sciences, social and behavioral sciences, and environmental sciences. As part of the assurance function, public health seeks to understand the medical care system in an area of study generally referred to as health policy and management or health administration, which also includes the administration and functioning of the public health system.

Epidemiology has been called the basic science of public health. As its name suggests, epidemiology is the study of epidemics. It focuses on human populations, usually starting with an outbreak of disease in a community. Epidemiologists look for common exposures or other shared characteristics in the people who are sick, seeking the causative factor.

Epidemiology often provides the first indications of the nature of a new disease. When AIDS was first recognized in the early 1980s, its cause was unknown. Doctors reported cases of this unusual disease to the Centers for Disease Control and Prevention, and epidemiologists began looking for common characteristics among the patients. Epidemiologic research indicated that it was an infectious disease spread through blood and body fluids and suggested a virus as the cause. This prompted the biomedical scientists to step in and look for the virus.

Epidemiology is important not only for deciphering the causes of exotic new diseases, but also for preventing the spread of old, well-understood diseases. Epidemiologists are mainstays of local health departments. In what is commonly known as "shoe-leather epidemiology," they may track down, for example, the source of a food-poisoning outbreak and force a restaurant to clean up its kitchen. Likewise, they may trace everyone who has been in contact with a college student diagnosed with meningitis so as to administer high doses of antibiotic and thereby prevent further spread of that dangerous disease. Epidemiologic studies have also been important in identifying the causes of chronic diseases such as heart disease and cancer.

Because public health deals with the health of populations, it depends very heavily on **statistics**. Governments collect data on births and deaths, causes of death, outbreaks of communicable diseases, cases of cancer, occupational injuries, and many other health-related issues. These numbers are diagnostic tools, informing experts how healthy or sick a society is, and where its weaknesses are. For example, the fact that the United States ranks 24th in infant mortality among the nations of the world, 28th in life expectancy of men, and 31st of women is one indication that the public health in the United States is not as good as that in many other countries.[11(Tables 13,14)]

To understand what the numbers mean, it is necessary to understand certain statistical concepts and calculations. The science of statistics is used to calculate risks from exposure to environmental chemicals, for example. Statistical analysis is an integral part of any epidemiologic study seeking the cause of a disease or a clinical study testing the effectiveness of a new drug.

Both public health and medicine depend on the **biomedical sciences**. A major proportion of human disease is caused by microorganisms. Prevention and control of these diseases in a population require an understanding of how these infectious agents are spread and how they affect the human body. Control of infectious diseases was a major focus of public health in the 19th and early 20th centuries. Biomedical research was very successful in gaining an understanding of the major killers of that period, providing the information and techniques by which successful public health measures could bring these diseases under control.

Biomedical research remains important to the understanding and control of newer diseases such as AIDS, which became the major epidemic of the late 20th and early 21st centuries worldwide. It has also contributed increasingly to an understanding of noninfectious diseases such as cancer and heart disease, which have become increasingly important as many infectious diseases have been effectively controlled. Recent progress in understanding human genetics is providing new insights into people's inherent susceptibility to various diseases, raising new hopes of cures as well as concerns about discrimination.

Environmental health science, a classic component of public health, is concerned with preventing the spread of disease through water, air, and food. Although it is not strictly a separate science, because it shares concerns about the spread of infectious organisms with biomedical sciences and depends on epidemiology to track environmental causes of disease outbreaks, it is usually considered a separate area of public health. Much of the great improvement in public health in the United States during the 20th century was due to improved environmental health, especially the fact that most Americans have safe drinking water. To address its concerns with safe water and waste disposal, environmental health depends on engineering to design, build, and maintain these systems.

Despite the fact that the importance of safe air, water, and food has been recognized for so many decades, many new challenges to environmental health continue to emerge. Not only do old systems fail, as occurred in Milwaukee, but new problems arise, brought about by modern lifestyles. Thousands of new chemicals enter the environment every year, and little is known about their effects on human health. Chemicals known to be toxic have accumulated in the environment, and methods must be devised to dispose of them safely. Other environmental threats to health include ultraviolet rays in sunlight and exposure to other kinds of radiation. In addition, human activities are causing changes in Earth's climate—changes that are permanently altering the environment and having important effects on human health.

Increasingly, public health is also concerned with social and behavioral sciences. As biomedical and environmental sciences have conquered many of the diseases that killed people of previous generations, people in modern societies are dying of diseases caused by their behavior and the social environment. Heart disease is related to nutrition and to exercise patterns; many forms of cancer are caused by smoking; abuse of drugs and alcohol is a notorious killer. Violence is a significant cause of death in our society and has attracted ongoing concern.

Some subgroups of the population have poorer health overall than others, for reasons that, while not completely understood, relate to social and behavioral factors. People with low incomes are less healthy than those with a higher socioeconomic status. Black Americans have lower life expectancy overall than white Americans, even when their incomes are similar. Other ethnic minority groups, including Hispanics, Asians, and American Indians, are at increased risk for a variety of health problems.

Social and behavioral sciences involve more unanswered questions than biomedical and environmental sciences do. Not enough is known about why racial and ethnic groups differ in their health-related behavior, why many people of all races behave in unhealthy ways, and how to prevent self-destructive behaviors. In the social and behavioral sciences, among all the areas encompassed by public health, research and application of its findings are most likely to make a difference in the future.

Until the beginning of the 20th century, public health and medicine overlapped substantially in their spheres of interest and activity. Both fields were concerned primarily with understanding the causes and prevention of infectious disease because medicine was relatively powerless to cure them. With the discovery of antibiotics, however, medicine gained the power to work miracles of healing, leading to a period in which its influence grew rapidly. Meanwhile, because of its less glamorous task of preventing disease, public health faded into obscurity.

Over the past few decades, it has become apparent that our society's emphasis on curing disease rather than preventing it has gone far out of balance. Medical care has become so expensive that a large proportion of the population cannot afford it, and spending for medical care has eaten up resources that could more profitably be used for education, housing, and the environment. Concerns about runaway costs, lack of access, and questionable quality of care have led to an increasing interest in studying the medical care system, its effectiveness, efficiency, and equity, leading to a science called health services research. Traditional categorization of public health fields puts this study into the area of health policy and management or health administration.

Prevention and Intervention

Public health's approach to health problems in a community has been described as a five-step process:

1. Define the health problem.
2. Identify the risk factors associated with the problem.
3. Develop and test community-level interventions to control or prevent the cause of the problem.
4. Implement interventions to improve the health of the population.
5. Monitor those interventions to assess their effectiveness.[6]

Thus, a main task of prevention is to develop interventions designed to prevent specific problems that have been identified either through an assessment process initiated by a public health agency or through community concern raised by an unusual course of events. For example, statistical data may show that a community has a high rate of cancer in comparison with other, similar communities, or a series of fatal crashes caused by drunk driving may mobilize a community to demand action to prevent further tragedies.

Public health has developed systematic ways of thinking about such problems that facilitate the process of designing **interventions** that prevent undesirable health outcomes. One approach is to think of prevention on three levels: primary prevention, secondary prevention, and tertiary prevention. **Primary prevention** prevents an illness or injury from occurring at all, by preventing exposure to risk factors. **Secondary prevention** seeks to minimize the severity of the illness or the damage due to an injury-causing event once the event has occurred. **Tertiary prevention** seeks to minimize disability by providing medical care and rehabilitation services.

As an example, interventions for primary prevention of cancer include efforts to discourage teenagers from smoking and efforts to encourage smokers to quit. In secondary prevention, screening programs are established to detect cancer early when it is still treatable. Tertiary prevention involves the medical treatment and rehabilitation of cancer patients.

This way of thinking was very effective in developing traffic safety programs that, over the past five decades, have significantly reduced the rates of injury from motor vehicle crashes. Primary prevention focused on preventing crashes by building divided highways and installing driver-assistance software in cars to correct lane departures and avoid collisions. Secondary prevention included the design of safer automobiles with stronger bumpers, padded dashboards, seat belts, and air bags. It also included laws requiring drivers and passengers to wear the seat belts. Tertiary prevention required the development of emergency medical services including ambulances, 911 calling networks, and trauma centers.

Another approach to designing interventions is to think of an illness or injury as the result of a chain of causation involving an agent, a host, and the environment. This approach is traditionally applied to infectious diseases: The agent may be a disease-causing bacterium or virus; the host is a susceptible human being; and the environment includes the means of transmission by which the agent reaches the host, which may be contaminated air, water, or food, or another human being who is infected. Prevention is accomplished by interrupting the chain of causation at any step. Rendering a potential host unsusceptible through immunization, for example, can interrupt the chain. Alternatively, the bacterium infecting a host can be killed through the use of antibiotics, or the environment can be sanitized through the purification of water and food.

The chain of causation model can be used for other kinds of illnesses or injuries as well. For example, suicide is the second leading cause of death in the 15- to 24-year-old age group.[11(Table 20)] In applying the model to prevention of youth suicide, the host is the susceptible young person; the agent is most often a gun or an overdose of pills; and the environment includes the young person's whole social environment, including family, school, and social media. A public health intervention could focus on how to make young people less susceptible to self-destructive thinking; it could try to change the messages presented by television and on Facebook and other social media that may lead a young person to think he or she is unattractive or otherwise inferior. However, the public health perspective tends to assume that the most effective target of intervention for youth suicide prevention is the agent, especially guns. Many adolescents are susceptible to depressed moods and think of killing themselves, but the best predictor of whether they will succeed is whether they have access to a gun.[12]

Public Health and Terrorism

Thankfully, there have been no large-scale terrorist events in the United States since 2001. Yet the means for causing mass injury and illness by individuals or groups who wish to cause harm to Americans have only increased. While prevention of violent acts such as hijacking airplanes or biological attacks such as distributing anthrax is primarily a responsibility of law enforcement, public health has an important role to play in controlling the damage caused by such events. In other words, primary prevention of terrorist acts may be out of the domain of public health, but secondary and tertiary prevention are very much a part of public health's mission. Success at these services depend on having well-designed plans in place before a disaster occurs.

The crashing of two planes into the World Trade Center triggered the activation of emergency response plans developed for New York City and New York State, plans designed as secondary prevention—minimizing the damage—and tertiary prevention—providing medical care to those injured in the disaster. Most critically important for saving lives was the ability for occupants of the buildings to get out as fast as possible. The fact that all but 2092 of the 17,400 people who were in the towers when the planes hit made it out is evidence that some aspects of the plans were effective.[13] However, studies done later found many flaws in the emergency planning. Plans for providing medical care to survivors were not seriously tested, because the capacity—including the arrival of numerous volunteers—exceeded the number of injured survivors. The greatest problem was a lack of coordination.

The public health response to the terrorist events that occurred on September 11, 2001, was essentially the same as the response needed for other emergencies and disasters: factory explosions, plane and train crashes, earthquakes, hurricanes, and so on. Public health was concerned not only with coordinating emergency medical care, but also with ensuring the safety of cleanup workers and area residents. Problems with polluted water, contaminated air, spoiled food, infestation of vermin, and so on had to be dealt with in downtown Manhattan just as they must be dealt with after a natural disaster.

The importance of public health became even more obvious in the aftermath of another terrorist event in 2001, in which anthrax was sent through the mail system. These **bioterrorism** attacks did not announce themselves in the dramatic fashion of the airplane hijackings. The first signs that a terrorist event had occurred were not recognized as such. No alarm bells rang when a few patients showed up in hospital emergency rooms with hard-to-diagnose illnesses. Anthrax announced itself in the same way that AIDS appeared, as an outbreak of something new that was reported to public health authorities, who then investigated.

The damage done by the anthrax mailings was relatively limited. However, the disaster that would result if a more infectious microorganism were used in a bioterrorist attack is potentially catastrophic. Bill Gates of the Bill and Melinda Gates Foundation, for example, recently warned that rapid advances in bioengineering have increased the possibility of an intentionally set pandemic on the scale of the 1918 flu that killed 50 to 100 million people.[14] In speculating about what would happen if a terrorist clandestinely released smallpox virus into a crowd, public health authorities realized that only the epidemiologic methods used for controlling natural epidemics could even begin to deal with such a crisis. Suddenly the media and politicians began talking about public health. Ironically, the threat of bioterrorism did more to teach the public about public health than any educational program. As Robert F. Meenan, then Dean of the Boston University School of Public Health, is quoted as saying, the anthrax attacks provided "a marketing campaign we could never have bought."[15] It appears, however, that the lessons learned about public health during those difficult times have not shifted the public's attention sufficiently from the more politically demanding concerns about paying for medical care.

Conclusion

This chapter has shown that public health is a broad term that is often misunderstood. It includes a goal—maximum health for all—as well as the means of attempting to achieve that goal. Public health is concerned with the prevention of disease and disability. It aims to benefit the entire population, in contrast to medicine, which focuses on the individual.

The functions of public health in a community can be compared with the functions of a physician in caring for a patient. Public health diagnoses and treats the community's ills by way of assessment, policy development, and assurance. It relies on the tools of science and politics. The public health sciences of epidemiology and statistics are applied in assessing a population's health. Policy is developed based on biomedical sciences, social and behavioral sciences, environmental health sciences, and the study of the medical care system. Public health depends on politics for decision making. Decisions on public health interventions to be taken by the community,

insofar as they require government action, are reached through politics.

Public health focuses on prevention of disease and disability. Preventive measures can be applied at three levels: Primary prevention aims to prevent a disease or injury from occurring at all; secondary prevention aims to minimize the damage caused by the illness or injury-causing event when it occurs; and tertiary prevention seeks to minimize any ensuing disability by providing medical care and rehabilitation.

Public health prevention programs function through interventions designed to interrupt the chain of causation that leads to an illness or an injury. Interventions can be directed toward eliminating or suppressing the agent that causes an illness or injury, strengthening the resistance of the host to the agent, or changing the environment in such a way that the host is less likely to encounter the agent.

Public health is an abstract concept that has often been misunderstood and neglected by politicians and the general public. The dramatic events in the fall of 2001 forced the government and the media to pay attention to the importance of public health, both in mitigating the effects of obvious disasters, and in recognizing and controlling the more insidious effects of bioterrorism. In the years since then, that attention has dwindled as public health has fallen out of the spotlight somewhat.

References

1. T. McKeown, *The Role of Medicine: Dream, Mirage or Nemesis?* (Oxford, UK: Basil Blackwell, 1979).
2. Centers for Disease Control and Prevention, "Public Opinion About Public Health—United States, 1999," *Morbidity and Mortality Weekly Report* 49 (2000): 258–260.
3. C.-E. A. Winslow, *The Evolution and Significance of the Modern Public Health Campaign* (New Haven, CT: Yale University Press, 1923); reprinted by the *Journal of Public Health Policy*, 1 (1984).
4. Institute of Medicine, Committee for the Study of the Future of Public Health, *The Future of Public Health* (Washington, DC: National Academy Press, 1988).
5. J. P. Leider, "The Problem with Estimating Public Health Spending," *Journal of Public Health Management and Practice* 22, no. 2 (2016): E1–E11.
6. Kaiser Family Foundation, "Summary of the Affordable Care Act," April 25, 2013, www.kff.org /health-reform/fact-sheet/summary-of-the-affordable -care-act/, accessed January 21, 2020.

7. Centers for Disease Control and Prevention, "Ten Great Public Health Achievements, 1900–1999," *Morbidity and Mortality Weekly Report* 48 (1999): 241–243.

8. Centers for Disease Control and Prevention. "Ten Great Public Health Achievements—United States, 2001–2010," *Morbidity and Mortality Weekly Report* 60, no. 19 (2011): 619.

9. T. Pilishvili, C. Lexau, M. M. Farley, J. Hadler, L. H. Harrison, N. M. Bennett, A. Reingold, et al., "Sustained Reductions in Invasive Pneumococcal Disease in the Era of Conjugate Vaccine," *Journal of Infectious Diseases* 201, no. 1 (2010): 32–41.

10. M. R. Moore, R. Link-Gelles, and W. Schaffner. "Impact of 13-Valent Pneumococcal Conjugate Vaccine Used in Children and Adults in the United States; Analysis of Multisite, Population-Based Surveillance," *Lancet Infectious Diseases* 15 (2015): 301–309.

11. U.S. National Center for Health Statistics, "Health, United States, 2017: With Special Feature on Mortality," 2018.

12. American Public Health Association, "Reducing Suicides by Firearms," Policy Number 20184, November 13, 2018, www.apha.org/policies-and -advocacy/public-health-policy-statements/policy -database/2019/01/28/reducing-suicides-by-firearms, accessed July 27, 2019.

13. R. R. M. Gershon, "Factors Associated with High-Rise Evacuation: Qualitative Results from the World Trade Center Evacuation Study," *Prehospital and Disaster Medicine* 22 (2007): 165–173.

14. B. Gates. "A New Kind of Bioterrorism Could Wipe out 30 Million People in Less Than a Year—And We Are Not Prepared," *Business Insider*, February 18, 2017, ewww.businessinsider.com/bill-gates-op-ed-bio -terrorism-epidemic-world-threat-2017-2, accessed July 27, 2019.

15. J. S. Smith, "The Personal Predicament of Public Health," *Chronicle of Higher Education*, June 27, 2003.

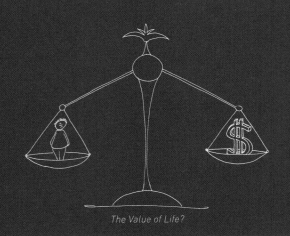
The Value of Life?

Why Is Public Health Controversial?

KEY TERMS

Economic impact
Individual liberty
Libertarian
Moralism

Paternalism
Political interference with
   science

Tragedy of the commons

The mission of public health as defined by the Institute of Medicine report, *The Future of Public Health*—"fulfilling society's interest in assuring conditions in which people can be healthy"[1(p.40)]—is very broad. These conditions include many factors that might not normally be perceived as relevant to public health. For example, the most significant factor in determining the health of a community is its economic status. People with higher incomes tend to be healthier for a variety of reasons. This expansive view of public health is not new. Winslow's 80-year-old definition specifically includes as part of public health's role, "the development of the social machinery which will ensure to every individual in the community a standard of living adequate for the maintenance of health."[2(p.1)]

Indeed, the early history of U.S. public health was closely tied to social reform movements. In addition to sanitary science and public hygiene, 19th-century reformers campaigned for improved housing, trade unions, the abolition of child labor, maternal and child health, and temperance. Winslow thought of public health as a military-style campaign and wrote of "whole populations mobilized for the great war against preventable disease."[3(p.27)]

Public health can be viewed as a broad social movement. Dan E. Beauchamp, a noted public health philosopher, has written that "public health should be a way of doing justice, a way of asserting the value and priority of all human life."[4(p.8)] In an influential 1974 paper entitled "Public Health as Social Justice," Beauchamp called on public health to challenge the ideology that prevails in the United States, an ideology that he dubbed "market justice." Market justice, he noted, emphasizes individual responsibility, minimal obligation to the common good, and the "fundamental freedom to all individuals to be left alone."[4(p.4)] Under market justice, powerful forces of environment, heredity, and social structure prevent a fair distribution of the burdens and benefits of society. Social justice, in contrast, suggests that minimal levels of income, basic housing, employment, education, and health care should be seen as fundamental rights. According to Beauchamp, "The historic dream of public health that preventable death and disability ought to be minimized is a dream of social justice."[4(p.6)]

Political conservatives have tended to resist this broad vision of public health. Many would prefer to limit public health to a technical enterprise focused on controlling communicable disease or as a safety net that provides medical care to the indigent. This restricted view of public health was long encouraged by physicians, who were concerned about government encroachment on their economic and professional independence; their political power helped to limit federal health funding in the 1930s and 1940s to programs, run by local health departments, which were narrowly focused on providing services for child health, control of venereal disease (i.e., sexually transmitted infection) and tuberculosis, and dental health.

Concerns about health threats from environmental pollution that arose in the 1960s were addressed independent of the traditional public health system, and separate agencies were set up to deal with them. Similarly, social problems such as homelessness, drug abuse, and violence were not thought of as public health problems, although they had adverse health consequences. It was this fragmentation of public health that led the Institute of Medicine committee to conclude in 1988 that public health was "in disarray"[1(p.19)] and to affirm the comprehensive view of public health expressed by Winslow and Beauchamp.

The broad view of public health's scope generates considerable controversy in the United States' individualistic, market-oriented society. The notion that government has an obligation to provide healthy conditions for citizens who are unwilling or unable to provide such conditions for themselves—and indeed to provide medical care for those who need it, as most other industrialized countries do—has often been attacked as socialist. Conservative politicians have won election to office by campaigning against taxes, starving governments of funds that could provide health services for all. Many Americans reflexively oppose being told what to do and resist the idea of governmental restrictions on their behavior, even when the intent is to protect their own health and that of others. Moreover, many health problems have their roots in unhealthy behaviors that are so personal and intimate that moralists oppose even discussing them. Three issues—economic, libertarian, and moral—tend to come up repeatedly in any debate over public health actions or activities.

Economic Impact

Most public health measures have some kind of negative **economic impact** on some segment of the population or industry. Consequently, any new proposal for a public health regulation is likely to inspire opposition from some quarter, on the grounds that it might cost jobs, add to the price of a product, or require a tax increase. It might also cut into a company's profits. Consequently, industries resist change: Milk producers resisted pasteurization; landlords resisted building codes; and automobile manufacturers resisted design changes to improve safety. These conflicts are particularly difficult to resolve, for a variety of reasons.

The difficulty in dealing with the economic impact of public health measures is illustrated by public health advocates' conflicts with the tobacco industry. Tobacco is clearly harmful to health, causing thousands of deaths and millions of dollars in medical costs annually. Yet it was only in 2009 that political leaders managed to assign to the Food and Drug Administration the power to regulate the tobacco industry, over the objection of politicians from tobacco-growing states such as Kentucky and North Carolina.[2] Tobacco is a major industry in the South, supporting jobs and providing profits for tobacco companies. Cigarette sales also are a significant source of income for many small businesses. Owners of bars and restaurants have fought laws restricting smoking on their premises, fearing that they would lose the patronage of smokers. Politicians are not eager to institute strong public health measures that would have such a major economic impact. Only in the past two or three decades, with the shift of public opinion against the tobacco industry, together with the industry's need to protect itself against a potentially bankrupting flood of lawsuits by injured smokers, have federal, state, and local governments begun to take serious steps to control smoking.

In many circumstances, controversy arises because those who pay for a public health measure are not the ones who benefit from it. Environmental regulations such as restrictions on timber harvesting in the Pacific Northwest regularly come under attack because they may cost jobs in the lumber industry, although they may preserve jobs in the fishing and tourist industries as well as contribute to a more stable climate in the long term. Regulations that protect the health and safety of workers may require expensive protective equipment, thus driving up the costs of the goods produced by those workers to consumers.

In times of economic difficulty, people are often unwilling to pay short-term costs to obtain a long-term benefit. For example, in both the fishing and lumber industries, stocks have become dangerously depleted, and there is a risk of killing off all the fish and cutting down all the timber, thereby destroying these industries altogether. Yet few workers in the fishing or lumber industries are willing to voluntarily cut back on their own harvests. Companies resist tough pollution control laws even though less-polluting technology may lead to

a long-term benefit not only for the environment but also for a company's competitiveness in international markets. This shortsightedness is often apparent at times of high gas prices, when U.S. automobile companies suddenly lose market share and profits because they invested so much of their production into formerly profitable gas-guzzling SUVs that Americans could no longer afford to drive.

The costs of public health measures are usually much easier to calculate than the benefits. For example, experts may know the cost of reducing smog in Los Angeles to a level that reduces deaths from lung disease by 10%. But how do they calculate whether this benefit is worth the cost? It is very difficult to put a dollar value on life and health. Furthermore, it is often difficult to quantify what the risk really is and how to balance it against other risks. People are concerned, for example, about farmers' use of pesticides, which may leave toxic residues on fruits and vegetables. Scientists can estimate the health risks that the average person faces by consuming these residues. But fruits and vegetables are an important part of a healthy diet. If the use of pesticides were forbidden, the crops might be less abundant, and the prices of produce might rise, perhaps discouraging some people from eating these nutritious foods. Thus, an effort to protect health might have a negative impact on health overall.

Individual Liberty

In the United States, one of the primary purposes of government is to "promote the general welfare," as called for in the U.S. Constitution. Health and safety, together with economic well-being, are the major factors that contribute to the general welfare. While the government cannot guarantee health and safety for each individual, its role is to provide for maximum health and safety for the community as a whole. One of the central controversies in public health is the extent to which government can and should restrict individual freedom for the purpose of improving the community's health.

There has long been general agreement that it is acceptable to restrict an individual's freedom to behave in such a way as to cause direct harm to others. Laws against assault and murder are found in the Bible and even in the Babylonian Code of Hammurabi, which dates to the 18th century B.C.E. When the harm is less direct, however, the issues become more controversial. Most controversial are governmental restrictions on people's freedom to harm themselves.

Government restrictions on behavior that causes indirect harm to others is the way to prevent what Garrett Hardin, in 1968, called the "**tragedy of the commons**."[5] Hardin describes a pasture open to all herdsmen in a community. The land can support a limited number of grazing cattle. If each herdsman tries to maximize his gain by keeping as many cattle as possible on the pasture—the commons—the pasture will be overgrazed. The cattle will starve, and the herdsmen will be ruined. The only way for the community to save the pasture is to agree to restrict the freedom of the herdsmen, placing fair and equitable limits on the number of cattle each can keep there.

In today's industrialized world, the "commons" comprises the air, water, and other elements of the environment that all people share. Because no individual has the power to control the quality of his or her own personal environment independent of the behavior of his or her neighbors, government action is required to protect these common resources. While the general principle of protecting the "commons" is accepted by most citizens, there

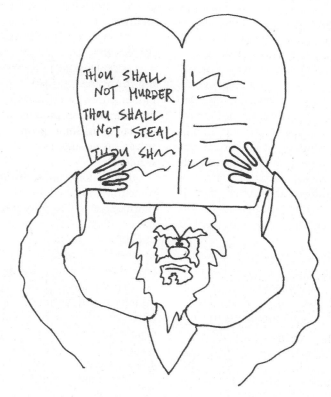

Restricting Individual Freedom

is plenty of room for controversy in defining what to include among the protected resources, as well as how extensive the protective measures should be.

The United States has made great progress over the past 50 years in cleaning up its air and water through the passage of federal legislation. Now questions are being raised as to whether the laws have gone too far in restricting the "freedom" to pollute. Companies have been required to limit emissions from their smokestacks; automobile makers have been required to install emission control devices on every car they manufacture. These regulations may have driven up the costs of automobiles and other products, but they have not limited anybody's freedom. Southern California, however, has continued to battle a serious air pollution problem. To help the city of Los Angeles to meet the federal mandates for clean air, officials there imposed regulations including a ban on gas-driven lawn mowers, elimination of drive-through windows in banks and fast-food restaurants (to cut the pollution that results from idling car engines), and a ban on charcoal lighting fluid. None of these activities on an individual basis—mowing a lawn, sitting in an idling car waiting for a hamburger, or lighting a few chunks of charcoal—contributes in any major way to the pollution of California's air, but when done by thousands of residents each day, they add up to a significant problem. Los Angeles's actions showed that Americans are willing to accept such significant limitations on their behavior to achieve the desirable goal of clean air to breathe.

The most controversial public health measures are requirements that restrict people's freedom for the purpose of protecting their own health and safety. Examples of such measures include requirements to wear seat belts when traveling in a car and helmets when riding a motorcycle. Such laws inspire allusions to "the tyranny of health"[6] and "the health police," although restrictions on use of many drugs, such as heroin, cocaine, LSD, and—during Prohibition in the early

20th century—alcohol have been generally accepted.

Such restrictions on individual behavior are often criticized as "**paternalism**." Libertarians, in the words of John Stuart Mill, argue that "the only purpose for which power can be rightfully exercised over any member of a civilized community, against his will, is to prevent harm to others . . . In the part [of his conduct] which merely concerns himself, his independence is . . . absolute."[7(p.90)] The one form of paternalism that is generally accepted is that children and young people can be restricted in their behavior on the basis that they are not yet mature enough to make considered judgments about their own best interests. Thus, laws prevent juveniles from buying tobacco and alcohol, require them to wear bicycle helmets and seat belts (even where adults are not required to wear them), and require parental permission to obtain birth control information or an abortion, or to go skydiving.

According to the **libertarian** view, which has a strong tradition in the United States, it is acceptable to outlaw drunk driving but not drunkenness itself. Similarly, smoking in indoor public places can be outlawed because the smoke bothers others (although strong resistance to this restriction persists in many places), yet smoking by adults cannot be regulated.

Restrictions on **individual liberty** are sometimes justified on the basis that their purpose is really to protect others, even when the argument is a bit strained. For example, unhelmeted motorcyclists could pose a threat to others because of the possibility of their losing control if hit by flying debris. Unhelmeted cyclists and unbelted motorists, when severely injured in road accidents, drive up insurance rates for others and in extreme cases may become expensive wards of the state. Alcoholics and drug users bring harm to their families and are a nuisance to their neighbors.

Most public health advocates believe that there are more fundamental justifications for restrictions on individual behavior for the sake of the public health. Beauchamp, the philosopher, explored the reasons in his book *The Health of the Republic*, arguing that such laws are needed most for behaviors that are common and carry small risks. Consistent use of seat belts, for example, prevents thousands of deaths and injuries in the population as a whole, although the risk people face on any one trip, when they must decide whether to buckle up, is quite small. While each individual's choice to take the risk of driving unbuckled may be rational, society's interest in preventing the thousands of deaths and injuries outweighs the minor inconvenience of obeying the seat belt law.

Beauchamp's argument in favor of limiting individual liberty for the common good is consistent with his view of public health as social justice. Death and disability are collective problems, he says, and collective action is needed to promote the common welfare. The U.S. tradition of supporting private liberty above all is wrong, as noted by an early critic of the American character, Alexis de Tocqueville, in that it "disposes [citizens] not to think of their fellows and turns indifference into a sort of public virtue."[8(p.16)]

Moral and Religious Opposition

Public health often arouses controversy on moral grounds, most often when it confronts sexual and reproductive issues. Acquired immunodeficiency syndrome (AIDS), other sexually transmitted diseases, teenage pregnancy, and low-birth-weight babies are major public health problems in the United States. The public health approach to these problems includes sex education in schools and the provision of contraceptive services, especially condoms. These measures are often vigorously opposed by members of certain religious groups who believe that they promote immoral behavior. Safe and legal abortion to terminate unwanted pregnancy is even more controversial. While clearly the safest and healthiest lifestyle is to abstain from sexual activity before marriage and then to be faithful to one's spouse, experience has long shown that preaching morality has limited efficacy in preventing sexually transmitted diseases and unwanted pregnancy.

AIDS has been an especially divisive issue because so many people with AIDS contracted the disease through behaviors that are often regarded as immoral—homosexual acts and intravenous drug use. Consequently, AIDS-related policy has been confounded by moral revulsion against the disease and its victims. While not supported by the evidence, it is commonly believed that education on how to protect oneself against contracting the virus that causes AIDS may encourage homosexuality and promiscuous sexual behavior in general. Similarly, moralists frown on the practice of providing clean needles to drug addicts because, while this intervention is effective in reducing the spread of the virus, they believe it condones the use of intravenous drugs.

Moralism also enters into discussions of alcohol and drug policy. Libertarians could argue against regulation of alcohol and bans on addictive drugs on the basis that consumption of drugs is private behavior that does not directly hurt others. Nevertheless, most members of the U.S. public accept the validity of such regulation. The power of government to limit drug and alcohol consumption is well established in the United States and corresponds with the tradition of limiting individual behavior for the common good.

While regulation for the common good may be viewed as a valid pursuit, trying to legislate morality has often proved to be ineffective, self-defeating, and a threat to liberty, in part because people differ in what they view as moral. When morality is the justification for banning certain behaviors, rational discussion is often impossible. Free speech is repressed, victims are demonized, practitioners of the behavior are driven underground, and the "epidemic"—whether AIDS, drug abuse, or teenage pregnancy—spreads more easily.[4]

Moral and religious concerns may also interfere with attempts to publicly discuss and carry out public health policy. This interference was brought to life in front of an audience at the New York Academy of Medicine on October 15, 2018, when four retired Surgeons General of the United States made plain the obstacles they faced in carrying out their duties. As Surgeon General in the George H. W. Bush White House, Dr. Antonia Novello recounted how she was blocked in 1992 from criticizing the Joe Camel cartoons in cigarette advertising that were aimed at children. During Bill Clinton's presidency, Dr. Joycelyn Elders described being forced to resign over her frank public statements on sex education, birth control, and drug policy; and Dr. David Satcher discussed being rebuked for promoting needle exchange programs aimed at limiting the spread of human immunodeficiency virus (HIV) and hepatitis. In the George W. Bush administration, Dr. Richard Carmona described being blocked from publicly discussing many issues, including the dangers of second-hand smoke, embryonic stem cell research, climate change, and emergency contraception. Across the board, these former government officials made clear the pressures they faced from conservative opposition to the public health policy that they were charged to promote.[9]

Political Interference with Science

While legitimate differences of opinion may arise about how to weigh the competing interests in making policy that affects public health, these decisions should be informed by science to the greatest extent possible. The George W. Bush administration was notorious for going beyond previous political practices in manipulating and distorting scientific evidence to fit its political agenda—that is, in engaging in **political interference with science**. In February 2004, the Union of Concerned Scientists (UCS), a nonprofit advocacy group, released a report called "Scientific Integrity in Policymaking," which was signed by more than 60 leading scientists, including 20 Nobel Prize winners.[10] The report documented many instances of the Bush administration's misrepresentation or suppression of scientific information and stacking of scientific advisory committees to obscure the fact that policy decisions were based on its political agenda, which usually favored right-wing constituencies and large corporations.

Global warming was an issue on which the Bush administration especially sought to suppress information and to discredit scientific evidence. According to the UCS, the political environment over this issue was so hostile that the Environmental Protection Agency (EPA) decided to omit an entire climate change section from a major report on the environment rather than compromise its credibility by misrepresenting the scientific consensus. A scientist from the National Oceanic and Atmospheric Administration reported that, when he organized a conference on carbon dioxide, he was told that the words "climate change" could not be used in the title of any presentation.

President Barack Obama by and large restored scientific integrity to federal policy making. His science advisor, physicist John Holdren, was one of the original signers of the UCS's report.[11] President Obama issued a scientific integrity directive in 2010, which was praised by the UCS, but the organization expressed reservations that the directive left an enormous amount of discretion to the agencies and departments that had to work out the details.[12]

The concerns that were raised about the second Bush administration returned in force during the presidency of Donald Trump. President Trump's first administrator of the EPA, Scott Pruitt, was a staunch supporter of the oil and gas industry and had sued the EPA over energy regulations repeatedly while in previous positions. Pruitt was on the record as stating that carbon dioxide may not be the primary contributor to global warming and that there was "tremendous disagreement" about the role of human activity in climate change—positions at odds with decades of scientific research.[13]

Once in office, Pruitt set to work reducing the influence of the scientific community and promoting the interests of the industries that the EPA is charged to regulate. Most worrisome, Pruitt pushed to change in fundamental ways how the EPA incorporates scientific research into the formulation of air pollution, water pollution, and toxic chemical use policy. Under the "Scientific Transparency" rule proposed by Pruitt, the EPA would be allowed to consider only research studies where the underlying data could be provided; this rule would apply retroactively to previously published studies. This seemingly innocuous proposal could lead to the exclusion of large swaths of relevant research, including studies that rely on data that cannot be made public, such as those using private medical records, and studies that were already published and for which the data may no longer be readily available. The consequences could be far-reaching, forcing the EPA to revisit and potentially revise many of the existing air, water, and chemical pollution rules currently on the books so that their formulation relies only on science that meets the proposed inclusion criteria.

The reaction from the scientific community was swift. Nearly all scientific and public health professional organizations, as well as the leading scientific journals *Science*, *Nature*, and *Proceedings of the National Academy of Science*, condemned the proposal. While the EPA's environmental regulation process over the years has created difficulties and tension between the scientific community and the regulated industries, there was at least a two-step process whereby the EPA's scientific staff reviewed and synthesized the existing research before handing it off to the political staff to decide on a course of action. The "transparency" proposal would bring politics into this first step—determining which research legally could and could not be considered during the evaluation of the scientific literature. Science legal expert Professor Wendy Wagner described this situation as "politics going to a place that should be off-limits," likening the proposal to that of the Indiana state legislature in the late 19th century that attempted to establish the value of pi as 3.2 rather than 3.14. Noted Wagner, even if the proposal did not become law, "what worries us in that we've gotten to this point—that this is even on the table."[14,15] Pruitt's replacement as EPA administrator, Andrew Wheeler, announced in November 2019 that the plan would indeed move forward.[16]

Conclusion

Public health is controversial because, depending on how it is defined, it may challenge people's values and demand sacrifices. The battle between an expansive perspective and a restrictive view of public health is ongoing. The expansive view asks people to give up a degree of personal liberty for the common good.

At its most idealistic, public health is a broad social movement—a campaign to maximize health for everyone in the population through distributing benefits and responsibilities in an equitable way. Health is therefore "a political endeavor as much as, or at times even more than, a medical one."[17(p.15)]

Public health measures are often controversial because they have an economic impact. The people or industries that must pay the price may not be the ones that will benefit from the new protections. Costs are usually more visible than benefits. Moreover, the price may need to be paid sooner, while the benefit may not be achieved until later.

Public health may be affected by personal and intimate behaviors, which are often embarrassing and even offensive to discuss.

Thus, some public health measures are controversial because they arouse moral or religious objections.

Although there are legitimate differences of opinion on how to weigh competing interests in making public health policy, the distortion and suppression of scientific evidence by politicians has been a long-standing problem. The concern was especially acute during the George W. Bush administration and has arisen again during the Donald Trump administration.

References

1. Institute of Medicine, Committee for the Study of the Future of Public Health, *The Future of Public Health* (Washington, DC: National Academy Press, 1988).
2. C.-E. A. Winslow, *The Evolution and Significance of the Modern Public Health Campaign* (New Haven, CT: Yale University Press, 1923); reprint, *Journal of Public Health Policy* (1984): 1.
3. C.-E. A. Winslow, "The Contribution of Hermann Biggs to Public Health: The 1928 Biggs Memorial Lecture," *American Review of Tuberculosis* 20 (1929): 1–28.
4. D. E. Beauchamp, "Public Health as Social Justice," *Inquiry* 13 (1976): 1–14.
5. G. Hardin, "The Tragedy of the Commons," *Science* 162 (1968): 1243–1248.
6. F. T. Fitzgerald, "The Tyranny of Health," *New England Journal of Medicine* 331 (1994): 196–198.
7. J. S. Mill, "On Liberty," quoted in D. E. Beauchamp, *The Health of the Republic: Epidemics, Medicine, and Moralism as Challenges to Democracy* (Philadelphia, PA: Temple University Press, 1988), 90.
8. A. de Tocqueville, *Democracy in America*, quoted in Beauchamp, *The Health of the Republic*, 16.
9. D. G. McNeil Jr., "Former Surgeons General Recount Political Pressure on the Job," *The New York Times*, October 24, 2018.
10. Union of Concerned Scientists, "Scientific Integrity in Policy Making," July 2004, www.ucsusa.org/sites /default/files/legacy/assets/documents/scientific _integrity/scientific_integrity_in_policy_making _july_2004_1.pdf, accessed August 15, 2019.
11. Union of Concerned Scientists, "2004 Scientist Statement on Restoring Scientific Integrity to Federal Policy Making," www.ucsusa.org/our-work /center-science-and-democracy/promoting-scientific -integrity/scientists-sign-on-statement.html, accessed August 15, 2019.
12. Union of Concerned Scientists, "Promoting Scientific Integrity," https://www.ucsusa.org/our-work/center -science-and-democracy/promoting-scientific -integrity, accessed August 15, 2019.
13. C. Davenport, "E.P.A. Chief Doubts Consensus View of Climate Change," *The New York Times*, March 9, 2017.
14. W. Wagner, E. Fisher, and P. Pascual, "Whose Science? A New Era in Regulatory 'Science Wars'," *Science* 362, no. 6415 (2018): 636–639.
15. R. Meyer, "Trump's Interference with Science is Unprecedented," *The Atlantic*, November 9, 2018.
16. L. Freedman, "E.P.A. to Limit Science Used to Write Public Health Rules," *The New York Times*, November 11, 2019."
17. L. Wallack et al., *Media Advocacy and Public Health: Power for Prevention* (Newbury Park, CA: Sage Publications, 1993), 15.

CHAPTER 3

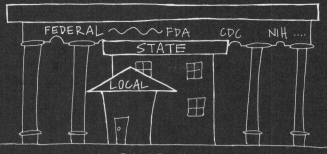

Federal, State, Local . . .

Powers and Responsibilities of Government

KEY TERMS

Centers for Disease Control and Prevention (CDC)
Environmental Protection Agency (EPA)
Federal role in public health
Food and Drug Administration (FDA)

Local public health agencies
Morbidity and Mortality Weekly Report (MMWR)
National Institutes of Health (NIH)
Nongovernmental organization (NGO)

Occupational Safety and Health Act
State health departments
Surgeon General

Governments ultimately have the responsibility of making the organized community efforts necessary to protect the health of the population, although many other organizations and community groups are also important participants. Government's role is determined by law; that is, government's public health activities must be authorized by legislation at the federal, state, or local levels. Public health law is further defined by decisions of the courts at the various levels. The broad decisions of the legislative and judicial branches of government are worked out in detail by the executive branch, usually by the agencies that issue regulations and carry out public health programs. The ultimate authority that allows the laws to

be written is a constitution or charter, whether federal, state, or local. Thus, the body of public health law is massive, consisting of all the written statements relating to health by any of the three branches of government at the federal, state, and local levels.

Many **nongovernmental organizations (NGOs)** play an important role in public health, especially through educational programs and lobbying. In recent years, stimulated in part by the Institute of Medicine's *The Future of Public Health* report,[1] there has been increasing emphasis on community involvement in public health planning and in generating support for and participation in public health activities. This process expands the concept of the public health system to include, for example, hospitals, businesses, and charitable and religious organizations.

Federal Versus State Authority

The U.S. Constitution does not mention health. Because the Tenth Amendment states that "the powers not delegated to the United States by the Constitution . . . are reserved to the States respectively," public health has been a responsibility primarily of the states. Most state constitutions provide for the protection of public health, and the original

states already had laws concerning health before the Constitution took effect.[2]

All states have laws such as mandates to collect data about the population, to immunize children before they enter school, to regulate the environment for purposes of sanitation, and to regulate safety. To a varying extent, responsibility for some public health activities may be delegated by the state to local governments. **Figure 3-1**, an organizational chart for a small state health department, shows public health activities typically provided for in state law.

The U.S. Constitution, in the Preamble, includes among the fundamental purposes of government, "to promote the general welfare." It gives the federal government authority to

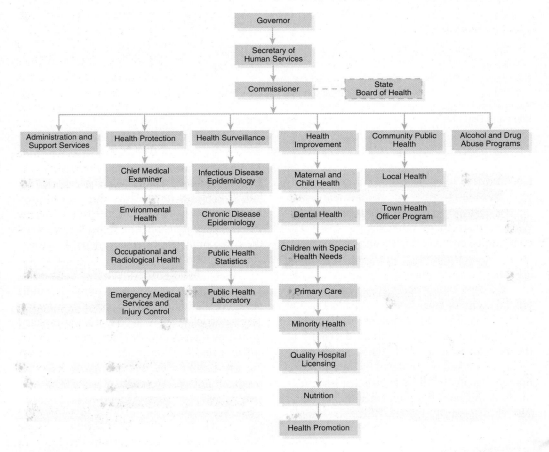

Figure 3-1 Organizational Chart of a State Health Department

regulate interstate commerce and to "collect taxes . . . to pay the debts and provide for the common defense and the general welfare." These powers are the basis for the **federal role in public health**.

The interstate commerce provision, for example, justifies the activities of the **Food and Drug Administration (FDA)**, which oversees extensive federal regulation of foods, drugs, medical devices, and cosmetics, most of which are distributed across state lines. It is obviously more efficient and economical for the industries that produce these products to be bound by uniform national rules rather than having to comply with 50 different sets of state regulations.

The power to tax and spend enables the federal government to achieve goals that it may lack the authority to address directly. Specifically, the federal government can provide funds to the states subject to certain requirements. For example, in 1967 the federal government mandated that, as a precondition for receiving highway construction funds, states must pass laws requiring motorcyclists to wear helmets. The effectiveness of the mandate was demonstrated by the fact that, by 1975, 47 states had passed such laws, with the result that motorcyclist deaths declined by 30% in these states.[3] Another example of federal influence over state health programs is the Medicaid program of providing health care for the poor. The federal government provides 65% of the funding for Medicaid.[4] States and counties administer the Medicaid program, providing the remaining funds, and must follow the guidelines established by Congress to receive the funds.[2]

example

Since World War II, the federal government has used these powers to steadily widen its role in public health, among other matters. That trend began to reverse in the 1980s. In a political climate hostile to government, especially the federal government, there was a strong movement in the U.S. Congress and the U.S. Supreme Court to cut government regulation and return more powers to the states. In an early example of the reversal, in 1976 Congress removed the financial penalty for lack of motorcycle helmet laws. By 1980, 27 states had repealed their helmet laws, and motorcycle deaths rose in those states by 38%.[3] The Medicaid program, which has become enormously expensive since it was established in 1965, has also been a target of Congress, which for some time threatened, without success, to hand it over to the states entirely.

In the 1990s, the U.S. Supreme Court under Chief Justice William Rehnquist began a trend known as New Federalism, which limited Congress's powers and returned authority to the states. For example, in 1995, the Court struck down a law making gun possession within a school zone a federal offense, rejecting the argument that gun possession was a matter of interstate commerce.[5] In 2001, it decided that the Americans with Disabilities Act could not be enforced against a state, ruling that a woman who was fired from her state job because she had breast cancer could not sue the state of Alabama.[6] However, New Federalism lost much of its momentum after 9/11 when, as *New York Times* reporter Linda Greenhouse noted, "suddenly the federal government looked useful, even necessary." In 2003, Rehnquist "gave up and moved on," writing the majority ruling that state governments could be sued for failing to give their employees the benefits required by the Family and Medical Leave Act.[7] The Supreme Court has since affirmed the priority of federal law over state law in decisions involving medical marijuana in California in 2005; gun control in Washington, D.C., in 2008; and same-sex marriage in 2015.[8]

How the Law Works

Governments have broad power to act in ways that curtail the rights of individuals. These police powers of governments are basic to public health, and are the reason why public health must ultimately be government's responsibility.[9] Police powers are invoked for three reasons: to prevent a person from harming others; to defend the interests of incompetent persons such as children or the mentally disabled; and, in some cases, to protect a person from harming himself or herself.[10]

Laws have been used to enforce compliance in health matters for more than a century. In 1905, a precedent was set for the state's police power in the area of health when the Massachusetts legislature passed a law that required all adults to be vaccinated against smallpox. A man named Jacobson refused to comply and went to court, arguing that the law infringed on his personal liberty. The trial court found that the state was within its power to enforce the law. Jacobson appealed his case all the way to the U.S. Supreme Court. He lost: The Supreme Court upheld the right of the state to restrict an individual's freedom "for the common good."[5]

Public health law has become more complex over the years, but it follows the same pattern. At any level of government, a legislature, perceiving a need, passes a statute. That statute may be challenged in court, and the decision of the court may be appealed to higher courts. Generally, on issues of constitutionality, a state court may overturn a local law or court decision, and a federal court may overturn a state law or court decision.

Since public health increasingly involves complex technical issues, legislatures at the several levels of government generally set up administrative agencies to perform public health functions. The legislature, recognizing that it lacks the necessary expertise, authorizes these agencies to set rules that define in detail how to accomplish the purpose of the legislation. The courts may then be called on to interpret the authority of the agencies under the laws and to determine whether certain rules or decisions of an agency are within its legal authority.

As an example of the interplay of legislation, agency rule making, and the role of the courts, consider the **Occupational Safety and Health Act**, passed by Congress in 1970. This legislation stated that "personal injuries and illnesses arising out of work situations impose a substantial burden upon . . . interstate commerce," and thus used the federal government's authority over interstate commerce to pass a public health statute.[11(p.180)] The law established the Occupational Safety and Health Administration (OSHA) within the Department of Labor. OSHA was authorized, among other things, to set standards regulating employees' exposure to hazardous substances. Representatives of industry challenged the constitutional authority of Congress to pass the law but were unsuccessful.

Industries that perceive themselves to be economically harmed by OSHA's standard setting have used other routes to weaken the agency's power. For example, OSHA decided to regulate benzene, which caused a variety of toxic effects among workers in the rubber and petrochemical industries. In 1971, OSHA set a standard limiting benzene exposure to 10 parts per million (ppm) in air, averaged over an 8-hour period. Epidemiologic evidence indicated, however, that exposure to lower concentrations of benzene over time might increase the risk of leukemia, and laboratory evidence supported those studies. In turn, in 1978, OSHA lowered the standard to 1 ppm over an 8-hour period. Representatives of the affected industries appealed the new regulations in court, claiming that evidence that benzene causes leukemia was not sufficiently strong, and that complying with the new standard would be too expensive. The court, in a ruling upheld later by the Supreme Court, agreed that OSHA did not have sufficient evidence to support the need for the new standard and had exceeded its authority in issuing the regulation.[11] The standard remained at 10 ppm until 1987, when evidence for the carcinogenicity of benzene was deemed convincing enough to justify the lower value.[12]

The courts did not rule on whether the cost of complying with a standard should be considered in the process of setting it. The act had specified that standards should ensure the health of workers "to the extent feasible."[11(p.180)] Industry argued that OSHA should have done a cost–benefit analysis before issuing the regulation. This issue was decided in another case, in which the courts determined that a formal cost–benefit analysis was not required under the law.[11] Usually, the expected cost of implementing regulations is considered together with the potential benefits when decisions are made—but plenty of room remains for controversy over the relative magnitudes of the costs and benefits.

Since regulatory activities of federal and state governments are so fundamental to public health, they are discussed throughout this text.

How Public Health Is Organized and Paid for in the United States

Local Public Health Agencies

The organization of public health at the local level varies from state to state and even within states. The most common local agency is the county health department. A large city may have its own municipal health department, and rural areas may be served by multicounty health departments. Some local areas have no public health department, leaving their residents to do without some services and to depend on state government for others.

Local health departments have the day-to-day responsibility for public health matters in their jurisdiction. These tasks include collecting health statistics; conducting communicable disease control programs; providing screening and immunizations; providing health education services and chronic disease control programs; conducting sanitation, sanitary engineering, and inspection programs; running school health programs; and delivering maternal and child health services and public health nursing services. Mental health may or may not be the responsibility of a separate agency.

In many states, laws assign **local public health agencies** the responsibility of providing medical care to the poor. While this task may be considered part of the assurance function defined in *The Future of Public Health*,[1] the Institute of Medicine found that this role tends to consume excessive resources and distract local health departments from performing their assessment and policy development functions. The provision of medical services by public health clinics has often been a source of friction with the medical establishment. Functions of a typical county health department are shown in the organizational chart in **Figure 3-2**.

The sources of funds for local health department activities vary widely among states. Some states provide the bulk of funding for local health departments, whereas others provide very little. The federal government may fund some local health department activities directly, or federal funds may be passed on from the states. A portion of the local health budget usually comes from local property and sales taxes, and from fees that the health department charges for some services. The extent to which local health departments are responsive to mandates from the state and federal government is likely to depend on how much of the local agency's budget is provided by these sources. When the bulk of a local health department's budget is determined by a city council or county legislature, the local agency's capacity to perform core functions may depend on its ability to educate the legislative body about public health and its importance.

State Health Departments

States have the primary constitutional responsibility and authority for the protection of the health, safety, and general welfare of the population, and much of this responsibility falls on

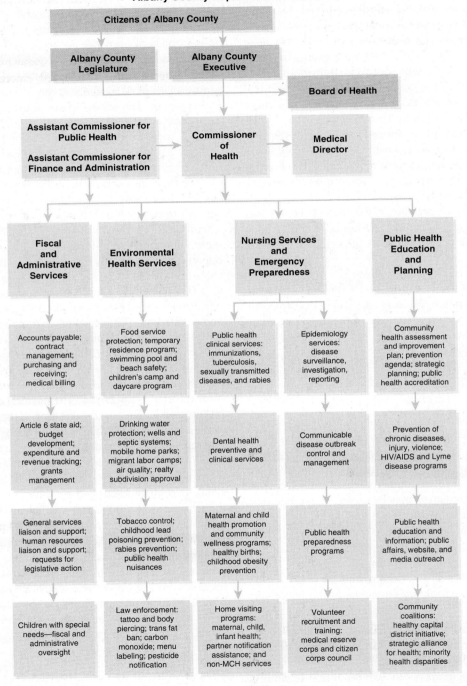

Figure 3-2 Organizational Chart of a County Health Department

Courtesy of the Albany County Department of Health.

state health departments. The scope of this responsibility varies: Some states have separate agencies for social services, aging, mental health, the environment, and so on. This may cause problems, for example, when the environmental agency makes decisions that impact the population's health without consulting the health agency, or—in one example described by the Institute of Medicine—when the Indian Health Service, the state health agency, and the state mental health agency argued about which was responsible for adult and aging services.[1] Some state health departments are strongly centralized, while others delegate much of their authority to the local health departments. State health departments depend heavily on federal money for many programs, so that their authority is limited by the strings attached to the federal funds.

State health departments define to varying degrees the activities of the local health departments. The state health department may set policies to be followed by the local agencies, and it generally provides significant funding, both from state sources and by channeling federal funds to local areas. The state health department coordinates activities of the local agencies and collects and analyzes the data provided by the local agencies. Laboratory services are often provided by state health departments. In addition, state health departments are usually charged with licensing and certification of medical personnel, facilities, and services, with the purpose of maintaining standards of competence and quality of care. An organizational chart for a typical state health department is shown in Figure 3-1.

People who lack private health insurance are generally the concern of state health departments, although many states pass this responsibility on to localities. Some of these people are covered by Medicaid, the joint federal–state program for the poor. States have significant—though not total—flexibility in how to administer the Medicaid program, determining eligibility rules for coverage as well as setting payment amounts for doctors, hospitals, and other providers of medical care to the Medicaid-covered population. Most states also provide some kind of funding to hospitals to reimburse them for treating uninsured patients who arrive in the emergency room and must be treated.

Funding for state health department activities comes mostly from state taxes and federal grants.

Federal Agencies Involved with Public Health

Most traditional public health activities at the federal level, other than environmental health, fall under the jurisdiction of the Department of Health and Human Services (HHS). **Figure 3-3** shows the HHS operating divisions. The predominant agencies are the **Centers for Disease Control and Prevention (CDC)**, the **National Institutes of Health (NIH)**, and the FDA. The **Surgeon General** is the nation's leading spokesperson on matters of public health. The position does not in itself carry much direct line authority, but it became very visible in the 1980s when C. Everett Koop spoke out with great courage and moral authority on the politically controversial subjects of acquired immunodeficiency syndrome (AIDS) and tobacco use.

The CDC is the main assessment and epidemiologic agency for the nation. Its mission, as its name implies, is to control and prevent human diseases. Traditionally, the CDC focused on infectious diseases and, therefore, engaged in crisis-oriented operations. In contrast, the NIH holds a longer view, as it functions as a research agency. The CDC is staffed with epidemiologists who travel throughout the country and the world to detect outbreaks of disease, to track down the causes of epidemics, and to halt their spread. It also has laboratories at its headquarters in Atlanta, where biomedical

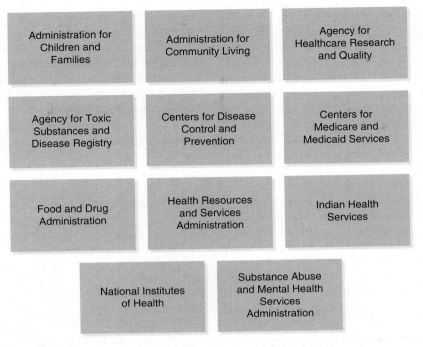

Figure 3-3 Health and Human Services Operating Divisions

Modified from U.S. Department of Health and Human Services, Organizational Chart, http://www.hhs.gov/about/agencies/orgchart/index.html, accessed August 3, 2019.

scientists study the viruses and bacteria linked with the epidemics. One of the 12 centers, institutes, and offices in the CDC is the National Center for Health Statistics, which is the national authority for collecting, analyzing, and disseminating health data for the United States.

The CDC has expanded its mission over recent decades to include chronic diseases, genetics, injury and violence, and environmental health. The CDC's change in focus is justified by the argument that infectious diseases are no longer the leading causes of death and disability in the United States, and that these other problems must be addressed to make further progress in preventing and controlling disease. However, the CDC's involvement in programs to prevent noninfectious diseases, injury, and violence is more controversial politically, in that it embroils the agency in discussions of health-related behavior, as well as of industries, such as tobacco

and firearms, that have supporters in Congress. **Figure 3-4** shows the organizational chart for the CDC.

The CDC issues a weekly publication called ***Morbidity and Mortality Weekly Report (MMWR)***, which is widely distributed in print and electronically via the Internet. *MMWR* reports on timely public health topics that the CDC deals with, such as outbreaks of infectious diseases and new environmental and behavioral health hazards. The first published report that heralded the onset of the AIDS epidemic appeared in *MMWR* on June 4, 1981.[13] The CDC's journal *Emerging Infectious Diseases*, published in print and online, discusses new infectious disease threats that occur naturally as well as potential bioterrorist threats.

The NIH is the largest biomedical research complex in the world, with its own research laboratories, most of which are located in Bethesda, Maryland, as well as a program that provides grants to biomedical

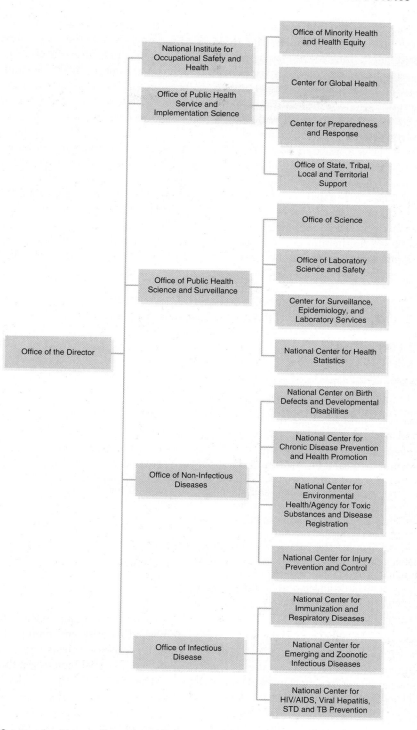

Figure 3-4 Centers for Disease Control and Prevention Organizational Chart

scientists at universities and research centers throughout the United States. The NIH supports research into topics ranging from basic cellular processes to the physiological errors that underlie human diseases, and its scientists publish more biomedical research than any other institution in the world except Harvard University.[14] The NIH's Clinical Center in Bethesda is a research hospital where medical researchers test experimental therapies. The NIH also includes the National Library of Medicine, which serves as a reference library for medical centers around the world. Its computerized bibliographic service can be accessed on the Internet. **Box 3-1** lists the NIH's institutes, centers, and offices.

NIH has enjoyed strong support from the U.S. Congress over the years. Research aimed at curing human diseases is a popular cause and, for the most part, is generally agreed to be a proper activity for the federal government. States and private companies have more limited resources to fund biomedical research. Even periodic budgetary constraints have usually spared NIH the worst of the axe.

Regulation of the food and drug industries has been difficult and controversial since Massachusetts passed the first American pure-food law in 1784. As recently as the late 19th century, milk was commonly watered down, then doctored with chalk or plaster of Paris to make it look normal.[15] The Pure Food and

---

Box 3-1 National Institutes of Health: Institutes, Centers, and Offices

- Office of the Director
- National Cancer Institute
- National Eye Institute
- National Heart, Lung, and Blood Institute
- National Human Genome Research Institute
- National Institute of Allergy and Infectious Diseases
- National Institute on Aging
- National Institute on Alcohol Abuse and Alcoholism
- National Institute of Arthritis and Musculoskeletal and Skin Diseases
- National Institute of Biomedical Imaging and Bioengineering
- Eunice Kennedy Shriver National Institute of Child Health and Human Development
- National Institute on Deafness and Other Communication Disorders
- National Institute of Dental and Craniofacial Research
- National Institute of Diabetes and Digestive and Kidney Diseases
- National Institute on Drug Abuse
- National Institute of Environmental Health Sciences
- National Institute of General Medical Sciences
- National Institute of Mental Health
- National Institute on Minority Health and Health Disparities
- National Institute of Neurological Disorders and Stroke
- National Institute of Nursing Research
- National Library of Medicine
- Center for Information Technology
- Center for Scientific Review
- Fogarty International Center
- National Center for Complementary and Alternative Medicine
- National Center for Advancing Translational Sciences
- NIH Clinical Center

Modified from National Institutes of Health, www.nih.gov/institutes-nih/list-nih-institutes-centers-offices, accessed August 3, 2019.

Drugs Act of 1906, a pivotal early consumer protection measure that led to the creation of the Food and Drug Administration, was opposed by the food-canning industry, drug and patent medicine manufacturers, whiskey interests, and the meatpacking industry. That law was passed soon after the publication of Upton Sinclair's best-selling novel *The Jungle*, an exposé of brutal and filthy conditions in the meatpacking plants in the Chicago stockyards.

The modern FDA was established in 1931, and the current law provides for the agency, in addition to ensuring that the food supply is safe and nutritious, to evaluate all new drugs, food additives and colorings, and certain medical devices, approving them only if they are proven safe and, in the case of drugs, effective. The agency also regulates vaccines and diagnostic tests, animal drugs, and cosmetics. Because FDA regulations affect major segments of the U.S. economy, this agency frequently comes under attack, either for being too restrictive or, when an approved product is found to cause harm, for being too lenient.

Other components of the HHS include the Centers for Medicare and Medicaid Services and the Agency for Healthcare Research and Quality, which supports research on healthcare quality and cost. The Indian Health Service agency operates hospitals and health clinics for Native Americans.

Responsibility for environmental health is scattered throughout the federal government, including the CDC's Center for Environmental Health and the NIH's National Institute of Environmental Health Sciences. The prime agency focused on the environment is the **Environmental Protection Agency (EPA)**, established in 1970 to carry out programs dealing with water pollution, air pollution, toxic substances control, and other issues of environmental contamination. The EPA is one of the most controversial federal public health agencies. It has often been attacked by Congress, and its policies were often watered down by both the George W. Bush and Donald Trump administrations.

Many other federal agencies have public health responsibilities. For example, although meat safety concerns were a major factor in the establishment of the FDA, standards focusing on meat safety are the province of the Department of Agriculture. The Department of Agriculture also oversees food and nutrition programs, including food stamps and school lunches. The Department of Education supervises health education and school health and safety programs. Among the responsibilities of the Department of Transportation is traffic safety, the purview of the National Highway Traffic Safety Administration, which has had great success in reducing deaths caused by motor vehicles. The Department of Labor has OSHA, which is concerned with occupational health and prevention of occupational injury. The Department of Veterans Affairs administers its own health and medical services. The Department of Defense, which provides medical care for the armed forces, has long had to deal with public health concerns relating to threats from infectious diseases in foreign climates as well as health effects from toxic chemicals and radiation. The Department of Homeland Security was created in 2003 to protect the public from acts of terrorism, natural disasters, and other emergencies.

Nongovernmental Role in Public Health

While government bears the major responsibility for public health, many nongovernmental organizations play important roles, especially in education, lobbying, and research. Organizations that focus on specific diseases, such as the American Heart Association, the American Cancer Society, the Alzheimer's Association, and the American Diabetes Association, lobby Congress for resources and policies to benefit their causes. They also conduct campaigns to educate the public and may sponsor research concerned with their disease. Professional membership organizations, such as the American Public

Health Association, the American Medical Association, and the American Nurses Association, also are active in lobbying Congress in support of public health issues such as research related to the health effects of smoking. However, the American Medical Association is also known for its opposition to some public health–related programs, such as the government-sponsored insurance option in President Obama's 2009 health reform plan, which contributed to its failure to be included. Other organizations that will play an important role in defining the future of public health include the National Association of City and County Health Officers, the Association of State and Territorial Health Officers, and the Association of Schools and Programs of Public Health.

A range of major philanthropic foundations provide funding to support research or special projects related to public health. For example, the Rockefeller Foundation focuses on world population issues; the Robert Wood Johnson Foundation on providing health care to the poor as well as on AIDS, alcoholism, and drug abuse; the Pew Charitable Trusts on health, AIDS, and drug abuse; the Kaiser Family Foundation on health and public policy; and the Commonwealth Fund on health and public policy, especially concerning minorities, children, and elderly people. The largest private foundation in the world is the Bill and Melinda Gates Foundation, whose mission is to improve global health.

Consumers groups organized around specific issues have sometimes had a major impact on national or regional policy related to public health. For example, Ralph Nader's traffic safety campaign in the 1960s forced Congress to pass legislation requiring the automobile industry to build safer cars. The Gay Men's Health Crisis played a critical role in the 1980s in starting up community health services for patients with AIDS in New York City.

One of the messages of the Institute of Medicine report was that governments alone cannot achieve the objectives of public health.[1] Organized community efforts to prevent disease and prolong life must involve all sectors of the community, including providers of healthcare services, local business, community organizations, the media, and the general public. In the words of one public health leader, "Public health, unlike virtually all other important social efforts, is dependent on its ability to obtain the participation of other agencies to solve its problems."[16(p.399)] Thus, public health leaders must be adept at negotiation and coalition building.

Some efforts—led by the federal government with the participation of other governmental and nongovernmental organizations—of the past decades are discussed elsewhere in this text to develop a framework for public health planning and action that involves all sectors of the community at the local, state, and national levels.

Conclusion

As an organized community effort, public health is primarily the responsibility of government, although a successful public health enterprise must involve all sectors of the community. Because the U.S. Constitution does not mention health, the states have the primary legal responsibility for public health. In turn, local governments, as the level of government closest to the people, provide the bulk of public health services. Despite the lack of explicit constitutional authority, the federal government has established a significant presence in public health. Federal agencies establish and enforce laws and regulations on issues with a national scope. Through its authority to tax and spend, the federal government leads and assists state and local governments in providing public health services.

References

1. Institute of Medicine, Committee for the Study of the Future of Public Health, *The Future of Public Health* (Washington, DC: National Academy Press, 1988).

2. T. Christoffel, *Health and the Law: A Handbook for Health Professionals* (New York: Free Press, 1982), 51–52.

3. G. S. Watson et al., "The Repeal of Helmet Use Laws and Increased Motorcyclist Mortality in the United States, 1975–1978," *American Journal of Public Health* 70 (1980): 579–585.

4. R. Rudowitz, R. Garfield, and E. Hinton, "10 Things to Know About Medicaid: Setting the Facts Straight," Kaiser Family Foundation, March 6, 2019, www.kff .org/medicaid/issue-brief/10-things-to-know -about-medicaid-setting-the-facts-straight/, accessed August 3, 2019.

5. L. O. Gostin, "Public Health Law in a New Century, Part II: Public Health Powers and Limits," *Journal of the American Medical Association* 283 (2000): 2979–2984.

6. W. E. Parmet, "After September 11: Rethinking Public Health Federalism," *Journal of Law, Medicine & Ethics* 30 (2002): 201–211.

7. L. Greenhouse, "2, 691 Decisions," *The New York Times*, July 13, 2008.

8. L. O. Gostin, "Medical Marijuana, American Federalism, and the Supreme Court," *Journal of the American Medical Association* 294 (2005): 842–844.

9. L. O. Gostin, "Public Health Law in a New Century, Part I: Law as a Tool to Advance the Community's Health," *Journal of the American Medical Association* 283 (2000): 2837–2841.

10. L. O. Gostin, "Public Health in a New Century, Part III: Public Health Regulation: A Systematic Evaluation," *Journal of the American Medical Association* 283 (2000): 3118–3122.

11. K. R. Wing, *The Law and the Public's Health* (Ann Arbor, MI: Health Administration Press, 1990), 180.

12. I. L. Feitshans, "Law and Regulation of Benzene," *Environmental Health Perspectives* 82 (1989): 299–307.

13. Centers for Disease Control and Prevention, "*Pneumocystis* Pneumonia—Los Angeles," *Morbidity and Mortality Weekly Report* 30 (1981): 1–3.

14. B. Crew, "The Top 10 Institutions in Biomedical Sciences in 2018," *Nature Index*, May 17, 2019.

15. R. M. Deutsch, *The New Nuts Among the Berries: How Nutritional Nonsense Captured America* (Palo Alto, CA: Bull Publishing, 1977).

16. G. Pickett, "Book Review: The Future of Public Health," *Journal of Public Health Policy* (Autumn 1989): 397–401.

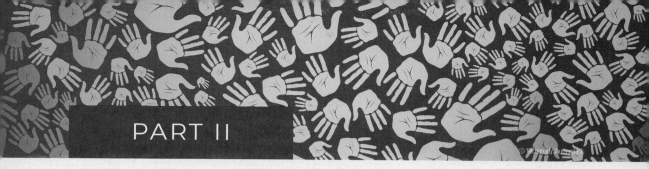

PART II

Analytical Methods of Public Health

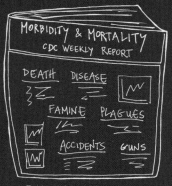

CHAPTER 4

Epidemiological Surveillance

Epidemiology: The Basic Science of Public Health

KEY TERMS

Chronic disease
Endemic rate
Epidemic
Epidemiologic investigation

Epidemiologic surveillance
Framingham Study
Notifiable diseases
Risk factors

Shoeleather epidemiology
Vital statistics

Charles-Edward Amory Winslow, the great public health leader of the early 20th century, called epidemiology "the diagnostic discipline of public health."[1(p.vii)] Epidemiologic methods are used to investigate causes of diseases, to identify trends in disease occurrence that may influence the need for medical and public health services, and to evaluate the effectiveness of medical and public health interventions. Epidemiology is used to perform public health's assessment function, as called for in the Institute of Medicine's report, *The Future of Public Health.*[2]

Epidemiology studies the patterns of disease occurrence in human populations and the factors that influence these patterns. The term is obviously related to epidemic (derived from a Greek word meaning "upon the people"). An **epidemic** is an increase in the frequency of a disease above the usual and expected rate, which is called the **endemic rate**. Thus,

epidemiologists count cases of a disease, and ask *who*, *when*, and *where* questions: Who is getting the disease? Where and when is the disease occurring? From this information, they can often make informed guesses as to why it is occurring. Their ultimate goal is to use this knowledge to control and prevent the spread of disease. This chapter aims to give a more intuitive sense of what epidemiology is and does. The science of epidemiology is examined in more detail in subsequent chapters.

How Epidemiology Works

The pioneering use of epidemiology to study and control a disease occurred in London between 1853 and 1854, and it stands as an illustration of what epidemiology is and how it works. This work was conducted by a British physician, John Snow, who is known as the father of modern epidemiology.

Snow was concerned about a cholera epidemic that had struck London in 1848. He noticed that death rates were especially high in parts of the city with water supplied by two private companies, both of which drew water from the Thames River at a point heavily polluted with sewage. Between 1849 and 1854, the Lambeth Company changed its source to an area of the Thames that was free of pollution from London's sewers. Snow noticed that the number of cholera deaths declined in the section of London supplied by the Lambeth Company, whereas there was no change in the sections supplied by the Southwark and Vauxhall Company. He formulated the hypothesis that cholera was spread by polluted drinking water.[3]

In 1853, a severe outbreak of cholera occurred that was concentrated in the Broad Street area of London, where some houses were supplied by one water company and some by the other. This provided an opportunity for Snow to test his hypothesis in a kind of "natural experiment," in which "people of both sexes, of every age and occupation, and of every rank and station . . . were divided into two groups without their choice, and, in most cases, without their knowledge."[4(pp.6–7)] Snow went to each house in which someone had died of cholera between August 1853 and January 1854 to determine which company supplied the water. When he tabulated the results, he found that in 40,046 houses supplied by the Southwark and Vauxhall Company, there were 1263 deaths from cholera. By comparison, in 26,107 houses supplied by the Lambeth Company, only 98 deaths occurred. The rate of cholera deaths was thus 8.5 times higher in houses supplied by the Southwark and Vauxhall Company than in those supplied by the Lambeth Company. This was convincing evidence that deaths from cholera were linked with the source of water (**Table 4-1**).

Snow would not have been able to test his hypothesis without the data on cholera deaths, which had been collected by the British government as part of a system for routine compilation of births and deaths, including cause of death, since 1839. Now, the governments of all developed countries collect data on births, deaths, and other **vital statistics**. These data are often used for epidemiologic studies.

Because it is preferable to recognize that an epidemic is occurring before many people start dying, governments also use a system called **epidemiologic surveillance**, requiring that certain **notifiable diseases** be reported as soon as they are diagnosed. These conditions are usually infectious diseases whose spread can be prevented by taking the appropriate actions. In the United States,

Table 4-1 Deaths from Cholera by Company Supplying Water to the Household, 1853–1854

Water Company	Number of Houses	Deaths from Cholera	Deaths from Cholera per 10,000 Houses
Southwark and Vauxhall Company	40,046	1263	315
Lambeth Company	26,107	98	37
Rest of London	256,423	1422	59

Data from J. Snow, "On the Mode of Communication of Cholera" (London: Churchill, 1855).

approximately 90 conditions have been identified by law as notifiable at the federal level, including anthrax, human immunodeficiency virus (HIV), measles, and Zika. Some states require reporting of additional infectious diseases. There may also be requirements for reporting birth defects, adverse reactions to immunizations, and other noninfectious conditions. For example, the state of Washington requires the reporting of gunshot wounds.[5] All physicians, hospitals, and clinical laboratories must report any case of a notifiable disease or condition to their local health department, which in turn reports to the state health department and the Centers for Disease Control and Prevention (CDC). The timely reporting of cases of notifiable diseases allows public health authorities to detect an emerging epidemic at an early stage. Measures can then be taken to control the spread of infectious diseases, as discussed later in this chapter.

Reporting of **chronic diseases** is less widespread, but some public health agencies have urged a system to monitor conditions such as birth defects, Alzheimer's disease, and asthma.[6] Such a system would help identify causes of these diseases, including environmental causes that could be controlled or eliminated, preventing further harmful effects. In 2010, nearly all types of cancer were added to the list of national notifiable diseases.

While the surveillance system was created to control the spread of known diseases, the established network of reporting can facilitate the recognition that a new disease may be emerging. The first step in recognizing that a community is facing a new problem is usually a report to the local or state health department or the CDC by a perceptive physician who notices something unusual that he or she thinks should be investigated further. This is how acquired immunodeficiency syndrome (AIDS) came to be recognized early in the epidemic.

A Typical Epidemiologic Investigation: Hepatitis Outbreak

Hepatitis A is a notifiable disease in all 50 states. Because it is caused by a virus that contaminates food or water, it is important to identify the source of any outbreak so that authorities can take steps to prevent wider exposure to the virus. Although hepatitis is not usually fatal to otherwise healthy people, it can make people quite sick for several weeks and can sometimes require hospitalization.

Because hepatitis is a notifiable disease, the local public health department is able to recognize when an outbreak occurs. A county may normally record only a few cases of hepatitis each year. This is the endemic rate, the background rate in a population. A sudden increase in the number of cases signifies an epidemic and calls for an **epidemiologic investigation** to determine why it is occurring.

The epidemiologic investigation requires asking the *who*, *where*, and *when* questions. This kind of medical detective work is nicknamed "**shoeleather epidemiology**." The investigator starts with the reported cases— the *who*—although other, unreported cases may turn up once the investigator starts asking questions. Each victim must be interviewed and asked the *when* question: On what date did the first symptoms appear? Knowing that hepatitis has an incubation period of approximately 30 days, it is possible to work back to an estimated date of exposure. The *where* question is the hardest to answer: Where did the victims obtain their food and water during the period of likely exposure and what sources did they have in common?

Perhaps all of the patients have eaten at the same restaurant. The epidemiologist would then visit this restaurant. If the investigator finds that the chef had developed hepatitis about a month earlier and been hospitalized, the contamination of the food will have stopped, and the epidemic will also stop. Alternatively, the chef may have had only a mild, perhaps unrecognized case and continued to work, thereby continuing to spread the infection. In this case, the health department might have to close the restaurant down, if necessary, until the chef is declared healthy.

Such investigations are a task frequently carried out by epidemiologists at local health departments. A large number of these investigations deal with food-poisoning outbreaks caused by contamination with *Salmonella* or *Shigella*, bacteria that commonly infect carelessly prepared or preserved food, and both of which cause notifiable diseases. The source of the Milwaukee cryptosporidiosis outbreak in 1993 was identified by such an epidemiologic investigation. Although cryptosporidiosis was not a notifiable disease, the epidemic was recognized because it was so severe and widespread. If the disease had been notifiable, it might have been recognized and halted earlier. Cryptosporidiosis was added to the national list of notifiable diseases in 1995. **Table 4-2** lists diseases that were reportable at the national level in 2017.

With some diseases, even a single case amounts to an epidemic. Measles, which is highly contagious, is preventable by vaccination. Although measles immunization for

Table 4-2 Infectious Diseases Designated as Notifiable at the National Level and Number of Cases Reported During 2017

Disease	Number of Cases
Anthrax	0
Arboviral diseases, neuroinvasive and non-neuroinvasive	344
Babesiosis	2368
Botulism, total	177
Brucellosis	140
Campylobacteriosis	67,537
Chancroid	7
Chlamydia trachomatis infection	1,708,569
Cholera	10
Coccidioidomycosis	14,364
Cryptosporidiosis	11,414
Cyclosporiasis	1194
Dengue virus infections	454
Diphtheria	0
Ehrlichiosis/anaplasmosis	7718
Giardiasis	15,193

Disease	Number of Cases
Gonorrhea	555,608
Haemophilus influenzae, invasive disease	5548
Hansen's disease/leprosy	94
Hantavirus infection, non-hantavirus pulmonary syndrome	2
Hantavirus pulmonary syndrome	33
Hemolytic uremic syndrome, post-diarrheal	338
Hepatitis	
A, acute	3365
B, acute	3409
B, perinatal infection	31
C, acute	4225
Human immunodeficiency virus diagnoses	33,938
Influenza-associated pediatric mortality	126
Invasive pneumococcal disease	19,780
Legionellosis (Legionnaires' disease)	7458
Leptospirosis	72
Listeriosis	887
Lyme disease	42,743
Malaria	2056
Measles	120
Meningococcal disease	353
Mumps	6109
Novel influenza A virus infections	66
Pertussis	18,975
Plague	5
Poliomyelitis, paralytic	0
Poliovirus infection, nonparalytic	0
Psittacosis	5
Q fever	193

(continues)

Table 4-2 Infectious Diseases Designated as Notifiable at the National Level and Number of Cases Reported During 2017 (*Continued*)

Disease	Number of Cases
Rabies	
Animal	4423
Human	2
Rubella	7
Rubella, congenital syndrome	5
Salmonellosis	54,285
Severe acute respiratory syndrome–associated coronavirus disease	0
Shiga toxin-producing *Escherichia coli*	8672
Shigellosis	14,912
Smallpox	0
Spotted fever rickettsiosis	6428
Streptococcal toxic-shock syndrome	372
Syphilis	101,567
Tetanus	33
Toxic shock syndrome (other than streptococcal)	30
Trichinellosis	15
Tuberculosis	9105
Tularemia	239
Typhoid fever	419
Vancomycin-intermediate and resistant *Staphylococcus aureus*	112
Varicella (chickenpox)	8777
Vibriosis	2085
Viral hemorrhagic fevers	0
Yellow fewer	0
Zika virus	1177

Data from Centers for Disease Control and Prevention, "National Notifiable Infectious Diseases and Conditions: United States," Table 1, 2017, wonder.cdc .gov/nndss/static/2017/annual/2017-table1.html, accessed August 7, 2019.

children was required by all states beginning in the 1970s, a number of measles epidemics occurred between 1989 and 1991 on college campuses. Each reported case triggered a need for mass immunizations on campus. When epidemiologists found that many of the affected students had been immunized as infants, they concluded that a second vaccination was necessary for older children. The new policy put a halt to measles epidemics on campuses. However, in recent years, parental resistance to immunization has led to outbreaks of this still dangerous disease.

Since the bioterrorist attacks in the fall of 2001, the CDC has added to the list of notifiable diseases several infectious diseases caused by potential agents of bioterrorism. The first sign of a bioterror attack could be the report of a single case identified in a hospital emergency room.

Legionnaires' Disease

In July 1976, the American Legion held a 4-day convention in Philadelphia. Before the event was over, conventioneers began falling ill with symptoms of fever, muscle aches, and pneumonia. By early August, 150 cases of the disease and 20 deaths had been reported to the Pennsylvania Department of Health, and the CDC was called in to help determine what was causing the epidemic. The investigation determined that the site of exposure was most likely the Hotel Bellevue-Stratford, one of four Philadelphia hotels where convention activities were held.[7,8] Delegates who stayed at the Bellevue-Stratford had a higher rate of illness than those who stayed at other hotels, and many of those who fell ill had attended receptions in the hotel's hospitality suites. However, cases also occurred in people who had only been near, not in, the hotel, suggesting that exposure could have occurred on the streets or sidewalks nearby. The evidence suggested that the causative agent was airborne, but it did not appear to spread in a person-to-person manner to the patients' families.

While the epidemiologists were conducting their investigation, they enlisted the help of the CDC's biomedical scientists to look for evidence of viruses or bacteria in the body tissues of the victims. They also considered the possibility of a toxic chemical, but no evidence of a cause could be found. It was not until the following January that the biomedical scientists found the bacteria responsible for the epidemic, which by then was called Legionnaires' disease. The hotel was searched for the source of the bacteria. It was eventually found in the water of a cooling tower used for air conditioning: *Legionella* bacteria had been pumped into the cooled air and inhaled by the victims.

Once the *Legionella* bacteria were identified, they were found to be responsible for a number of other outbreaks of pneumonia around the country. The bacteria were also identified in preserved blood and tissue samples collected in 1965 from victims of a previously unsolved outbreak of pneumonia that affected some 80 patients at St. Elizabeth's psychiatric hospital in Washington, DC, killing 14 of them.[8] Thus Legionnaires' disease had probably been around but had gone unrecognized as a specific disease at least since the invention of air conditioning. Federal air-conditioning standards were changed after the Philadelphia epidemic, with stringent requirements for cleaning of cooling towers and large-scale air-conditioning systems being introduced. Although most of the 5000-plus Legionnaires' disease cases that occur in the United States each year are isolated incidents, significant outbreaks still occur, including one associated with the Sheraton Atlanta Hotel in the summer of 2019 that sickened an estimated 73 people and led to a 4-week closure of the hotel.[9] Because legionellosis is now a notifiable disease, outbreaks are recognized more quickly and control measures implemented more rapidly.

Eosinophilia–Myalgia Syndrome

Although infectious agents are usually suspected first in any outbreak of a new disease, epidemiologists must also consider exposure to a toxic substance as an alternative cause. Physicians and epidemiologists found this to be the case in a puzzling outbreak first reported in New Mexico. In October 1989, several Santa Fe doctors were comparing notes on three patients suffering from a novel condition involving fatigue, debilitating muscle pain, rashes, and shortness of breath. Blood tests performed on all three patients had revealed very high counts of white blood cells called eosinophils. The doctors knew of no known condition that could explain these findings. However, they were struck by the fact that all three patients, when questioned about drugs or medications they were taking, had mentioned a health food supplement called L-tryptophan. L-Tryptophan is a "natural" substance, a component of proteins, that had been publicized as a treatment for insomnia, depression, and premenstrual symptoms. Believing that more than coincidence was involved in these three cases, the doctors reported them to the New Mexico State Health Department.[10]

The State Health Department reported the cases to the CDC and began an investigation to determine whether additional cases existed and whether they shared a consistent link with L-tryptophan. By searching the records of clinical laboratories in Santa Fe, Albuquerque, and Los Alamos, the investigators discovered 12 additional patients whose blood had exhibited high white cell counts since May 1. A team of health department investigators interviewed these 12 people and found that they all had used L-tryptophan. They also interviewed 24 people of the same age and sex as the patients who lived in the same neighborhoods—a control group—and found that only two had taken the supplement. This strongly suggested the existence of a link between L-tryptophan exposure and the illness. The CDC notified other state health departments, which conducted their own investigations. By November 16, the CDC had received reports from 35 states of 243 possible cases of the new disease, called eosinophilia–myalgia syndrome (EMS). On November 17, the Food and Drug Administration announced a nationwide recall of products containing L-tryptophan. The publicity brought forth a flood of new reports of the syndrome, but then new cases began to drop off. By August 1, 1992, 1511 cases had been reported by all 50 states. Many patients were left with permanent disabilities and 38 people had died, but the epidemic was over.[11]

Why had this natural substance caused such severe consequences? L-Tryptophan is an amino acid, which is naturally present in many foods including meat, fish, poultry, and cheese. It is also added to infant formulas, special dietary foods, and intravenous and oral solutions administered to patients with special medical needs. No cases of EMS had been reported from these products. Tests on the recalled tablets indicated that a toxic contaminant, formed as a result of a recent change in one factory's method of production, may have been responsible for the epidemic of 1989. However, other evidence suggested that earlier, unrecognized cases had occurred since the product was introduced in 1974.[12] The fact that many people took the supplements with no apparent harm suggests that individual variations in susceptibility may exist.

Serious outbreaks of illness caused by toxic contamination of food, owing to production errors or outright fraud, have occurred numerous times over the past few decades. It is usually epidemiologists who identify the source of the problem. To many public health experts, the EMS epidemic of 1989 resembled an illness with similar symptoms that affected some 20,000 people in Spain in 1981, killing more than 300 of them within a few months. An infectious agent had first been suspected, but epidemiologists noted an odd geographic distribution of the outbreak. The affected individuals lived either in a localized area south of Madrid or in a corridor along a road north of the city. The epidemiologists found that the affected households had bought oil for cooking from itinerant salespeople, who were illegally selling oil that had been manufactured for industrial use.[13] Laboratory scientists investigating the nature of the contaminants and how they might have caused the symptoms did not specifically identify a single chemical as being responsible. They now suspect that a range of chemicals, even at very low concentrations, may induce autoimmune responses in susceptible people, causing the body's immune system to attack its own tissues. Such outbreaks caused by toxic contamination of foods and drugs may be much more common than is generally recognized.[14] In the cases of toxic oil syndrome and EMS, government action to remove the contaminated product put an end to the epidemic. However, survivors still suffer from symptoms.

Epidemiologic surveillance is a major line of defense in protecting the public against disease. It is the warning system that alerts the community that something is wrong, that a gap has opened in the protective bulwark against preventable disease or that a new disease has appeared on the horizon. The sooner the surveillance system kicks in, the sooner action can be taken to stop the epidemic. Before the health department is notified, individual doctors are trying to cure individual patients, often unaware that the problem is more widespread. After the epidemic is recognized, all the resources of the community—local, state, or national—can be mobilized to prevent the disease's spread. Whether it uses vaccination campaigns against measles, isolation of hepatitis-infected food workers, new regulations on air-conditioning systems, or recall of contaminated food or drugs, the government must act to protect the health of the public. Epidemiologic surveillance has become even more important as concerns about bioterrorism have increased.

Epidemiology and the Causes of Chronic Disease

Epidemiology has had a different role to play in investigating the causes of the diseases common in older age, such as cancer and heart disease, which are quite different from infectious diseases and acute poisoning. Until the mid-20th century, these conditions were thought of as a natural part of aging, and no one thought to look for causes or tried to prevent them.

Cancer, heart disease, and other diseases of aging do not have single causes. They tend to develop over a period of time, are often chronic and disabling rather than rapidly fatal, and cannot be prevented or cured by any vaccine or "magic bullet." The best hope for protecting the public against these diseases is to learn how to prevent them, or at least how to delay their onset. Prevention, however, requires an understanding of the cause or causes of a disease and the factors that influence its progression. Epidemiology has made major contributions to the current understanding of the causes of heart disease and some cancers and what can be done to prevent them. Epidemiologic studies will continue to yield information on how people can protect themselves against cancer, Alzheimer's disease, and other afflictions of aging.

Epidemiologic studies of these chronic diseases are much more complicated and difficult than investigations of acute outbreaks of infectious diseases or toxic contamination. Except for the clear link between smoking and lung cancer (discussed later in this chapter), most chronic diseases cannot be attributed to a single cause. Indeed, many different **risk factors** may play a part in causing a disease. The long period over which these diseases develop also contributes to the difficulty of determining the causative factors. Epidemiologists must determine which of a person's many experiences over the previous decades are relevant, and what significant exposures might have occurred 10 or 20 years ago that may have increased the person's risk of developing the disease today.

Epidemiology has developed a number of methods to study chronic diseases and to address the difficult questions related to them. The rest of this chapter describes a few of the best-known studies that have had major impacts on understanding the causes of heart disease and lung cancer.

Heart Disease

Since the 1920s, when infectious disease mortality dropped to approximately its current low levels, heart disease has been the leading cause of death in the United States for both men and women. Deaths from heart disease increased dramatically during the first half of the 20th century (**Figure 4-1**). After World War II, one in every five men was affected with heart disease before the age of 60, and little was known about why. In 1948, an epidemiologic study was launched in Framingham, Massachusetts, to investigate factors that might be causing the

problem. It was the first major epidemiologic study of a chronic disease. More than half of the middle-aged population of the town, more than 5000 healthy people, were examined, and data were recorded on their weight, blood pressure, smoking habits, the results of various blood tests, and other characteristics. Two years later, the same people were examined again, and these tests have been and continue to be repeated every two years for the rest of their lives.[15]

As early as 10 years later, the Framingham Heart Study had revealed a great deal about how to predict which of the study participants were likely to develop heart disease. The study identified three major risk factors: high blood pressure, high blood cholesterol, and smoking. As a result of the findings, concepts of "normal" blood pressure and cholesterol levels changed significantly. Doctors had previously believed that blood pressure naturally increased as people aged and that this increase was normal and healthy. The **Framingham Study** found that some people maintained their youthful blood pressure and cholesterol values as they got

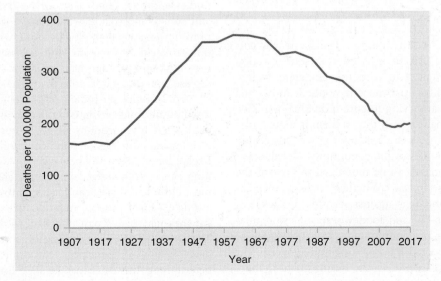

Figure 4-1 Death Rates for Heart Disease in the United States, 1907–2017

Data from Centers for Disease Control and Prevention, National Vital Statistics System, "Historical Data, 1900–1998," www.cdc.gov/nchs/data/dvs/lead1900_98.pdf, accessed August 7, 2019; and detailed tables of the National Vital Statistics Report 68(9), "Deaths: Final Data for 2017," www.cdc.gov/nchs/data/nvsr/nvsr68/nvsr68_09-508.pdf, accessed August 7, 2019.

older and that these people remained healthier. Weight gain and lack of exercise were found to be associated with increased blood pressure and cholesterol values and with an increased risk of heart disease.[16]

The Framingham findings have had a major impact on the course of the heart disease epidemic. Publicity on the information obtained through this study, confirmed and supported by other studies, persuaded some people to change their behavior and formed the basis of public health programs to encourage others to do the same. By the 1970s, it was clear that death rates from heart disease were falling in the United States. By 1970, this decline was picked up in the Framingham Study itself.[16] This improvement was associated with a reduction in risk factors: In 1970, blood cholesterol levels were lower; blood pressure was lower; and smoking was less common. These beneficial trends have continued. In 2015, the age-adjusted death rate from cardiovascular disease in the United States was 71% lower than it was in 1970.[17]

Meanwhile, the Framingham Study has continued and expanded, and much more has been learned. For example, a smoker's risk of heart disease rapidly drops back to that of a nonsmoker soon after the smoker quits—but low-tar, low-nicotine cigarettes are no better than the old-fashioned kind in their effects on risk of heart disease.[16] Various forms of cholesterol have been identified, including high-density lipoprotein (HDL) cholesterol—the "good" kind that is protective—and low-density lipoprotein (LDL) cholesterol—the "bad" kind. Exercise has been found to increase HDL cholesterol and to protect against heart disease. Recent findings indicate that an individual's social network has a significant effect on his or her health. For example, friends, siblings, spouses, and sometimes coworkers and neighbors can influence the risk of becoming obese, the decision to quit smoking, and the tendency to be happy. In fact, having a happy friend living within a mile increases the probability of being happy oneself by 25%.[18–20] The scope of the Framingham Study has also expanded: In 1978, the subjects began to be given neurologic examinations in addition to tests for cardiac risk factors. The investigators were watching for the development of Alzheimer's disease in the aging study population, hoping that they would be able to detect risk factors for this increasingly common and tragic condition.[21]

An offshoot of the original study, the Framingham Offspring Study, was created in 1971; it included about 5000 children of the original participants and their spouses. Investigators have sought to compare risk factors both within families and across generations, hoping to sort out the roles of genetics and environment in heart disease and other common disorders. The younger study population is being tested with more advanced medical technologies and more sophisticated blood tests, including genetic tests. In 1994, a more diverse sampling of Framingham residents, called the Omni Cohort, was added. Another expansion to form the Third Generation Study, which enrolled grandchildren of the study's original participants, was added in 2002; and a Second Generation Omni Cohort, as well as a New Offspring Spouse Cohort, was established in 2003. Much of the recent research has focused on finding genetic connections to the longstanding Framingham topic of heart disease, but recent work has continued to expand the study's scope to topics such as flu susceptibility and the effects of air pollution.[22]

Lung Cancer

Epidemiologic studies seeking causes of cancer began soon after the Framingham Study. However, studies of most kinds of cancer had much less success than the studies of heart disease; epidemiologists had few strong clues about possible causes or risk factors.

An exception was the link between smoking and lung cancer. Mortality from lung cancer began increasing dramatically after the 1930s

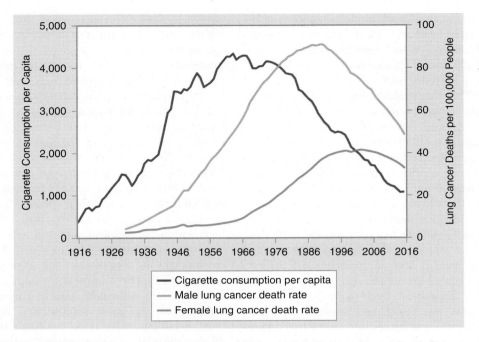

Figure 4-2 Per Capita Cigarette Consumption and Male and Female Lung Cancer Death Rates per 100,000 People in the United States, 1916–2016
Cigarette consumption is through 2015. Age-adjusted based on 2000 U.S. standard population.

Data from Cigarette Consumption, 1900–1994: Centers for Disease Control and Prevention, "Surveillance for Selected Tobacco-Use Behaviors—United States, 1900–1994," www.cdc.gov/mmwr/preview /mmwrhtml/00033881.htm, accessed August 7, 2019. 1995–1999: American Lung Association, "Overall Tobacco Trends," www.lung.org/finding-cures/our-research/trend-reports/Tobacco-Trend-Report.pdf, accessed August 7, 2019. 2000–2015: T. W. Wang et al., "Consumption of Combustible and Smokeless Tobacco—United States, 2000–2015," www.cdc.gov/mmwr/volumes/65/wr/mm6548a1.htm#T1_down, accessed August 7, 2019. Lung Cancer, 1930–2011: American Cancer Society, "Cancer Facts & Figures 2015," www.cancer.org/research/cancerfactsstatistics/cancerfactsfigures2015/index, accessed August 7, 2019. 2012–2014: American Cancer Society, "Cancer Facts & Figures 2017," www.cancer.org/research/cancer-facts-statistics/all-cancer-facts-figures/cancer-facts-figures-2017.html, accessed August 7, 2019. 2016: Centers for Disease Control and Prevention, "United States Cancer Statistics: Data Visualizations," gis.cdc.gov/Cancer/USCS/DataViz.html, accessed August 7, 2019.

(**Figure 4-2**). Because it was logical to suppose that the cause might be something that was inhaled, the two main hypotheses proposed to explain this increase were tobacco smoking and air pollution, as both had increased during the same period that lung cancer rates were rising. Several early studies conducted in England and the United States beginning in the late 1940s questioned patients with lung cancer about their smoking habits. All of these studies found that a high proportion of these patients were heavy smokers.

In late 1950 and early 1952, two major epidemiologic studies were started that convincingly established a link between lung cancer and tobacco smoking. The British epidemiologists Richard Doll and A. Bradford Hill sent out a questionnaire to all physicians in the United Kingdom, asking whether they were smokers, past smokers, or nonsmokers. Smokers and ex-smokers were asked to provide additional information on their age at starting to smoke and the amount of tobacco smoked, and ex-smokers were asked when they had quit smoking. More than 40,000 doctors responded to the survey.[23]

During the following years, Doll and his collaborators, by arrangement with the British Medical Association and the Registrar General of the United Kingdom, gathered information on which doctors had died each year and what their cause of death was. A little more than four years after the survey began, several important conclusions became apparent. First, the death rate from lung cancer was approximately 20 times higher among smokers than among nonsmokers, increasing as the amount smoked increased. Second, the death rate among ex-smokers was lower than that among smokers and declined as the length of time increased since the doctor had quit smoking. Third, the contrast in lung cancer mortality between smokers and nonsmokers was the same whether the doctors lived in rural or urban areas. Therefore, the difference could not be attributed to air pollution. Fourth, deaths from heart attacks were also significantly higher among heavy smokers aged 35 to 54 than among nonsmokers.[24]

A similar study on a much larger group of people was started shortly after the Doll and Hill study in the United States by epidemiologists E. Cuyler Hammond and Daniel Horn. They obtained smoking histories from almost 188,000 men aged 50 to 69 and followed them over a period of 3 years and 8 months. For all the study participants who died, they obtained the cause of death from death certificates. Their findings confirmed and extended the results of the Doll and Hill study of British doctors. First, cigarette smokers were more than 10 times more likely to die of lung cancer than were nonsmokers. Second, cigarette smokers were about five times more likely to die of cancer of the lip, tongue, mouth, pharynx, larynx, and esophagus than were nonsmokers. Several other types of cancer were also more common among smokers. Third, heavy smokers (two or more packs per day) were 2.4 times more likely to die of heart disease than were nonsmokers.[25]

The British study continued until 1971, tracking all the doctors for 20 years, by which time approximately 33% of them had died. The longer period of observation confirmed the results obtained earlier. An interesting finding was that many physicians reacted to the earlier reports by quitting smoking. By 1971, the average number of cigarettes smoked per day by the physicians in the study was less than half what it had been in 1951, and as a result, lung cancer became relatively less common as a cause of death in this group.[24]

The Framingham Study and the two lung cancer studies are examples of prospective cohort studies, following large numbers of people over extended periods of time. These are considered among the most reliable kinds of epidemiologic studies for investigating causes of chronic diseases. Other such studies have been done and continue at present, with many of them seeking causes of various kinds of cancer.

Conclusion

Epidemiology is an important component of the assessment function of public health. Epidemiologists investigate epidemics of known and unknown diseases by counting the number of cases and identifying how they are distributed by person, place, and time. Using this information, they can often determine a probable cause of a new disease or a reason for an outbreak of a previously controlled disease. This knowledge allows public health workers to institute measures aimed at preventing and controlling the spread of the disease.

An early achievement of epidemiology was the recognition in the 19th century that cholera was spread by polluted water. In 1993, similar epidemiologic methods determined that polluted water had caused an outbreak of cryptosporidiosis in Milwaukee. The same approach has been successful in halting outbreaks of illness caused by toxic contaminations. "Shoeleather epidemiology" by local health departments provides the frontline defense against acute diseases. Epidemiologic surveillance, including mandatory reporting of notifiable diseases, alerts a local health department that an epidemic is beginning in time for an agency to investigate the reasons and take preventive action.

Epidemiology also sheds light on the causes of chronic disease. Formal, long-term studies of heart disease and lung cancer provided the earliest information on the risk factors that contributed to these diseases. The Framingham Study, which has tracked citizens of Framingham, Massachusetts, for more than six decades, identified high blood pressure, high blood cholesterol, and smoking as risk factors for heart disease. Two epidemiologic studies conducted through the 1950s and 1960s—one on the smoking habits of British doctors and a similar study on a group of 188,000 American men—indicated a clear link between smoking and lung cancer.

Epidemiology's role in identifying causes of disease leads directly and indirectly to prevention and control. In some cases, regulatory action by a local government is necessary to eliminate disease-causing conditions. Sometimes, simply publicizing the results of a study allows people to modify their behavior to avoid risk factors for a disease. For example, information released in the 1950s on results from the Framingham Study and the studies regarding smoking and lung cancer contributed to a significant decline in smoking in the United States, which has subsequently led to a drop in mortality from both heart disease and lung cancer since the 1960s. To achieve additional improvements in public health, health agencies build on epidemiologic information to develop policy and plan programs aimed at reducing risk and promoting health in the population.

References

1. C.-E. A. Winslow et al., quoted in R. C. Brownson and D. B. Petitti, eds., *Applied Epidemiology: Theory to Practice* (New York: Oxford University Press, 1998), vii.
2. Institute of Medicine, *The Future of Public Health* (Washington, DC: National Academy Press, 1988).
3. C. J. Hennekens and J. F. Buring, *Epidemiology in Medicine* (Boston, MA: Little, Brown, 1987).
4. J. Snow, "On the Mode of Communication of Cholera" (London: Churchill, 1955). Quoted in Hennekens and Buring, *Epidemiology in Medicine*.
5. Washington State Department of Health, "Washington State Communicable Disease Report 2017," November 2018, www.doh.wa.gov/Portals/1/Documents/5100/420 -004-CDAnnualReport2017.pdf, accessed August 7, 2019.
6. P. J. Hilts, "Panel Urges Monitoring of Chronic Diseases," *The New York Times*, September 12, 2000.
7. D. W. Fraser et al., "Legionnaires' Disease," *New England Journal of Medicine* 297 (1977): 1189–1197.
8. L. Garrett, *The Coming Plague: Newly Emerging Diseases in a World out of Balance* (New York: Farrar, Straus, and Giroux, 1994).
9. H. Oliviero, "First Legionnaires' Death Linked to Atlanta Outbreak Confirmed," *The Atlanta Journal-Constitution*, August 6, 2019, www.ajc.com/lifestyles /first-legionnaires-death-linked-sheraton-atlanta -confirmed/ZHRqHIpOczM1eTfVTSoA3L/, accessed August 6, 2019.
10. Centers for Disease Control and Prevention, "Eosinophilia–Myalgia Syndrome—New Mexico," *Morbidity and Mortality Weekly Report* 38 (1989): 765–767.
11. S. L. Nightingale, "Update on EMS and l-Tryptophan," *Journal of the American Medical Association* 268 (1992): 1828.
12. T. A. Medsger Jr., "Tryptophan-Induced Eosinophilia–Myalgia Syndrome," *New England Journal of Medicine* 322 (1990): 926–928.
13. E. M. Kilbourne et al., "Clinical Epidemiology of Toxic-Oil Syndrome: Manifestations of New Disease," *New England Journal of Medicine* 309 (1983): 1408–1414.
14. M. Posada de la Paz , R. M. Philen, and I. A. Borda, "Toxic Oil Syndrome: The Perspective After 20 Years," *Epidemiology Reviews* 23 (2001): 231–247.
15. Boston University and National Heart, Lung, and Blood Institute, "Framingham Heart Study," 2019, www .framinghamheartstudy.org/, accessed August 7, 2019.
16. W. B. Kannel, "The Framingham Experience," in M. Marmot and P. Elliott, eds., *Coronary Heart Disease Epidemiology: From Aetiology to Public Health* (New York: Oxford University Press, 1992).
17. G. A. Mensah, G. S. Wei, P. D. Sorlie, L. J. Fine, Y. Rosenberg, P. G. Kaufmann, et al., "Decline in Cardiovascular Mortality: Possible Causes and Implications," *Circulation Research* 120, no. 2 (2017): 366–380.
18. N. A. Christakis and J. H. Fowler, "The Spread of Obesity in a Large Social Network over 32 Years." *New England Journal of Medicine* 357, no. 4 (2007): 370–379.
19. N. A. Christakis and J. H. Fowler, "The Collective Dynamics of Smoking in a Large Social Network," *New England Journal of Medicine* 358, no. 21 (2008): 2249–2258.

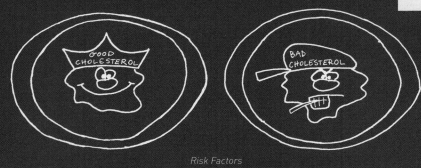

Risk Factors

Epidemiologic Principles and Methods

KEY TERMS

Association
Case-control study
Cases
Cohort study
Common-source outbreak
Control group
Controls

Determinant
Double-blind
Epidemic curve
Incidence
Intervention study
Mortality rate
Odds ratio

Placebo
Prevalence
Probability
Propagated-source outbreak
Randomized
Relative risk
Treatment group

This chapter examines epidemiology more closely, defining some of its basic terms and describing how epidemiologists use these terms to describe the patterns of disease occurrence. The chapter also explains the different kinds of epidemiologic studies, providing examples of the types of information that each form of epidemiologic study can provide.

Epidemiology is defined as "the study of the distribution and determinants of disease frequency in human populations."[1(p.1)] Each of these terms must be clearly understood.

First, the epidemiologist must define the disease in a clear way so that there is no doubt about whether an individual case should or should not be counted. Some diseases are easier to identify than others. In a hepatitis outbreak, the symptoms are fairly nonspecific, and not every patient who comes to an emergency

room with vomiting and diarrhea has hepatitis. Therefore, the epidemiologist must include the results of blood tests for liver function in his or her case definition. In a study of deaths from gunshot wounds, by contrast, the cases are fairly easy to count because virtually 100% of deaths are reported, and the cause of death is usually identified easily and listed on the death certificate. With an emerging disease like eosinophilia–myalgia syndrome, working out the case definition might be the most important part of the investigation.

In defining a disease to be studied, epidemiologists use the term "disease" broadly: "Health outcome" is a more accurate but cumbersome description of what is to be studied. For example, epidemiologists might study the frequency and distribution of high blood cholesterol, which is not a disease but is related to the risk of heart attack, or they might study injuries due to traffic accidents, which are not diseases but are certainly significant to health. In both cases, an epidemiologic study may point to ways of preventing the negative health outcome.

In measuring disease frequency, it is necessary not only to count the number of cases but also to relate that number to the size of the population being studied, yielding a rate. Seventy-three cases of Legionnaires' disease among a few thousand visitors to an Atlanta hotel, as happened in July 2019, is of much greater concern than if the same number of cases were diagnosed in the whole country. In calculating a rate, the denominator is generally the population at risk. The rate of ovarian cancer in a city with 1 million residents, for example, would be calculated by dividing the number of cases by the female population, not the total population of the city.

Two kinds of frequency measures are commonly used in epidemiology: incidence rates and prevalence rates. **Incidence** is the rate of new cases of a disease in a defined population over a defined period of time. For notifiable diseases, it is ascertained by counting cases reported to the local or state health departments and dividing by the population at risk. Incidence measures the **probability** that a healthy person in that population will develop the disease during that time. Incidence rates are useful in identifying causes of a disease. For example, the incidence of birth defects in Europe rose dramatically in 1960 after the introduction of thalidomide, a drug used in sleeping pills. This sudden increase and its timing aroused suspicions that thalidomide use by pregnant women was the cause of limb deformities in their infants—a suspicion that was soon confirmed by epidemiologic studies.[2]

Prevalence is the total number of cases existing in a defined population at a specific time. It is generally measured by doing a survey. Incidence and prevalence are related to each other, but the nature of this relationship depends on how long people live with the disease. A disease with high incidence could have a low prevalence if people recover from it rapidly, or if they die from it in a short period of time. In contrast, for chronic diseases that are not lethal—arthritis, for example—the prevalence will be much higher than the incidence. For most diseases, prevalence rates change slowly and are less useful for epidemiologic studies. They are most useful in assessing the societal impact of a disease and planning for healthcare services.

Death rates, or **mortality rates** (the incidence of death), are often used as a measure of frequency for diseases that are usually fatal. Death rates are close to incidence rates for the most lethal diseases, such as pancreatic cancer. For diseases such as breast cancer, which many women survive, the mortality rate will be much lower than the incidence rate. Death rates are not at all useful as a measure of frequency for diseases that are rarely fatal, such as arthritis.

The distribution of disease consists of the answers to the *who, when*, and *where* questions. The *who* question characterizes the disease victims by such factors as age, sex, race, and economic status. For example, the incidences of cancer and heart disease are greater in older people; measles and chickenpox occur more often in the young. Old women and young men are more likely to suffer broken bones than are old men and young women. During the early months of the acquired immunodeficiency syndrome (AIDS) epidemic, the answer to the *who* question was gay men and intravenous drug abusers—information that led to some obvious hypotheses as to how the disease was transmitted.

The *when* question looks for trends in disease frequency over time: Is the incidence increasing, decreasing, or remaining stable? The incidence of lung cancer in American men, for example, increased steadily from the 1930s to about 1990, when it peaked and began to decrease. Meanwhile, the incidence of stomach cancer has been declining. Posing another kind of *when* question, epidemiologists look for seasonal variations in incidence. The incidence of respiratory infections, for example, is always higher in the winter.

The *when* question is crucial in tracking an outbreak of infectious diseases such as hepatitis and legionellosis. Epidemiologists construct **epidemic curves** by plotting the number of cases identified over a period of time. **Figure 5-1** shows the epidemic curve for the 1976 outbreak of Legionnaires' disease in Philadelphia. It is clear from this epidemic curve that most of the victims were exposed to the virus at about the same time and, therefore, probably from a common source. This figure represents a type of **common-source outbreak**. Comparing the dates of onset with the dates of possible exposure, epidemiologists calculated an incubation period of 2 to 10 days. An epidemic curve such as the one shown in **Figure 5-2** is typical of a disease that has been passed from one person to another, and represents a **propagated-source outbreak**.[3]

The *where* question compares disease frequency in different countries, states, counties, or other geographic divisions. It may also compare disease frequencies in urban and rural populations. The hypothesis that fluoride protects against tooth decay arose from the observation that dental cavities were less common in children who lived in parts of the country that had high concentrations of fluoride in the water. Statistics on causes of death in different countries can be very suggestive in generating hypotheses about the causes of disease. The wide international variation in death rates from heart disease has been interpreted in a variety of ways, including that diet is a factor and exposure to air pollution has a negative effect on health.

Thus, information on the distribution of disease gives clues about the **determinants** of disease. International comparisons of cancer incidence, such as those shown in **Figure 5-3**, have led to hypotheses on causes of various kinds of cancer. For example, cancer of the

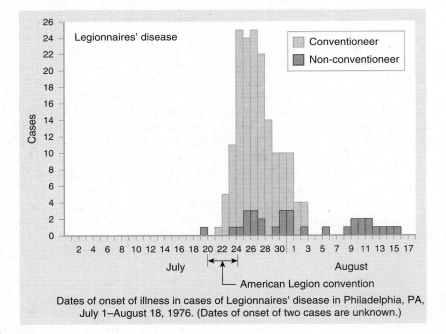

Dates of onset of illness in cases of Legionnaires' disease in Philadelphia, PA, July 1–August 18, 1976. (Dates of onset of two cases are unknown.)

Figure 5-1 Epidemic Curve for Legionnaires' Disease Outbreak

Data from Centers for Disease Control and Prevention, "Steps of an Outbreak Investigation, 2004," www.cdc.gov/publichealth101/documents/introduction-to-epidemiology.pdf, accessed August 25, 2019.

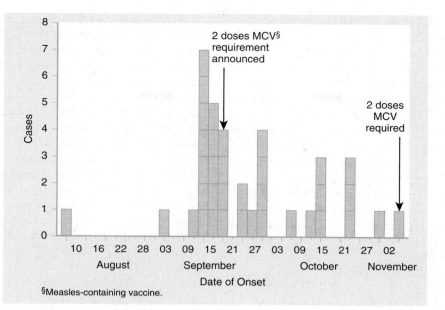

§Measles-containing vaccine.

Figure 5-2 Number of Confirmed Measles Cases by Date of Rash Onset and Three-Day Interval—Anchorage, Alaska, August 7–November 23, 1998

Reproduced from Centers for Disease Control and Prevention, *Morbidity and Mortality Weekly Report* 47 (1999): 1110, www.cdc.gov/mmwr/preview/mmwrhtml/00056144.htm, accessed August 8, 2019.

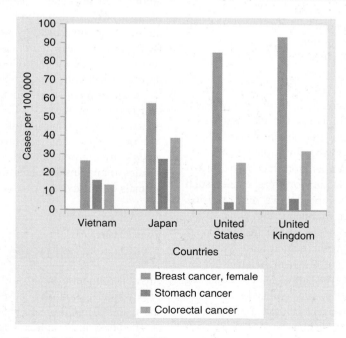

Figure 5-3 Cancer Rates in Four Countries, 2018
Age-standardized incidence rates, cases per 100,000 population.

Data from World Health Organization, International Agency on Research on Cancer, *Cancer Today*, "Fact Sheets, 2018," gco.iarc.fr/today/fact-sheets-populations, accessed August 8, 2019.

colon and rectum is much more common in industrialized countries than in developing countries, which led to the hypothesis that the difference is due to differences in diet: Americans eat meals rich in fat, meat, and dairy products, whereas diets in Vietnam are traditionally high in fiber, cereals, and vegetables. Evidence that environmental factors rather than genetics are to blame comes from studies of people who move from a low-rate country to a high-rate country. They tend to develop higher rates of the disease as they acquire the habits of the host country. In Japan, the rates of colorectal cancer have more than doubled since the 1950s as Japanese adopted more Western-style diets.[4] In contrast, in the United States, colon cancer rates have fallen dramatically since 1980—a decline attributed to increased use of colonoscopy screening, during which precancerous polyps may be removed. Nevertheless, while the screening rate of people aged 50 or older, for whom the tests are recommended, had reached 63% as of 2015, more progress is needed to reach the National Colorectal Cancer Roundtable goal of 80%, the screening level at which an estimated 203,000 deaths can be averted.[5]

International patterns of breast cancer are somewhat similar to those of colorectal cancer—that is, higher in the West and lower in Asia—suggesting that similar dietary factors may play a role in the development of breast cancer.[6,7] However, as more has been learned about other risk factors for breast cancer, such as hormonal and reproductive history, it has become clear that diet is not the whole story.[7] The incidence of breast cancer in Japan is far lower than that in the United States. Rates of stomach cancer are much higher in Vietnam and Japan than in the United States, indicating that different dietary factors may be involved: Diets high in smoked foods, salted meat or fish, and pickled vegetables increase the risk of stomach cancer. However, *Helicobacter pylori*, the bacterium that causes ulcers, also plays an important role in causing stomach cancer.[8]

The relevance of the *who* and *when* questions is clearly illustrated in the evidence that smoking is a determinant of lung cancer. Men began smoking cigarettes early in the 20th century, and lung cancer rates began rising 20 years later. Women did not begin smoking in large numbers until the 1940s and 1950s. Lung cancer rates for women did not begin to rise sharply until the 1960s.

Why are broken bones more common in males in younger age groups, yet more common in females in elderly populations? This question leads to an investigation of the determinants of broken bones. In boys and young men, these injuries are usually the result of accidents stemming from reckless behavior, in which males are more likely to engage than females. In the elderly, however, broken bones usually result from osteoporosis, or weakening of the bones, which is more common in older females.

Epidemiology studies human populations, usually using observational rather than experimental methods. The alternative approach to investigating causes of disease is the biomedical approach, which often relies on animal models of the disease. Each approach has both advantages and disadvantages. Experiments done on animals can yield clear answers as to cause and effect, while for ethical reasons experiments cannot usually be done on humans. However, uncertainties always arise about the relevance of animal studies to humans and whether the findings in animals can be extrapolated to people.

Kinds of Epidemiologic Studies

Answers to the *who, when*, and *where* questions provide clues about the causes of a disease or the source of an outbreak. This type of analysis is called descriptive epidemiology. The hypotheses generated by descriptive epidemiology are tested by formal epidemiologic studies, designed to confirm or disprove the hypothesis.

For example, in investigating the eosinophilia–myalgia syndrome (EMS) outbreak in New Mexico, epidemiologists found an apparent link with the use of L-tryptophan. To test the hypothesis, they conducted a study comparing 12 cases of EMS with 24 controls, a case-control study (described later in the chapter) that confirmed the link.[9]

Epidemiologic studies are sometimes referred to as being prospective or retrospective. Prospective studies start in the present and monitor groups of people into the future, or they may start at a point in time in the past and look forward from there. Retrospective studies look into the past for causes of diseases from which people currently suffer. In both cases, investigators are looking for **associations** between exposure to the suspected causative factor and the disease (or other health outcome).

Intervention Studies

Intervention studies are the exception to the rule that epidemiologists do not perform experiments. These studies are conducted in very much the same way as laboratory experiments on animals. They are usually undertaken to test a new treatment for a disease, such as a chemotherapy drug for cancer, or a preventive measure, such as a vaccine. In a clinical trial, a **treatment group** is exposed to the intervention, while a **control group** is not exposed. The investigators then watch and wait to see whether the response of the treatment group differs from that of the control group. Of course, only a limited number of interventions lend themselves to being tested in clinical trials for ethical reasons or because a trial is too difficult to conduct. In testing treatments for serious diseases, there must be enough doubt about the effectiveness of the intervention to justify withholding it from people who could be helped and enough evidence that it will not harm the people on whom it is tested.

The control group may be given a **placebo**—an inactive substance similar in appearance to the drug or vaccine being tested. When a treatment for a disease is already known to exist, trials may compare the new treatment with the existing treatment. The purpose of the placebo is to prevent subjects from knowing whether they are receiving the intervention. Many trials over the years have found that as many as one-third of patients respond to a placebo as if it were the intervention, reporting that they feel better or that they suffered side effects—a phenomenon called the placebo effect. The drug being tested must show a higher response rate than the placebo if it is to be considered effective.

The most convincing clinical trials are conducted in a randomized, double-blind manner. **Randomized** means that each subject is assigned to the treatment group or the control group at random. This helps equalize the groups with respect to unknown and known factors that might affect the results. **Double-blind** means that both the patient and the physician (researcher) are blind as to whether the patient is receiving the drug or a placebo. One reason that the doctor should also be blinded is that studies have shown patients to respond more favorably to a treatment that the doctor believes in. Another reason is to prevent the possibility that doctors might interpret the patient's condition differently if they know how the patient is being treated.

In a therapeutic clinical trial, both the treatment group and the control group are composed of patients who have the disease for which a therapy is being tested. Thousands of therapeutic trials are being conducted each year by pharmaceutical companies testing new drugs. The Food and Drug Administration (FDA) requires that the safety and effectiveness of any new drug must be demonstrated in a properly conducted clinical trial before it can be approved for marketing.

A classic example of a randomized, double-blind clinical trial of a preventive intervention is the field trial of the polio vaccine in 1954. Polio, then a greatly dreaded disease in the United States, killed and paralyzed both children and adults. President Franklin Roosevelt, for example, had paralysis of the legs from polio, which he had contracted at the age of 39 when he was already active in politics and public service.[10] In 1952, 21,269 cases of paralytic polio were reported in the United States.[11] The development of a vaccine by Jonas Salk offered great hope for prevention of this scourge. Preliminary tests had shown that the vaccine was safe and stimulated formation of disease-fighting antibodies in the blood of people who had been vaccinated. Before the vaccine could be approved for widespread use, however, it had to be tested in a clinical trial to determine if it really could protect a large number of people against the disease. In 1954, some 400,000 schoolchildren in 11 states were given the Salk vaccine or a "dummy" vaccine (the placebo); they were then tracked through the end of the year to see whether they became ill with polio. The incidence of polio among the children who had received the vaccine turned out to be less than half that of those given the placebo vaccine.[12] This result demonstrated that polio immunization could reduce the incidence of disease; in fact, the use of the vaccine (or an oral vaccine developed by Albert Sabin in the 1960s) has virtually eliminated polio in the United States.

Another randomized controlled trial of a preventive intervention is the Physicians' Health Study, in which 22,000 U.S. physicians participated. Two hypotheses were being tested: whether aspirin reduced mortality from heart disease and whether beta-carotene decreased the incidence of cancer. The physicians were randomly divided into four groups: those who took aspirin and beta-carotene, those who were given one or the other and a placebo, and those who were given placebos only. The trial began in 1983 and was scheduled to run until 1995. The aspirin part of the trial was halted in 1988, however, because it was clear by that time that the physicians taking aspirin had a much-reduced risk of suffering a heart attack.[13] They were only 56% as

likely to have a heart attack as the group taking the placebo. The beta-carotene part of the trial, which continued until 1995, found no significant difference in the incidence of cancer between the group receiving beta-carotene and the placebo group.[14]

The Kingston–Newburgh study of fluoride for the prevention of tooth decay was another form of **intervention study**—a community trial. Before the study began, the schoolchildren of these two small cities on the Hudson River in New York State were similar in general health and in the prevalence of tooth decay. For the study, fluoride was added to the water supply of Newburgh, beginning in 1945, while Kingston's water was not fluoridated. Ten years later, dental examinations were conducted on the schoolchildren in both cities. The children of Newburgh were found to have approximately half as many decayed, missing, or filled teeth as the children of Kingston had. No adverse health effects were found in the Newburgh children. This evidence was strongly supportive of the value of fluoridation in preventing tooth decay.[15]

Cohort Studies

Since such experiments are not possible for most hypotheses that epidemiologists want to test, methods have been devised by which investigators can link the exposure to some factor, such as a behavior like smoking, to an outcome, such as a disease like lung cancer, by simply observing the study subjects, without any actual experimenting or intervening in their lives. Often the most accurate of these methods is the **cohort study**. In a typical cohort study, large numbers of people—all healthy at the time the study begins—are questioned concerning their exposures. They are then observed over a period of time to see whether those who were exposed to the factor being studied are more likely to develop the disease than those who were not. This approach is similar to performing an experiment, except that, instead of the researcher assigning (usually through randomization) the participants to the exposed or control groups, the people themselves have chosen whether they belong to the "exposed" group or the control group through their actions, such as their decision to smoke.

The Framingham Heart Study is a cohort study, as were the Doll–Hill and Hammond–Horn studies of smoking and lung cancer. Another well-known cohort study, still under way, is the Nurses' Health Study, which started in 1976 with some 120,000 married female nurses, looking for factors that may be related to the development of breast cancer and other diseases. The participating nurses, since expanded to included male nurses, have been sent questionnaires every two years, asking about their diet, drinking and smoking habits, and use of drugs. The study found that nurses had a 50% higher risk of breast cancer while they were taking oral contraceptives, but the risk fell back to normal after they stopped taking these medications. Another finding was that regular consumption of alcohol increases the risk of breast cancer by 10% to 40%.[16,17] Most recently, the Nurses' Health Study has shown that eating gluten is not associated with an increased risk of coronary heart disease, and that gluten-free diets offer little benefit for people without celiac disease.[18]

Epidemiologic studies are designed to determine not only the existence of an association between an exposure and a disease, but also the strength of that association.

The measure of the strength of association obtained by cohort studies and intervention studies is the **relative risk**—that is, the ratio of the incidence rate for persons exposed to the factor to the incidence rate for persons in the unexposed group. A relative risk of 1.0 means that there is no association between the exposure and the disease. A value greater than 1.0 indicates an increased risk from exposure, while a value less than 1.0 indicates a decreased risk.

Doll and Hill, in their study of British physicians, found that the relative risk of lung cancer in heavy smokers compared to nonsmokers was 23.7, a major effect.[19] The calculation that led to this conclusion is shown in **Table 5-1**. In the Nurses' Health Study, the relative risk of breast cancer for current contraceptive use is 1.5, while that for past use is 1.0. These findings are much less dramatic. In the Physicians' Health Study, the relative risk of a heart attack for men taking aspirin was 0.56.[13] This decrease was significant enough to recommend that most older men might benefit from this preventive measure, but the recommendation would carry much less weight than a recommendation to stop smoking.

Case-Control Studies

In contrast with cohort studies, which start out by measuring exposure to some factor of interest among a population of healthy people and then watching for the development of

Table 5-1 Relative Risk of Lung Cancer in Heavy Smokers Compared to Nonsmokers

Lung Cancer Death Rates	
Exposure Category	Per 100,000 Persons
Heavy smokers	166
Nonsmokers	7
Relative risk	166/7 = 23.7

Data from R. Doll and A. B. Hill, "Lung Cancer and Other Causes of Death in Relation to Smoking: A Second Report on the Mortality of British Doctors," *British Medical Journal* 2 (1956), 1071–1081.

disease among those people, **case-control studies** start with people who are already ill and look back in time to determine their exposure. Case-control studies are much more efficient than cohort studies in that they focus on a smaller number of people and can be completed relatively quickly. In a case-control study, **cases**, people who have the disease, are compared with **controls**, healthy individuals chosen to match the cases as much as possible in age, sex, and other factors that might be relevant to the disease. The investigator asks all participants the same questions concerning the extent of their exposure to factors hypothesized to have caused the disease. Small case-control studies are commonly done to follow up a hypothesis generated by shoeleather epidemiology, as was done in the investigation of EMS and L-tryptophan described earlier.

An important case-control study conducted in the mid-1980s sought the cause of Reye syndrome, a deadly disease of children that occurred a few weeks after a child had recovered from a viral infection such as chickenpox. The study tested the hypothesis that the development of Reye syndrome was linked to medications the child was given during the viral illness.[20] The cases were children who had been diagnosed with Reye syndrome and reported a previous respiratory or gastrointestinal illness or chickenpox. Controls were children who did not have Reye syndrome but who had recently been diagnosed with chickenpox or a respiratory or gastrointestinal illness. Parents of the children in both groups were asked which medications their children had received during the viral illness. The results of this study are shown in **Table 5-2**.

It is not possible to calculate the relative risk in a case-control study because this calculation requires knowing the rate of new cases in the exposed versus unexposed groups—but the starting point of a case-control study is a group that already has the disease, which does not directly reveal the rate of new cases in a broader population. Instead, case-control studies estimate the strength of the association between exposure and disease by calculating the **odds ratio**. The odds ratio, which is actually a ratio of two ratios, is calculated as follows: The numerator of the odds ratio is the ratio of exposed subjects to nonexposed subjects in the case group; the denominator is the ratio of exposed subjects to nonexposed subjects in the control group. In the Reye syndrome study, the odds ratio has as the numerator the ratio of the children with Reye syndrome who took aspirin to children with Reye syndrome who did not take aspirin, and as the denominator the ratio of children without Reye syndrome who took aspirin to children without Reye syndrome who did not

Table 5-2 Use of Aspirin and Other Salicylates and Reye Syndrome

	Cases of Reye Syndrome	Controls
Used salicylates	26	53
Did not use salicylates	1	87
Total	27	140
Odds ratio:	$\dfrac{26/1}{53/87} = \dfrac{26 \times 87}{53 \times 1} = \dfrac{2262}{53} = 42.7$	

Data from D. E. Lilienfeld and P. D. Stolley, *Foundations of Epidemiology* (New York: Oxford University Press, 1994), and E. S. Hurwitz et al., *Journal of the American Medical Association* 257 (1987): 1905–1911.

take aspirin. From Table 5-2, this calculation is 26 to 1 divided by 53 to 87, yielding an odds ratio of 42.7, indicating a strong link between the use of aspirin and Reye syndrome.

Thus, this study indicates that children who are given aspirin to treat a viral infection are much more likely to develop Reye syndrome than are children who do not take aspirin. As a result of this study, the FDA required drug producers to put warning labels on aspirin containers and told pediatricians to advise parents to give their children acetaminophen (Tylenol) rather than aspirin to treat infections. After peaking in the United States in 1980 at 555 pediatric cases per year, the Reye syndrome incidence has been no higher than 36 cases per year since 1987.[21]

A case-control study was also effective in determining the cause of an outbreak of microcephaly that emerged among infants born in northeast Brazil in 2015. Microcephaly is a rare, devastating condition in which babies are born with abnormally small heads and often severe brain damage. Researchers suspected that the outbreak was related in some way to the Zika virus infection, which had recently been reported in Brazil.

Epidemiologists considered three hypotheses for the cause of the microcephaly: (1) Zika virus infection contracted by the mother and fetus during pregnancy; (2) the mother's exposure to a newly introduced larvicide that had been used to control mosquitoes, which carry and transmit the virus; and (3) use of the tetanus, diphtheria, and pertussis vaccine (Tdap), which had recently been introduced to expectant mothers in the region. The study population consisted of newborns from women in eight hospitals in the region. Cases were those babies born with microcephaly (a total of 91); for each case baby, two control babies (a total of 173) were chosen (individual controls for several cases were not available). The control babies were chosen as the first two newborns born after 8:00 a.m. on the day after the associated case baby who had the same gestational age as the case baby, so that conception

of the case and control babies occurred at the same stage of the epidemic, and they were born in one of the same hospitals.

When the case-control results were analyzed, it become obvious which of the three hypotheses was correct. The mothers of 45 of the 91 case babies had received the Tdap vaccine, while 107 of the 173 control babies are received the vaccine. The associated odds ratio was 0.6, indicating that the Tdap vaccine, if anything, was associated with less microcephaly. Similarly, 49 of 91 case babies came from neighborhoods that had recently introduced larvicide at the water storage site, whereas 92 of the 173 control babies did so; the associated odds ratio was 1.0, indicating no impact at all. In contrast, 32 of 91 cases were Zika-positive (including 19 of 26 of the severe microcephaly cases) compared to 0 of 173 of the controls. The odds ratio was 189.5, an extremely strong association (because the denominator of the odds ratio contained a 0 for the control, a simple adjustment in this case was to add 0.5 to all counts so as to avoid an odds ratio of an infinity, as shown in **Table 5-3**). The researchers suspected that false-negative Zika test results explained many of the remaining microcephaly cases that tested negative for Zika infection (the test does produce false negatives). Overall, the data pointed directly to the cause of the microcephaly epidemic in northeast Brazil—congenital Zika virus infection—and allowed the researchers to rule out the two competing hypotheses—the introduction of larvicide and the Tdap vaccine.[22]

Consumers of public health research sometimes refer to relative risk and odds ratio interchangeably, but the two are not the same. Relative risk is a ratio of probabilities and is easier to interpret: It simply represents how much higher or lower is the incidence for one group versus another. The odds ratio is less intuitive for most people. Fortunately, the odds ratio is an excellent approximation of relative risk when the disease has an incidence of less than approximately 10%. Reye syndrome is quite rare, occurring in fewer than 0.1% of children who take aspirin, so the odds ratio of 42.7 is a

Table 5-3 Odds Ratios of Zika Virus Infection, Larvicide, and Vaccine Versus Microcephaly in Brazilian Newborns

	Cases (91)	Controls (173)	Odds Ratio
Vaccine	45 (57%)	107 (70%)	(45/46)/(107/66) = 0.6
Larvicide	49 (54%)	92 (53%)	(49/42)/(92/81) = 1.0
Zika-positive	32 (35%)	0 (0%)	(32.5/59.5)/(0.5/173.5) =189.5

Note: Because Zika-positive has zero exposed subjects in the control group, 0.5 is added to all cells in the odds ratio calculation for Zika-positive in order to avoid an odds ratio of infinity.

Data and calculations from T. de Araújo et al., "Association between microcephaly, Zika virus infection, and other risk factors in Brazil: final report of a case-control study," *The Lancet Infectious Diseases* 18 (2018), 328–336.

good approximation of the relative risk, indicating that children who use aspirin are approximately 42.7 times more likely to develop Reye syndrome than children who do not. For more common diseases, relative risk and odds ratio can diverge quite significantly. In that situation, it is more accurate to say that the odds (rather than the risk or the probability) is higher or lower by a certain amount under the exposure, or simply that there is a strong (or weak) positive (or negative) association.[23]

Conclusion

Epidemiologists study the distribution and determinants of frequency of disease in humans. Disease frequency is usually expressed as the incidence rate—the number of new cases in a defined population at risk over a defined period of time—or as the prevalence rate—the number of existing cases in a defined population at a single point in time. Incidence is most useful in identifying causes of disease.

Descriptive epidemiology looks at the distribution of disease by characteristics of the person (e.g., age, sex, ethnicity, personal habits), the place (e.g., variations by geographic areas), and the time (e.g., changes in incidence over the long term, seasonal variations, or time since an epidemic began). This information on the distribution of disease may lead to hypotheses about the determinants, or causes, of disease.

Hypotheses generated through descriptive epidemiology can be tested through systematic epidemiologic studies. Several types of epidemiologic studies can be performed. Intervention studies are true experiments in which subjects are assigned to either a treatment group (people who receive the intervention) or a control group (people who do not receive the intervention). The most common and rigorous type of intervention study is the randomized, double-blind clinical trial used to test new drug treatments or preventive measures.

For most situations in which epidemiologists wish to investigate whether a certain exposure causes a certain disease, it would be unethical to conduct an intervention study. The next best option is a cohort study, in which subjects are questioned about their exposures and then tracked over time, comparing the exposed group with the unexposed group to see whether the exposed group is more likely to develop the disease. The third major type of study is the case-control study, which begins with cases of the disease and asks questions about their previous exposures, comparing their answers with those of a healthy control group.

Epidemiologists study human populations, which limits the types of studies that can be done. However, epidemiology has provided some of the most useful information about factors that affect human health.

References

1. B. MacMahon and D. Trichopoulos, *Epidemiology: Principles and Methods* (Boston, MA: Little, Brown, 1996).

2. C. G. Hennekens and J. F. Buring, *Epidemiology in Medicine* (Boston, MA: Little, Brown, 1987).

3. Centers for Disease Control and Prevention, "Lesson 1: Introduction to Epidemiology, Section 11: Epidemic Disease Occurrence," in *Principles of Epidemiology in Public Health Practice*, 3rd ed., www.cdc.gov/csels/dsepd/ss1978/lesson1/section11.html, accessed August 8, 2019.

4. R. Doyle, "Colorectal Cancer Mortality Among Men," *Scientific American* (January 1996): 27.

5. American Cancer Society, "Colorectal Cancer Facts & Figures 2017–2019," www.cancer.org/content/dam/cancer-org/research/cancer-facts-and-statistics/colorectal-cancer-facts-and-figures/colorectal-cancer-facts-and-figures-2017-2019.pdf, accessed August 8, 2019.

6. World Health Organization, International Agency for Research on Cancer, "Cancer Today: Population Fact Sheets," gco.iarc.fr/today/fact-sheets-populations, accessed August 15, 2019.

7. P. Porter, "'Westernizing' Women's Risks? Breast Cancer in Lower-Income Countries," *New England Journal of Medicine* 358 (2008): 213–216.

8. N. Uemura, S. Okamoto, S. Yamamoto, N. Matsumura, S. Yamaguchi, M. Yamakido, et al., "*Helicobacter pylori* Infection and the Development of Gastric Cancer," *New England Journal of Medicine* 345 (2001): 784–789.

9. Centers for Disease Control and Prevention, "Eosinophilia–Myalgia Syndrome—New Mexico," *Morbidity and Mortality Weekly Report* 38 (1989): 765–767.

10. J. P. Lash, *Eleanor and Franklin: The Story of Their Relationship* (New York: W. W. Norton, 1971).

11. M. B. Gregg and B. M. Nkowane "Poliomyelitis," in J. Last, ed., *Maxcy-Rosenau Public Health and Preventive Medicine* (Norwalk, CT: Appleton-Century-Croft, 1986), 173–176.

12. G. D. Friedman, *Primer of Epidemiology* (New York: McGraw-Hill, 1994).

13. Steering Committee of the Physicians' Health Study Research Group, "Final Report on the Aspirin Component of the Ongoing Physicians' Health Study," *New England Journal of Medicine* 321 (1989): 129–135.

14. C. H. Hennekens, J. E. Buring, J. E. Manson, M. Stampfer, B. Rosner, N. R. Cook, et al., "Lack of Effect of Long-Term Supplementation with Beta Carotene on the Incidence of Malignant Neoplasms and Cardiovascular Disease," *New England Journal of Medicine* 334 (1996): 1145–1149.

15. E. R. Schlesinger, D. E. Overton, H. C. Chase, and K. T. Cantwell, "Newburgh–Kingston Caries: Fluorine Study XIII. Pediatric Findings After Ten Years," *Journal of the American Dental Association* 52 (1956): 296–306.

16. R. J. Lipnick, J. E. Buring, C. H. Hennekens, B. Rosner, W. Willett, C. Bain, et al., "Oral Contraceptives and Breast Cancer: A Prospective Cohort Study," *Journal of the American Medical Association* 255 (1986): 58–61.

17. M. P. Longnecker, "Alcoholic Beverage Consumption in Relation to Breast Cancer: Meta-Analysis and Review," *Cancer Causes and Control* 5 (1994): 73–82.

18. B. Lebwohl, Y. Cao, G. Zong, F. B. Hu, P. H. R. Green, A. I. Neugut, et al., "Long Term Gluten Consumption in Adults Without Celiac Disease and Risk of Coronary Heart Disease: Prospective Cohort Study," *British Medical Journal* 357 (2017): j1892.

19. R. Doll and A. B. Hill, "Lung Cancer and Other Causes of Death in Relation to Smoking: A Second Report on the Mortality of British Doctors," *British Medical Journal* 2 (1956): 1071–1081.

20. D. E. Lilienfeld and P. D. Stolley, *Foundations of Epidemiology* (New York: Oxford University Press, 1994), 227–228.

21. E. D. Belay, J. S. Bresee, R. C. Holman, A. S. Khan, A. Shahriari, and L. B. Schonberger, "Reye's Syndrome in the United States from 1981 Through 1997," *New England Journal of Medicine* 340 (1999): 1377–1382.

22. T. de Araújo, R. A. A. Ximenes, D. B. Miranda-Filho, W. V. Souza, U. R. Montorroyos, A. P. L. de Meio, et al., "Association Between Microcephaly, Zika Virus Infection, and Other Risk Factors in Brazil: Final Report of a Case-Control Study," *The Lancet Infectious Diseases* 18 (2018): 328–336.

23. A. J. Viera, "Odds Ratios and Risk Ratios: What's the Difference and Why Does It Matter?", *Southern Medical Journal* 101 (2008): 730–734.

CHAPTER 6

The Study of Humans

Problems and Limits of Epidemiology

KEY TERMS

Bias
Conflict of interest
Confounding variables

Dose–response relationship
Institutional review board
Random variation

Selection bias

The ultimate goal of many epidemiologic studies is to determine the causes of disease. This is generally done first by observing a possible association between an exposure and an illness, second by developing a hypothesis about a cause-and-effect relationship, and third by testing the hypothesis through a formal epidemiologic study. While the formal study can strongly support the conclusion that a certain exposure causes a certain disease, many potential sources of error arise when drawing such a conclusion. Studies of chronic diseases, which often have multiple determinants and develop over long periods of time, are especially prone to error.

Problems with Studying Humans

All epidemiologic studies have the advantage of studying humans rather than experimental animals—but all are also limited by that fact.

Each type of epidemiologic study has its own strengths and weaknesses.

Consider the design of an epidemiologic study to test the hypothesis that a low-fat diet reduces the risk of heart disease. The average American already eats a high-fat diet and has a high risk of heart disease compared with residents of many other countries, so it should be possible, ethically, to compare the health of people who eat this diet with others who have other dietary patterns.

The randomized controlled trial—the most rigorous form of intervention study—is the most similar study in concept to a biomedical scientist's experiment with rats. Suppose researchers choose a group of subjects who have been eating an average American diet and divide them randomly into an experimental group, who will be instructed to eat a strict low-fat diet over the next five years, and a control group, who will be told to continue eating their usual diet. Researchers will monitor both groups, watching for signs of heart disease, and they expect that, if their hypothesis is correct, fewer people in the low-fat group will become ill.

Most likely, the researchers will be disappointed with the results. The problem is that it is impossible to control the behavior of human beings under such circumstances. If the experiment was being conducted using rats, researchers would feed them the assigned diets and, therefore, could be certain of the relative exposures of the two groups. With people, however, even if researchers could find enough of them who would agree to participate in the experiment, it is questionable whether they would remain on the appropriate diet over the necessary length of time. People in the experimental group might succumb to temptation and drop out of the study or lie about what they have eaten. People in the control group might become concerned about their health and voluntarily cut back on the amount of fat they eat. It is unrealistic to expect to successfully implement a randomized controlled trial that requires people to alter their behavior over a significant period of time, unless the subjects have a special motivation to participate—if they are suffering from a serious disease, for example—and participation in a trial is their only chance to have access to a new, potentially more effective treatment.

Instead of using a randomized controlled trial to test the dietary hypothesis, researchers might try a cohort study. With this approach, they would choose a large group of people who are free of heart disease, ask them detailed questions about their diets, and then, over the next five years, compare the health of those who already eat a low-fat diet with those who eat an average American diet. This design would not require people to change their behavior. The problem with this scenario is that the people who have voluntarily chosen to eat a low-fat diet may differ in other respects from the group who eat the average diet. The low-fat group members are likely to be more health conscious in general. They may be less likely to smoke and more likely to exercise, for example. As a consequence, these people would have a reduced risk of heart disease even if a low-fat diet did not have a protective effect.

The third type of study, the case-control study, has its own difficulties. When using this design, researchers would choose a group of people who already have heart disease; perhaps they would go to a hospital and interview patients recovering from a heart attack. A comparable group of people who do not have heart disease would serve as the control group. Researchers would question people in both groups about their diets over the past five years and decide whether the diets should be classified as high-fat or low-fat. If the researchers' hypothesis is correct, the patients who have had heart attacks will report a diet higher in fat than the control group. This approach also has obvious problems. People are not likely to remember what they ate in the past, they might be embarrassed to admit how self-indulgent they have been, or the controls may be different from the cases in ways that the researchers may not have anticipated or may be hard to account for in the comparison. The information that researchers obtain concerning exposure in the case-control trial may not be reliable.

These difficulties do not mean that researchers cannot draw valid conclusions from any kind of epidemiologic study. However, they demonstrate the types of errors to which different kinds of studies may be prone and alert researchers about what to watch out for in choosing a study design and in interpreting the results.

Sources of Error

News reports of new health studies can often be confusing. Sometimes conflicting reports are published on the health effects of various substances. Coffee is reported to cause heart disease; then it is reported that there is no such effect. Oat bran is reported to prevent cancer; then it is reported to make no difference. Fish is good for your heart; fish is full of toxic chemicals that may cause harm. All of these contradictions tend to make people distrustful of the news and uncertain about how to protect their health. Given that most of these news reports are based on epidemiologic studies, it is useful to understand possible sources of error in such studies and how to look for the truth in the reports.

One of the most common reasons that a study might lead to a wrong conclusion is that the reported result is merely a **random variation** and the association is merely due to chance. As a general rule, epidemiologic studies of chronic diseases require large numbers of subjects to draw valid conclusions. Causes of these diseases are usually complex, and long periods may pass between the exposure to a possible cause and the development of illness, making it difficult to draw conclusions about associations between exposure and disease. The cause-and-effect relationship is not obvious—unlike, for example, when a bullet in the heart causes death, or exposure of an unvaccinated child to the measles virus causes the child to develop measles in 10 to 12 days. The weaker the relationship between exposure and disease, the larger the group of people who must be studied to clarify the relationship. If the group being studied is too small, a cause-and-effect relationship is likely to be missed or a spurious relationship will show up by chance alone. One of the reasons that the Doll–Hill and Hammond–Horn results (*Epidemiology: The Basic Science of Public Health*) concerning smoking and lung cancer are so convincing is that they involved such large numbers of subjects.

Well-designed studies may be able to avoid a number of other possible sources of error. For example, the cohort study of a low-fat diet proposed previously may be invalidated by the presence of confounding variables, such as smoking and exercise. **Confounding variables** are factors associated with the exposure that may independently affect the risk of developing the disease. Such an error may have occurred in a 1980s study that suggested coffee drinking could cause pancreatic cancer, a finding that has not been replicated in other studies. Since many heavy coffee drinkers were also smokers, the cancer was more likely caused by the smoking rather than the coffee.[1] To eliminate the errors caused by smoking as a confounding variable, researchers might conduct the study only on nonsmokers. Alternatively, statistical techniques may be used to adjust the results and compensate for confounding variables—as long as the investigator is clever enough to think of possible factors that may affect the results and take them into consideration when collecting the data and calculating the results. While the investigators in the study of coffee corrected for smoking over the five-year period before the cancer was diagnosed, their correction may have been inadequate.

An interesting example of confounding occurred in a study, published in 1999 and widely publicized, suggesting that small children were more likely to become myopic—nearsighted—if they slept in a lighted room. In a follow-up study, investigators asked the children's parents about their own vision. It turned out that myopic parents were more likely to leave lights on in their children's rooms than parents with better vision. Their children, therefore, were more likely to be nearsighted because they inherited the condition from their parents, not from the light exposure.[2]

Bias, or systematic error, may be introduced into a study in a number of ways. **Selection bias** can arise when the control group is insufficiently similar to the treatment group. For example, consider the finding of an increased rate of heart disease among individuals with osteoarthritis, a common musculoskeletal disease in which the protective cushioning between bones wears down so that joints become painful and stiff. People with this condition often take nonsteroidal anti-inflammatory drugs

(NSAIDs) to treat the pain. It was natural to wonder, then, if the elevated rate of heart disease among patients with osteoarthritis was due to the pain medicine they were taking, which had been associated with heart disease in other contexts.

A prospective study published in 2019 tracked individuals with osteoarthritis over time to see if they developed heart disease.[3] To create a control group, each individual with osteoarthritis was matched with three individuals of the same age and gender who did not have osteoarthritis. For all individuals, the researchers knew their histories of prescription NSAID use and certain other characteristics, such as income, and health conditions, such as hypertension. After controlling for these possible confounding variables, the authors found 23% more heart disease events in the osteoarthritis group compared to the control group, largely due to NSAID use.

The researchers acknowledged, however, that confounding variables not included in their data set might explain at least some of this elevated rate. For example, the researchers did not know individuals' family histories of heart disease, or their levels of smoking and physical activity. Might the osteoarthritis group have scored worse on these dimensions than the control group? The data suggested this was the case: The researchers reported that 29.4% of the osteoarthritis group were obese compared to 19.8% of the control group; the researchers also found rates of hypertension and chronic obstructive pulmonary disease (COPD) in the osteoarthritis group that were 5.5 percentage points and 3 percentage points higher, respectively, than those in the control group. Almost certainly, then, the osteoarthritis group was generally less healthy than the control group, which may explain some (or all) of the elevated heart disease in a way that is unrelated to NSAIDs. As a result, it seems reasonable to worry that the process by which the control group was chosen introduced some degree of selection bias.

Selection bias may also occur when there is a systematic difference between people who choose—or are chosen—to participate in a study and those who do not. For example, in a 1988 case-control study that found exposure to high electromagnetic fields (EMF) from power lines increased the risk of childhood cancer, the controls were chosen by a process of telephone random-digit dialing until a child was located who matched a case by age and sex. Cases and controls were compared, and cases were found to have had a higher exposure to EMF. However, the cases were also found to have lower socioeconomic status; they were more likely to live in areas of high traffic density, and their mothers were more likely to smoke. The random-digit dialing had created a bias: Because poor families were less likely to have a telephone, or less likely to have an answering machine and to return calls, the control group was more affluent and consequently was less exposed to confounding poverty-associated factors.[1]

An extreme example of selection bias—and a mistake that no well-trained epidemiologist would make—was seen in author Shere Hite's report on male and female relationships. Hite distributed 100,000 questionnaires on women's attitudes about men and sex, but received only 4500 replies. Hite reported that 84% of the women in the study were dissatisfied with their intimate relationships, results that were widely publicized. The low response rate suggests that selection bias was operating and that the most dissatisfied women preferentially responded to the survey.[4]

Cohort studies, which tend to extend over many years, often suffer from a form of bias caused by people dropping out or being untraceable when the time comes to tally the results. If people who get sick drop out at a different rate from those who remain healthy, the results will be compromised. Subjects who are lost to follow-up may be more likely than those who are traceable to have entered an institution or to have moved in with family, indicating a serious health problem. A high dropout rate poses a serious threat to the validity of any epidemiologic study.

Reporting bias or recall bias is a common problem in case-control studies. It occurs when the case group and the control group systematically report data differently, even if they had the same exposure. Subjects' reports of their dietary intake are notoriously unreliable. For example, underweight individuals consistently overreport their fat intake, while obese individuals underreport it.[1] Similarly, studies attempting to relate certain diseases to alcohol consumption may suffer from reporting bias because people who drink heavily tend to underreport their consumption. Case-control studies that attempt to determine causes of birth defects are especially subject to recall bias, since the mother of a child born with a malformation is likely to have thought a great deal about what might have caused the problem, whereas mothers of healthy children would be less likely to notice an unusual exposure.

Proving Cause and Effect

For the most part, epidemiologic studies, no matter how well designed to avoid error, cannot prove cause and effect. In fact, that is why epidemiologists usually speak of "risk factors" rather than "causes." However, several factors can be combined to strengthen the cause-and-effect inference.

First, as discussed previously, a study with a large number of subjects is more likely to yield a valid result than is a small study. Second, the stronger the association measured between exposure and disease—the higher the relative risk or odds ratio—the more likely that there is a true cause-and-effect relationship. For example, a Reye syndrome case-control study found a 42.7 odds ratio from exposure to aspirin during a viral infection. By contrast, a case-control study of Brazilian babies, tested for an association between pregnant women being vaccinated for measles, mumps, and rubella and their babies developing microcephaly, found an odds ratio of 1.1. The much stronger association found in the Reye syndrome study makes it highly probable that aspirin causes the syndrome in children, whereas the much weaker vaccination result could be due to some error or alternative explanation.

Third, a **dose–response relationship** between exposure and risk of disease is evidence supporting exposure as a cause of the disease. Some of the earliest evidence that long-term exposure to low levels of x-rays had adverse health consequences came from a study comparing the mortality rates of different types of physicians were systematically exposed to different amounts of radiation. Radiologists had the highest exposure to radiation and the lowest life expectancy. Ophthalmologists and otolaryngologists had very little exposure and the highest life expectancy. Internists, whose exposure was intermediate, had intermediate life expectancy, confirming a dose–response effect: The higher the dose of radiation, the greater the effect on lifespan.[5]

Fourth, epidemiologic evidence is more convincing if there is a known biological explanation for an association between an exposure and a disease. Studies suggesting that EMF causes leukemia and other forms of cancer have been viewed with skepticism because of the lack of a known mechanism by which such low energy fields could have a biological effect. The question is unresolved. However, a number of other exposures have been identified by epidemiologic studies as causes of disease before a biological explanation was found. For example, strong epidemiologic evidence that cigarette smoking was a major cause of heart disease existed long before there was any biological explanation, and the mechanism is still not well understood.

A good indication that an epidemiologic result is valid is that it is consistent with other investigations. If several independently designed and conducted studies lead to the same conclusion, it is unlikely that the conclusion resulted from bias or other error. If the reports are conflicting, however, people must be wary of accepting any of the results.

"4/20" Day and Fatal Accidents: Doobie-ous Results

A 2018 study published in a leading medical journal examined whether motor vehicle fatalities spiked during the informal but popular holiday known as "4/20 Day" or "Weed Day."[6] On this holiday, which begins at 4:20 p.m. on April 20, marijuana enthusiasts gather to publicly celebrate and use the drug. A reasonable hypothesis, then, is that the rate of traffic accidents is higher between 4:20 p.m. and midnight on April 20 as a result of stoned drivers having a higher risk of an accident and more of this "drugged driving" occurring at this time.

The researchers set out to test this hypothesis by gathering data on all traffic fatalities in the United States between 1992 and 2016. They then compared the fatality rates on April 20 between 4:20 p.m. and midnight for these years with the fatality rates on April 13 and April 27 for the same years. If drugged driving is more prevalent on April 20 and increases the risk of accidents, then perhaps a spike in traffic fatalities would appear in the data on this day. The

two "control" days near in time to April 20, on the same day of the week as April 20, would address the possibility of weekly and annual seasonality—for example, if accident rates were higher in the spring or on certain days of the week unrelated to drugged driving.

Indeed, the authors found a relative risk of fatal accidents on April 20 of 1.12, a 12% increase relative to the control days. They concluded that "policy makers may wish to consider these risks when liberalizing marijuana laws, paying particular attention to regulatory and enforcement strategies to curtail drugged driving."[6]

Naturally, these results garnered significant media attention. *The Los Angeles Times*, for example, printed the headline, "Drivers Beware: Risk of Fatal Car Crashes Spikes on the 4/20 Marijuana 'Holiday,' Study Says."[7] This is all seemed reasonable until two other epidemiologists posted a critique of the study.[8] They ran the same test but for all days of the year—that is, they compared fatalities for each day of the year to fatalities one week before and one week after that day of the year—and found that April 20 did not look particularly unusual. In fact, as **Figure 6-1** shows, at least some (if not all) of the April 20 effect seemed to be due to

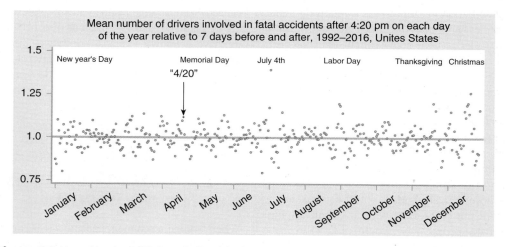

Figure 6-1 Mean Number of Drivers in Fatal Accidents per Day: Relative to 7 Days Before and After

Data from the Fatal Analysis Reporting System, National Highway Transportation Safety Administration, as organized by S. Harper and A. Palayew, https://osf.io/ncdvg/, accessed August 20, 2019. The figure is modified from Figure 2 of S. Harper and A. Palayew, "The annual cannabis holiday and fatal traffic crashes," *Injury Prevention* (2019): injuryprev-2018.

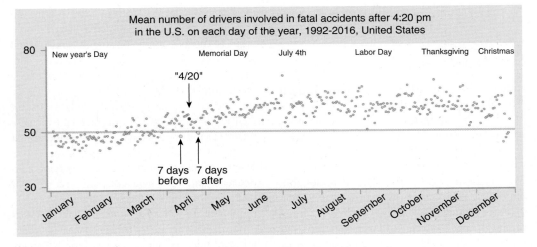

Figure 6-2 Mean Number of Drivers in Fatal Accidents per Day: Absolute Counts

Data from the Fatal Analysis Reporting System, National Highway Transportation Safety Administration, as organized by S. Harper and A. Palayew, https://osf.io/ncdvg/, accessed August 20, 2019. Figure created by H. Schneider.

random variation. Digging deeper, **Figure 6-2** suggests the April 20 effect may have more to do with unusually low fatality rates on the two control days, April 13 and 27, than with an unusually high fatality rate on April 20 itself.

This case illustrates how several sources of error could enter a study. First, the original study had only 15 April 20 outcomes to work with (one for each year between 1992 and 2016). This represents a relatively small sample—and one that does not allow for a particularly confident conclusion. Second, as we saw earlier with the study of osteoarthritis, the choice of control group can be all important. Using the fatality rate seven days before and after April 20 as the control group certainly seems reasonable, but as Figure 6-2 shows, it may not have worked as intended.

A third source of error comes from assumptions about marijuana smoking. It is almost certainly the case that drugged driving is more dangerous than sober driving, but it might not be as dangerous as drunk driving. Perhaps people who would otherwise drink and drive used use marijuana as an alternative, leading to a lower accident rate. It is also possible that marijuana users tend to consume the drug at home and, therefore, are less likely to drive. In the end, the evidence from the original study is inconclusive. More importantly, the extent of the danger from drugged driving remains uncertain.

Finally, the figures in the study critique show a spike in fatalities on July 4 that is far larger than that occurring on any other day. This is almost certainly a real effect, not only because the effect is so large and persists when viewed from a range of analytical perspectives (as in Figures 6-1 and 6-2), but also because we have a known explanation: July 4 brings together one of the busiest driving days of the year and one of the highest drinking days of the year. This is evidently a deadly combination.

Epidemiologic Studies of Hormone Replacement Therapy: Confusing Results

When women reach menopause at age 50 or so, their natural production of the hormone estrogen drops significantly. Many women at this stage of life begin to have menopausal symptoms that can be troubling: hot flashes that disturb their well-being during the day and their sleep at night, and vaginal dryness that causes discomfort and interferes with sexual activity. Prescription of estrogen supplements relieves these symptoms, and this treatment became popular in the 1960s. Estrogen was promoted as a means to help keep women "feminine forever"—as promised in a best-selling book of that title by Robert Wilson, published in 1966.[9] Large numbers of postmenopausal women took the hormone in the hope that it would keep them looking and feeling younger, improve their memory, and stave off other effects of aging. When evidence appeared in the 1970s that women taking estrogen had an increased risk of uterine cancer, the problem was averted by adding another hormone, progesterone, to the prescription. Progesterone countered the effect of the estrogen on the uterus without appearing to diminish its positive effects on other organs. Clinicians had good reason to believe that these female hormones would protect women. Rates of cardiovascular disease are well known to be much lower among women than men until middle age, but then to increase after menopause to match the rates among men. Also, older women are much more likely to suffer from osteoporosis, a thinning of the bones that leads to fractures. It was reasonable to think that hormone supplements might also protect women against these problems.

Numerous epidemiologic studies over the years supported the protective role of estrogen for bones and hearts. Most notably, the Nurses' Health Study—a large cohort study ongoing since 1976—found that women taking hormone therapy had a 61% lower risk of heart disease and a 75% lower risk of hip fractures.[10] These studies found small increases in breast cancer risk, but the trade-off seemed worthwhile for many women. In 1999, approximately 38% of postmenopausal women in the United States were using hormone replacement therapy (HRT).[11]

Then, in July 2002, the news broke that HRT was not as beneficial as it had seemed. The previous positive evidence had all come from observational studies. Meanwhile, a huge clinical trial, called the Women's Health Initiative (WHI), had been under way since 1991. The researchers announced in 2002 that the WHI had been stopped early on the basis that the risks had been found to outweigh the benefits.[12] Women randomly assigned to take a combination pill of estrogen plus progesterone were found to have a higher risk of breast cancer than were women taking a placebo, which was not surprising. The surprise was that women taking the combination pill were also found to have higher risks of heart attack, stroke, and blood clots. The women in the experimental group had fewer hip fractures and fewer cases of colorectal cancer than the control group did, but this protective effect was not enough to outweigh the risks.

The news from the WHI study seemed to contradict the overwhelming evidence from cohort studies that HRT protected women against heart disease. However, the WHI was a clinical trial, the gold standard of epidemiologic studies, so it was much less likely to be subject to bias. Many women stopped taking HRT when the news came out, and the drug's sales fell by 50% within six months.[13]

After the results of the WHI study were published, epidemiologists struggled to understand why the Nurses' Health Study and the WHI study produced such conflicting results. There are still many unanswered questions, but one important factor seems to be selection bias. Women in the observational studies who chose to take hormones were healthier to begin with and had healthier habits than the women who did not take the hormones. Many other factors appear to be involved, including biologic differences between the women in the two types of studies: Women in the Nurses' Health Study were younger and thinner than the women in the WHI. There is also a bias stemming from the fact that cohort studies tend to miss adverse events that occur very soon after a therapy is begun, and the cardiovascular risk from HRT is highest during the first year after beginning therapy.[14,15] Evidence supporting some of the WHI conclusions emerged in 2006 when routinely collected cancer data revealed that breast cancer incidence in the United States had dropped significantly in 2003 and 2004, apparently the result of so many women discontinuing use of HRT.[13] Nevertheless, a 2017 analysis of the long-term outcomes of the WHI participants showed no impact of HRT on mortality overall, nor on cardiovascular mortality or total cancer mortality in particular.[16] Current recommendations call for HRT to be used only short-term for postmenopausal symptoms.

Ethics in Epidemiology

Most epidemiologic studies are observational and have little potential for harm. Exceptions do occur, however, especially in the conduct of intervention studies. Nowadays, strict ethical limitations apply in any study involving humans. These rules were developed in reaction to abuses such as those carried out by Dr. Joseph Mengele, who conducted medical experiments on concentration camp prisoners during World War II. Ethical abuses have not been limited to Nazi war criminals, however. At one time, medical researchers in the United States were not overly concerned with the rights of the experimental subjects, who were often poor patients or captive populations such as prisoners or inmates of mental institutions. That situation changed in 1972, when news of the Tuskegee syphilis study shocked the nation.

Syphilis was a dread disease for hundreds of years, inspiring some of the same moral revulsion as AIDS has sometimes done more recently. Spread by sexual contact, syphilis had an unpredictable course that, over a variable number of years, could lead to a range of grim symptoms, including blindness, heart disease, dementia, and paralysis. It was sometimes treated with an arsenic-containing drug called salvarsan, which had been shown to cure syphilis in rabbits but which was not always effective in human patients and sometimes killed them. Some scientists suspected that the disease was not as uniformly dire as its reputation suggested and that the treatment might be worse than the disease. This conclusion was supported by the results of a Norwegian study of untreated syphilis done during the early part of the 20th century, which found that as many as 75% of the patients were symptom-free when examined more than 20 years after contracting the disease.[17]

In 1932, the U.S. Public Health Service and scientists from Tuskegee Institute began a similar study of about 400 black men in Macon County, Alabama, where syphilis was rampant: 40% of the population suffered from the disease. The purpose was to observe the course of the disease in these men, who were not to receive treatment. In part because it was not common practice at the time, and in part because the subjects were poor, black, and uneducated, the investigators did not try to explain what they intended to do or ask the subjects' permission. The men were told they had "bad blood" and were enticed to participate with free "treatments" and physical examinations, free hot lunches, and free burials. In the 1940s, penicillin was discovered and became standard treatment for syphilis, but the Tuskegee subjects did not receive the antibiotic until after the story broke in 1972.[17]

There is some question about whether the men were physically harmed by the researchers' withholding of antibiotic treatment. The course of syphilis is complicated, and the surviving subjects were in a late, noninfectious stage by the time penicillin was discovered—perhaps too late to help most of them. Nevertheless, this study raised a number of ethical issues, with the major one being that the men were deceived. They were not told what syphilis was or that they were part of a study, and they were led to believe that they were receiving treatment. Furthermore, one test done on the subjects was a spinal tap, a painful procedure that uses a needle to withdraw spinal fluid, and that has the potential of causing harmful side effects, including—rarely—paralysis. This treatment would not likely have been tolerated by white, middle-class Americans, and many critics have concluded that the study was racist. In fact, revelations about the study led many African Americans to distrust medical research. The misconception still lingers that the men were deliberately infected with syphilis.[18]

The outcry that followed the publicity about the Tuskegee study in 1972 led directly to the establishment of rules for the conduct of human experimentation. All institutions that receive federal funds must follow these rules. The rules require that every research subject must be informed of the purpose of a study and its risks and benefits. The subjects must freely consent to participate. In addition, any such study must be approved in advance by an **institutional review board**, a committee that includes representatives of the community as well as other scientists, who must agree that the study is well designed, that its benefits outweigh its risks, and that the subjects are truly given the opportunity for informed consent. Clinical trials are halted if the treatment group is clearly showing better or worse results than the control group. This was done, for example, in the portion of the Physicians' Health Study that looked at aspirin's effectiveness in preventing heart attacks when it became clear that subjects taking aspirin were suffering fewer heart attacks than those in the placebo group.[19] It was also done in the WHI study of HRT, described earlier in this chapter.

Even with the current strict ethical guidelines, a number of controversial issues surround clinical trials, including whether such trials should be conducted at all, who should participate, whether informed consent is truly possible, and whether unproven treatments should be available outside of clinical trials. All of these controversies came to the foreground in the early days of the AIDS epidemic. People with AIDS knew they had a fatal disease that had no known cure and they were desperate. Many of them were very politically active. People with AIDS argued that they did not have time to wait for clinical trials to test the efficacy of every promising new drug. They wanted immediate access to any new drug that showed promise in the laboratory, because they would prefer to try something—anything that had the slightest chance of working—rather than face certain death. On the other side of the argument is the history of useless therapies that have been employed for years or decades because no one had ever done a scientific test of whether they worked. This is a true ethical dilemma pitting the individual against society. Can we deny today's patient a treatment that "can't hurt" and might help so that future patients will have access to a treatment with proven effectiveness? The pressure for untested therapies for AIDS has now been eased by the development of drugs that have been found effective in clinical trials.

The use of bleeding by 18th-century physicians as a treatment for almost any illness is well known. The argument for this therapy appears foolish to us today, but the absence of curative power was not obvious to the people of the time. Similarly, tonsillectomies were performed on more than half of all children in the 1930s through the 1950s in the belief that the operation prevented rheumatic fever and other complications of strep throat. In fact, there was no evidence for this benefit, and it is now believed that a tonsillectomy may make strep infection more difficult to diagnose and treat.[20] Unfortunately, it can be difficult to do a randomized controlled study of a treatment that is already in wide use, because people do not want to risk being randomized to a placebo treatment if they suspect the active therapy is effective.

Such was the case in the 1990s with bone marrow transplant as a treatment for advanced breast cancer. With conventional chemotherapy, a patient had a 40% to 45% chance of living for five more years. A procedure that removed a woman's bone marrow, administered a much higher dose of chemotherapy than usual, and then replaced the bone marrow, in theory gave her a better chance of surviving the cancer. However, the procedure was itself arduous and risky, subjecting the woman to a 5% chance of dying from complications of the treatment. It was also expensive, costing as much as $200,000. The National Cancer Institute sponsored three large, national trials of bone marrow transplants for breast cancer. The trials required women to be randomly assigned to the transplant group or to conventional therapy. Many were reluctant to participate in a trial because they wanted the most aggressive treatment, perceiving that this offered them their last best hope for survival. Some people also questioned whether it was ethical to deny women the chance to choose the procedure, forcing them into a trial. Conversely, might the practice of offering the transplant outside of a trial be unethical because surgeons and hospitals have a **conflict of interest**, perhaps influencing patients to choose a treatment from which they—the surgeons and hospitals—stand to profit financially? Insurance companies were forced through lawsuits and political pressure to pay for these expensive and arduous procedures without evidence that they saved lives.[21]

Ultimately, enough women enrolled in clinical trials in the United States and in other countries to test the hypothesis, and negative results began to appear in 1999. An analysis of results from several studies published in 2004 strongly suggested that the intensive procedure did not lead to better survival for women who underwent it and, in fact, led to more treatment-related deaths and adverse side effects than those experienced by the controls. As the authors of *False Hope: Bone Marrow Transplant for Breast Cancer* point out, 23,000 to 40,000 American women with breast cancer had the procedure done outside of clinical trials, while only 1000 were recruited to participate in the clinical trials.[22] "Although there was no deliberate effort to deceive women," they write, "the combined effect of salesmanship by physicians, lawyers, legislators, entrepreneurs,

and the press led one of our respondents to say, 'We were all sold a bill of goods.'"[22(p.286)] If the clinical trials had not been completed, bone marrow transplant might have become the standard treatment, although, like bleeding and tonsillectomies, it appears to do more harm than good.

Conflicts of Interest in Drug Trials

Epidemiologic studies are complicated enough, with many opportunities to make honest errors in interpreting them (as described earlier in this chapter), but when millions of dollars are at stake—which is the case with clinical trials of new prescription drugs—it is increasingly obvious that conflicts of interest often affect reported results. The U.S. Food and Drug Administration (FDA) requires drug developers to study their products in randomized controlled trials before any new drug can be approved for use in the United States. Pharmaceutical companies conduct these studies to establish the safety and efficacy of a drug and then submit the results to the FDA in search of the agency's approval. Often, the results of these studies are also submitted for publication to medical journals; such a publication in a reputable journal adds to the credibility of a drug's effectiveness.

Because randomized controlled trials are considered the best way to test drugs, and because FDA scientists review the results of the companies' studies, FDA approval has generally been considered evidence that a drug was indeed safe and effective. However, in the late 1990s and early 2000s, a rash of publicity about harm caused by FDA-approved drugs raised questions about the clinical trials that supported their approval. Some of these drugs were removed from the market after news of their harmful side effects came out; others were required to post "black-box warnings" on their packaging, indicating that they should be prescribed with caution. Questions were raised about the arthritis drugs Vioxx and Bextra, and the diabetes drug Avandia, which were suspected of raising the risk of heart attacks; the cholesterol-lowering drug Baycol, which caused sometimes fatal muscle damage and was removed from the market in 2001; the asthma drugs Serevent and Advair, which appeared to exacerbate asthma attacks in some patients; and the psychotropic drug Paxil and other antidepressants, which increase the risk of suicidal behavior in children and young people.[23]

Harmful side effects may be missed in a clinical trial because they are rare and the number of subjects studied may be too small for them to be noted. However, the case of Vioxx demonstrated that a company may purposely suppress negative information about a drug during the approval process. In fact, evidence now shows that companies may purposely bias their studies in ways that make the drugs appear safer and more effective than they are.

Vioxx was the first of a new class of drugs called cyclooxygenase-2 (COX-2) inhibitors to be introduced in the late 1990s. These drugs are a class of nonsteroidal anti-inflammatory drugs (NSAIDs) that are used for pain relief—especially arthritis pain—and are designed to be less irritating to the digestive system than the established, over-the-counter NSAIDs, such as aspirin, ibuprofen, and naproxen.

Soon after the FDA approved Vioxx, the *New England Journal of Medicine* published a report of a clinical trial conducted by drug company scientists that had found a 50% reduction of serious gastrointestinal side effects in patients taking Vioxx compared with those taking naproxen.[24] The same article reported that Vioxx caused a five-fold increase in the risk of heart attacks and strokes, but the drug company, Merck, claimed that this result occurred because naproxen protected the heart, as aspirin was known to do. Meanwhile, Pfizer introduced its own COX-2 inhibitors, Celebrex and Bextra. There were high hopes for these drugs, which were also being studied

for prevention of colon cancer and Alzheimer's disease. However, the evidence mounted that all the COX-2 inhibitors increased the risk of heart attacks. A later study found that naproxen was not protective of the heart, although it was not harmful either.[25] In 2004, Merck removed Vioxx from the market; Bextra was withdrawn in 2005. Celebrex and several newer COX-2 inhibitors are still being sold, although they are required to carry warnings of cardiovascular risk.

These events raised many questions about the way the clinical trials were conducted and reported. In 2005, the *New England Journal of Medicine* published an "Expression of Concern" accusing the Merck authors of providing misleading information in the 1999 article.[26] Information that came out during lawsuits by patients who had been harmed by Vioxx revealed that the scientists knew of three heart attacks and other cardiovascular problems among the subjects taking the drug but had not included them in the data submitted to the journal.

It turns out that the pharmaceutical industry uses many tricks to prejudice the conclusions of clinical trials. Marcia Angell, a former editor of the *New England Journal of Medicine*, describes them in her book, *The Truth About the Drug Companies: How They Deceive Us and What to Do About It.*[27] She lists seven strategies the industry uses to bias research. One of the most common is to test a new drug in a clinical trial against a placebo. This seems reasonable, but the results may be misleading if older, well-established drugs are already in use for the same condition. The new drug will inevitably be more expensive than the older ones—a benefit to the company—but there is no benefit for patients unless the new drug works better, something the trial does not test.

Drug companies may also use financial incentives to influence physician-researchers to come up with results favorable to the companies. In the extreme case, companies sometimes design clinical trials and seek academic scientists to carry them out, paying the scientists for their work; then the companies analyze and interpret the results and decide what should be published. Even when the scientists conduct their own research, they may be paid as consultants to companies whose products they are studying, or they may become paid members of advisory boards or speakers' bureaus, or they may own stock in the company. These arrangements tend to bias the researchers in favor of the companies' products. One survey found that industry-sponsored research was nearly four times as likely to be favorable to the company's product than research sponsored by the National Institutes of Health (NIH).[27(p.106)] Another study found that researchers with financial ties to the pharmaceutical industry—through consultancy payments, speaker fees, stock ownership, or patents related to the study drug—were more likely to report positive outcomes compared to researchers without financial ties. The study reported an odds ratio of 3.6, indicating a relatively strong association between financial ties and positive study outcomes.[28]

Until recently, when a company sponsored a study, it often had the last word on whether the results could be published at all. This led to strong publication bias: Trials with positive results were published, whereas those with negative results were never revealed. In fact, this tendency was reinforced by the preference of medical journals, which tend not to be interested in publishing articles about treatments that do not work. Since 2005, however, many reputable journals have adopted a policy of refusing to publish reports of clinical trials unless they have been registered at the beginning in a database of clinical trials, meaning that negative results cannot be hidden. The 2007 Food and Drug Administration Revitalization Act now requires registration of all such trials in a public database sponsored by the National Library of Medicine, ClinicalTrials.gov.[29] However, a 2017 review of compliance with this requirement found that much work remains before a fully effective system is in place. For example, a significant number of studies are still registered only after the trials have begun, often 12 months or more late, continuing to allow for the possibility of selectively registering studies that seem more promising.[30]

Conclusion

Epidemiologic studies are susceptible to many sources of error. Confounding factors may influence the results, suggesting an association where none exists. Bias may be introduced in the selection of cases or controls, in the reporting of exposures or outcomes, or in the disproportionate loss to follow-up of exposed or unexposed groups. Nevertheless, epidemiology is the basic science of public health. It is the only science of disease that focuses on human experience.

Certain design characteristics of epidemiologic studies can make them less or more convincing. Studies with large numbers of subjects are more likely to be valid than are smaller studies. A strong measure of association between exposure and disease, in the form of a high relative risk or odds ratio, is likely to indicate a true cause-and-effect relationship. A dose–response relationship that shows increasing risks from higher exposures adds to the validity of a study. A known biological explanation for an association between an exposure and a disease makes epidemiologic evidence more convincing than in situations where there is no known mechanism.

While observational studies have little potential for harming people, many ethical questions have been raised about clinical trials. In response to well-publicized abuses of the past, clinical trials and many other epidemiologic studies are required to be approved by committees, called institutional review boards, which ensure that the subjects' rights are protected. Other ethical concerns have been raised about the availability of treatments that have not been tested in clinical trials. At the same time, conflicts of interest in clinical trials testing the safety and efficacy of new drugs, which are required of pharmaceutical companies, have raised questions about the integrity of the research. Drug companies, which have vast amounts of money at stake in the outcomes of these trials, have found ways to manipulate the research to make drugs look better than they are.

Despite its flaws, epidemiology is still of necessity the basic science of public health. Epidemiologic data, when confirmed by repeated, well-designed studies and supported by the results of biomedical experiments in the laboratory, provide the best certainty as to the causes and cures of human disease.

References

1. G. Taubes, "Epidemiology Faces Its Limits," *Science* 269 (1995): 164–169.

2. A. Aschengrau and G. R. Seage III, *Essentials of Epidemiology in Public Health* (Sudbury, MA: Jones and Bartlett, 2003), 286.

3. M. Atiquzzaman, M. E. Karim, J. Kopec, H. Wong, and A. H. Anis, "Role of Non-steroidal Anti-Inflammatory Drugs (NSAIDs) in the Association Between Osteoarthritis and Cardiovascular Diseases: A Longitudinal Study," *Arthritis & Rheumatology* 71 (2019): 1835–1843.

4. S. Hite, *Women and Love: A Cultural Revolution in Progress* (New York: Alfred A. Knopf, 1987), described in V. Cohn and L. Cope, *News and Numbers: A Guide to Reporting Statistical Claims and Controversies in Health and Other Fields*, 2nd ed. (Ames, IA: Iowa State University Press, 2001), 154–156.

5. R. Seltser and P. E. Sartwell, "The Influence of Occupational Exposure to Radiation on the Mortality of American Radiologists and Other Medical Specialists," *American Journal of Epidemiology* 81(1965): 2–22.

6. J. A. Staples and D. A. Redelmeier, "The April 20 Cannabis Celebration and Fatal Traffic Crashes in the United States," *JAMA Internal Medicine* 178 (2018): 569–572.

7. K. Kaplan, "Drivers Beware: Risk of Fatal Car Crashes Spikes on the 4/20 Marijuana 'Holiday,' Study Says," *Los Angeles Times*, February 12, 2018.

8. S. Harper and A. Palayew, "Is 4/20 Deadly?" April 19, 2018, http://samharper.org/new-blog/2018/4/17/is-420-deadly, accessed August 20, 2019.

9. R. A. Wilson, *Feminine Forever* (New York: M. Evans and Company, 1966).

10. G. Kolata, "Hormone Studies: What Went Wrong?" *The New York Times*, April 22, 2003.

11. J. E. Manson and K. A. Martin, "Postmenopausal Hormone-Replacement Therapy," *New England Journal of Medicine* 345 (2001): 34–40.

12. G. Kolata, "Citing Risks, U.S. Will Halt Study of Drugs for Hormones," *The New York Times*, July 9, 2002.

13. G. Kolata, "Reversing Trend, Big Drop Is Seen in Breast Cancer," *The New York Times*, December 15, 2006.

14. F. Grodstein, T. B. Clarkson, and J. E. Manson, "Understanding the Divergent Data on Postmenopausal Hormone Therapy," *New England Journal of Medicine* 348 (2003): 645–650.

15. M. Stampfer, "Commentary: Hormones and Heart Disease: Do Trials and Observational Studies Address Different Questions?" *International Journal of Epidemiology* 33 (2004): 454–455.

16. J. E. Manson, A. K. Aragaki, J. E. Rossouw, G. L. Anderson, R. L. Prentice, A. Z. LaCroix, et al., "Menopausal Hormone Therapy and Long-Term All-Cause and Cause-Specific Mortality: The Women's Health Initiative Randomized Trials," *Journal of the American Medical Association* 318 (2017): 927–938.

17. G. E. Pence, *Classic Cases in Medical Ethics: Accounts of the Cases That Shaped and Define Medical Ethics*, 5th ed. (Boston, MA: McGraw-Hill, 2008).

18. S. M. Reverby, "More Than Fact and Fiction: Cultural Memory and the Tuskegee Syphilis Study," *Hastings Center Report* (September–October 2001): 22–28.

19. Steering Committee of the Physicians' Health Study Research Group, "Final Report on the Aspirin Component of the Ongoing Physicians' Health Study," *New England Journal of Medicine* 321 (1989): 129–135.

20. E. Braunwald et al., eds., *Harrison's Principles of Internal Medicine* (New York: McGraw-Hill, 1987).

21. G. Kolata, "Women Resist Trials to Test Marrow Transplants," *The New York Times*, February 15, 1995.

22. R. Rettig, P. Jacobson, C. M. Farquhar, and W. M. Aubry, *False Hope: Bone Marrow Transplantation for Breast Cancer* (Oxford, UK: Oxford University Press, 2007).

23. U.S. Food and Drug Administration, "Index to Drug-Specific Information," March 30, 2015, https://www.fda.gov/Drugs/DrugSafety/PostmarketDrugSafety InformationforPatientsandProviders/ucm111085.htm, accessed August 22, 2019.

24. C. Bombardier, L. Laine, A. Reicin, D. Shapiro, R. Burgos-Vargas, B. Davis, et al., "Comparison of

Upper Gastrointestinal Toxicity of Rofecoxib and Naproxen in Patients with Rheumatoid Arthritis," *New England Journal of Medicine* 343 (2000): 1520–1528.

25. D. J. Graham, "COX-2 Inhibitors, Other NSAIDs, and Cardiovascular Risk: The Seduction of Common Sense," *Journal of the American Medical Association* 296 (2006): 1653–1656.

26. G. D. Curfman, S. Morrissey, and J. M. Drazen, "Expression of Concern: Bombardier et al., 'Comparison of Gastrointestinal Toxicity of Rofecoxib and Naproxen in Patients with Rheumatoid Arthritis,'" *New England Journal of Medicine* 353 (2005): 1520–1528.

27. M. Angell, *The Truth About the Drug Companies: How They Deceive Us and What to Do About It* (New York: Random House, 2004).

28. R. Ahn, A. Woodbridge, A. Abraham, S. Saba, D. Korenstein, E. Madden, et al., "Financial Ties of Principal Investigators and Randomized Controlled Trial Outcomes: Cross Sectional Study," *British Medical Journal* 356 (2017): i6770.

29. J. M. Drazen, S. Morrissey, and G. D. Curfman "Open Clinical Trials," *New England Journal of Medicine* 357 (2007): 1756–1757.

30. D. A. Zarin, T. Tse, R. J. Williams, and T. Rajakannan, "Update on Trial Registration 11 Years After the ICMJE Policy Was Established," *New England Journal of Medicine* 376 (2017): 383–391.

CHAPTER 7

Understanding Uncertainty

Statistics: Making Sense of Uncertainty

KEY TERMS

Adjusted rate
Confidence interval
Cost–benefit analysis
Cost-effectiveness analysis
Crude rate
False negative

False positive
Lead-time bias
Overdiagnosis bias
p value
Power
Rates

Risk assessment
Screening
Sensitive
Specific
Statistical significance
Statistics

The science of epidemiology rests on statistics. In fact, all public health, because it is concerned with populations, relies on statistics to provide and interpret data. The chapter on the role of data in public health discusses the kinds of data that governments collect to assess the need for public health programs and evaluate public health progress. The term **statistics** refers to both the numbers that describe the health of populations and the science that helps to interpret those numbers.

The science of statistics is a set of concepts and methods used to analyze data with the purpose of extracting information. The public health sciences discussed in this text depend on the collection of data and the use of statistics to interpret those data. Statistics makes possible the translation of data into information about causes and effects, health risks, and disease cures.

Because health is determined by many factors—genes, behavior, exposure to infectious organisms or environmental chemicals—that interact in complex ways in each individual, it is often not obvious when or whether specific factors are causing specific health effects. Ethical and logistical limits affect the kinds of studies that can be conducted on human populations and the conclusions that can be drawn from biomedical studies on animals. Only by systematically applying statistical concepts and methods can scientists sometimes tease out the one influence among many that may be causing a change in some people's health. Often, however, statistics indicates that an apparent health effect may be simply a random occurrence.

The problems and limits of epidemiology are defined in large part by the uncertainties that are the subject of the science of statistics.

This chapter discusses the science of statistics in more detail, describing how it is used to clarify conclusions from a study or a test, to put numbers into perspective so that researchers can make comparisons and discern trends, and to show the limits of human knowledge.

The Uncertainty of Science

People expect science to provide answers to the health questions that concern them. In many cases, science has satisfied these expectations. Nevertheless, the answers provided by science are not always as definitive as people want them to be. For example, science has shown that the human immunodeficiency virus (HIV) causes acquired immunodeficiency syndrome (AIDS). But that does not mean that a woman will definitely contract AIDS from having sex with an HIV-positive man. Her chance of becoming infected with the virus from one act of unprotected intercourse is about one in 1000.[1] Similarly, scientific studies show that as a treatment for early breast cancer, a lumpectomy followed by radiation is as effective as a mastectomy—but a woman who chooses the lumpectomy still has a 10% chance of cancer recurrence.[2] Both the woman who had unprotected intercourse and the woman who chose the lumpectomy would dearly like to believe that they will be one of those in the majority of cases who will have a positive outcome, but science cannot promise them that. It can only say, statistically, that if 1000 women have unprotected sex with an HIV-positive man, 999 probably will fare well while one will not, and if 100 women with early breast cancer have a lumpectomy with radiation, 90 probably will be cancer-free after 15 years while 10 will have a recurrence.

In many cases, not enough data are available to give us even that degree of certainty, or the data that exist are too ambiguous to allow a valid conclusion. In 1995, the *New England Journal of Medicine* published a report that the Nurses' Health Study (a cohort study), which had monitored 122,000 nurses for 14 years, found a 30% to 70% increased risk of breast cancer in women who had taken hormone replacement therapy after menopause.[3] One month later, the *Journal of the American Medical Association* published the results of a case-control study that found no increased risk from the hormones. Some 500 women who had newly diagnosed breast cancer were no more likely to have taken postmenopausal hormones than a control group of 500 healthy women.[4] In *The New York Times* article reporting on these studies, each researcher is quoted as suggesting possible flaws in the other study.[5] There was little comfort in these results for women seeking certainty on whether the therapy would improve their health. According to one view, postmenopausal estrogen was clearly worth the possible risk of cancer because it appeared to decrease a woman's risk of heart disease and osteoporosis. The opposing argument suggested that women could achieve similar benefits without the possible risk through exercise, avoiding smoking, eating a low-fat diet, maintaining a normal weight, and taking aspirin. The latest analysis of clinical trial results has contradicted some of the findings of each of these studies; reassuringly, hormone replacement therapy has been found not to affect the mortality rates from cancer or heart disease.[6]

Contradictory results from epidemiologic studies are common. This kind of research has many possible sources of error, including bias and confounding, which are factors irrelevant to the hypothesis being tested that may affect a result or conclusion. Later in this chapter, we address additional factors to be considered in assessing the credibility of a study's conclusions.

People sometimes demand certainty even when science cannot provide it. For example, in 1997, controversy arose over the issue of whether women ages 40 through 49 should be screened for breast cancer using mammography. Studies had shown that routinely testing women age 50 and older with breast x-rays could reduce breast cancer mortality in the population. However, studies done on younger women had not demonstrated a life-saving benefit overall for this group. Routine screening of these women increases their radiation exposure, perhaps raising their risk of cancer. It also yields many false alarms, leading to unnecessary medical testing and major expense. The follow-up testing itself may cause complications, and many of the women remain anxious even after cancer is ruled out.[7]

In early 1997, Dr. Richard Klausner, the director of the National Cancer Institute (NCI), called together a panel of experts to advise him on the issue. The panel concluded that, for younger women, the benefit did not justify the risks and costs, and recommended that each woman make the decision in consultation with her doctor, considering her own particular medical and family history. The public and political response was heated: After a barrage of media publicity, the U.S. Senate voted 98 to 0 to endorse a nonbinding resolution that the NCI should recommend mammography for women in their 40s. A letter signed by 39 congresswomen stated that, "without definitive guidelines, the lives of too many women are at risk to permit further delay," assuming that screening could save lives despite the lack of evidence.[8(p.1104)] In the end, director Klausner, with the support of President Bill Clinton and Secretary of Health and Human Services Donna Shalala, recommended that women in their 40s should be screened. It seems clear that pressure from politicians eager to get credit for supporting women's health led to a pretense of scientific certainty where none existed.

On this question, further analysis supported the politicians, although the benefit is weaker for the younger age group. While the "melee that followed the meeting will not qualify for a place in the history of public health's most distinguishing scientific or policy moments," in the words of one analyst, there is now a far better understanding of the issue and evidence that screening may be life-saving for some younger women.[9(p.331)] However, because the incidence of breast cancer is lower in women in their 40s, and the effectiveness of mammography is also lower in the denser breasts of the younger women, the benefit of screening is less for them. In a review of the evidence published in 2007, the conclusion seemed to echo the NCI's original recommendation that individual women, in consultation with their doctor, should decide whether to be screened. The authors suggested that, "a woman 40 to 49 years old who had a lower-than-average risk for breast cancer and higher-than-average concerns about false-positive results might reasonably delay screening. Measuring risks and benefits accurately enough to identify these women remains a challenge."[10p.522)]

Remarkably, the whole political uproar was repeated in 2009, when an independent panel of experts, appointed by the Department of Health and Human Services, issued a recommendation that routine breast cancer screening begin at age 50, not 40. Because the recommendation was published in the midst of the public debate over healthcare reform, conservative politicians cried "rationing." As science reporter Gina Kolata pointed out in a *New York Times* article, the dispute gives many people "a sense of déjà vu."[11] The data had not changed much since the earlier debate, except that new evidence was published in 2008 suggesting that some invasive breast cancers may spontaneously regress, supporting the argument that screening may lead to unnecessary treatment.

Many people concerned about how to protect their health find it frustrating when today's news seems to contradict yesterday's reports. As this example shows, science is a work in progress. In the words of Dr. Arnold Relman, former editor of the *New England Journal of Medicine*, "Most scientific information is of a probable nature, and we are only talking about probabilities, not certainty. What we are concluding is the best opinion at the moment, and things may be updated in the future."[12(p.11)] Returning to the question of breast cancer screening, even among women aged 50, an important element of uncertainty remains: It has been estimated that for every 10,000 women offered annual screening over a 20-year period, 681 cancers would be diagnosed, of which 129 would represent overdiagnosis, while 43 deaths from breast cancer would be avoided. The overdiagnoses are instances where the cancer would not otherwise have presented over the woman's lifetime, but the apparent discovery of disease may lead to invasive treatment that could significant reduce the woman's quality of life. For a woman receiving a cancer diagnosis from screening, then, it is not possible to know if her life would be saved or she would experience unnecessary treatment. We must weigh the probabilities, which given the available data for this age group of women, favor screening.[13]

Probability

Scientists quantify uncertainty by measuring probabilities. All events, including all experimental results, can be influenced by chance. Thus, probabilities are used to describe the variety and frequency of past outcomes under similar conditions as a way of predicting what should happen in the future. Aristotle said that, "the probable is what usually happens." Statisticians know that the improbable happens more often than most people think.[12(p.19)]

One concept that scientists use to express the degree of probability or improbability of a certain result in an experiment is the **p value**. The p value expresses the probability that the observed result could have occurred by chance alone. A p value of 0.05 means that if an experiment were repeated 100 times, the same answer would result 95 of those times, while 5 times would yield a different answer. If a person tosses a coin 5 times in a row, it is improbable that it will come up the same—heads or tails—every time. However, if each student in a class of 16 conducts the experiment, it is probable

that 1 student will get the identical result in all 5 tosses. The probability of that occurrence is 1 chance in 16, or 0.0625 ($p = 0.0625$). Thus a p value of 0.05 says that the probability that an experimental result occurred by chance alone is less than the probability of tossing 5 heads or 5 tails in a row. A p value of 0.05 or less has been arbitrarily taken as the criterion for a result to be considered statistically significant.

Another way to express the degree of certainty of an experimental result is by calculating a **confidence interval**—that is, a range of values within which the true result probably falls. The narrower the confidence interval, the lower the likelihood of random error. Confidence intervals are often expressed as margins of error, as in political polling, when a politician's support might be estimated at 50% plus or minus 3%. In such a case a case, the confidence interval would be 47% to 53%.[12]

While p values and confidence intervals are useful concepts in deciding how seriously to take an experimental result, it is wrong to place too much confidence in an experiment just because it yields a low p value or a narrow confidence interval. There may be 10,000 clinical trials of cancer treatments under way at any time. If a p value of 0.05 is taken to imply **statistical significance**, 5 out of every 100 ineffective treatments would appear to be beneficial—errors caused purely by chance.[12] Thus, large numbers of cancer treatments could be in clinical use that are actually not effective. Other reasons that a study with a low p-value result could lead to an erroneous conclusion are bias or confounding, which are systematic errors. For example, the results of the study that linked coffee drinking with pancreatic cancer were statistically significant with a p value of 0.001.[14] The conclusion is thought to be wrong—not because of random error, but rather because the cancer was caused by smoking rather than coffee drinking.[15]

The fact that the probable is not always what happens leads to the Law of Small Probabilities.[12] The most improbable things are bound to happen occasionally, such as throwing heads 5 times in a row, or even—very rarely—99 times in a row. This means, for example, that a few people with apparently fatal illnesses will inexplicably recover. They may be convinced that their recovery was caused by something they did, giving rise—if their story is publicized—to a new vogue in quack therapies. But because their recovery was merely a random deviation from the probable, other patients will not get the same benefit.

Another consequence of the Law of Small Probabilities is the phenomenon of cancer clusters. Every now and then a community will discover that it is the site of an unusual concentration of some kind of cancer, such as childhood leukemia, causing residents to become highly alarmed. Is a carcinogen in the air or the drinking water causing the problem? Under great political pressure, the local and state government will investigate, but no acceptable explanation may be found. Most such clusters are due to statistical variation, akin to an unusual run of tails in a coin toss. Such an explanation tends to be unsatisfactory to community residents, who may accuse the government of a cover-up. After the investigation, however, the number of new cases usually returns to more or less normal levels, and the sense of alarm subsides.

If a cluster is very large, it is likely not to be a random variation—just as in coin tossing, 50 heads in a row is a much less likely outcome than 5 heads in a row unless there is something wrong with the coin. A large number of cases is said to confer **power** to a study. Power is the probability of finding an effect if there is, in fact, an effect. Thus, an epidemiologic study that includes large numbers of subjects has more power than a small study, and the results are more likely to be valid, although systematic errors due to bias or confounding can be present in even the largest studies.

In designing studies of any kind, statisticians can calculate the size of the study population necessary to find an effect of a certain size if it exists. Studies with low power are likely to produce **false-negative** results—that is, to find no effect when there actually is one. **False-positive** results occur when the study finds an effect that is not real—that is, when a random variation appears to be a true effect. In a study of epidemiologic studies, a statistician examined the power of each of 71 clinical trials that reported no effect. He concluded that 70% of the studies did not have enough patients to detect a 25% difference in outcomes between the experimental group and the control group. Even a 50% difference in outcomes would have been undetectable in half of the studies.[12] This common weakness in epidemiologic studies is one reason for the contradictory results so often reported in the news.

In a review of high-dose chemotherapy and bone marrow transplant as treatments for advanced breast cancer, the authors addressed the question of whether the studies had enough power to detect a significant improvement in survival for the treated women. They concluded that at least one of the individual studies did have sufficient power, and that the systematic review of all studies combined had the power to detect a 10% difference after five years.[16] Although some subgroups of women appeared to have benefited slightly from the high-dose treatment, further studies would be necessary to demonstrate this relation, and no such studies are planned. Thus, the question remains of how much difference would be clinically relevant. Would it be acceptable for a woman to undergo the arduous treatment if her chance of survival was only 10% better? Such a question cannot be answered by statisticians.

The Statistics of Screening Tests

In public health's mission to prevent disease and disability, secondary prevention—that is, early detection and treatment—plays an important role. When the causes of a disease are not well understood, as in breast cancer, little is known about primary prevention. In such a case, the best public health measure is to screen the population at risk so as to detect the disease early, when it is most treatable. **Screening** is also an important component of programs to control HIV/AIDS by identifying HIV-infected individuals so that they can be treated and counseled about how to avoid spreading the virus to others. As discussed later in this text in the context of genetic diseases, newborn babies are routinely screened for certain congenital diseases that can be treated before they do permanent damage to the infants' developing brains and bodies.

Ideally, laboratory tests to be used in screening programs should be highly accurate. Unfortunately, most tests are likely to yield either false positives or false negatives. Tests may be highly **sensitive**, meaning that they yield few false negatives, or they may be highly **specific**, meaning that they yield few false positives. Many highly sensitive tests are not very specific, and vice versa. For most public health screening programs, sensitive tests are desirable to avoid missing any individual with a serious disease who could be helped by some intervention. However, inexpensive, sensitive tests chosen to encourage testing of as many at-risk individuals as possible are often not very specific. When a positive result is found, more specific tests are then conducted to determine if the first finding was accurate. For example, if a sensitive mammogram finds a suspicious spot in a woman's breast, the test is usually followed up with a biopsy to determine whether the spot is indeed cancerous.

When screening is done for rare conditions, the rate of false positives may be as high as or higher than the number of true positives, leading to a lot of follow-up testing on perfectly normal people. Such a situation occurred in 1987 when the states of Illinois and Louisiana mandated premarital screening for HIV.[17] As the rate of HIV infection in the general, heterosexual population is quite low, a great many healthy people were unnecessarily alarmed and subjected to further tests, while very few HIV-positive people were identified. Some couples went to neighboring states to marry to avoid the nuisance. The programs were discontinued within a year. The problem of false positives is also the reason why mammography screening is questionable for women in their 40s, and it still creates problems for women age 50 and older, as discussed earlier.

For some other conditions, screening may not be as beneficial as expected. One of these conditions is prostate cancer, discussed later in this text. Another is lung cancer screening of smokers. Lung cancer is usually a fatal diagnosis; by the time most patients experience symptoms, it is too late for medicine or surgery to make a difference. The idea of screening smokers so that cancers can be detected and treated earlier in the course of the disease has been around since the 1970s and 1980s. However, at that time, the only method of screening was to use chest x-rays, and it turned out that cancers detected by x-ray screening were almost always too far advanced to be treatable.

In fall 2006, a paper published in the *New England Journal of Medicine* reported that screening with spiral computed tomography (CT) scans (a kind of three-dimensional x-ray) could detect lung cancers early enough that treatment allowed 80% of patients to survive for 10 years, compared to a 10% survival rate for patients who had been diagnosed the usual way.[18] A few months later, the *Journal of the American Medical Association* published another study, concluding that spiral CT scanning does not save lives and may actually cause more harm than good.[19] An analysis of the findings of the first trial revealed two sources of bias: **lead-time bias** and **overdiagnosis bias**.[20] The former may occur in all cancer screening and must be taken into consideration before concluding that screening saves lives. Lead-time bias occurs when increased survival time after diagnosis is counted as an indicator of success. If early detection of a cancer does not lead to a cure, the only result of early diagnosis is that patients will live longer with the knowledge that they are sick before dying at the same time they would have died anyway. This appears to be the case in the *New England Journal of Medicine* study of lung cancer screening. In fact, the effects of the additional diagnostic tests and surgeries that follow the early diagnosis may hasten the patient's death.

Overdiagnosis bias occurs when the tumors detected by the screening are not likely to progress to the stage that they cause symptoms and become life-threatening. Such small tumors had also been found in the earlier lung cancer screening trials using x-rays. Overdiagnosis bias is also a problem with prostate cancer screening, and perhaps with breast cancer screening, as discussed earlier in this chapter. The only way to be sure that screening actually saves lives is to conduct randomized controlled trials, comparing mortality among patients who are screened with that of patients who are not screened. Such trials, together with data showing that age-adjusted breast cancer mortality has fallen in the United States by 38% since 1992, have shown that mammography does save lives.[9,10,21]

Rates and Other Calculated Statistics

Epidemiology makes extensive use of rates in studies of disease distribution and determinants. **Rates** put the raw numbers into perspective by relating them to the size of the population being considered. Vast quantities of health-related data are collected on the U.S. population—data that are used to assess the people's health and to evaluate the effectiveness of public health programs. For these purposes, the raw numbers are subjected to statistical adjustments that yield various rates useful in making comparisons and identifying trends.

For example, knowing that a city has 500 deaths per year is not very informative unless the population of the city is known. Death rates are often expressed as the number of deaths per 1000 people. Thus, 500 deaths per year is a low number for a city of 100,000, yet is high for a city of 50,000. The overall death rate in the United States was 8.2 per 1000 people in 2013.[22] The same data may yield different rates depending on the population used as the basis for comparison. Rates are usually calculated using the population at risk for the denominator. In the case of death rates, the whole population is at risk. The birth rate is an exception; like the death rate, the birth rate is defined as the number of live births per 1000 people. The fertility rate, by contrast, does use the population at risk, giving the number of live births per 1000 women ages 15 to 44. Two communities with the same fertility rate may have quite different birth rates if one contains many young women and the other is older and has a higher proportion of men. Both rates start with the same raw number—the number of live births—but use a different population for reference. In 2018, the birth of 3,788,235 babies in the United States led to a fertility rate of 59.0 births per 1000 women aged 15 to 44. The fertility rate ranged from 67.9 births per 1000 women aged 20 to 24, to 99.6 births per 1000 women aged 30 to 34, to 11.9 births per 1000 women aged 40 to 44.[23]

Other rates commonly used as indicators of a community's health are the infant mortality rate and the maternal mortality rate. The infant mortality rate is the number of infants who die before their first birthday in a year, divided by the number of live births in that year. The maternal mortality rate is the number of deaths among women associated with pregnancy and delivery in a year, divided by the number of live births in that year.

For some purposes, the numbers can be made still more useful by converting **crude rates** into **adjusted rates**. Death rates are often adjusted for the age of the population. The adjustment uses a statistical calculation to make the populations being examined equivalent to one another. For example, the crude mortality rate in Florida is much higher than

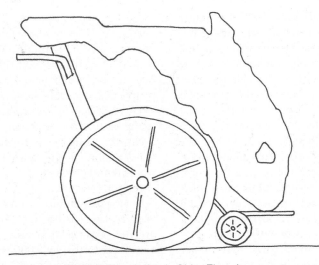

Florida's Population Is Older Than Average

the crude mortality rate in Alaska. There is no cause for alarm in Florida, however. Since the average age of Floridians is significantly higher than the average age of Alaskans—in fact, many residents of other states retire to Florida and die there, whereas people who move to Alaska are likely to be young—it is to be expected that a higher percentage of Floridians would die each year. After adjusting the mortality rate to what it would be if the average ages of the two populations were the same, the age-adjusted mortality rate for Alaska is higher than that in Florida (**Table 7-1**). Rates may also be adjusted for other factors relevant to health, such as gender, race, ethnicity, and so forth. For example, because males have higher mortality rates at all ages than females, it may sometimes be useful to calculate a gender-adjusted mortality rate for a population that has a higher proportion than average of one gender.

Rates are also calculated on a group-specific basis. For instance, researchers may calculate rates for males alone or females alone, blacks, whites, Hispanics, members of other racial or ethnic groups, and people in defined age groups. This kind of data informs us, for example, that males have higher mortality rates than females in the same age group, and that blacks have higher mortality rates than whites of the same sex and age. It is common to break down death rates from various causes by age group, revealing that different age groups

Table 7-1 **Mortality Rates for Florida and Alaska, 2017**

	Florida	Alaska
Crude death rate per 100,000	970.4	596.2
Age-adjusted death rate per 100,000	672.1	708.8

Data from Centers for Disease Control and Prevention, National Center for Health Statistics, "Underlying Cause of Death 1999–2017" on CDC WONDER Online Database, released December, 2018. Data are from the Multiple Cause of Death Files, 1999–2017, as compiled from data provided by the 57 vital statistics jurisdictions through the Vital Statistics Cooperative Program. Accessed at http://wonder.cdc.gov/ucd-icd10.html on August 22, 2019.

are more likely to die of different causes. For example, death rates from cancer, stroke, and heart disease increase steadily with age, except for a small peak in deaths of infants because of congenital heart defects.[24(Tables 24–26)] Death rates from AIDS, however, are highest for the 45-to-54 age group and fall to almost zero for those older than 85 years.[24(Table 29)] Death rates from firearms injuries and motor vehicle injuries are highest in the 20-to-24 age group, except that death rates from motor vehicle injuries are higher for people older than age 85.[24(Tables 31,34)]

Further calculations can be done using age-specific death rates to yield life expectancies, which are intuitively meaningful in describing the health of a population. Life expectancy is the average number of years of life remaining to people at a particular age, and it reflects the mortality conditions of the period when the calculation is made. Life expectancies may be determined by race, sex, or other characteristics using age-specific death rates for the population with that characteristic. The most common figure used in comparing the health

of various populations is the life expectancy at birth. As seen in **Figure 7-1**, life expectancies at birth in the United States increased steadily from 1900 until around 2014, when this trend was broken by small declines over the latter part of the 2010s. **Table 7-2** shows the life expectancy at birth for males and females of selected countries, highlighting the low life expectancy of Americans relative to people of other wealthy countries. In 2017, life expectancy for American males ranked 25th out of the 31 listed countries, while life expectancy for American females ranked 27th out of the 31 listed countries.

Another calculated concept that is sometimes used as a measure of premature mortality is years of potential life lost (YPLL). This measure gives greater weight to deaths of young people, as is appropriate given the priorities of public health: The goal of public health is not to eliminate death entirely, but rather to enable people to live out their natural lifespan with a minimum of illness and disability.

Calculation of YPLL arbitrarily chooses 75 as the age before which a death is considered

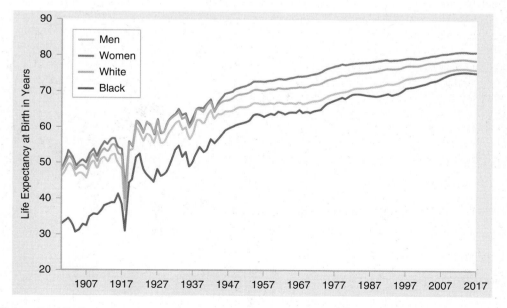

Figure 7-1 Life Expectancy at Birth According to Race and Sex in the United States, 1900–2017

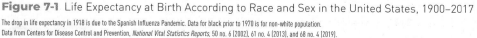

The drop in life expectancy in 1918 is due to the Spanish Influenza Pandemic. Data for black prior to 1970 is for non-white population.
Data from Centers for Disease Control and Prevention, *National Vital Statistics Reports*, 50 no. 6 (2002), 61 no. 4 (2013), and 68 no. 4 (2019).

Table 7-2 **Life Expectancy at Birth for Males and Females of Selected Countries, 1980 and 2017**

Country	Male			Female		
	1980	2017	2017 Rank	1980	2017	2017 Rank
Australia	71	80	9	78	85	7
Austria	69	79	17	76	84	13
Belgium	70	79	19	77	84	17
Canada	72	81	6	79	84	10
Czech Republic	67	77	24	74	83	24
Denmark	71	79	18	77	83	23
Estonia	64	73	29	74	82	25
Finland	69	79	22	78	84	9
France	70	80	15	78	86	4
Germany	70	79	21	76	84	19
Greece	73	79	20	78	84	16
Hungary	66	73	31	73	80	30
Iceland	79	80	10	80	84	14
Ireland	70	80	11	76	84	18
Israel	82	81	5	76	85	8
Italy	80	81	3	77	86	6
Japan	73	81	2	79	87	1
Korea	62	80	14	70	86	3
Mexico	64	75	26	70	80	29
Netherlands	73	80	13	79	83	21
New Zealand	70	80	12	76	86	20
Norway	72	81	4	79	84	12
Poland	66	74	27	74	82	26
Portugal	68	78	23	75	84	11
Slovak Republic	67	74	28	74	81	28
Spain	72	81	8	79	86	2
Sweden	73	81	7	79	84	15

Country	Male				Female		
	1980	2017	2017 Rank		1980	2017	2017 Rank
Switzerland	72	82	1		79	86	5
Turkey	56	73	30		60	79	31
United Kingdom	70	79	16		76	83	22
United States	70	76	25		77	81	27

Data from Centers for Disease Control and Prevention, *Health, United States, 2014*, Table 15; and The World Bank, "Life expectancy at birth," https://data.worldbank.org/indicator/SP.DYN.LE00.IN, accessed August 20, 2019.

premature (age 65 was used before 1996). As an example, the death of a person 15 to 24 years of age counts as 55.5 YPLL before age 75. Homicides rank relatively high in YPLL because they are likely to kill young people, who have more years to lose, despite not being one of the top 15 causes of death overall in the United States. **Table 7-3** shows a comparison of the leading causes of death in the United States with the leading causes of YPLL.

Table 7-3 **Years of Potential Life Lost (YPLL) Before Age 75 by Cause of Death, 2016, and Number of Deaths, 2017**

Cause of Death	YPLL	Rank by YPLL	Number of Deaths	Rank by Number of Deaths
Unintentional injuries	1,334	1	169,936	3
Cancer	1,262	2	599,108	2
Heart Disease	959	3	647,457	1
Suicide	439	4	47,173	10
Homicide	275	5	19,510	>15
Chronic liver disease and cirrhosis	188	6	41,743	11
Diabetes	178	7	83,564	7
Chronic lower respiratory disease	176	8	160,201	4
Cerebrovascular disease	164	9	146,383	5
Influenza and Pneumonia	80	10	55,672	8
Nephritis, nephrotic syndrome, and nephrosis	70	11	50,633	9
HIV disease	47	12	5,698	>15
Alzheimer's disease	14	13	121,404	6

Data from Centers for Disease Control and Prevention, *Health, United States, 2017*, Table 18, and *National Vital Statistics Report* 68 no. 9 (2019), "Deaths: Final Data for 2017," Table 8.

Risk Assessment and Risk Perception

While some statistical concepts might seem difficult and confusing, people have an intuitive understanding of statistics affecting their everyday lives. They understand that the future is full of uncertainties, and they naturally try to minimize risks or at least weigh risks against expected benefits. Their intuitive judgment of risks, however, often does not coincide with the more scientific estimates of statisticians. It turns out that while judgments of risk by the average person include statistical estimates that are often fairly accurate, they are also influenced by psychological factors that public health professionals should perhaps take into consideration.

Public health's mission to protect the population from disease and injury requires governments to minimize risks or at least weigh risks against expected benefits, just as individuals do in their own lives. The formal process of **risk assessment** identifies events and exposures that may be harmful to humans and estimates the probabilities of their occurrence as well as the extent of harm they may cause.

Risk assessment is often done on the basis of historical data. For example, one may predict that the number of motor vehicle crashes next year will be similar to the number this year, increasing or decreasing according to the trend established over the past several years. Risks that certain chemicals will cause cancer in humans are usually estimated by analogy with data obtained from animal studies. For many situations, however, there is little basis on which to make comparisons. In such cases, assessing risks involves making many assumptions, some of which may be little better than guesses. To estimate the probability of a mishap related to a new technology, various possible chains of events are considered, and a risk for something going wrong is estimated for each step, perhaps by analogy with conventional technology. The risks for the individual steps are then added or multiplied to obtain a risk for the whole. This approach was used, for example, when nuclear power plants were first introduced, and it helped engineers to identify what kind of safety devices should be incorporated to reduce the probability of failure.[25] Even so, the assessment appears to have underestimated the risk at Three Mile Island, Pennsylvania, as discussed later in this chapter.

Using such methods, scientists calculate probabilities that various injurious events will occur and rank them in order, as shown in **Table 7-4**. According to an analysis published in 1987, experts said that the most risky activities and technologies were motor vehicles, smoking, alcoholic beverages, handguns, and undergoing surgery. When members of the general public were asked about their perceptions of risks, however, their list was headed by nuclear power, which was ranked 20th by the experts. Other risks that people tended to rank higher than the experts did included electromagnetic fields, genetic engineering, and radioactive waste.[26]

As a result of the apparent irrationality of the public in response to risks that the experts estimated to be small, a field of study has developed concerning risk perception. While experts assess risk on the basis of expected mortality as predicted from historical data, the general public includes other considerations in its assessments. When these additional criteria are analyzed, it appears that the public's perception may not be so irrational after all.

Risk perception researchers have found that people's concern about a risk is affected by certain associated factors. For example, familiar risks are more acceptable than unfamiliar ones. Risks that people perceive they have control over are more acceptable than those that are uncontrollable. A risk with potentially catastrophic consequences is unacceptable, even if it is highly unlikely to occur. People are more likely to accept a risk from an activity that is perceived as beneficial, but they want the risks and benefits to be distributed equitably.

Table 7-4 Ordering of Perceived Risk for 30 Activities and Technologies

Activity or Technology	League of Women Voters	College Students	Experts
Nuclear power	1	1	20
Motor vehicles	2	5	1
Handguns	3	2	4
Smoking	4	3	2
Motorcycles	5	6	6
Alcoholic beverages	6	7	3
General (private) aviation	7	15	12
Police work	8	8	17
Pesticides	9	4	8
Surgery	10	11	5
Firefighting	11	10	18
Large construction	12	14	13
Hunting	13	18	23
Spray cans	14	13	26
Mountain climbing	15	22	29
Bicycles	16	24	15
Commercial aviation	17	16	16
Electric power (nonnuclear)	18	19	9
Swimming	19	30	10
Contraceptives	20	9	11
Skiing	21	25	30
X-rays	22	17	7
High school and college football	23	26	27
Railroads	24	23	19
Food preservatives	25	12	14
Food coloring	26	20	21
Power mowers	27	28	28
Prescription antibiotics	28	21	24
Home appliances	29	27	22
Vaccinations	30	29	25

The ordering is based on the geometric mean risk ratings within each group. Rank of 1 represents the most risky activity or technology.
Reprinted with permission from P. Slovic, "Perception of Risk," *Science* 236 (1987): 280–285. Copyright 1987, AAAS.

Risk perception researchers classify risks based on two scales: dread and knowability. The more dreaded the risk, the less acceptable it is; similarly, unknown risks are less acceptable than known risks. **Figure 7-2** maps various risks according to the concern they evoke on the two scales. Thus, although driving an automobile is, from a statistical perspective, one of the most risky activities, it does not arouse great anxiety because it is neither dreaded nor unknown. Moreover, people perceive that they have control when

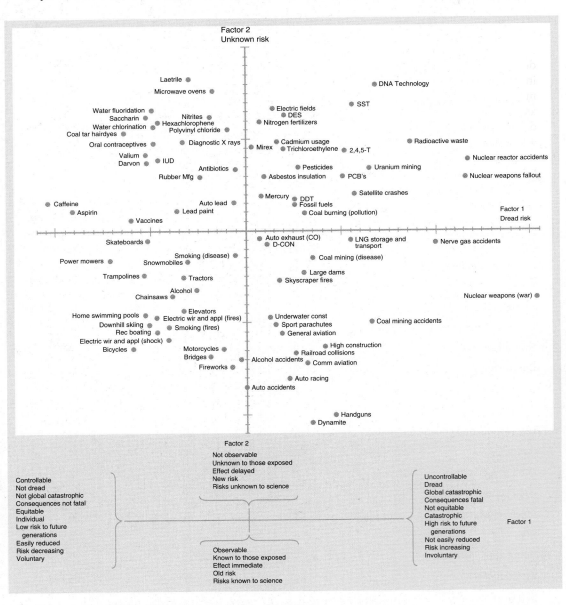

Figure 7-2 Location of 81 Hazards on Factors 1 and 2

Reproduced from P. Slovic et al., in R. W. Kates et al., ed., *Perilous Progress: Managing the Hazards of Technology* (Boulder, CO: Westview Press, 1985), 108.

they are driving, and the benefit is obvious to them. Conversely, a nuclear reactor accident is highly dreaded and, therefore, is perceived by the public as more risky than the experts believe it to be. People perceive that they lack control over nuclear reactors, and the benefits of nuclear power may not be clear to people who live in their vicinity.

The public's perception about nuclear power gained credibility after the 1979 accident at the Three Mile Island nuclear reactor in Pennsylvania. According to the experts, numerous safeguards were in place to prevent an accident, and the chance of a serious breakdown was remote. In fact, the safety systems worked during the 1979 incident to the extent that no disaster actually happened: No one was killed, and there was no significant radiation leak. Nevertheless, the fact that the breakdown occurred at all sent a signal that the experts may have underestimated the risks. Public opposition to nuclear power increased dramatically, and stricter requirements for reactor safety were imposed, raising construction and operating costs. The 1986 reactor meltdown at Chernobyl, Ukraine, further squelched interest in nuclear energy in the United States, as did the 2011 accident at the Fukushima Daiichi plant in Japan. Only one new plant has opened in the United States since 1996 (the Watts Barr Nuclear Plant in Tennessee), although at least one other is currently under construction.[27,28] Concern about climate change caused by the burning of fossil fuels alters the risk–benefit balance for nuclear power.

An interesting example of anomalous risk perception—one that is of great relevance to public health—is the paradox that adolescents so often engage in activities that they "know" to be dangerous, such as smoking, drunk driving, drug use, and unprotected sex. Studies aimed at understanding why teens engage in health-threatening behaviors can help public health practitioners design interventions to prevent such behaviors. In the case of smoking, for example, surveys have shown that teenagers can fairly accurately predict the probability that smokers will die of lung cancer and other diseases. However, the same surveys have found that teenage smokers perceive themselves to be at little or no risk. It turns out that they plan to quit smoking in the next few years—an inaccurate perception because they underestimate the addictive nature of nicotine and the difficulty of quitting once they are addicted.[29] Tobacco control programs, then, have focused on convincing adolescents that tobacco companies are trying to lure them into addiction.

Cost–Benefit Analysis and Other Evaluation Methods

Other types of statistical calculations are frequently carried out as part of public health decision making. One of these is **cost–benefit analysis**, which weighs the estimated cost of implementing a policy against the estimated benefit, usually in monetary terms. For example, when the U.S. government sought to set occupational exposure limits for benzene, the industry argued that setting a low exposure limit would be very expensive and that the benefit in lives saved would be small. Part of the difficulty in conducting such an analysis is the determination of what monetary value to place on a life saved. In other situations, the analysis provides a clearer justification for a program. For example, an analysis of the costs and benefits of immunizing children against measles, mumps, and rubella—comparing the costs of the immunization program with the costs of caring for the thousands of patients whose disease would not have been prevented if no immunizations had been done—yielded a 13-to-1 ratio of benefits to costs.[30]

Another evaluation technique is **cost-effectiveness analysis**, which compares the efficiency of different methods of attaining the same objective. For example, it may be so expensive to prevent heart attacks in healthy men by prescribing cholesterol-lowering drugs that a cost-effectiveness analysis would conclude that it is cheaper to skip the drugs and provide cardiac care for the men who do suffer an attack. Cost–benefit analysis and cost-effectiveness analysis "cannot serve as the sole or primary determinant of a health care decision," according to a congressional report, but the process of identifying and considering all the relevant costs and benefits can improve decision making.[31(p.211)]

Conclusion

The world is full of uncertainty. Science may not always be able to provide answers to people's questions. Statistics offers a way to learn, at least, how certain people can be about what they think they know.

Statistics is a tool widely used in public health. Most epidemiologic studies and most studies in the other public health sciences depend on statistics to analyze data and interpret findings. Statistical analyses can establish the probability that what was observed occurred by chance alone. A measure commonly used to indicate the probability that a study finding is the result of chance is the *p* value. Even when a low *p* value indicates that a result is statistically significant, there is still a chance that the result may not be valid, even if all sources of bias are ruled out. Studies with large numbers of subjects are more likely to be valid than small studies, although sources of error other than random variation are still possible in large studies.

Knowledge of statistics is also important in evaluating screening tests, which are used as a secondary prevention approach to detect diseases so that they can be treated at an early stage. Tests that are highly sensitive tend to yield false positives, whereas tests that are highly specific tend to yield false negatives. Most screening programs use sensitive tests and follow up positive results with more expensive tests that are both highly sensitive and highly specific. For conditions that are rare in the population being screened, the rate of false positives may be higher than the rate of true positives. Screening programs are also subject to biases, such as lead-time bias and overdiagnosis bias, which may make them less useful for saving lives than expected.

To put numbers into perspective, they are often converted into rates. Rates are useful in epidemiology and as a way of understanding the importance of the vast quantities of data used for assessment of the public's health and evaluation of public health programs. Rates commonly used as public health indicators include mortality (death) rates, birth rates, fertility rates, infant mortality rates, and maternal mortality rates. Rates may be statistically adjusted to make them comparable from one population to another. Age-specific rates can be calculated as well. Other statistical concepts useful as public health indicators include life expectancy and years of potential life lost.

Public health's efforts to protect the population may require calculations of risk. Risk assessment is a formal process of calculating the probabilities of various injurious events. The scientific assessment of risk sometimes conflicts with people's perception of risk.

Public health is based on science, including the science of statistics, which is the science of uncertainty. To paraphrase statistician and author Robert Hooke, scientific studies are often the only way to answer people's questions, but the studies do not produce "unassailable, universal truths that should be carved on stone tablets." Instead, they produce statistics, which must be interpreted.[12(p.64)]

References

1. R. A. Royce, A. Seña, W. Cates, Jr., and M. S. Cohen, "Sexual Transmission of HIV," *New England Journal of Medicine* 336 (1997): 1072–1078.

2. I. L. Wapnir, J. J. Dignam, B. Fisher, E. P. Mamounas, S. J. Anderson, T. B. Julian, et al., "Long-Term Outcomes of Invasive Ipsilateral Breast Tumor Recurrences After Lumpectomy in NSABP B-17 and B-24 Randomized Clinical Trials for DCIS," *Journal of the National Cancer Institute* 103, no. 6 (2011): 478–488.

3. G. A. Colditz, S. E. Hankinson, D. J. Hunter, W. C. Willett, J. E. Manson, M. J. Stampfer, et al., "The Use of Estrogens and Progestins and the Risk of Breast Cancer in Postmenopausal Women," *New England Journal of Medicine* 332 (1995): 1589–1593.

4. J. L. Stanford, N. S. Weiss, L. F. Voigt, J. R. Daling, L. A. Habel, and M. A. Rossing, "Combined Estrogen and Progestin Hormone Replacement Therapy in Relation to Risk of Breast Cancer in Middle-Aged Women," *Journal of the American Medical Association* 274 (1995): 137–142.

5. G. Kolata, "Cancer Link Contradicted by New Hormone Study," *The New York Times*, July 12, 1995.

6. J. E. Manson, A. K. Aragaki, J. E. Rossouw, G. L. Anderson, R. L. Prentice, A. Z. LaCroix, et al., "Menopausal Hormone Therapy and Long-Term All-Cause and Cause-Specific Mortality: The Women's Health Initiative Randomized Trials," *Journal of the American Medical Association* 318, no. 10 (2017): 927–938.

7. H. C. Sox, "Benefit and Harm Associated with Screening for Breast Cancer," *New England Journal of Medicine* 338 (1998): 1145–1146.

8. V. L. Ernster, "Mammography Screening for Women Aged 40 Through 49: A Guidelines Saga and a Clarion Call for Informed Decision Making," *American Journal of Public Health* 87 (1997): 1103–1106.

9. R. A. Smith, "Breast Cancer Screening Among Women Younger Than 50: A Current Assessment of the Issues," *CA: A Cancer Journal for Clinicians* 50 (2000): 312–336.

10. K. Armstrong, E. Moye, S. Williams, J. A. Berlin, and E. E. Reynolds, "Screening Mammography in Women 40 to 49 Years of Age: A Systematic Review for the American College of Physicians," *Annals of Internal Medicine* 146 (2007): 516–526.

11. G. Kolata, "Get a Test. No Don't. Repeat," *The New York Times*, November 22, 2009.

12. V. Cohn and L. Cope, *News and Numbers: A Guide to Reporting Statistical Claims and Controversies in Health and Other Fields*, 2nd ed. (Ames, IA: Iowa State University Press, 2001), 11.

13. M. G. Marmot, D. G. Altman, D. A. Cameron, J. A. Dewar, S. G. Thompson, and M. Wilcox, "The Benefits and Harms of Breast Cancer Screening: An Independent Review," *British Journal of Cancer* 108, no. 11 (2013): 2205.

14. B. MacMahon, S. Yen, D. Trichopoulos, K. Warren, and G. Nardi, "Coffee and Cancer of the Pancreas," *New England Journal of Medicine* 304 (1981): 630–633.

15. G. Taubes, "Epidemiology Faces Its Limits," *Science* 269 (1995): 164–169.

16. C. Farquhar, J. Marjoribanks, A. Lethaby, and M. Azhar, "High-Dose Chemotherapy and Autologous Bone Marrow or Stem Cell Transplantation Versus Conventional Chemotherapy for Women with Early Poor Prognosis Breast Cancer," *Cochrane Database of Systematic Reviews* 5 (2016):CD003139. doi: 10.1002/14651858.CD003139.pub3.

17. R. Bayer, *Private Acts, Social Consequences: AIDS and the Politics of Public Health* (New York: Free Press, 1989).

18. International Early Lung Cancer Action Program Investigators, "Survival of Patients with Stage I Lung Cancer Detected on CT Screening," *New England Journal of Medicine* 355 (2006): 1763–1771.

19. P. B. Bach , J. R. Jett, U. Pastorino, M. S. Tockman, S. J. Swenson, and C. B. Begg, "Computed Tomography Screening and Lung Cancer Outcomes," *Journal of the American Medical Association* 297 (2007): 953–961.

20. H. G. Welch, S. Woloshin, and L. M. Schwartz, "How Two Studies on Cancer Screening Led to Two Results," *The New York Times*, March 13, 2007.

21. National Institutes of Health, National Cancer Institute, "Cancer Stat Facts: Female Breast Cancer," https://seer.cancer.gov/statfacts/html/breast.html, accessed August 20, 2019.

22. Centers for Disease Control and Prevention, "Deaths: Final Data for 2013," *National Vital Statistics Report* 64, no. 2, http://www.cdc.gov/nchs/data/nvsr/nvsr64/nvsr64_02.pdf, accessed March 15, 2015.

23. Centers for Disease Control and Prevention, "Births: Provisional Data for 2018," *National Vital Statistics Report* 007, May 2019, www.cdc.gov/nchs/data/vsrr/vsrr-007-508.pdf, accessed August 20, 2019.

24. Centers for Disease Control and Prevention, "Health, United States, 2014," http://www.cdc.gov/nchs/data/hus/hus14.pdf, accessed September 9, 2015.

25. R. Wilson and E. A. C. Crouch, "Risk Assessment and Comparisons: An Introduction," *Science* 236 (1987): 267–270.

26. P. Slovic, "Perception of Risk," *Science* 236 (1987): 280–285.

27. M. L Wald, "Nuclear Plants, Old and Uncompetitive, Are Closing Earlier Than Expected," *The New York Times*, June 14, 2013.

28. M. Blau, "First New US Nuclear Reactor in 20 Years Goes Live," CNN, October 21, 2016, www.cnn.com /2016/10/20/us/tennessee-nuclear-power-plant/index .html, accessed August 20, 2019.

29. P. Slovic, "Do Adolescent Smokers Know the Risks?" in P. Slovic, *The Perception of Risk* (London: Earthscan Publications, 2000), 363–371.

30. C. C. White et al., "Benefits, Risks and Costs of Immunization for Measles, Mumps and Rubella," *American Journal of Public Health* 75 (1995): 739.

31. G. Pickett and J. J. Hanlon, *Public Health: Administration and Practice* (St. Louis, MO: Times Mirror/Mosby, 1990), 211.

Collecting Data

The Role of Data in Public Health

KEY TERMS

Behavioral Risk Factor
    Surveillance Survey (BRFSS)
National Center for Health
    Statistics (NCHS)

Public health informatics
Surveillance systems

United States Census
Vital statistics

Just as a doctor monitors the health of a patient by taking vital signs—blood pressure, heart rate, and so forth—public health workers monitor the health of a community by collecting and analyzing health data. These data, called health statistics, play a vital role in public health's assessment function. They are used to identify special risk groups, to detect new health threats, to plan public health programs and evaluate their success, and to prepare government budgets. The statistics collected by federal, state, and local government serve as the raw material for research on epidemiology, environmental health, social and behavioral factors in health, and for the medical care system.

At the federal level, the primary agency that collects, analyzes, and reports data on the health of Americans is the **National Center for Health Statistics (NCHS)**, which is part of the Centers for Disease Control and Prevention (CDC). The NCHS collects its data in two main ways. First, states periodically transmit data they have compiled from local records; vital statistics, including virtually all births and deaths, are routinely collected this way. Second, the NCHS conducts periodic surveys of representative samples of the population, seeking information on certain characteristics such as health status, lifestyle and health-related behavior, onset and diagnosis of illness and disability, and the use of medical care. Some of these surveys are conducted on a state-by-state basis, so the data they collect are useful to states and local communities. In addition, other federal agencies that collect data for their own purposes share it with the NCHS.

Vital Statistics

Births and deaths are the most basic, reliable, and complete data collected. Virtually every birth and every death in the United States are recorded on a birth certificate and a death certificate, respectively. Certificates are filed with the local registrar by the attending physician, midwife, undertaker, or other attendant. The state health department is generally responsible for collecting these reports and transmitting them periodically to the NCHS.

Birth certificates contain information supplied by the mother about the child's family, including names, addresses, ages, race and ethnicity, and education levels. Medical and health information is supplied by the hospital, doctor, or other birth attendant concerning prenatal care, birth weight, medical risk factors, complications of labor and delivery, obstetrical procedures, and abnormalities in the newborn. In the past few decades, many states have added a question about the mother's use of tobacco to the birth certificate. Much of the information on the certificate is confidential, withheld even from the person represented by the certificate. Its main use is for public health research, providing the data that can be used to relate features of the mother and her pregnancy to the health of the child.

The information on death certificates is subject to a number of uncertainties, depending on how well the informant knew the deceased and the circumstances of the death. For example, information on parents, education, and occupation may not be known if the decedent is an elderly person with no surviving relatives. The accuracy and consistency with which causes of death are specified are also subject to uncertainty. Incorrect diagnoses are common; in the absence of an autopsy, the exact cause of death may not be known. If a number of conditions contribute to the fatal process, underlying causes and immediate causes may be confused. For some conditions, such as acquired immunodeficiency syndrome (AIDS) or suicide, the cause of death may be misstated deliberately by the local official because of social stigma.

In addition to births and deaths, **vital statistics** include marriages and divorces,

spontaneous fetal deaths, and abortions. Data on marriages and divorces are legal events that require universal reporting, but they are less interesting from a public health point of view. Reporting of spontaneous fetal deaths is incomplete, especially for those that occur relatively early in a pregnancy; many may go unrecognized. Induced abortions are also probably somewhat underreported. In some states, the name of the woman who had the abortion is not included in the report for reasons of confidentiality.

Because infant mortality is an important public health issue, the NCHS has set up a special computer system that links vital records of infants born during a given year who died before their first birthday. The linkage allows researchers to compare information on the death certificates with that on the birth certificates, providing insight into factors that contribute to infant deaths.

The United States Census

The data collected through the vital statistics system and other methods must be converted into rates if they are to be useful for many public health purposes. These calculations require information on the number of people in the population being referred to, the number that serves as the denominator when a vital statistic is used as the numerator. To calculate age-adjusted or age-specific rates, it is necessary to know how many people are in each age group. To determine sex-specific or race-specific rates, one needs to know how many males and females there are and how many blacks, whites, Hispanics, and people of other races are in each sex and each age group. This information is collected by the U.S. Census Bureau, which is part of the Department of Commerce. Without an accurate count of the U.S. population and all its characteristics, the government's health statistics would not be accurate.

As every schoolchild knows, the U.S. Constitution requires that the population of the United States be counted every 10 years to determine each state's representation in the House of Representatives. Based on that simple mandate, the Census Bureau has developed the **United States Census**, a national survey that provides data not only on the geographic distribution of the population and its sex, age, and ethnic characteristics, but also on a wide variety of social and economic characteristics, including education, housing, and health insurance status. Furthermore, because the population is always in flux and its characteristics tend to change fairly quickly, the Census Bureau tracks trends in the population between the decennial censuses, using polls and surveys and other sources of data such as birth and death records, immigration and emigration records, and school statistics. Census Bureau data are vital for the operation of the nation's social, political, economic, and industrial systems, and they are essential for the practice of public health.

The 2020 census is the first to allow responses by Internet and telephone. As in previous years, every person living in the United States, including citizens and noncitizens here legally or not, is counted. Troops deployed overseas, students away at college, individuals in prison, and others outside their usual living residence are also counted. Data collection for the 2020 census began in January 2020 in the westernmost parts of Alaska, and by March 2020 nearly all U.S. households were contacted by the Census Bureau. Households that did not respond by April 2020 began receiving in-person visits by trained census interviewers.[1]

Because census data can determine the political composition of the U.S. Congress and the distribution of federal funds to states and communities, various interest groups carefully monitor how the data are collected. An issue that was particularly controversial for the 2020 census was whether to include a question on citizenship status; such a question had been absent from the questionnaire since 1950. The Donald Trump administration's stated reason for insisting on the inclusion of this question was to help enforce voting rights protections for racial and language minorities. This explanation was thrown out in federal court as a "sham justification," and in July 2019 the U.S. Supreme Court agreed, stating that the administration's reasoning was "contrived." The actual motivation, the courts stated, was to suppress response rates in immigrant communities, where undocumented individuals live in fear of deportation and might prefer to remain unnoticed by the government. Cities and states with large immigrant communities fought against the inclusion of the citizenship question because a population undercount would reduce their political power and access to federal funds. In the end, after much debate and legal wrangling, the citizenship question was excluded from the 2020 census.[1]

In a win for the gay and lesbian community, the 2020 census included new household categories that allowed individuals to identify their relationship as "same-sex" or "opposite-sex." After the new data are released in 2021, it should be possible to calculate detailed public health statistics for homosexual couples and families.[1]

Inevitably, some people are missed or counted twice in the census. The missing ones are likely to be the poorest and most marginal members of the population—the homeless, illegal immigrants, fugitives from the law. In contrast, wealthy people who own more than one home might be counted twice. The Census Bureau estimates that the 2010 census missed approximately 10 million people and counted about 36,000 people twice.[2] Such errors can lead to systematic inaccuracies in health statistics. For example, blacks tend to be undercounted in the census, whereas black births and deaths are more accurately recorded.

In turn, birth and death rates calculated for blacks tend to be higher than their true value would be if correct population numbers were used for the denominator.

Starting in 2010, the way the census was conducted underwent a major change: Only the most basic data would be collected from everyone, using what used to be called the short form, which asks for name, age, sex, race and ethnicity, and relationship of everyone living in the household. Previous censuses had sought to gain a fuller understanding of population characteristics by using a long form for about one in six addresses, asking questions about education, housing, employment, transportation, language, ancestry, and other issues useful for governments and businesses. In an attempt to make the collection of this detailed information more efficient and more timely, the Census Bureau in 2005 launched the American Community Survey (ACS), a new ongoing survey collects the same kind of information previously collected on the long form. The long form is no longer being used in the decennial census. Instead, the ACS is sent each year to approximately 3 million households selected to be representative of the populations of local jurisdictions. It is designed to help communities plan transportation systems, zoning, schools, healthcare facilities, and housing, as well as estimate the need for social services.[3]

Republican Party hostility to the ACS broke out in May 2012, when the Republican-led House of Representatives voted to eliminate the ACS entirely on the grounds that it is too intrusive. A number of business groups, including the U.S. Chamber of Commerce and the National Association of Home Builders, were able to save the ACS, which provides important economic data for business planning as well as government decision making.[4] In 2015, however, Republicans in the U.S. Congress again declared their hostility to the ACS.[5] Defenders of the ACS continue to successfully beat back these attacks.

NCHS Surveys and Other Sources of Health Data

As noted previously, the NCHS, in addition to collecting data from the states, actively conducts a number of surveys to gather additional information on the health of the U.S. population.[6] Two ongoing NCHS surveys aim to assess the health of the population as a whole, estimate the prevalence of selected diseases and risk factors, and look for trends. In most years, interviewers for the National Health Interview Survey (NHIS) contact approximately 35,000 households and ask questions about illnesses, injuries, impairments, chronic conditions, access to health care, utilization of medical resources, and other health topics.[7] The National Health and Nutrition Examination Survey (NHANES) is designed to obtain even more detailed and accurate information; doctors and nurses are sent in vans to conduct physical and dental examinations and laboratory tests on a carefully selected sample of the population. Each year, 15 counties are visited, and approximately 5000 individuals of all ages are selected to undergo the tests. Data are collected on the prevalence of chronic conditions, including cardiovascular disease, diabetes, kidney disease, respiratory disease, osteoporosis, and hearing loss, as well as risk factors for those conditions, such as smoking, alcohol consumption, sexual practices, physical fitness and activity, weight, and dietary intake.[8] In the summer of 2019, for example, NHIS and NHANES data were used to study the amount of whole grains in the diets of Americans, how many teenagers were attempting to lose weight, and the ways in which Americans were trying to reduce their prescription drug expenditures.[9]

The NCHS also administers the National Health Care Survey, which gathers information on how health care is organized and provided in the United States. An important function of these surveys is to gather data on the operations of doctors' offices, community health centers, hospitals, nursing homes, hospice organizations, and other health facilities. Data from the National Health Care Survey, for example, were recently analyzed to learn about adoption rates of electronic health records: In 2017, 86% of office-based physicians used such health records, though only about 42% communicated these records with other facilities electronically—indicating the U.S. healthcare system as a whole has a long way to go in terms of achieving full interoperability of electronic data systems. Data from the National Health Care Survey also recently showed the degree of overcrowding at hospital emergency rooms, finding an average wait time of 24 minutes at lower-volume facilities, compared to 49 minutes at higher-volume facilities. The longer wait times sometimes had serious consequences, including delayed treatments for heart attacks.[10]

The **Behavioral Risk Factor Surveillance Survey (BRFSS)**, which is conducted by the federal government in collaboration with the states, also obtains information on health-related behaviors. It asks questions about health; risk factors, including high blood pressure, high blood cholesterol, diabetes, and weight; and health-related behaviors such as diet and physical activity, cigarette smoking, alcohol use, seat belt use, and drinking and driving. In addition, it asks whether people get preventive medical care such as mammograms, Pap smears, colon cancer screening, and immunizations. The BRFSS gathers some of the same information as NHANES, but has the notable advantage of surveying many more people—it is the largest continuously conducted health survey in the world, completing more than 400,000 interviews per year—and it allows analysis of how the factors vary from one state to another.[11] However, the information is self-reported and may be less reliable than that obtained in NHANES. For example, the BRFSS found that, according to people's own reports, approximately 28% of adults were obese in 2011,[12] whereas the NHANES survey, using direct measurements, found a rate of about

35%.[13] This discrepancy accords with previous observations that overweight people generally report that they weigh less than they do.

The NCHS has conducted a variety of other surveys, including the National Youth Fitness Survey, the National Survey of Family Growth, and the National Immunization Survey. Some surveys are done in collaboration with other agencies, such as the National Asthma Survey, in collaboration with the CDC's National Center for Environmental Health; the National Infant Feeding Practices Study, in collaboration with the Food and Drug Administration; and the National Health Interview Survey on Disability, in collaboration with several other agencies including the Social Security Administration.

Other governmental agencies collect health-related data according to the focus of their responsibilities. For example, the Environmental Protection Agency carries out surveillance for health hazards in the environment, including air pollutants and releases of toxic chemicals. The National Cancer Institute coordinates a program called Surveillance, Epidemiology, and End-Results (SEER), used to monitor long-term trends of cancer incidence and mortality. The Centers for Medicare and Medicaid Services has billing records for the Medicare program, which are useful for research on utilization and outcomes of medical care. The Food and Drug Administration collects reports of adverse reactions to drugs after they have been approved and are on the market, and it sometimes recommends recalls of pharmaceutical products if a serious problem appears that was not noted during preapproval testing. Surveillance for product-related injuries is conducted by the Consumer Product Safety Commission.

Is So Much Data Really Necessary?

While it might seem that the government collects enormous amounts of information on its citizens, public health can never have too much data. These data are critically important in developing the **surveillance systems** that form the basis of effective public health practice as well as the planning and evaluation efforts that are increasingly being used in public health programming.

The statistics collected by federal, state, and local agencies are used in all areas of public health. Early notification of communicable disease cases is a classic use of public health information to protect the public's health. The need for public health interventions to control other problems may not be obvious without an analysis of data. This explains the Institute of Medicine's insistence on the importance of assessment as a core function of public health.[14] Public health leaders are increasingly stressing the importance of planning, setting goals, and managing public health programs to meet these goals—a process that requires data at the local, state, and federal levels. For example, a community may not recognize that it has a problem with unintended pregnancy and low-birth-weight babies unless it analyzes the data from birth certificates, comparing local data with statewide or national averages. Recognition of such a problem might persuade local public health leaders to consider school-based birth control education and services.

Throughout this text, during discussions of public health issues (including biomedical, social and behavioral, environmental, and medical care issues), problems are defined according to the data that are available. In any area of public health, problems are identified in terms of statistics. The success of intervention programs in confronting a problem is evaluated based on whether they improve the statistics.

In an era when people tend to frown on "big government" and yearn for lower taxes, there is always pressure to cut back fiscal support for data collection and analysis, as these activities might seem less urgent than fighting a known epidemic, for instance. Yet without data, experts cannot recognize that an epidemic is beginning. Inspired by the recommendations

of *The Future of Public Health*,[14] the CDC has taken the lead in coordinating and encouraging the use of data in public health assessment. Recent events, including the emergence and resurgence of infectious diseases and the fear of bioterrorism, have stimulated the development of new surveillance systems within the United States and around the world.

With or without adequate data, decisions affecting public health policy and the allocation of scarce resources from government budgets must be made. It is increasingly important that these policy and fiscal decisions be based on timely and accurate information.

Accuracy and Availability of Data

British economist Sir Josiah Stamp (1880–1941) wrote in 1929:

> The Government [is] very keen on amassing statistics. They collect them, add them, raise them to the nth power, take the cube root and prepare wonderful diagrams. But you must never forget that every one of those figures comes in the first instance from the village watchman, who just puts down what he damn well pleases.[15]

The process of data collection is always imperfect. Even data for births and deaths—the most accurately reported health events—may be flawed. The decennial census produces errors, and political difficulties arise when trying to rectify them. Most other sources of health information, which rely on surveys or voluntary reports, are even more incomplete or subject to bias. For example, the Youth Behavioral Factor Risk Survey of high school students, conducted by states and reported to the CDC, misses adolescents who have the highest risks—those who have dropped out of school.

Errors in reporting the cause of death on death certificates are a prime example of the errors about which Stamp warns. They are especially worrisome for public health, in that mortality data have such a strong influence on planning and priority setting for public health programs. Autopsies are being done with declining frequency, in part because of cost concerns, but also because doctors may believe that sophisticated diagnostic technology has rendered autopsies obsolete. In 1972, autopsies were performed in 19.3% of deaths; in 2007 (the most recent year for which data are available), that proportion had fallen to 8.5%.[16,17] Cause-of-death information is still subject to uncertainty in many cases, and several studies have found that evidence obtained from an autopsy contradicted the clinical judgment of doctors in 15% to 32% of cases. Information gained from an autopsy answers the question, Did the patient receive the correct treatment for the correct disease? This information can improve the quality of medical care for future patients as well as improve the accuracy of vital statistics.

Because some of the inaccuracies on birth and death certificates may result from carelessness on the part of the busy health professionals who file them, new electronic methods of filing that are being introduced in some states are expected to improve the quality of the data. For example, maternal deaths are suspected of being underreported because doctors often fail to check off on a women's death certificate whether she was pregnant or gave birth in the time period prior to her death. If an electronic death certificate is used, the computer will refuse to accept the form—it will not "send" it—until that question is answered.[18]

Computers are extensively used in the analysis of public health data, of course, and new applications are continually improving the timeliness and accessibility of the data. Weekly reports of notifiable diseases from state and local health agencies are transmitted electronically to the CDC, allowing for a prompt response to new outbreaks. Laboratory results are also reported electronically, facilitating the rapid identification of bacterial and viral strains that may be causing illness in scattered locations around the country. Databases that are kept up-to-date by electronic filings can provide rapid feedback on the effectiveness of new public health interventions as well as help detect emerging problems.

The new information technology—or **public health informatics**, as it is sometimes called—has vastly improved the accessibility of public health information to public health workers and the general public. The CDC and most other federal and state public health agencies make information available over the Internet. For example, *Morbidity and Mortality Weekly Reports* are searchable online, and articles can be downloaded from the CDC's Web page. The National Cancer Institute provides the latest information on cancer therapies and prognoses tailored for doctors and for patients. Most of the information is freely available to all, although some data sets require users to have special passwords before they are allowed access; others are available to authorized users only on CDs or other media.

Confidentiality of Data

When anyone collects information on other people, questions always arise about how the information will be used and who will be allowed access to it. In general, all information collected from individuals by governments for whatever purpose is considered confidential and cannot be divulged without the consent of the individual. In most cases, the information is entered into a massive database from which individual names and addresses are removed. For research purposes, an identifying number may remain attached to the data to enable researchers to match information in one database with that in another. This technique is used, for example, in matching birth and death records to learn more about the factors that contribute to infant mortality.

For the U.S. Census, individual records are kept sealed for 72 years—so, for example, records from the 1950 census are set to be released in 2022. One major breach of these confidentiality rules has occurred: Under the Second War Powers Act of 1942, the administration of President Franklin Roosevelt allowed access to individualized census data to assist in the identification and internment of Japanese Americans.[19] No significant violations of confidentiality have occurred since then.

On a more decentralized level, there is always concern that a determined snoop who works in an agency or knows an employee could obtain confidential information on an individual and use it to that individual's detriment. Agencies that handle confidential data impose stringent rules on access. Researchers must explain and justify their need for the data and promise to safeguard its confidentiality. Most agencies have an institutional review board or data protection committee, often including members from the community, which weighs the researchers' claims and decides whether to grant permission for access. Other than its use for research, the only exception made to the promise of confidentiality is when people must be notified that they have been exposed to a communicable disease.

The conflict between the need for confidentiality and the need for open access to information has played out over various aspects of the AIDS epidemic. Because human immunodeficiency virus (HIV)–positive individuals feared (with good reason) that they might face discrimination if employers, landlords, and others learned of their infection, public health practitioners were concerned that patients would refuse to be tested unless confidentiality was ensured. Hence, the rules for reporting HIV were handled differently from other communicable diseases: Anonymous testing was allowed, and the system for reporting cases to many state health departments and the CDC was modified to maintain anonymity. More recently, with the advent of new drugs that can clearly help AIDS patients and slow the onset of AIDS in HIV-infected individuals, HIV's exempt status has, for the most part, been discontinued, and it is now treated like other communicable diseases.

Conclusion

Statistics are the vital signs of public health. Local, state, and federal governments collect data on their citizens, starting with birth certificates and ending with death certificates. The U.S. Census, conducted every 10 years, provides information on the age, sex, and ethnic composition of communities—information that allows the calculation of birth rates, death rates, infant mortality rates, life expectancies, and other data that form the basis for public health's assessment function.

The NCHS is the repository for the vital statistics data received from the states. This federal agency also conducts a number of periodic and ongoing surveys to collect additional information on Americans, including information on family structure, specific health conditions, behavioral risk factors, and other data useful in planning public health intervention programs.

Health statistics are used for all aspects of public health policy development and evaluation. Uses of such data include health needs identification, analysis of problems and trends, epidemiologic research, program evaluation, program planning, budget preparation and justification, administrative decision making, and health education.[20]

Electronic means have become the primary way to collect, transmit, store, and analyze data and to make the data available to public health workers and the general public. Strict precautions are taken to ensure confidentiality of information about individuals.

References

1. H. Lo Wang, "What You Need to Know About the 2020 Census," National Public Radio, March 31, 2019 (updated July 18, 2019), www.npr.org/2019/03/31/707899218/what-you-need-to-know-about-the-2020-census, accessed August 26, 2019.

2. U.S. Census Bureau, "Census Bureau Releases Estimates of Undercount and Overcount in the 2010 Census," News Release, May 22, 2012, www.census.gov/newsroom/releases/archives/2010_census/cb12-95.html, accessed August 26, 2019.

3. C. Holden, "New Annual Survey Brings Census into the 21st Century," *Science* 295 (2002): 2202–2203.

4. C. Rampell, "The Beginning of the End of the Census," *The New York Times*, May 19, 2012.

5. "Editorial: Don't Starve the Census," *The New York Times*, March 10, 2015.

6. National Center for Health Statistics, "NCHS Fact Sheet: Summary of Current Surveys and Data Collection Systems," June 2019, www.cdc.gov/nchs/data/factsheets/factsheet_summary.pdf, accessed August 28, 2019.

7. National Center for Health Statistics, "About the National Health Interview Survey," www.cdc.gov/nchs/nhis/about_nhis.htm, accessed August 28, 2019.

8. National Center for Health Statistics, "About the National Health and Nutrition Examination Survey," www.cdc.gov/nchs/nhanes/about_nhanes.htm, accessed August 28, 2019.

9. National Center for Health Statistics, "NCHS Data Briefs," www.cdc.gov/nchs/products/databriefs.htm, accessed August 27, 2019.

10. National Center for Health Statistics, "National Health Care Surveys," June 2019, www.cdc.gov/nchs/data/factsheets/factsheet_nhcs.pdf, accessed August 28, 2019.

11. Centers for Disease Control and Prevention, "Behavioral Risk Factor Surveillance System: About BRFSS," https://www.cdc.gov/brfss/about/index.htm, accessed August 28, 2019.

12. Centers for Disease Control and Prevention, "BRFSS Prevalence & Trends Data," www.cdc.gov/brfss/brfssprevalence/, accessed August 28, 2019.

13. C. L. Ogden et al., "Prevalence of Childhood and Adult Obesity in the United States, 2011–2012," *Journal of the American Medical Society* 311 (2014): 806–814.

14. Institute of Medicine, Committee for the Study of the Future of Public Health, *The Future of Public Health* (Washington, DC: National Academy Press, 1988).

15. J. Stamp, *Some Economic Factors in Modern Life* (London: P. S. King, 1929), 258–259, quoted in R. Goodman and R. Berkelman, "Physicians, Vital Statistics, and Disease Reporting," *New England Journal of Medicine* 258 (1987): 379.

16. D. L. Hoyert, National Center for Health Statistics, "The Changing Profile of Autopsied Deaths in the United States, 1972–2007," *NCHS Data Brief* 67 (August 2011), www.cdc.gov/nchs/data/databriefs/db67.pdf, accessed August 28, 2019.

17. National Center for Health Statistics, "The Autopsy, Medicine, and Mortality Statistics," *Vital and Health Statistics* 3, no. 32 (October 2001), www.cdc.gov/nchs/data/series/sr_03/sr03_032.pdf, accessed August 28, 2019.

18. M. Zdeb and M. Applegate, personal communication.

19. J. R. Minkel, "Confirmed: The U.S. Census Bureau Gave Up Names of Japanese-Americans in WW II," *Scientific American*, March 30, 2007.

20. G. Pickett and J. J. Hanlon, *Public Health: Administration and Practice* (St. Louis, MO: Times Mirror/Mosby, 1990), 151–153.

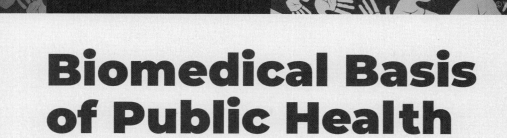

Biomedical Basis of Public Health

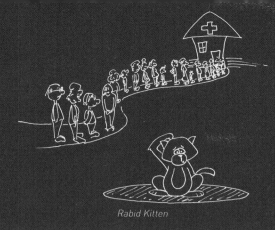
Rabid Kitten

CHAPTER 9

The "Conquest" of Infectious Diseases

KEY TERMS

Aerosols
Bacteria
Carrier state
Chain of infection
Contact tracing
Herd immunity

Immunization
Method of transmission
Parasites
Pathogen
Quarantine
Reservoir

Susceptible host
Vector
Vaccination
Viruses

Throughout history, until the beginning of the 20th century, infectious diseases were the major killers of humans. Bubonic plague, the "Black Death," is said to have wiped out as much as 75% of the population of Europe and Asia in the 14th century. Tuberculosis was the number one killer in England in the mid-19th century. An example of the toll of infectious diseases is seen in **Figure 9-1**, which provides death rates for the population of New York City over the period 1804 to 2017. Epidemics of smallpox and cholera swept through the city every few years, killing many people in each wave. In the mid-19th century, background mortality rates—largely from tuberculosis, typhoid, and miscellaneous respiratory and gastrointestinal diseases—were double what they became by 1930.

These infectious diseases were largely conquered through public health measures, including purification of water, proper disposal of sewage, pasteurization of milk, and immunization, as well as improved nutrition and personal hygiene. The discovery and introduction of antibiotics in the 1940s also played a role. In fact, by the 1960s, the threat of infectious diseases seemed to have been reduced to a minor nuisance.

In contrast to the fear, drama, and excitement that accompanied efforts to understand and control infectious diseases in the late 19th and early 20th centuries, public health in the 1960s and 1970s seemed to have become routine and boring. This period in the history of public health corresponds to the time when, according to the Institute of Medicine, public health was falling into disarray because of complacency.[1] This chapter focuses on the battles that public health practitioners have won. It discusses the causes of infectious diseases, how they are transmitted, and how classic public health measures have brought them under control.

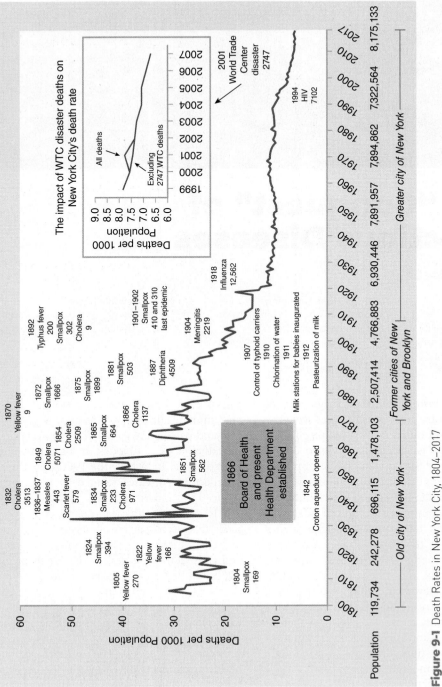

Figure 9-1 Death Rates in New York City, 1804–2017

Infectious Agents

The major epidemic diseases are caused by **bacteria**, **viruses**, or **parasites**. The fact that each of these diseases is caused by a specific microbe was established in the 1880s and 1890s, at a time of great scientific excitement, when almost every year marked a discovery of a new disease-causing bacterium.

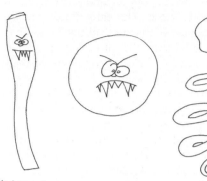

BACILLI   COCCI   SPIROCHETE

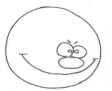

ROUNDWORM   HOOKWORM

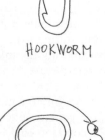

PINWORM   TAPEWORM

Robert Koch, a German physician, developed techniques to classify bacteria by their shape and their propensity to be stained by various dyes. As billions of bacteria—most of them harmless to humans—inhabit the skin, throat, mouth, nose, large intestine, and vagina, scientists needed to develop a set of rules that could be used to prove that a specific organism caused a specific disease. These rules are called "Koch's postulates":

1. The organism must be present in every case of the disease.
2. The organism must be isolated and grown in the laboratory.
3. When injected with the laboratory-grown culture, susceptible test animals must develop the disease.
4. The organism must be isolated from the newly infected animals and the process repeated.[2]

Koch applied these rules in his proof that tubercle bacilli were the cause of tuberculosis, the leading cause of death in Europe at that time. Bacilli are bacteria that appear rod-shaped when observed under the microscope. Koch identified another bacillus, *Vibrio cholera*, as the cause of cholera. Other disease-causing bacilli identified during that period included those that cause plague, typhoid, tetanus, diphtheria, and dysentery.

Round-shaped bacteria, called cocci, include streptococci, which cause strep throat and scarlet fever; staphylococci, which cause wound infections; and pneumococci, which cause pneumonia. Syphilis is caused by a corkscrew-shaped bacterium called a spirochete. All these bacteria were identified by the beginning of the 20th century.

For some infectious diseases, however, no bacterial agent could be found. Smallpox, for example, was known to be transmitted from a sick person to a healthy one by something in the pus of the patient's lesions. Early attempts to isolate a causative microorganism proved unsuccessful. The agent that caused the disease could pass through the finest available filters and could not be observed in any existing microscope. Smallpox was recognized to be one of a number of diseases caused by such "filterable agents" or viruses. It was not until 1935, when the American scientist W. M. Stanley crystallized tobacco mosaic virus, that the true nature of viruses was demonstrated.

Whereas bacteria are living, single-celled organisms that can grow and reproduce outside the body if given the appropriate nutrients, viruses are not complete cells. These complexes of nucleic acid and protein lack the machinery to reproduce themselves. Various kinds of viruses infect not only animal cells but also plant cells—as tobacco mosaic virus infects tobacco—and even bacteria. They can survive extreme conditions such as treatment with alcohol and drying in a vacuum and become active again when they are injected into a living cell. They reproduce themselves by taking control of the cell's machinery, often killing the cell in the process. The human diseases caused by viruses include smallpox, yellow fever, polio, hepatitis, influenza, measles, rabies, and acquired immunodeficiency syndrome (AIDS), as well as the common cold.

Human diseases can also be caused by protozoa, or single-celled animals that can live as parasites in the human body. Malaria, spread by mosquitoes; cryptosporidiosis, which caused the Milwaukee diarrhea epidemic in 1993; and giardiasis, also known as "beaver fever," are examples of protozoal diseases. Other parasites, such as roundworms, tapeworms, hookworms, and pinworms, are the most common source of human infection in the world. Except for pinworms, however, they are not common causes of disease in the United States today.

Means of Transmission

Infectious diseases are spread by a variety of routes, either directly from one person to another or indirectly by way of water, food, or **vectors** such as insects and animals. Bacteria and viruses that cause respiratory infections, including colds, influenza, and tuberculosis, are transmitted through the air on **aerosols**, water droplets produced when an infected person coughs or sneezes. They can also be transmitted from an infected person to objects he or she touches, such as doorknobs, utensils, or towels; from there, they can be picked up by the next person who touches the contaminated object and transferred by hand to the nose. The early European settlers made use of this route of transmission to inflict a primitive form of biological warfare on the Native American people, giving them blankets that had been used by patients suffering from smallpox. The disease decimated Native American populations because they had no immunity to the virus.

Gastrointestinal infections such as cholera, cryptosporidiosis, and diphtheria are generally spread by the fecal–oral route, by which fecal matter from an infected person reaches the mouth of an uninfected person. This may occur as a result of poor personal hygiene or by contamination of drinking water because of inadequate sanitary systems. Vector-borne diseases, including malaria, yellow fever, and West Nile encephalitis, generally use a more complex route from one person to another, most often through an insect.

Each disease has its own pattern of development after a person is infected, and the time during which the patient is capable of transmitting the infection to others varies from one disease to another. Some diseases are most likely to be transmitted during the most symptomatic phase—for example, when a patient suffering from tuberculosis or the common cold is most actively coughing and sneezing. Others, such as measles and mumps, are most communicable during the day or two before noticeable symptoms develop. A few diseases can exist in a **carrier state**, in which the infected person can transmit the disease without having symptoms, as demonstrated by the infamous case of Typhoid Mary.[3]

Mary Mallon worked as a cook in a series of wealthy New York homes at the beginning of the 20th century. After an increasing number of family members in these homes became sick with typhoid fever, some of them fatally, suspicion fell on the cook. Because she was healthy, and because cooking was the only way she knew to support herself, Mary resisted medical tests; when finally proven to be a carrier of the bacteria, she refused to accept the results. Eventually she had to be incarcerated to prevent her from taking jobs where she might spread the disease by the fecal–oral route. She remained in the custody of the New York City Health Department for the rest of her life. It was Mary's occupation, of course, that made her such a threat to the public health. The discovery of antibiotics, which came too late to help Mary, made it possible to eliminate the bacteria in typhoid carriers. Other viruses, such as herpes and hepatitis B, can persist in carrier states, and no treatment is known to eliminate them.

Chain of Infection

Control of infectious diseases remains an important component of public health. The public health approach to controlling infectious diseases is to interrupt the **chain of infection**. Many methods used to accomplish this interruption have now become routine, but vigilance is always required.

The chain of infection, which comprises the pattern by which an infectious disease is transmitted from person to person, is composed of several links (**Figure 9-2**):

1. **Pathogen**. The pathogen is a virus, bacterium, or parasite that causes the disease in humans.
2. **Reservoir**. The reservoir is a place where the pathogen lives and multiplies. Some pathogens spread directly from one human to another and have no other reservoir. Others may infect nonhuman species, spreading from them to humans only occasionally. Plague, for example, is a disease of rodents that is transmitted to

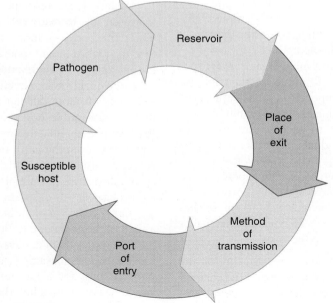

Figure 9-2 Chain of Infection

humans by the bite of a flea. Rats are the reservoir of plague. Raccoons and bats are reservoirs for rabies, which spreads to humans only through the bite of a rabid animal. Contaminated water or food may also serve as reservoirs for some human diseases.

3. **Method of transmission**. The pathogen must have a way to travel from one host to another, or from a reservoir to a new host. The flea is a vector for plague, transferring the plague bacillus from rat to human by sucking it up when it bites the rat and then injecting it into a human host with a second bite. Food-borne diseases are transmitted when a person eats contaminated food; water-borne diseases are transmitted when someone drinks contaminated water. Many respiratory diseases are transmitted by aerosols. AIDS, syphilis, gonorrhea, and a number of other diseases are transmitted by sexual contact.

4. **Susceptible host**. Even if the pathogen gains entry, a new potential host may not be susceptible because that host has immunity to the pathogen. Immunity may develop as a result of previous exposure to the pathogen, or the host may naturally lack susceptibility for a variety of reasons. Most microorganisms are specifically adapted to infect certain species. Canine distemper virus, for example, does not infect humans. Even within species, susceptibility to specific viruses varies among individuals. Scientists have been puzzled about why a very few people who have been repeatedly exposed to the human immunodeficiency virus (HIV) do not become infected; recent studies have found a genetic mutation that makes them resistant to the virus.

Public health measures to control the spread of disease aim to interrupt the chain of infection at whichever links are most vulnerable. At link 1, the pathogen could be killed, for example, by using an antibiotic to destroy the disease-causing bacteria. At link 2, one could eliminate a reservoir that harbors the pathogen. For example, controlling rat populations in cities by picking up garbage is a way of preventing the spread of plague to humans. Adequate water and sewage treatment prevents the spread of water-borne diseases, and proper food-handling methods eliminate reservoirs of food-borne pathogens.

At link 3, transmission from one host to another could be prevented by quarantining infected individuals, for example, or by warning people to boil their water if the water supply becomes contaminated. Hand washing is an important way to prevent the spread of disease: It prevents restaurant workers from contaminating food, prevents hospital workers from carrying pathogens from one patient to another, and allows all individuals to protect themselves against pathogens they may pick up from the environment and put in their mouth. The spread of sexually transmitted diseases can be prevented by use of a condom, which blocks the movement of the pathogens to the uninfected person.

At link 4, the resistance of hosts can be increased by **immunization**, which stimulates the body's immune system to recognize the pathogen and to attack it during any future exposure. **Vaccination** not only keeps the individual from contracting a disease, but also makes it more difficult for the pathogen to find susceptible hosts. In some cases, it may even be possible to completely eliminate a pathogen from the Earth by eliminating the susceptibility of its potential hosts. This was accomplished in the case of smallpox, as discussed later in this chapter.

Other links are often included separately as part of the chain of infection when it is useful to consider them as sites for public health intervention. For example, the port of entry into the host for a mosquito-borne disease would be the skin—a link that could be interrupted if the potential host wears long sleeves and gloves. Similarly, the place of exit is the route by which the pathogen leaves the host.

Public health measures to control the spread of infectious disease include both routine prevention measures and emergency measures to control an outbreak once it has begun. Many of the measures mentioned earlier—especially those concerning links 2 and 3—belong to the category of "environmental health." Immunization (link 4) is a major weapon that has had great success against the dread diseases that created the epidemics of the past. However, vaccines do not exist for all diseases: Notably, a vaccine against AIDS has not yet been developed. Even when vaccines do exist, some diseases are too rare to justify the trouble and expense of vaccinating everyone. In such cases, surveillance becomes especially important.

Epidemiologic surveillance is the system by which public health practitioners watch for disease threats so that they may step in and break the chain of infection, halting the spread of disease. In the early history of public health, the solution was often **quarantine**—isolation of the patient to prevent him or her from infecting others. Quarantine is still used occasionally, when the disease is serious and no effective vaccine is available. For example, a patient diagnosed with tuberculosis—which is slow to respond to medication—might be ordered to stay home for 2 to 4 weeks after treatment starts until the disease is no longer infectious.

More often, the public health response when an outbreak is detected by surveillance is to locate people who have had contact with the infected individual and to immunize them or give them medical treatment, as appropriate. For tuberculosis, **contact tracing** is used in addition to quarantine: People who have been exposed to the patient are given prophylactic doses of antibiotics. Tuberculosis has presented new and more difficult problems to the public health system in recent years because of the development of drug-resistant strains of the causative bacteria.

Contact tracing is also routinely used for controlling sexually transmitted diseases, such as syphilis and gonorrhea. Syphilis, which tends to affect the poor, the homeless, drug users, and prostitutes, can be diagnosed by a blood test. Because it has few symptoms in the early stages, it may go untreated and is easily spread. The challenge for public health is to identify those persons with the disease through screening programs carried out, for example, in a city jail. Once a case is identified, public health workers try to discreetly alert those who have been exposed. The public health worker asks the person who has been diagnosed to identify sexual contacts; the worker then notifies the contacts that they have been exposed without identifying the source of the exposure. Syphilis is readily cured by penicillin. If untreated, it may cause long-term damage to the heart and brain; congenital syphilis in infants born to infected mothers can be lethal.

The classic public health measures of surveillance and quarantine were key components in combating severe acute respiratory syndrome (SARS), a highly infectious new disease that first emerged in southern China in November 2002. Because China did not at first report the disease, it was not recognized as a major threat until March 2003, when the World Health Organization (WHO) issued a global alert and a travel advisory. WHO had been alerted by Dr. Carlo Urbani, an infectious disease specialist working in Vietnam, who noticed that a patient who had recently arrived in Saigon from Hong Kong was suffering from an atypical form of pneumonia. Dr. Urbani himself soon contracted the disease and died. Epidemiologic detective work found that the patient in Saigon, as well as patients soon identified in Toronto and Singapore, had all stayed in the same hotel in Hong Kong where a traveler from southern China had spent one night before falling ill with the syndrome. More than a dozen guests at the hotel had been infected by that one traveler, and they carried the disease to several other countries.[4]

By July 5, 2003, when WHO declared that SARS had been contained, the disease had infected 8439 people in 30 countries and had killed 812 people.[5] Although a virus was identified, lab tests could not diagnose the disease until weeks after a patient had developed symptoms. No drug has been found effective against the virus; instead, treatment requires intensive respiratory therapy during extended hospital stays. SARS was contained by old-fashioned measures: quickly isolating patients who were suspected to have the disease—because of fever, cough, and previous contact with a known SARS patient—and quarantining anyone who had come in contact with them. The epidemic had severe economic impact wherever it broke out, keeping business and vacation travelers from affected areas and even scaring away visitors from Chinatowns in American cities.

Public health officials voiced concerns that the disease might be seasonal and break out again in 2004, but this did not occur. A few small outbreaks in 2004 stemmed from inadequate safety measures in research laboratories, but alert health workers kept the disease from spreading. Since 2004, no known cases of SARS have occurred anywhere in the world.[6] However, in late 2019, a related virus, called SARS-CoV-2, emerged, also in China. It spread rapidly around the world, causing a pandemic. The disease is similarly being fought by traditional public health measures.

Rabies

Rabies, a fatal disease of the nervous system caused by a virus, kills an estimated 59,000 people around the world each year. This infection is usually contracted through a dog bite. In the United States, transmission of the disease to humans is very effectively prevented by routine public health measures. Although there is an effective human vaccine against rabies, routine immunization of everyone is not recommended. Human exposure to the rabies virus in the United States is relatively rare, and the vaccine is expensive and inconvenient to deliver, requiring several injections over a period of approximately a month.

The rabies virus infects only mammals, and it is almost always transmitted when a rabid animal bites another animal or a human. Since the animal most likely to bite a human is the dog, mandatory immunization of dogs against rabies is the first line of defense in the protection of people. Wild animals serve as the reservoir of rabies, and dogs are most likely to be exposed by being bitten by a rabid wild animal. Domestic cats are also at risk for exposure to rabies from wildlife, and immunization is recommended for them as well.

The public health system has defined clear guidelines for responding to a report of a person's being bitten by a domestic or wild animal, depending on the likelihood that the animal is rabid. Because immunization of dogs is widespread in the United States, fewer than 100 cases of rabies occur annually in the 60 million dogs in this country, and a dog bite is considered unlikely to transmit the disease. If the biting dog (or cat) appears to be healthy, it need only be observed for 10 days to ensure that it remains healthy. Rabies virus affects the brain; from there, it travels to the salivary glands and is secreted in saliva. An animal capable of transmitting the virus in its saliva will already have brain involvement, exhibit symptoms, and be dead within a few days. That is sufficient time for the bitten person to be given the series of vaccinations that will protect him or her from the disease.

If the biting animal is wild, or if there is other reason to suspect that it is rabid, it must be killed and its brain tested for signs of rabies virus infection. There is no way to determine definitively whether a living animal has rabies. If the test shows the animal to be rabid, the bite victim receives the vaccinations. If no sign of rabies is found, no vaccinations are given. There is no room for error in these tests: Once symptoms of rabies appear, it is too late to save the victim. Public health laboratories take this responsibility very seriously. Generally, immunizations are given to anyone who is bitten by a wild animal that cannot be captured and tested.

To control rabies, public health practitioners conduct surveillance for rabies in wildlife. When raccoons, skunks, and foxes in a geographic area are infected with the virus, they are likely to pose a threat to humans and domestic animals. In Europe and in some parts of the United States, public health officials are attempting to control rabies in wildlife by distributing bait containing an oral rabies vaccine. Unfortunately, scientists have not yet figured out how to vaccinate bats in this way.

Bats are the most dangerous rabies threat to humans. Even in parts of the United States where the disease is not endemic among most wildlife, rabid bats are likely to be found. Because these animals are nocturnal and elusive, contact with bats may go unnoticed. During 2017, state and regional public health departments in the United States reported 4454 rabid animals to the Centers for Disease Control and Prevention (CDC). Nearly all were wildlife: 32% were bats, 29% were racoons, and 21% were skunks, while 6% were cats and 1% each were dogs and cows. Four human rabies fatalities occurred in 2017 and 2018: a 65-year-old Virginia woman who contracted rabies from a dog while traveling in India; a 56-year-old Florida woman who was bitten by a rabid bat; a 6-year-old boy who was also bitten by a bat; and a 69-year-old Delaware woman who lived in an area where rabid racoons had been found.[7]

The rabies surveillance system has been remarkably successful. The cost of rabies control is significant, however. Testing the brain of an animal for rabies costs about $100, and a series of vaccinations for a person suspected of being exposed may cost as much as $1500. In 1994, after a kitten in a New Hampshire pet store tested positive for rabies, 665 people received post-exposure treatment at a cost of more than $1 million for the vaccines alone.[8] In 2008, a rabid puppy was among a group of 24 dogs and 2 cats that were brought to the United States in a rescue mission aimed at reuniting American soldiers with pets they had adopted in Iraq. By the time the puppy was diagnosed, the animals had been dispersed to 16 states around the country. Concerned that the puppy might have bitten other animals in the group, federal and state public health workers tracked them all down,

vaccinated them, and placed them in quarantine for 6 months.[9] As a result of this incident, the CDC issued new regulations on the importation of animals to the United States.[10]

Smallpox and Polio

While constant vigilance is required to protect people from rabies because wild animals serve as a reservoir of the disease, some pathogenic viruses, including measles and polio, have no nonhuman reservoir. Universal immunization against these diseases, therefore, might potentially eliminate the measles and polio viruses from the Earth. This has been achieved with smallpox, one of public health's greatest victories.

Smallpox

Smallpox was a particularly feared disease that is believed to have first emerged in Asia about the time of Christ and tended to spread in major epidemics that claimed millions of lives in China, Japan, the Roman Empire, Europe, and the Americas.[2] It was highly contagious, spread by aerosol or by touch. The concept of vaccination originated with smallpox: The observation that survivors of the disease were immune to future infection inspired the idea that people could be protected against serious illness by inoculating them with small amounts of infected matter from a person suffering a mild case. While the procedure was not entirely safe, the practice became widespread in the American colonies, and George Washington ordered his entire army to be inoculated. In 1796, the practice of immunization became less risky when the British physician Edward Jenner—inspired by the observation that milkmaids appeared to be immune to smallpox—proved that inoculation with cowpox matter, which was harmless to humans, provided immunity against smallpox.[11]

By 1958, routine immunization had eliminated smallpox in the United States and other industrialized countries. However, the disease remained widespread in 33 underdeveloped countries, killing 2 million people per year. With support from both the United States and the Soviet Union, WHO developed plans for a program to eliminate smallpox. Between 1967 and 1977, medical teams traveled all over the world in search of outbreaks of the disease. Local governments were mobilized to vaccinate residents of areas where an outbreak was occurring. Because the lesions of smallpox were so conspicuous, the investigators could track outbreaks by showing pictures of victims and asking people if they knew of anyone with this disease. Once a patient was located, he or she could be quarantined and everyone in the vicinity vaccinated, sometimes by force. The last case was found in Somalia in October 1977.[2]

Today, the smallpox virus officially remains in only two places, stored in laboratories at the CDC and in a Russian laboratory in Siberia. By international agreement, genetic studies were conducted, after which both stocks of the virus were scheduled to be destroyed in 1999. The decision to destroy the virus was controversial, with some scientists believing that valuable information might be gained in future studies using techniques that were not yet known. In 1999, WHO decided to defer the destruction for a few more years.[12]

Meanwhile, word began leaking out of the former Soviet Union that the Soviets had been working on smallpox as a bioweapon. Fears arose that they had shared their stocks of the virus with rogue states such as Iraq and North Korea. The anthrax attacks of 2001 further raised fears about bioterrorism. Plans for destruction of the smallpox virus were put on hold, and research priorities have focused on developing an improved vaccine and finding drugs that would be effective against the virus.

As of 2019, the debate over smallpox virus destruction was still ongoing. Some scientists believe that valuable lessons remain to be learned by studying the virus. Others agree with D. A. Henderson, leader of the WHO's eradication effort, who says, "Let's destroy the virus and be done with it. . . . We would be better off spending our money in better ways." One concern is that the molecular sequence of the virus is publicly known, meaning that, even if all smallpox viruses are eliminated, someone could synthesize it in a laboratory and loose it on the world. In fact, in 2017, Canadian scientists were able to reconstruct the extinct horsepox virus using genetic material ordered through the mail. The same process could be used to reconstruct the smallpox virus regardless of whether the last known stocks have been destroyed, perhaps making the question of whether to destroy remaining smallpox stocks moot.[13]

Polio

Poliovirus, like smallpox virus, infects human beings only, and polio similarly has the potential to be eradicated. In 1988, at a time when 350,000 children were being paralyzed each year, WHO set a goal of eradicating polio by the year 2000.[14] This goal was not met, but substantial progress has been made against this crippling disease: Polio has been essentially eliminated from the Western Hemisphere, Europe, Southeast Asia, and the Western Pacific, and by 1999, annual polio cases were reduced by 99% worldwide.[15]

Only two countries continue to have endemic polio—Afghanistan and Pakistan—and only 33 cases were identified in these countries in 2018. Eradication is near at hand but has proved extremely difficult to achieve. In 2003, rumors spread among Muslims, especially in Nigeria, that the polio vaccine had been deliberately contaminated to cause AIDS or infertility. Several Nigerian states halted vaccinations, the number of cases in Nigeria jumped to 800 in 2004, and the virus spread to several other African countries that had previously been polio free. Under pressure from WHO, Nigeria resumed polio immunizations the following year.[14] Much of the remaining endemic areas are extremely remote, making them hard to reach by technicians attempting to immunize children. In Afghanistan, immunization programs have also faced state bans on house-to-house campaigns. Nevertheless, complete eradication may be achieved within the next few years, with progress on this front being led by a joint collaboration of WHO, the Bill and Melinda Gates Foundation, CDC, the United Nations, and several other groups.[16]

Polio is proving more difficult to eradicate than smallpox for several reasons.[17] Unlike with smallpox, many "invisible" cases of polio occur, in which children may be infected and able to spread the virus by the fecal–oral route, yet not show any symptoms. Thus it is not possible to focus on small outbreaks as targets for polio eradication, as was done with smallpox. In addition, the polio vaccine is imperfect and must be administered several times to become effective. Furthermore, political upheaval has interfered with immunization campaigns in some countries. In Pakistan and Nigeria, for example, polio vaccinators have been killed by Islamic extremists.

Backsliding: Measles and Malaria

Measles, another viral disease that could in theory be eradicated, offers an example of what happens when public health relaxes its vigilance. Before a vaccine became available, almost all children contracted measles, with this disease causing 400 to 500 deaths per year in the United States and 4000 cases of chronic disability from measles encephalitis annually.[18] After a vaccine became available in 1963, the number of cases in the United States dropped precipitously. **Figure 9-3** shows this drop, illustrating the seemingly miraculous power

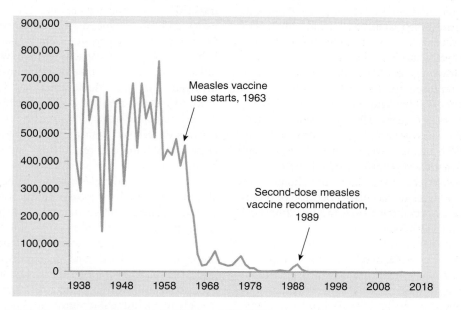

Figure 9-3 Measles Cases in the United States, 1938–2018

1938-1943: Data from U.S. Census Bureau, "Statistical Abstract of the United States 1944-45," https://www.census.gov/library/publications/1945/compendia/statab/66ed.html, accessed September 3, 2019.

1944-1993: Data from Centers for Disease Control and Prevention, *Morbidity and Mortality Weekly Report* Annual Supplement Summary 1993 Vol. 42, No. 53.

1994-1999: Data from Centers for Disease Control and Prevention, *Morbidity and Mortality Weekly Report* 48 no. 53 (2001), https://www.cdc.gov/mmwr/preview/mmwrhtml/mm4853a1.htm, accessed September 3, 2019.

2000-2005: Data from Centers for Disease Control and Prevention, *Morbidity and Mortality Weekly Report* 54 no. 53 (2005), https://www.cdc.gov/mmwr/preview/mmwrhtml/mm5453a1.htm, accessed September 3, 2019.

2006-2010: Data from Centers for Disease Control and Prevention, *Morbidity and Mortality Weekly Report* 59 no. 53 (2010), https://www.cdc.gov/mmwr/preview/mmwrhtml/mm5953a1.htm, accessed September 3, 2019.

2011-2012: Data from Centers for Disease Control and Prevention, *Morbidity and Mortality Weekly Report* 61 no. 53 (2012), https://www.cdc.gov/mmwr/preview/mmwrhtml/mm6153a1.htm, accessed September 3, 2019.

2013-2017: Data from Centers for Disease Control and Prevention, *Nationally Notifiable Diseases: Infectious Weekly Tables 2018*, accessed September 3, 2019.

2018: Data from Centers for Disease Control and Prevention, "Weekly cases of notifiable diseases, United States, U.S. territories, and Non-U.S. Residents weeks ending August 24, 2019," Table 1, https://stacks.cdc.gov/view/cdc/80997, accessed September 3, 2019.

of vaccines over certain diseases. In 1978, the U.S. Department of Health and Human Services set a goal to eradicate measles from the United States by 1982. Even though humans are the only reservoir for measles and measles does not exist in a carrier state,[19] that ambition proved overly optimistic.

One problem was that outbreaks of measles began to occur among high school and college students who had been vaccinated as babies. It became clear that the immunity conferred by vaccination in infancy wears off and that a booster vaccination is necessary in older children—a practice that is now recommended at the age of 4 to 6. The booster should be given to adolescents if they did not receive it earlier. Implementation of the new recommendations was widespread in the 1990s, and measles cases in the United States declined to low levels. In fact, measles was declared eliminated from the United States in 2000, meaning that all cases could be traced to individuals who contracted the disease outside the country and brought it here.[18]

However, in 2011, 222 measles cases were reported to the CDC, compared to a median of 60 per year during 2001 to 2010.[20] Of those 222 cases, 196 were American residents, the majority of whom were children, and 86% of them were unvaccinated or had unknown vaccination status. Of the 66 children who were unvaccinated but should have been, 50 were unvaccinated because of philosophical or religious beliefs (a topic discussed later in this chapter).

The year 2014 proved to be a bad year for measles. A total of 644 cases were reported from 27 states, with more than half of them occurring among unvaccinated Amish children in Ohio.[21] Then in December, a large outbreak began in California that spread across the country.[22] The first reported case was an 11-year-old girl who had visited a Disney theme park in southern California during the exposure period and was hospitalized; she had not been vaccinated. The source of the exposure has not been identified, but the strain of the virus was the same as one that had recently caused a large outbreak in the Philippines and has also been detected in other countries. Disney theme parks attract many international visitors, one of whom presumably carried the virus to California in 2014. After the outbreak, California changed the law to remove the religious exemption from the vaccination requirement, leading to an increase in the vaccination rate from 90% to 96%, and allowing many more communities to reach herd immunity status.[23]

One of the largest recent measles outbreaks in the United States began in October 2018 within a community of Orthodox Jews in the village of New Square, just north of New York City. Patient Zero, the originator of the outbreak, was a 14-year-old boy who had acquired measles recently in Israel (he had, in turn, acquired it from an Israeli who had traveled to Ukraine, where measles is rampant), and then attended a holiday service at the community synagogue. The synagogue had a 7000-person capacity, which was in full use that particular day. This circumstance involved a case of bad luck rather than a resistance to vaccines: Patient Zero had happened to be home sick from school on the day his classmates received their measles vaccine; his twin brother and the rest of his family had been vaccinated.

Patient Zero's measles case was recognized almost immediately by local public health officials, though not before transmission to others at the synagogue could be prevented. The New York State epidemiologist assigned to the case, Robert McDonald, teamed up with a local rabbi, Yitzchok Sternberg, to conduct the painstaking work of contact tracing: They quickly mapped the interior of the synagogue, and identified who had attended services that day, where everyone sat, who interacted with whom, and which paths and through which doors in the building they walked. To identify susceptible hosts, the team worked to contact those who might have been exposed and determine their vaccination status.

Over the following week, two additional community members returning from Israel presented with measles, and the first domestic transmission occurred. Six additional cases from the synagogue exposure also appeared.[23] In total, 654 measles cases occurred in New York City and 414 occurred in other parts of New York State, largely within the Orthodox Jewish community in the area of New Square.[24]

Public health leaders had hoped that when and if polio is eradicated, the organizational and medical resources that had been mobilized in that campaign could then be used in a vaccination campaign against measles. Given the uncertainties with polio eradication and the difficulties with achieving universal immunization in the United States, the prospect for measles eradication worldwide appears doubtful. Measles is still endemic in some European countries and is present at higher levels in Africa and Southeast Asia. Nevertheless, progress has clearly been made: The number of estimated deaths from measles was reduced from 562,000 in 2000 to 110,000 in 2017.[24]

An attempt to eradicate an eradicable disease can backfire if it is not conducted with sufficient political will, knowledge, and resources. This was the case with malaria, which was the target of an international eradication campaign in the 1950s and 1960s. There is no nonhuman reservoir for the malaria-causing parasites, and the route of transmission is a vector, a certain species of mosquito. The primary weapon in the eradication effort was the pesticide DDT, which was widely applied in an effort to kill the mosquitoes. Although the campaign produced dramatic results, funding ran out before the ultimate objective was achieved, and the disease's resurgence had a greater impact than ever. A combination of factors contributed to the calamity: DDT-resistant mosquitoes emerged; the pathogen developed resistance to the main antimalarial drug, chloroquine; and populations in former malarial areas lost their immunity to the disease because of lack of exposure.[25] Today, malaria remains one of the most widespread potentially fatal infectious diseases in the world, killing an estimated 1 million people annually, mainly children.[26] The disease occurs mainly in tropical and subtropical areas and has been largely eliminated in the United States, but global climate change and international travel could contribute to the reemergence of malaria as a public health problem in the South.

Fear of Vaccines

The benefits of vaccination are obvious to public health and medical professionals. However, just as Muslim leaders in Nigeria resisted polio vaccination owing its rumored link with infertility, so suspicion has spread in the United States that measles immunization causes autism. Autism often becomes apparent at about the age when the vaccine is given. Consequently, some parents refused to allow their children to be vaccinated against measles. Similarly, unfounded stories about side effects of the pertussis (whooping cough) vaccine—that it might cause sudden infant death syndrome (SIDS)—led many parents to resist that vaccine.[27]

Suspicions about the safety of vaccines were exacerbated by the actions of British surgeon Andrew Wakefield, who in 1998 published a fraudulent paper claiming that the measles/mumps/rubella (MMR) vaccine was linked to the onset of autism. Wakefield's paper was published in a highly regarded journal, *The Lancet*. Many other scientists doubted the claims, however, and a thorough investigation eventually found that Wakefield was guilty of misconduct. He had misrepresented the facts about the children he claimed to have studied and had cooked up a scheme to profit by filing lawsuits against the drug companies that manufactured the vaccine.[28] *The Lancet* retracted the paper in 2010, stating that the journal had been deceived. Wakefield's medical license was withdrawn and he was barred from practicing medicine in the United Kingdom.

Because parental concerns became so widespread, the Institute of Medicine has conducted periodic reviews of the latest evidence on vaccine safety. In 2003, it published a review on SIDS and concluded that "the evidence favors rejection of a relationship between some vaccines and SIDS."[29] In 2004, the Institute of Medicine reviewed evidence on a possible link between the vaccine and autism; again, it concluded that "the body of epidemiological evidence favors rejection of a causal relationship between the MMR vaccine and autism."[30] In both cases, the review committees acknowledged that the concern about the vaccines was understandable because the diseases are poorly understood, and they recommended more research on the causes of SIDS and autism.

The evidence cited in the autism report included a major study done in Denmark, in which records of a half million children were analyzed. About one in five children had not received the vaccine, and the researchers found that these children developed autism at the same rate as children who had been vaccinated.[31] Some vaccines do have real risks, including fever and seizures that occur in a small number of infants after they are vaccinated for pertussis and rare cases of polio caused by the oral polio vaccine, which contains the live, weakened virus. These risks are much smaller than the risks of the diseases in an unvaccinated population. However, many American parents are too young to remember the fears aroused by polio in the past, and they may be unaware that formerly common childhood diseases such as measles and chickenpox sometimes have serious complications. Whooping cough, for example, can be fatal in infants exposed to unvaccinated older siblings who contract the disease. Because of the success of vaccinations, people have never seen these diseases and, therefore, no longer fear them.

All states have laws requiring that children be immunized before starting school, but there are always exemptions for children with medical conditions that make immunization harmful to them. Some states also have exemptions for religious reasons or "personal belief exemptions."

The measles outbreaks in 2011, 2014, and 2018–2019 illustrate the dangers of leaving children unvaccinated. In these outbreaks, most of the cases were linked to people who had traveled abroad or visited from another country and spread the virus to unvaccinated children in this country. It is often in wealthy communities that parents refuse to subject their children to the small risk of immunization. They count on the fact that most other children are vaccinated to protect their own children from being exposed. For example, the Garden of Angels private school in the wealthy area of Santa Monica has a lower vaccination rate compared to other parts of California. The school's website states, "Our Garden Ideology aspires to accurately mirror an environment where students are limited by nothing and liberated by everything." In response, the *New Yorker* reporter Nick Paumgarten sarcastically remarked, "Nothing says 'liberation' like pertussis."[23] Indeed, much of the protection afforded by a high rate of immunization in a population comes from **herd immunity**, the phenomenon by which even infants too young to be vaccinated and people with weakened immune systems for various reasons, as well as those who refuse to be immunized, are unlikely to be exposed to a disease because the majority of the population is immune. If the percentage of immunity in the population falls too low, however, outbreaks are likely. In such a case, even vaccinated people are at risk, because no vaccine is perfect.

In Orange County, California, where Disneyland is located, some private schools have immunization rates as low as 60%. Parents of children with cancer and other conditions that preclude vaccination are becoming increasingly angry at the risk their children are being exposed to as a result of other parents' refusal to vaccinate their children.[32] Fortunately, according to a 2016 Pew Research Center survey, the vast majority of Americans (82%) support requiring the measles vaccine for healthy schoolchildren, and 88% believe the vaccine's benefits outweigh the risks. Perhaps unsurprisingly, the survey also found a strong relationship between vaccine support and science knowledge: 55% of those with limited science knowledge believed in the vaccine's benefits, while 91% with high science knowledge recognized the benefits.[33] The news about the Disneyland measles outbreak led California to put an end to the personal belief exemption in 2015.[33] Similarly, the 2018–2019 New York outbreak led the state to revoke all nonmedical exemptions from the vaccine requirement to attend schools and childcare centers: Starting with the 2019–2020 school year, all New York State children without a medical contraindication must be vaccinated or else be homeschooled or move out of state.[34]

Another drawback of people's fear of vaccines is that pharmaceutical companies have become reluctant to invest in developing them. Parents' tendency to blame a recent immunization for any serious health problem suffered by their children often prompts them to sue the company that made the vaccine. This experience, together with the fact that prices charged for vaccines tend to be low, has caused many companies to end their vaccine production altogether. While immunization is considered the most effective intervention for preventing disease and promoting health, it is not clear that even the current vaccines will continue to be available. The example of the former Soviet Union offers a stark warning for what can happen in this situation: Diphtheria is virtually unknown in the West now, but in the 1980s, when the public health system in Russia was in chaos and immunizations stopped, the disease surged, leading to 200,000 cases and 5000 deaths there.[35]

It has been suggested that anti-vaccination sentiment is a social media phenomenon, spread through rumors and false news stories on Facebook and other platforms. However, as the Amish and Orthodox Jewish outbreaks show, it is really a broader social network phenomenon. In the Amish community, the use of electronics is almost nonexistent; in the Orthodox Jewish community, women are discouraged from using computers and smartphones. In these circumstances, anti-vaccination sentiment primarily spreads the old-fashioned way, by word of mouth.[23]

Public health in the United States can celebrate success in the fight against many common diseases. In 2016, data from the CDC showed that age-adjusted death rates for many infectious diseases were at all-time lows. For example, influenza and pneumonia (for which vaccines are available) killed only about half as many Americans in 2016 compared to 2000, and only about one-fourth as many as in 1960: the death rate from HIV (for which a vaccine is not available) has fallen by more than 80% since its peak around 1990; and the rates of new hepatitis, diphtheria, rubella, and tuberculosis cases were at or near all-time lows. In contrast, measles has beaten back eradication efforts even in rich countries like the United States, and rates of new syphilis and chlamydia cases have more than doubled over the last 20 years.[36] Meanwhile, the devastating disease caused by poliovirus persists in a number of poorer countries. So, while great gains have been made, infectious diseases are far from being conquered.

Conclusion

Public health has had great success in controlling infectious diseases. Classic public health measures prevent transmission of disease-causing bacteria, viruses, and parasites by interrupting the chain of infection. Measures employed at various links in the chain include killing the pathogen, eliminating the reservoir that harbors the pathogen, preventing transmission from one host to another or from the reservoir to hosts, and increasing the resistance of hosts by immunization.

Rabies is an example of a disease that has been successfully controlled in the United States by public health measures. Immunization of dogs is the primary barrier protecting humans from the reservoir of the virus, which is wild animals. By maintaining surveillance and intervening with vaccination when a person has been exposed to a possibly rabid animal, public health has kept the number of human deaths from rabies very low. SARS, a new, highly communicable disease first recognized in Asia in 2003, was successfully controlled by the classic public health measures of surveillance, isolation, and quarantine.

Smallpox, measles, and polio are viral diseases against which effective vaccines have been developed and that have no nonhuman reservoir. In theory, they could be eliminated from the Earth. This goal has been accomplished with smallpox, with only two known stocks of the virus remaining. Polio has been eliminated from the United States and many other parts of the world, and a campaign is under way to eradicate it, although progress has been erratic and some experts doubt that the goal is realistic. The prospects for measles eradication are less clear. The United States has experienced periodic epidemics of measles, including one in 2014–2015, when infected people entered the country from endemic areas. Reluctance by some parents to vaccinate their children weakens herd immunity and threatens to cause outbreaks of infectious diseases that could have otherwise been controlled.

Success in controlling infectious diseases requires adequate resources and political will to maintain effective immunization programs and ongoing epidemiologic surveillance.

References

1. Institute of Medicine, Committee for the Study of the Future of Public Health, *The Future of Public Health* (Washington, DC: National Academy Press, 1988), 19.

2. L. Garrett, *The Coming Plague: Newly Emerging Diseases in a World out of Balance* (New York: Farrar, Straus & Giroux, 1994), 403.

3. G. Pickett and J. J. Hanlon, *Public Health: Administration and Practice* (St. Louis, MO: Times Mirror/Mosby, 1990).

4. J. M. Hughes, "The SARS Response: Building and Assessing an Evidence-Based Approach to Future Global Microbial Threats," *Journal of the American Medical Association* 290 (2003): 3251–3253.

5. K. Bradsher, "SARS Declared Contained, with No Cases in Past 20 Days," *The New York Times*, July 6, 2003.

6. Centers for Disease Control and Prevention, "Severe Acute Respiratory Syndrome (SARS)," www.cdc.gov/sars/index.html, accessed September 9, 2019.

7. X. Ma, B. P. Monroe, J. M. Cleaton, L. A. Orciari, Y. Li, J. D. Kirby, et al., "Rabies Surveillance in the United States During 2017," *Journal of the American Veterinary Medical Association* 253 (2018): 1555–1568.

8. D. L. Noah, M. G. Smith, J. C. Gotthardt, J. W. Krebs, D. Green, and J. E. Childs, "Mass Human Exposure to Rabies in New Hampshire: Exposures, Treatment, and Cost," *American Journal of Public Health* 86 (1996): 1149–1151.

9. Centers for Disease Control and Prevention, "Rabies in a Dog Imported from Iraq—New Jersey, June 2008," *Morbidity and Mortality Weekly Report* 57 (2008): 1076–1078.

10. Centers for Disease Control and Prevention, "Importation," www.cdc.gov/importation/index.html, accessed September 9, 2019.

11. G. Rosen, *A History of Public Health* (Baltimore, MD: Johns Hopkins University Press, 1993).

12. L. Altman, "Killer Smallpox Gets a New Lease on Life," *The New York Times*, May 25, 1999.

13. K. Kupferschmidt, "How Canadian Researchers Reconstituted an Extinct Poxvirus for $100,000 Using Mail-Order DNA," *Science*, July 6, 2017.

14. L. Roberts, "Polio Eradication: Is It Time to Give Up?" *Science* 312 (2006): 832–835.

15. Centers for Disease Control and Prevention, "CDC's Work to Eradicate Polio," September 2014, www.cdc.gov/polio/pdf/cdcs-work-to-eradicate-polio_508.pdf, accessed September 9, 2019.

16. World Health Organization, Polio Global Eradication Initiative, "Polio Endgame Strategy 2019–2023: Eradication, Integration, Certification and Containment," 2019.

17. I. Arita, M. Nakane, and F. Fenner, "Is Polio Eradication Realistic?" *Science* 312 (2006): 852–854.

18. Centers for Disease Control and Prevention, "Measles History," February 5, 2018, www.cdc.gov/measles /about/history.html, accessed September 9, 2019.

19. Centers for Disease Control and Prevention, "Measles," in *Epidemiology and Prevention of Vaccine-Preventable Diseases*, 13th ed., www.cdc.gov /vaccines/pubs/pinkbook/downloads/meas.pdf, accessed September 4, 2019.

20. Centers for Disease Control and Prevention, "Measles—United States, 2011," *Morbidity and Mortality Weekly Report* 61 (2012): 253–257.

21. Centers for Disease Control and Prevention, "Measles Cases and Outbreaks," www.cdc.gov/measles/cases -outbreaks.html, accessed September 9, 2019.

22. J. Zipprich, K. Winter, J. Hacker, D. Xia, J. Watt, K. Harriman et al., "Measles Outbreak—California, December 2014–February 2015," *Morbidity and Mortality Weekly Report* 64 (2015): 153–154.

23. Nick Paumgarten, "The Message of Measles," *The New Yorker*, August 26, 2019.

24. World Health Organization, "New Measles Surveillance Data for 2019," www.who.int/immunization/newsroom /measles-data-2019/en/, accessed September 2, 2019.

25. Centers for Disease Control and Prevention, "The History of Malaria, an Ancient Disease," November 9, 2012, www.cdc.gov/malaria/about/history/index. html, accessed September 9, 2019

26. Centers for Disease Control and Prevention, "Malaria's Impact Worldwide," www.cdc.gov/malaria /malaria_worldwide/impact.html, accessed September 9, 2019.

27. E. W. Campion, "Suspicions About the Safety of Vaccines," *New England Journal of Medicine* 347 (2002): 1474–1475.

28. F. Godlee, J. Smith, and H. Marcovitch, "Wakefield's Article Linking MMR Vaccine and Autism Was Fraudulent," *British Medical Journal* 342 (2011): c7136.

29. Institute of Medicine, Immunization Safety Review Committee, *Vaccinations and Sudden Unexpected Death in Infancy* (Washington, DC: National Academies Press, 2003).

30. Institute of Medicine, Immunization Safety Review Committee, *Vaccines and Autism* (Washington, DC: National Academies Press, 2004).

31. K. M. Madsen, A. Hviid, M. Vestergaard, D. Schendel, J. Wohlfahrt, P. Thorsen, et al., "A Population-Based Study of Measles, Mumps, and Rubella Vaccination and Autism," *New England Journal of Medicine* 347 (2002): 1477–1482.

32. J. M. Sharfstein, "Of Mouse and Measles," *Journal of the American Medical Association* 313 (2015): 1504–1505.

33. Pew Research Center, "Vast Majority of Americans Say Benefits of Childhood Vaccines Outweigh Risks," February 2, 2017.

34. S. Otterman, "Get Vaccinated or Leave School: 26,000 New York Children Face a Choice," *The New York Times*, September 3, 2019.

35. R. Rappuoli, H. I. Miller, and S. Falkow, "The Intangible Value of Vaccination," *Science* 297 (2002): 937–939.

36. Centers for Disease Control and Prevention, National Center for Health Statistics, "Health, United States, 2017—Data Finder," Table 017 and Table 033, www.cdc.gov/nchs/hus/contents2017.htm, accessed September 3, 2019.

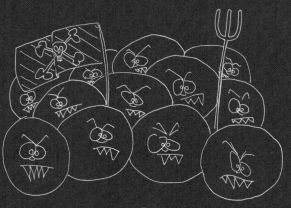

CHAPTER 10

Bacterial Resistance

The Resurgence of Infectious Diseases

KEY TERMS

Acquired immunodeficiency
  syndrome (AIDS)
Antibiotic resistance
Antibody
Directly observed therapy (DOT)
Ebola

Emerging infectious diseases
Extensively drug-resistant
  tuberculosis (XDR TB)
Highly active antiretroviral
  therapy (HAART)
Influenza

Multidrug resistance (MDR)
Outbreak
Prions
Retrovirus
West Nile virus
Zika virus

The appearance of **acquired immunodeficiency syndrome (AIDS)** in the early 1980s challenged the widely held belief that infectious diseases were under control. However, there had been intimations during the previous few decades that the microbes were not as controllable as generally believed. The influenza virus was proving stubbornly unpredictable, deadly new variants of known bacteria were beginning to crop up, and the familiar old bacteria were becoming strangely resistant to antibiotics. That trend has continued, and the importance of public health in combating these growing problems has become increasingly apparent.

The Biomedical Basis of AIDS

By the turn of the 21st century, the exotic disease that seemed to strike only gay men had turned into a worldwide scourge: The human immunodeficiency virus (HIV) now infects more than 38 million individuals and kills more than 750,000 people each year around the globe.[1] In the United States as of 2016, some 675,000 people had died of AIDS.[2] Since the **outbreak** was first recognized, a great deal has been learned about HIV, how it causes AIDS, and how it is spread.

HIV is a **retrovirus**, a virus that uses RNA as its genetic material instead of the more usual DNA. Retroviruses have long been known to cause cancer in animals, and they were extensively studied for clues to the causes of human cancer; this research proved helpful for understanding the immunodeficiency virus when it was identified. Two human retroviruses—causing two types of leukemia—were known before HIV was discovered. Retroviruses infect cells by copying their RNA into the DNA of the cell, penetrating the genetic material like a "mole" in a spy agency. This DNA may sit silently in the cell, being copied normally along with the cell's genetic material for an indefinite number of generations. Alternatively, it may take over control of the cell's machinery, causing the uncontrolled reproduction typical of cancer.

The target of HIV is a specific type of white blood cell called the CD4-T lymphocyte, or T4 cell. T4 cells are just one of many components of the complicated immune machinery that becomes activated when the body recognizes a foreign invader such as a bacterium or a virus. The T4 cell's role is to divide and reproduce itself in response to such an invasion and to attack the invader. In a T4 cell that is infected with HIV, activation of the cell activates the virus as well, which then produces thousands of copies of itself in a process that kills the T4 cell. The T4 cells are a key component of the immune system because, in addition to attacking foreign microbes, they regulate other components of the immune system, including the cells that produce **antibodies**, the proteins in the blood that recognize foreign substances. Thus destruction of the T4 cells disrupts the entire immune system.[3]

The course of infection with HIV takes place over a number of years. After being exposed to HIV, a person may or may not notice mild, flu-like symptoms for a few weeks, during which time the virus is present in the blood and body fluids and may be easily transmitted to others by sex or other risky behaviors. The body's immune system responds as it would to any viral infection, producing specific antibodies that eliminate most of the circulating viruses. The infection then enters a latent period, with the virus remaining mostly hidden in the DNA of the T4 cells, although a constant battle is taking place between the virus and the immune system. Billions of copies of the virus are produced, and millions of T4 cells are destroyed daily.[4] During this time, the person is quite healthy and is less likely to transmit the virus than during the early stage of infection (although transmission is still possible). Eventually, after several years, the immune system begins to lose the struggle, and so many of the T4 cells begin to die that they cannot be replaced rapidly enough. When the number of T4 cells drops below 200 per cubic millimeter of blood, or approximately 20% of the normal level, symptoms may appear, and the person is vulnerable to opportunistic infections and certain tumors. At the same time, the number of circulating copies of the virus increases, and the person again becomes more capable of transmitting the infection to others.[5] At this stage, the person meets the criteria for AIDS, which is defined based on the T4 cell count and/or the presence of opportunistic infections.

The development and licensing of a screening test in 1985 was a major step forward in the fight against HIV. This test measures antibodies to the virus, which begin to appear 3 to 6 weeks after the original infection. This test is relatively fast and inexpensive, yet sensitive enough to give the first indication that the individual may be HIV positive. The test is used for three purposes: (1) diagnosing individuals at risk to determine whether they are infected so that they may be appropriately counseled and, if necessary, treated; (2) monitoring the spread of HIV in various populations via epidemiologic studies; and (3) screening donated blood or organs to ensure that they do not transmit HIV to a recipient of a transfusion or transplant. A major drawback of the antibody screening test is the absence of antibodies in the blood during the initial 3- to 6-week period after infection. This "window" of non-detectability may give newly infected people a false sense of security.

More accurate tests that look for the virus itself in the blood are now available. These tests are used to confirm infection in people who have tested positive with the screening test. In the United States, they are also performed on all donated blood to ensure that no virus-infected blood is used for transfusions.

Tests that directly measure a virus in the blood have contributed a great deal to our understanding of the biomedical basis of HIV infection. Measurement of "viral load"—the concentration of virus in the blood—is a valuable tool for evaluating the effectiveness of therapeutic drugs. Viral load has also been found to influence an individual's chances of transmitting the virus by sexual and other means. Thus a therapy that is effective in reducing viral load can help control the spread of HIV.

The major pathways of HIV transmission vary in different populations. Homosexual relations between men are still the leading route of exposure for men in the United States, but injection drug use accounts for 10% of new HIV infections in Americans.[2] Transmission by heterosexual relations, especially from male to female, is becoming increasingly common in this country; it is the leading route of infection for females. In the developing countries of Asia and Africa, where HIV infection is still spreading rapidly—there were 1.4 million new cases of HIV in these regions in 2018[1]—heterosexual relations are the most common means of transmission. Several studies have found that circumcision protects men against contracting HIV from infected women; conversely, circumcision does not appear to protect women against contracting HIV from infected men. Studies of the effect of circumcision on male-to-male transmission have yielded mixed results.[6]

The sharing of needles is a common route of transmission in developing countries because of insufficient supplies of sterile equipment for medical use. In poor countries, medical personnel often use one syringe repeatedly for giving immunizations or injections of therapeutic drugs. If one of the patients is HIV positive, this practice may transmit the infection to future patients who later receive an injection with the same needle. Transfusion with HIV-contaminated blood is no longer a significant source of HIV infection in the United States, but it still occurs in countries too poor to screen donated blood.

A special case of HIV transmission occurs from an infected mother to her infant, in utero or during delivery; such transmission may occur in 25% to 33% of births unless the mother takes antiretroviral drugs. The virus can also be transmitted to breastfed babies in their mother's milk. All infants of HIV-positive women will test positive during the first few months after birth, because fetuses in the womb receive some of their mothers' antibodies. This transfer of antibodies provides natural protection against disease (though not HIV) during infants' first months of life. Many states in the United States routinely perform HIV screening tests on newborns' blood as part of their newborn screening programs; these tests of a baby's blood for HIV antibodies therefore provide evidence of the mother's HIV status. The special issues raised by maternal–fetal transmission of the virus have been the subject of ethical, legal, and political controversy at the national and state levels. Drug therapies are now capable of preventing transmission of the virus from mother to infant in 99% of cases.[7] Similar drug treatment of mothers and/or infants can prevent transmission in breast milk.

In the United States, HIV/AIDS has become a disease of minorities. Although African Americans account for only 12% of the U.S. population, this group represents more than 40% of new cases of HIV/AIDS that have been diagnosed in recent years.[8] According to the Centers for Disease Control and Prevention (CDC), the rate of infection was almost 7 times higher in black men than in white men and 15 times higher in black women than white women.[2] Hispanics are diagnosed at 3 times the rate of whites, and represented 27% of new cases of HIV/AIDS in 2016. Among the factors that contribute to the higher rates among minorities are the fact that people tend to have sex with partners of the same race and ethnicity; minorities' tendency to experience higher rates of other sexually transmitted diseases, which increase the risk of transmission of HIV; socioeconomic issues associated with poverty; lack of awareness of HIV status; and negative perceptions about HIV testing.[8]

Progress in treating HIV/AIDS over the past two decades has been dramatic. Early therapy focused on treating opportunistic infections, which were often the immediate cause of death in patients with AIDS. The first antiretroviral therapy, zidovudine (AZT), was approved by the Food and Drug Administration (FDA) in 1987.[9] This drug interfered with the replication of HIV by inhibiting the enzyme that copies the viral RNA into the cell's DNA. However, the virus's tendency to mutate rapidly leads to the development of resistance to the drug, meaning that its effectiveness can wear off.

As scientists gained a better understanding of the virus, they developed drugs that target different stages of viral replication. Protease inhibitors, which interfere with the ability of newly formed viruses to mature and become infectious, were introduced in 1995.[9] At the same time, scientists recognized that treating patients with a combination of drugs that attack the virus in different ways reduces the opportunity for HIV to mutate and develop resistance. The introduction of these drug combinations, called **highly active antiretroviral therapy (HAART)**, led to dramatic improvements in the survival of HIV-infected patients. As a result, the number of AIDS deaths fell by more than half between 1996 and 1998 and has continued to decline slowly but steadily since then.[10]

The development of effective treatments for HIV/AIDS has had many beneficial consequences. HAART can reduce viral load to undetectable levels in the blood and body fluids of many patients, which greatly reduces the likelihood that the virus will be transmitted to others

through sexual contact and other means. The availability of effective therapy also encourages at-risk people to be tested and counseled on ways to protect themselves and to prevent transmission of the virus to others. Scientists had initially hoped that HAART would be able to completely eradicate HIV from the body, but this hope has not been realized. The virus manages to survive in protected reservoirs of the body, rebounding into active replication when the drugs are withdrawn. For some patients, side effects of HAART can be severe and even fatal; approximately 40% of patients treated with protease inhibitors develop lipodystrophy, characterized by abnormal distributions of fat in the body, sometimes accompanied by other metabolic abnormalities.[11] Moreover, the virus can develop resistance to these drugs if used improperly. A survey of blood samples taken between 1999 and 2003 found that 15% of patients receiving HAART were resistant to at least one drug.[12]

New drugs continue to be developed, including a class called "fusion inhibitors," introduced in 2003, that interfere with HIV's ability to enter a host cell, and a class called "integrase inhibitors," introduced in 2002, that prevent the virus from becoming integrated into the genetic material of human cells.[13] A totally new approach, published in 2014 but not ready for clinical application, uses genetic engineering to knock out a receptor on the membrane of T cells, making these cells resistant to HIV.[14,15] Thus, for many patients, HIV infection has become a chronic disease, necessitating lifelong therapy but enabling them to live relatively normal lives. The drugs are expensive, however, costing as much as $39,000 per year per patient, and many insurance plans cover only some of the cost.[16]

The greatest hope for controlling AIDS—especially in the developing world, where the new drugs are often unaffordable—is to develop an effective vaccine. Prevention through immunization has been the most effective approach for the viral scourges of the past, including smallpox, measles, and polio. Early hopes for the rapid availability of a vaccine against AIDS have faded, however. In fact, after several promising vaccine candidates failed in clinical trials, the National Institutes of Health (NIH) held a meeting of vaccine researchers in March 2008, to reassess whether a vaccine will ever be possible and determine which new approaches could be tried.[17] Perhaps not surprisingly, a virus well adapted to disabling the immune system is also highly effective at eluding attempts to employ that same immune system against it. Part of the difficulty in developing an effective vaccine is that the virus constantly changes its appearance, making it unrecognizable to the immune mechanisms mobilized against it by a vaccine. This characteristic is common to RNA viruses. Another difficulty is the lack of a good animal model for studying HIV/AIDS.[18] As of 2019, several HIV vaccines were in Phase 3 efficacy trials, including the Inbokodo and Mosaico clinical trials that include thousands of volunteers in countries around the world.[19]

At present, the most effective way to fight AIDS is to prevent transmission (step 3 in the chain of transmission, as described in the *"Conquest" of Infectious Diseases* chapter). This requires education and efforts at motivating people to change their high-risk behavior, an exceedingly difficult task.

HIV seems to have appeared from nowhere and to have spread over the entire world within a decade. Where did the virus come from? Genetic studies of HIV show that it is related to viruses that commonly infect African monkeys and apes, and it seems likely that a mutation allowed one of these viruses to infect humans. Some evidence indicates that this type of event—cross-species transmission of viruses—may occur fairly frequently. Monkeys and chimpanzees are killed for food in parts of Africa, which could explain how humans were exposed.[9] HIV is remarkable, however, for the speed with which it has spread into the human population worldwide.

Scientists conjecture that the human form of the virus may have existed in isolated pockets of Africa for some time, but that its rapid spread was the result of social conditions in Africa and the United States in the late 1970s. Because symptomatic AIDS does not appear until several years after the original infection, the first patients recognized in the 1980s were probably infected in the early and mid-1970s. The earliest case in the United States is suspected to have been Robert Rayford, who died in 1969 at the age of 16, after exhibiting (now recognized in retrospect) many of the tell-tale symptoms of AIDS, including numerous internal lesions knowns as Kaposi's sarcoma.[20] Investigators trying to track the spread of the epidemic even further back have tested stored blood samples drawn in earlier times; they have found HIV-infected samples from as early as 1966, in the blood of a widely traveled Norwegian sailor who died of immune deficiency. The sailor's wife and one of his three children later died of the same illness, and their stored blood, when tested, was also found to be infected with HIV.[21] An even older blood sample drawn from a West African man in 1959 has been found to contain fragments of the virus, but it is not known whether the man developed AIDS.[22] This evidence implies that sporadic early outbreaks of the disease occurred in isolated African villages, going undetected for decades.

The reasons for the recent emergence of HIV disease as a significant problem include the disruption of traditional lifestyles by the movement of rural Africans to urban areas, trends magnified by population growth, waves of civil war, and revolution. The apparent worldwide explosion of AIDS then occurred because of changing patterns of sexual behavior and the use of addictive drugs in developed and developing countries, together with the ease of international air travel.

Ebola

In 1976, before the AIDS epidemic was recognized but while, as scientists now believe, the virus was spreading silently into African cities, another viral illness broke out with much more dramatic effect in Zaire and Sudan. Symptoms caused by the previously unidentified **Ebola** virus include fever, vomiting, diarrhea, and severe bleeding from various bodily orifices. Several hundred people became ill from the disease, and as many as 90% of its victims died. The disease spread rapidly from person to person, affecting especially family members and hospital workers who had cared for patients. Investigators from the CDC and the World Health Organization (WHO) identified the virus and helped devise measures, including quarantine, to limit the spread of the disease, which eventually disappeared. The Ebola virus broke out again in Zaire in the summer of 1995, killing 244 people before it again seemed to vanish.[23] Since then, repeated outbreaks have occurred in West and Central Africa. According to CDC data, more than 800 Africans died of Ebola between 1996 and early 2013.[24]

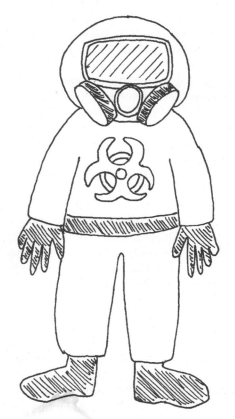

Ready to Treat an Ebola Patient

The Ebola virus infects monkeys and apes as well as humans, and on a number of occasions infected monkeys have been imported into the United States. In 1989, a large number of monkeys imported from the Philippines died of the viral infection at a primate quarantine facility in Reston, Virginia. In that episode, which served as the basis for Richard Preston's book *The Hot Zone*, several laboratory workers were exposed to the virus, which fortunately turned out to be a strain that did not cause illness in humans.[25] Fruit bats, common in African jungles, are thought to serve as the reservoir for the virus between outbreaks in the human population.[26] Like HIV, Ebola may spread to humans when they handle the carcasses of apes used for food. However, unlike HIV, the Ebola virus kills the apes it infects, leading at times to significant declines in populations of gorillas and chimpanzees[27]; outbreaks in humans have been preceded by the discovery of dead animals near villages where those outbreaks occur.[28]

In 2014, a major Ebola epidemic spread through the populations of several countries in West Africa. Hardest hit were Liberia, Guinea, and Sierra Leone—all poor countries that have been plagued by political unrest and inadequate medical care systems. Ebola spread easily to healthcare workers and to family members who cared for patients. The corpses of people who died of the disease teemed with the virus, and the West African funeral customs of touching and kissing the dead contributed to the contagiousness of the disease. In Sierra Leone, an explosion in the number of cases was triggered by the funeral of a traditional healer in early summer.[29] Medical workers learned to don protective clothing that covered all surfaces of their bodies. Unfortunately, in the heat of the West African summer, it was hard for workers to spend much time in such cumbersome garb.

More than 28,600 cases, with about 11,300 deaths, were reported in the West African epidemic, though those numbers are thought to be undercounts.[26] Notably, the virus came to the United States during the 2014 epidemic. The first patient was a Liberian man who became ill while visiting relatives in Dallas, Texas, in September 2014. Thomas Eric Duncan was taken to a hospital, examined, and sent home with antibiotics. Although hospital staff were told he had been in Guinea, the information did not trigger alarm, and Ebola was not suspected. Three days later, Duncan's condition worsened and he was taken back to the hospital, where he died on October 8.[30] Two nurses who cared for him contracted the disease within days of his death. They were treated at two of four hospitals in the United States that have special units for treating dangerous infectious diseases: Emory University Hospital and the National Institutes of Health Clinical Center. Both women recovered.[31] Another American patient, Dr. Craig Spencer, arrived in New York in late October after treating patients in Guinea during his service with Doctors Without Borders. He had been monitoring himself and was hospitalized at Bellevue Medical Center when he developed a fever. Dr. Spencer also recovered.[32]

The better outcomes achieved by American patients compared with the high death rate among West Africans—more than 70% in some West African countries—is due in part to excellent supportive care provided them in U.S. hospitals. One measure that some of them received was transfusion with serum from survivors, which contains antibodies to the virus. Some patients were treated with ZMapp, an experimental drug. Whether either of these treatments contributed to their survival is not certain and became hard to evaluate when the epidemic waned, leaving fewer patients on whom to test the approaches. A surprising finding has been that, even after a patient appears to be fully recovered, the virus may linger in his or her body. Male survivors have been warned to use condoms because their semen contains Ebola virus for a still unknown period after recovery. Dr. Ian Crozier, who contracted the disease when working with WHO in Sierra Leone and was evacuated to Emory University

Hospital in September 2014, learned after his discharge that one eye was badly infected with virus and he was in danger of losing his sight. He was treated with an experimental drug and gradually recovered his vision. Many of the survivors have also reported other aftereffects of the disease, including extreme fatigue, joint and muscle pain, and hearing loss.[33]

Researchers have achieved significant breakthroughs since the 2014 outbreak. In 2016, an vaccine called rVSV-ZEBOV was created that provides near-complete protection against the disease if given at least a week before exposure.[34] Two new experimental treatments, REGN-EB3 and mAb-114, showed cure rates of approximately 90% in patients who were enrolled in trials in 2018 and 2019. These drugs act as synthetic versions of human antibodies, attaching themselves to the disease-causing viruses and preventing them from entering cells. Preliminary outcomes for the drugs were so strong—the mortality rate was only 10% with these treatments, compared to 70% without them—that the overseeing committee recommended making the treatments available immediately and ending trials of ZMapp, which had been used with moderate success in the earlier outbreak. These new treatments provided enormous hope when addressing the 2019 outbreak in the Democratic Republic of Congo, which killed 1800 people.[35]

Publicity about Duncan (the Texas patient) and healthcare workers who were exposed to Ebola through contact with him or in West Africa caused alarm in the United States. The fact that Dr. Spencer had spent several days in New York City on his return from Africa, dining out, bowling, and taking the subway before he began to feel ill also raised concerns, although no one was infected by his actions.[36] In October 2014, the governors of New York and New Jersey announced that all healthcare workers returning from West Africa would be quarantined. The first person affected by this policy was Kaci Hickox, a nurse who had worked with Doctors Without Borders in Sierra Leone treating patients infected with Ebola. After a grueling two-day journey from Africa, she was greeted at Newark Liberty Airport by a frenzy of fear and disorganization. After being detained for hours among officials who had donned coveralls, gloves, and face shields, Hickox was sent to a nearby hospital. There, she was placed in a tent with a toilet but no shower and told she would be kept there for a 21-day mandatory quarantine.[37]

Hickox appeared on a Sunday talk show to criticize Governor Christie's policy. She noted that Ebola is infectious only after a patient begins to show symptoms and stated that she had not had symptoms. Moreover, a blood test had found no evidence of Ebola infection. Hickox hired a legal team to defend her civil rights, and Christie, after four days, freed her from the quarantine and arranged for her to be driven to her home in Maine. She never developed the disease.[38]

After the Hickox fiasco, policies on quarantine eased in most of the United States as science began to guide policy. It was recognized that mandatory isolation would discourage medical volunteers from going to West Africa to help eradicate the epidemic at its source. Most returning workers were willing to endure a milder form of quarantine at home, being monitored by public health workers, taking their temperature twice a day, and keeping a distance of three feet from others when in public.[39]

West Nile, Zika, and Other Emerging Viruses

Other new or resurgent viruses have appeared in various parts of the world, including the United States, in the recent past. In May and June 2003, for example, public health authorities in Illinois and Wisconsin received reports of a disease similar to smallpox among people who had had direct contact with prairie dogs. Prompt investigation by state officials and the CDC identified the cause as monkeypox virus, which was known from outbreaks in Africa. Although this virus infects monkeys, the primary hosts for monkeypox are rodents.[40]

The outbreak in the United States spread to 72 people in six Midwestern states. Fortunately, monkeypox is not highly contagious in humans, and it is a less severe disease than smallpox. Although no one died in the outbreak, the incident raised alarms about exotic pets. The illness in the prairie dogs was traced back through pet stores and animal distributors to an Illinois distributor, which in April had imported several African rodents, including a Gambian giant rat that had died of an unidentified illness. In June 2003, the U.S. government banned the import of all rodents from Africa. Careful surveillance and isolation of exposed people and animals halted the outbreak by the end of July, and no further cases of monkeypox have been reported since then.[41]

In 1993, the CDC was called in when two healthy young New Mexico residents living in the same household died suddenly within a few days of each other of acute respiratory distress, their lungs filled with fluid. Within three weeks, biomedical scientists had recognized that the illness, which had claimed several other victims in the Four Corners area of the Southwest, was caused by hantavirus. Named after the Hantaan River in Korea, the hantavirus had been responsible for kidney disease among thousands of American soldiers in Korea during the 1950s. In New Mexico, the virus was found to be carried by deer mice, which had been especially plentiful in the Four Corners area because of an unusually wet winter. All of the human victims of hantavirus had had significant exposure to mouse droppings, either in their homes or in their places of work.[42]

The CDC declared hantavirus pulmonary syndrome (HPS) a notifiable disease in 1995, and as of 2017, 728 cases had been reported in 36 states.[43] More than one-third of the victims have died, often in a matter of hours.

By adding HPS to the list of notifiable diseases, the CDC hoped to help medical workers recognize it more readily. In the case of a Rhode Island college student who may have contracted the disease in 1994 from exposure to mouse droppings while making a film at his father's warehouse, the hospital did not recognize that he was seriously ill and sent him home from the emergency room the first time he appeared there; two days later he returned much sicker, and he died five hours after being hospitalized.[44]

Rodents are suspected as carriers of several hemorrhagic fevers characterized by symptoms similar to those caused by hantavirus or the Ebola virus: Bolivian hemorrhagic fever (caused by the Machupo virus), Argentine hemorrhagic fever (caused by the Junin virus), and Lassa fever in Sierra Leone are all carried by rats. In recent years, well-known insect-borne viruses, such as yellow fever and equine encephalitis, have resurged in areas of South and Central America where they had been thought to be vanquished.[23] Dengue fever, also spread by mosquitoes, has become one of the most widespread mosquito-borne illnesses in the world, infecting as many as 400 million people per year globally, and causing 22,000 deaths annually. Four different viruses can cause dengue fever, so a person, once recovered, can actually contract the disease up to three more times. As of September 2019, 408 cases of dengue, a nationally notifiable disease, were reported in the United States, although 404 of them were associated with travel abroad.[45]

In the summer of 1999, the United States first experienced the effects of **West Nile virus**, which spread rapidly across the country over the next few years. The first sign of the new disease was a report to the New York City Health Department by an infectious disease specialist in Queens, New York, that an unusual number of patients had been hospitalized with encephalitis, an inflammation of the brain. The disease was suspected to be St. Louis encephalitis, a mosquito-borne disease that is endemic in the southern United States, and the diagnosis was supported by the patients' reports that they had been outdoors in the evenings during peak mosquito-bite hours. Soon, however, a great number of dead crows began to be found in the New York area, and a veterinarian at the Bronx Zoo reported unprecedented deaths among the zoo's exotic birds. Lab tests confirmed that the virus causing the human disease was the same as the one that was killing the birds, but St. Louis encephalitis virus was not known to infect birds. West Nile virus was well known in Africa, West Asia, and the Middle East. It is known to be fatal to crows and several other species of birds, but also infects horses. Ultimately, 56 patients were hospitalized in the New York epidemic, 7 of whom died.[46,47]

How the West Nile virus came to New York is not known. The most likely explanation is that it came in an infected bird, perhaps a tropical bird that was smuggled into the country. The virus is easily spread among birds by several species of mosquitoes, some of which also bite humans. Although the threat disappeared with the mosquitoes after the first frost in the fall, the next summer saw a spread of the disease to upstate New York and surrounding states. Carried by migratory birds, the virus has now arrived in all 48 contiguous states.[48] It appears that West Nile virus is here to stay. In 2018, it caused illness in 2647 people, making it the most common mosquito-borne disease in the United States.[49] Although most cases are not serious, resulting in a fever and other moderate symptoms (if any), about 1 in 150 infected people develop a serious reaction that can prove fatal or result in long-term impairments, including fatigue, weakness, depression, personality changes, gait problems, and memory deficits.[50,51]

Public health professionals fight the virus by educating the public about eliminating standing water where mosquitoes breed, wearing long sleeves, and using repellant. A vaccine is available for horses, and scientists are working on developing a vaccine that will be effective for humans.

The **Zika virus** was first identified in 1947 among monkeys in the Zika Forest of Uganda. This virus was not given much thought until a major outbreak occurred on the Micronesian island of Yap that infected 70% of the human population. Worldwide attention focused on Zika for the first time in 2015, when a massive outbreak in Brazil infected approximately 1 million people, having likely arrived via a traveler visiting for the 2014 World Cup. While the infection causes only mild symptoms in adults, it was (and continues to be) devastating for unborn fetuses, often causing microcephaly or small and misshapen heads and severe neurologic damage.[52]

The global public health response to the 2015–2016 Zika outbreak received mixed reviews. WHO was praised for very publicly declaring a global health emergency, drawing worldwide attention to the problem. The response that followed led to advisories that kept pregnant women from traveling to affected regions, new diagnostic tests for Zika, and research into a vaccine that is now in Phase 2 clinical trials. A small outbreak that occurred in 2016 in the Wynwood section of Miami was quickly contained due to the astute response of local public health authorities.[53] But there were also failings. Most notably, many poor Brazilian women did not receive the important advisory to postpone pregnancy and, due to conservative religious concerns, did not receive counseling on the option of abortion when an affected fetus was discovered.[54] These shortcomings undoubtedly contributed to the 8165 cases of microcephaly (likely a large undercount of the true number) that were reported in Brazil in the wake of the 2015–2016 outbreak.[55]

A variety of environmental factors are responsible for the recent emergence of so many new pathogens. Human activities that cause ecological changes, such as deforestation and dam building, bring people into closer contact with disease-carrying animals. Modern agricultural practices, such as extreme crowding of livestock, intensify the risk that previously unknown viruses will incubate in crowded herds and become widely dispersed to human consumers. International distribution of meat and poultry may help to spread new pathogens. The popularity of exotic pets in the United States also can lead to the spread of pathogens, such as monkeypox and perhaps West Nile virus, from animals or birds to people. A breakdown of public health efforts such as mosquito control programs because of complacency or insufficient funding has resulted in the reappearance of insect-borne diseases. Spread of the viruses in developing countries is facilitated by urbanization, crowding, war, and the breakdown of social restraints on sexual behavior and intravenous drug use. U.S. residents will not be able to escape the effects of these new pathogens. The ease and speed of international travel mean that a new infection first appearing anywhere in the world could traverse entire continents within days or weeks. This possibility was dramatically illustrated by the emergence and rapid spread of severe acute respiratory syndrome (SARS). The SARS virus is believed to have been transmitted to humans from an animal species used for food in China, possibly the civet cat.

In 2020, the SARS-Cov-2 coronavirus (closely related to the previously known virus, now called SARS-Cov-1) has caused a worldwide pandemic being compared to the 1918 flu pandemic, described later in this chapter. Scientists are just beginning to learn about the behavior of the virus, testing drugs to treat the disease, and trying to develop a vaccine.

Influenza

Influenza—the "flu"—may seem like an old and familiar infectious disease. In reality, it can be a different disease from one year to the next and has the capacity to turn into a major killer. This happened in the winter of 1918–1919, when the flu killed 20 million to 40 million people worldwide, including 196,000 people who died in the United States in October 1918.[53] Even in an average year, approximately 8% of the U.S. population gets the flu, and about 40,000 Americans die from the disease.[54] Although most deaths from flu usually occur in people older than age 65, the 1918 epidemic preferentially struck young people.

Influenza virus has been studied extensively, and vaccination can be effective, but constant vigilance is necessary to protect people from the disease. Like HIV, influenza is an RNA virus, constantly changing its appearance and adept at eluding recognition by the human immune system. Because of the year-to-year variability of the flu virus, flu vaccines must be changed annually to be effective against the newest strain. Each winter, viral samples are collected from around the world and sent to WHO, where biomedical scientists conduct experiments designed to predict how the virus will mutate into next year's strain. The vaccine takes more than six months to develop each year, so these educated guesses form the basis for the next year's vaccine.

At unpredictable intervals, however, a lethal new strain of the flu virus can come along, as it did in 1918. A strain that caused the Asian flu emerged in 1957, and a third strain, called Hong Kong flu, arrived in 1968. Neither of these outbreaks was as deadly as the 1918 epidemic, although 70,000 Americans—not an insignificant number—died from the Asian flu. In 1976, CDC scientists thought they had evidence that another deadly strain, called swine flu, was emerging, and the country mobilized for a massive immunization campaign. That time, the scientists had made a mistake: The anticipated epidemic never occurred. Infectious disease experts have for decades been expecting a new epidemic, which did occur in 2009, as discussed later in this section.

New strains of influenza virus, especially those that have undergone major changes, tend to arise in Asia, particularly China, and then spread around the world from there. One of the reasons China is an especially fertile source of new flu strains is that animal reservoirs for influenza—pigs and birds—are common there, living in close proximity to humans. Human and animal influenza viruses can incubate in a pig's digestive system, forming new genetic combinations, and then are spread by ducks as they migrate. While such hybrid viruses, containing human and animal genes, are only rarely capable of infecting humans, those that are able to do so are the most likely to be deadly.

Until recently, little was known about what made the 1918 strain of influenza so deadly, or how to predict the lethality of newly emerging strains. Recently, however, genetic studies have become possible using samples of the 1918 virus. Tissue taken from soldiers who died in 1918 had been stored at the Armed Forces Institute of Pathology in Washington, D.C.; other tissue samples were taken from victims in an Alaskan village who were buried in permanently frozen ground. Scientists have found that the 1918 virus has features in common with avian flu viruses that make them especially dangerous to humans, and they also resemble the human virus enough that they can spread easily among people.[56] Similar avian features were found in the viruses that caused epidemics in 1957 and 1968.

In 1997, influenza experts became alarmed when a 3-year-old Hong Kong boy died from a strain of influenza virus that normally infects chickens. An epidemic of the disease had occurred among the birds a few months earlier. Antibodies to the virus were found in the blood of the boy's doctor, although he did not become ill, and public health authorities watched for more cases with great concern. Two dozen other people became sick by December, and six died. To prevent further transmission from chickens to humans, the Hong Kong government ordered that all 1.5 million chickens in the territory be killed. That action seems to have been effective in halting the epidemic in humans.[57]

Bird flu emerged again in 2003 and has become widespread in Asia, Africa, Europe, and the Middle East, despite efforts to eliminate it by killing millions of birds. Between 2003 and the early 2017, more than 1500 human cases were reported, with approximately half dying of the disease.[58,59] Thus far it appears that most of the human victims of the bird flu caught the virus from chickens, rather than from other humans. There is great concern that mixing of the viral genes could occur in a person infected with both the bird virus and a human flu virus, resulting in a much more virulent strain capable of spreading among humans. Such a new virus could start a global pandemic of a lethal form of the disease, as occurred in 1918.

In spring 2015, an outbreak of avian influenza struck the United States. Millions of turkeys and chickens died or were culled in Midwestern states. No humans have caught this flu, but concern remains that it might happen. This virus, which shares some genes with the avian flu that infected poultry in Asia and Europe, is believed to have been carried to the North American continent by migrating ducks, geese, and swans. When it arrived in the new world, the virus then mixed with genes from North American viruses. The National Institutes of Health developed an experimental vaccine against the bird flu when it first affected humans in Asia, and the CDC is considering whether it might provide some protection to workers dealing with infected flocks. The CDC is also working on a vaccine against the new virus.[60]

Even a "normal" year of the flu can have a spike in fatalities. The 2017–2018 flu season was the deadliest in the Unites States in more than a decade, with this disease killing approximately 79,000 Americans. While most were older than the age of 65, 180 children and teenagers also died.[54,61]

In late 2011, controversy arose over research funded by the National Institutes of Health that created a highly transmissible form of the avian flu virus. This work was done in ferrets, which are a good model of how flu viruses behave in humans. Two groups of researchers, at the University of Wisconsin and a Dutch university, created mutations in the virus that enabled it to spread by aerosol. The National Science Advisory Board for Biosecurity asked that details of the experiments be withheld from publication to prevent terrorists from replicating them.[62] Later, at a WHO meeting

in February 2012, officials concluded that the risk of the virus's use by bioterrorists was outweighed by the danger that changes might occur naturally in the wild that would give the virus the ability to cause a pandemic.[63] Full publication will allow scientists to recognize warning signals that the virus is becoming more dangerous, which also might lead to better treatments.

The public health approach to influenza control can serve as a model for how to predict and possibly prevent the spread of other new viral threats. As the AIDS epidemic has shown, a new virus can come from "nowhere" and wreak havoc all over the world within a few years. Complacency over the "conquest" of infectious diseases has led governments to cut budgets and reduce efforts at monitoring disease. That should not happen again. The public health information-gathering network is more important than ever.

New Bacterial Threats

Bacteria, which a few decades ago seemed easily controllable because of the power of antibiotics to wipe them out, have, like viruses, emerged in more deadly forms in recent years. Previously unknown bacterial diseases such as Legionnaires' disease and Lyme disease have appeared with greater frequency. More baffling is the fact that some ordinary bacterial infections have turned unexpectedly lethal. A great cause for concern is the development of resistance to drugs. Resistance can spread among pathogens of the same species and even from one bacterial species to another.

Legionnaires' disease and Lyme disease are not caused by newly emerging bacteria, but only recently have they become common enough to be recognized as distinct entities and for their bacterial causes to be identified. *Legionella* bacteria are able to flourish in water towers used for air conditioning. Regulations requiring antimicrobial agents in the water have been effective in limiting the spread of

Legionnaires' disease. The conditions that promote the spread of Lyme disease, however, are more difficult to change. The pathogen that causes Lyme disease was identified in 1982 as a spirochete that is spread by the bite of an infected deer tick.[64] The reservoir for Lyme disease is the white-footed mouse, on which the deer tick feeds and becomes infected. Deer, on which the ticks grow and reproduce, are an important step in the chain of infection. The recent explosion in the deer population in suburban areas has, in turn, meant that Lyme disease has now become a problem for humans.

In the past, infection with streptococci, the bacteria that cause strep throat, had been easily cured with penicillin. However, for reasons that are not well understood, a more lethal strain of the bacteria, called group A *Streptococcus*, has become increasingly common. The sudden death of Muppets puppeteer Jim Henson in 1990 from fulminating pneumonia and toxic shock was caused by this new, virulent strain. The headline-grabbing "flesh-eating bacteria" that infect wounds to the extent of necessitating amputations and even causing death are also group A streptococci. The group A strain, which produces a potent toxin, was prevalent in the early part of the 20th century, when it caused scarlet fever, which frequently proved fatal in children, and rheumatic fever, which often caused damage to the heart. For decades, the group A strain was superseded by strains B and C, which were much milder in their pathogenic effects. Now, for reasons that are not clear, the group A strain has become much more prevalent.[65,66]

Another bacterium that has recently become more deadly is *Escherichia coli*, which is normally present without ill effect in the human digestive tract. In 1993, the new threat gained national attention when a number of people became severely ill after eating hamburgers at a Jack in the Box restaurant in Seattle, and four children died of kidney failure. The culprit was found to be a new strain of *E. coli*, which had acquired a gene for shiga toxin

from a dysentery-causing bacterium. The toxin, which has no treatment, causes kidney failure, especially in children and the elderly. The shiga toxin gene had "jumped" from one species of bacteria to another while both were present in human intestines. The resulting strain, called *E. coli* serotype O157:H7, is now quite common in ground beef, leading public health authorities to recommend or require thorough cooking of hamburgers.[21(p.427)] The "jumping gene" phenomenon has also been found in cholera and diphtheria bacteria, with bacterial strains being either benign or virulent depending on the presence or absence of genes that produce toxins.

Since the finding that *E. coli* O157:H7 is common in hamburger, this pathogen has been discovered to cause illness through a number of other exposures, including unpasteurized apple cider and alfalfa sprouts.[67(pp.160–161)] In 1999, an outbreak occurred in upstate New York among people who had attended a county fair. The bacteria were found in the water supplied to food and drink vendors. It turns out that *E. coli* O157:H7 is widespread in the intestines of cattle, especially calves, which excrete large quantities of the bacteria in manure. The manure may contaminate apples that fall from trees or other produce; if not thoroughly washed before being consumed, these foods may then spread the disease to people. At the New York State county fair, the water was contaminated because heavy rain washed manure from the nearby cattle barn into a well.[68] A vaccine against the toxic bacteria has been approved for cattle in the hope of reducing the risk of human exposure.[69]

Perhaps the most disturbing development in infectious diseases is **antibiotic resistance** among many species of bacteria, a development that leaves physicians powerless against many diseases they thought to be conquered. The process by which bacteria become resistant to an antibiotic is a splendid example of evolution in action. In the presence of an antibiotic drug, any mutation that allows a single bacterium to survive confers on it a tremendous selective advantage. That bacterium can then reproduce without competition from other microbes, transmitting the mutation to its offspring. The result is a strain of the bacteria that is resistant to that particular antibiotic. The mutated gene can also "jump" to other bacteria of the same or different species through the exchange of plasmids, small pieces of DNA that can move from one bacterial organism to another. Different mutations may be necessary to confer resistance to different antibiotics. Some bacteria become resistant to many different antibiotics, making it very difficult to treat patients infected with those bacteria.

Improper use of antibiotics also favors the development of resistance, and the current widespread existence of resistant bacteria testifies to the carelessness with which these life-saving drugs have been used. For example, antibiotics are powerless against viruses, so the common practice of prescribing these drugs for a viral infection merely affords stray bacteria the opportunity to develop resistance. Another example of improper use is patients' practice of stopping antibiotic use when they feel better instead of continuing to take the full prescribed course. The first few days' dose may have killed off all but a few bacteria, the most resistant; those bacteria may then survive and multiply, becoming much more difficult to control. In some countries, antibiotics are available without a prescription, increasing the likelihood that they will be used improperly.

A practice that significantly contributes to antibiotic resistance is the widespread use of low doses of antibiotics in animal feeds for the purpose of promoting the growth of livestock and to prevent disease among animals living in crowded, unsanitary conditions. More antibiotics are used in this manner than in medical applications, and this practice has clearly led to the survival of resistant strains of bacteria that may not only contaminate the meat but also spread the antibiotic resistance genes to other bacteria.[70] Studies have shown that these "superbugs" can be transmitted to humans.[71]

Because the agricultural industry benefits from the practice and has fought restrictions against antibiotic use in animals, the government has found it difficult to impose regulations on it. In 2013, the FDA took the step of asking antibiotics manufacturers to modify their labels in a way that discourages overuse of the drugs. The FDA also called for all use of antibiotics in farm animals to be overseen by veterinarians.[72]

The bacteria *Salmonella* and *Campylobacter* cause an estimated 2.5 million cases of food-borne illness in the United States each year.[73,74] In a 1999 study, in 26% of *Salmonella* cases and 54% of *Campylobacter* cases, the bacteria were found to be resistant to at least one antibiotic, probably because of antibiotic use in animal feed.[75] Resistance to erythromycin and other common antibiotics is increasingly found in group A streptococci, the lethal strain discussed previously.[76] Infection with methicillin-resistant *Staphylococcus aureus* (MRSA) is a major problem in hospitals, burn centers, and nursing homes, where hospital staff may carry the bacteria from one vulnerable patient to another. Intensive efforts succeeded in reducing the rates of MRSA infections in hospitalized patients by 54% between 2005 and 2011, though this progress has since stalled.[77,78] Healthcare-associated infections, many of which are caused by drug-resistant bacteria, are estimated to contribute to some 100,000 deaths annually in the United States.[79]

Multidrug-Resistant Tuberculosis

Tuberculosis (TB), which is spread by aerosol, was once a major killer in the United States. Between 1800 and 1870, it accounted for one out of every five deaths in this country; in 1900, it killed 194 of every 100,000 Americans and was the second leading cause of death, behind pneumonia/influenza. Worldwide, TB is still the leading cause of death among infectious diseases; in 2017, an estimated 10 million people developed the disease and 1.6 million died of it worldwide.[80] It is a disease associated with poverty, thought to be conquered in the affluent United States, where the incidence of TB has steadily declined since 1882. While better living conditions and improved nutrition appear to explain most of the early reduction in TB rates in the Unites States, two specific anti-TB measures also contributed to these gains: the required reporting of TB cases to local health officials, who were then able to take responsive steps, and the opening of state-run sanatoriums, where sick individuals could not as easily infect others.[81] With the introduction of antibiotics in 1947, mortality from TB was dramatically reduced, sanatoriums were closed, and TB seemed vanquished.

In the decade beginning in 1985, however, the trend reversed. There were several reasons for the increased incidence of TB, which was particularly concentrated in cities and among minority populations. The HIV epidemic was certainly a major factor. People with defective immune systems are more susceptible to any infection, but HIV-positive people are especially vulnerable to TB. A growing homeless population and the rise in intravenous drug use, both of which are associated with HIV infection, were other factors in increasing TB rates. Homeless shelters, prisons, and urban hospitals are prime sites for the transmission of this infection.

However, TB is not limited to the "down and out" or those who participate in high-risk behavior. "The principal risk behavior for acquiring TB infection is breathing," as one expert says.[82(p.1058)] People have been infected with TB bacilli in the course of a variety of everyday activities: a long airplane trip sitting within a few rows of a person with active TB,[83] hanging out in a Minneapolis bar frequented by a homeless man with active TB,[84] and, most frighteningly, attending a suburban school with a girl whose TB went undiagnosed for 13 months.[85]

When a healthy person inhales TB bacilli, these pathogens do not usually cause illness in the short term. Most often, the immune system responds by killing off most of the bacilli and walling off the rest into small, calcified lesions in the lungs called tubercles, which remain dormant indefinitely. Evidence that a person has been exposed shows up in tuberculin skin tests, which cause a conspicuous immune response when a small extract from the bacillus is injected under the exposed person's skin. For reasons that are not well understood, but probably relate to individual immune system variations, a small percentage of people develop active disease soon after exposure; others may harbor the latent infection for years before it becomes active, if ever. Infected people have a 10% lifetime risk of developing an active case. The risk for people who are HIV positive is much higher: as much as 50%.[67] Most cases of active TB are characterized by growth of the bacilli in the lungs, causing breakdown of the tissue and the major symptom—coughing—which releases the infectious agents into the air.

Before the introduction of antibiotics, approximately 50% of all patients with active TB died. Antibiotics dramatically reduced not only the mortality rate but also the incidence rate, because the medication relieved coughing and, therefore, inhibited the spread of disease. However, the development of **multidrug resistance (MDR)** in some strains of TB bacilli has meant that the disease is much more difficult and expensive to treat, and the mortality rate is much higher.

The increased prevalence of the antibiotic-resistant strains in all parts of the United States during the 1980s is thought to be due to the fact that many patients did not take their medications regularly. The TB bacillus is a particularly difficult pathogen to manage from a medical standpoint because it grows slowly and because diagnostic testing can take several weeks. Once the disease is diagnosed, even the most potent antibiotic must be taken for several months to wipe out the pathogens. Patients commonly begin to feel better after 2 to 4 weeks of taking an effective prescribed drug. However, if they stop taking the medication at that point, they may relapse with a drug-resistant strain.

The threat posed by MDR TB to all strata of society was made clear by an epidemic that was finally recognized in a suburban California school in 1993. The source of the outbreak was a 16-year-old immigrant student who had contracted the disease in her native Vietnam.[85] She had developed a persistent cough in January 1991, but her doctors had failed to diagnose the cause as TB until 13 months later. Even then, they did not report the case to the county health department, as required by law, and when the case was reported by the laboratory that had analyzed her sputum, the doctors refused to cooperate with the health department. By the time the county authorities took over her case in 1993, the girl had developed a drug-resistant strain. In accordance with standard public health practice, the health department then began screening all of the girl's contacts for TB infection. Some 23% of the 1263 students given the tuberculin skin test were found to be positive for exposure to the infection. Of those, 13 students had active cases of the drug-resistant strain of the disease. Fortunately, no one died.[86]

It is clearly in the community's best interests to ensure that all patients with TB are properly diagnosed and provided with a full course of medications, whether or not they can afford to pay for those drugs, to prevent them from spreading the disease. New York City has proven that, by applying public health measures, it is possible to reverse the trend of increasing incidence of MDR TB. In 1992, the number of TB cases diagnosed in the city had nearly tripled over the previous 15 years, and 23% of new cases were resistant to drugs. The city and state began intensive public health measures, which included screening high-risk populations and providing therapy to everyone diagnosed with active TB. A program of **directly observed therapy (DOT)** was instituted for patients who were judged unlikely to take their medications regularly. Outreach workers traveled to patients' homes,

workplaces, street corners, park benches, or wherever necessary to observe that each patient took each dose of his or her medicine. As a result of these measures, the number of new cases of TB fell in 1993, 1994, and 1995, and the percentage of new cases that involved MDR strains also declined by 30% in a 2-year period.[87] New York's success has been echoed by the national trend (**Figure 10-1**), giving hope that concerted public health efforts will eventually eliminate TB as a serious public health threat in the United States. DOT is recognized all over the world as the most effective approach to dealing with TB.

The majority of TB cases reported in the United States occur among foreign-born persons. This reflects the fact that TB infection is widespread throughout the world, especially in developing countries and in countries with high rates of HIV infection. The prevalence of MDR TB strains is a major concern: Worldwide, 458,000 people are estimated to have MDR TB. The proportion of TB cases that involve MDR strains can reach 20% in some countries, with India, China, and the Russian Federation accounting for almost half of these cases.[80] In the United States, the proportion of MDR cases among all patients with TB is only about 1%, with these cases mainly occurring among foreign-born persons.[88] Because of immigration and international travel, the United States will need to continue TB control programs domestically and also actively participate in global efforts to control the disease around the world to avoid future outbreaks in this country.

In 2007, the CDC revised its requirements for overseas medical screening of applicants for immigration to the United States.[89] Federal agencies also developed measures to prevent individuals with certain communicable diseases, including active TB, from traveling on commercial aircraft. Names of these individuals are placed on a Do Not Board list by federal, state, or local public health agencies and distributed to international airlines. A similar list is distributed to border patrol authorities

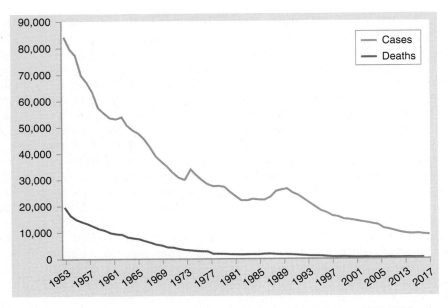

Figure 10-1 Numbers of Tuberculosis Cases and Deaths in the United States, 1953–2017

Data from Centers for Disease Control and Prevention, "Reported Tuberculosis in the United States, 2017," Table 1, www.cdc.gov/tb /statistics/reports/2017/table1.htm, accessed September 8, 2019.

in an effort to prevent individuals deemed dangerous to the public health from entering the country through a seaport, airport, or land border. These lists are managed by the CDC and the Department of Homeland Security.[90,91]

In the 1990s, even more threatening strains of TB began to appear around the world—namely, **extensively drug-resistant tuberculosis (XDR TB)**. While strains of MDR TB are resistant to the most common anti-TB drugs, some drugs remain effective against them, although they are more expensive and are difficult to administer. XDR TB is resistant to virtually all anti-TB drugs, leading to a mortality rate of 50% or more among patients infected with these strains. According to one expert, this raises "concerns about a return to the pre-antibiotic era in TB control."[92]

The most deadly form yet emerged in 2006, when doctors in South Africa learned that 52 of 53 patients with a particular strain had died within a month of diagnosis. Only a small proportion of new TB cases involve XDR (approximately 30,000 cases annually),

but until recently diagnosis with such a strain represented a death sentence. However, a major breakthrough occurred in 2019 when a three-antibiotic cocktail was discovered to have a 90% success rate among 109 patients with XDR TB who had enrolled in a last-ditch trial to save their lives. In August 2019, the FDA approved this approach, and WHO and other aid groups are expected to adopt it quickly.[93]

Public health measures to protect airline passengers and U.S. residents from exposure are far from perfect. The CDC reports that despite the State Department's requirement that immigrants and refugees undergo screening overseas, dozens or hundreds of individuals with active TB arrive in the United States each year—mainly foreign visitors, foreign students, and temporary workers. One example cited by the CDC occurred in 2011, when the Ohio Department of Health reported to the CDC that a college student from China had arrived with active TB. She had traveled from Japan on a flight to California that lasted more than 8 hours, and then took two connecting flights to reach Ohio. As required in such a situation, the airlines were asked to identify passengers who were potentially exposed by sitting in the same row or two rows in front of or in back of the infected person. The CDC then contacts state health departments, which are expected to notify individuals in their jurisdictions of their potential exposures. In this case, 15 people were identified as being at risk.[94]

Clearly, there is an ongoing struggle between microbes' ability to evolve new variations and human ingenuity in devising new defenses against them. A high-profile 2019 report by the United Nations on antimicrobial resistance declared that "alarming levels of resistance have been reported in countries of all income levels, with the result that common diseases are becoming untreatable, and lifesaving medical procedures riskier to perform."[95] Without changes to the serious overuse of these medicines in humans, livestock, and agriculture, the report predicted a dramatic increase in the rate of drug-resistant infections, with devastating consequences, in the coming decades.[95] The arrival of such an era would force public health professionals back to more emphasis on prevention of disease transmission through classical public health measures such as surveillance, immunization, sanitation, and infection control procedures.

Prions

As if new viruses and drug-resistant bacteria were not worrisome enough, a novel form of infectious disease grabbed headlines in the 1990s. Creutzfeldt–Jakob disease (CJD) is a rare and devastating disorder in which the patient develops dementia and ultimately dies, and the brain appears spongy on autopsy because many brain cells have died. Similar diseases in animals can be transmitted by injecting brain tissue from an infected animal into the brain of a previously healthy one. However, no virus or bacteria has been found responsible for causing the condition. In 1997, Stanley Prusiner, a scientist at the University of California Medical

School in San Francisco, won the Nobel Prize for his controversial theory that this type of disease is caused by particles called **prions**, which contain protein but no nucleic acid and, therefore, no traditional genetic material.

In 1996, a paper appeared in a British medical journal reporting that 10 persons in the United Kingdom younger than 45 years of age had been diagnosed with a CJD-like condition, an unusually high incidence in a group much younger than those usually struck by the disease.[96] The authors suggested a link with an epidemic of bovine spongiform encephalopathy (BSE), known as "mad cow disease," which had killed more than 160,000 cattle in Britain over the previous decade. The disease was spread by the (now discontinued) practice of grinding up discarded animal parts and adding them to feed for other cattle. A flurry of alarm and a European ban on British beef led the British government in 1996 to order the mass slaughter of all at-risk cattle to prevent the possibility of human exposure to infected beef.[97]

The evidence is strong that consumption of contaminated beef is the cause of new variant CJD (vCJD). As of March 2017, 231 cases had been reported worldwide, of which 178 occurred in the United Kingdom. Most of the affected individuals had lived in the United Kingdom during the years of the BSE outbreak among cattle.[98] Four cases have been reported in the United States, two of whom probably contracted the disease in the United Kingdom and one of whom probably contracted it in Saudi Arabia.[99] The fourth case, confirmed after a patient died in Texas in 2014, occurred in a man who had traveled widely in Europe and the Middle East.[100] Americans have little chance of being exposed to BSE in the United States. Regulations on cattle feed have been tightened, and certain ruminant parts are prohibited from entering the food supply. Restrictions have been introduced that prohibit importation of live ruminants, such as cattle, sheep, and goats, except from Canada, which also implemented stricter feed regulations.

Although controversy persists about whether enough is being done to protect cattle in North America from BSE, only 6 cases in American cows and 20 cases in Canadian cows had been identified as of August 2018.[101,102] No cases of vCJD have been attributed to consumption of American beef.

Other prion diseases have been identified in humans and animals. Two of them, Gerstmann–Straussler–Scheinker syndrome and fatal familial insomnia, are extremely rare genetic diseases. A third prion disease, kuru, was endemic in certain tribes in Papua New Guinea, where it was recognized and studied in the mid-20th century. A tribal custom in that region was for mourners to eat the internal organs of dead family members; in consequence, kuru would spread within families.[103] The only prion disease that might potentially threaten human health in the United States is chronic wasting disease (CWD), which affects North American deer, elk, and moose. The CDC warns hunters to consult with state or provincial wildlife agencies to identify areas where CWD occurs—it is currently found in states including Wisconsin and Colorado, and in Canada. Where it does occur, the CDC recommends that hunters consider having an animal tested before eating its meat and using care in handling carcasses. For nonhunters, local public health organizations discourage people from using birdfeeders that attract deer, as this may also facilitate transmission to humans.[104,105]

Public Health Response to Emerging Infections

The U.S. public health system has taken many steps toward responding to the emerging threats of infectious diseases. While still underfunded and challenged from all sides, U.S. public health agencies have devoted significant resources to developing plans and identifying priorities for confronting the threats.

The Institute of Medicine (recently renamed National Academy of Medicine) has undertaken several studies to address the environmental, demographic, social, and other factors leading to the emergence or reemergence of infectious diseases. One of its conclusions is that most of the emerging infectious disease events have been caused by zoonotic disease pathogens—that is, infectious agents that are transmitted from animals to humans. Factors that contribute to the risk of this animal-to-human transmission include human population growth, changing patterns of human–animal contact, increased demand for animal protein, increased wealth and mobility, environmental changes, and human encroachment on farmland and previously undisturbed wildlife habitat. Clearly, these diseases are an international problem, and dealing with them requires an international response.[106]

Global surveillance for infectious diseases is critically important for identifying potential epidemics early enough to bring them under control. In the past, diseases that went unnoticed in animals but spread to humans included AIDS, Ebola, avian influenza, and SARS. Effective control of **emerging infectious diseases** requires worldwide disease surveillance focusing not only on human populations, but also on domestic animals and wildlife. Thus, the CDC is collaborating with, in addition to WHO, the World Organisation for Animal Health and the Food and Agricultural Organization of the United Nations. In addition, the United States helped launch the Global Health Security Agenda in 2014 to promote international efforts to monitor and control public health threats.

Other priorities that the Institute of Medicine has identified for controlling emerging infections include reducing inappropriate use of antibiotics by banning their use for growth promotion in animals and developing improved diagnostic tests for infectious diseases so that antibiotics are not used for viral diseases. The Institute of Medicine also recommends developing new vaccines, new antimicrobial drugs, and measures aimed at vector-borne diseases.[107]

Public Health and the Threat of Bioterrorism

In the late 1990s, concern increased in the United States about the possibility that biological organisms could be used as agents of warfare and terrorism. The anthrax attacks of 2001 demonstrated that this concern was well founded. Earlier incidents had raised awareness of the possible threat, including revelations by a Russian defector that the Soviets had developed systems for loading smallpox virus on ballistic missiles.[108] Concern was heightened by evidence that Iraq had produced missile warheads and bombs containing anthrax spores and botulinum toxin. The Aum Shinrikyo cult that in 1995 released sarin gas in a Tokyo subway was found later to have experimented with releases of aerosolized anthrax and botulinum toxin throughout the city.[109] Closer to home, a 1984 outbreak of salmonellosis that sickened 751 people in The Dalles, Oregon, was eventually traced to intentional contamination of salad bars in several restaurants, details of which were revealed much later in a criminal prosecution of the Baghwan religious cult that was responsible for the incident.[110]

Even before the anthrax attacks of 2001, the CDC had developed plans for dealing with biological terrorism. After 2001, awareness of the possibility of biological attacks increased, and planning of means to prevent and/or cope with such attacks has continued. In contrast to bombings or chemical attacks, dissemination of biological agents is likely to be done in a covert way. Thus, the first signs of an attack are likely to be seen by physicians and hospital emergency rooms. Local health departments will carry out the initial investigations of unusual disease outbreaks, and good surveillance is vital for recognizing outbreaks as early as possible. In sum, the approach to bioterrorism preparedness is much the same as the response to an epidemic of any other origin. Although concerns about bioterrorism have subsided in recent years, a strong public health system remains vital to U.S. national security.

Conclusion

Infectious diseases have increasingly threatened the health of Americans over the past few decades, challenging the earlier view that infectious diseases were under control. The appearance of AIDS in the 1980s was an early sign that a new disease could appear out of "nowhere" and rapidly become a lethal, worldwide epidemic. Other viruses such as Ebola and Zika have emerged in tropical areas and have threatened the United States when conditions were right. A deadly hantavirus appeared in the United States in 1993 and has been reported in 34 states. West Nile virus was first recognized in New York City in 1999 and has spread across the country to almost all states. Zika infected more than 1 million people in Brazil by 2015 and emerged as a concern for pregnant women traveling to tropical areas and even residents in southern United States. Influenza is a highly infectious disease that can spread rapidly all over the world. While the public health system has worked collaboratively on an international scale, adapting vaccines to keep up with the rapidly mutating viruses, everyone is frightened by the prospect of another worldwide flu epidemic like the one in 1918 that killed 20 to 40 million people.

New bacterial diseases have also been appearing in the United States as ecological and cultural conditions change. Lyme disease and Legionnaires' disease have been significant problems in the past few decades. *Streptococcus* and *E. coli* have become much more deadly in recent years. Many bacteria, including *Mycobacterium tuberculosis*, have developed resistance to antibiotics, making them much less vulnerable to treatment.

To combat today's emerging infectious threats, public health professionals must continually update the measures that proved successful in conquering infectious diseases in the early part of the 20th century. Plans are in place to fortify the public health system to improve surveillance and response to the new threats. As with many other aspects of public health, however, political controversy and economic concerns tend to impede the implementation of effective measures, such as those needed to deal with antibiotic resistance stimulated by agricultural practices and, in the case of Zika, to advise women on family planning and the option of abortion. Concerns about the threat of biological terrorism have added urgency to the call for strengthening the public health system in the United States.

References

1. United Nations Programme on HIV and AIDS (UNAIDS), "Global HIV & AIDS Statistics: 2019 Fact Sheet," www.unaids.org/en/resources/fact-sheet, accessed September 5, 2019.
2. Centers for Disease Control and Prevention, "CDC Fact Sheet: Today's HIV/AIDS Epidemic," August 2016, www.cdc.gov/nchhstp/newsroom/docs/factsheets/todaysepidemic-508.pdf, accessed September 5, 2019.
3. W. C. Greene, "AIDS and the Immune System," *Scientific American* (September 1993): 99–103.
4. M. Pope and A. T. Haase, "Transmission, Acute HIV-1 Infection and the Quest for Strategies to Prevent Infection," *Nature Medicine* 9 (2003): 847–852.
5. M. A. Nowak and A. J. McMichael, "How HIV Defeats the Immune System," *Scientific American* (August 1995): 58–65.
6. Centers for Disease Control and Prevention, "Male Circumcision," August 17, 2012, http://stacks.cdc.gov/view/cdc/13546/, accessed September 9, 2019.
7. Centers for Disease Control and Prevention, "HIV and Pregnant Women, Infants, and Children," March 2019, www.cdc.gov/hiv/pdf/group/gender/pregnantwomen/cdc-hiv-pregnant-women.pdf, accessed September 9, 2019.
8. Centers for Disease Control and Prevention, "HIV Among African Americans," www.cdc.gov/nchhstp/newsroom/docs/factsheets/cdc-hiv-aa-508.pdf, accessed September 9, 2019.
9. A. S. Fauci, "HIV and AIDS: 20 Years of Science," *Nature Medicine* 9 (2003): 839–843.
10. Centers for Disease Control and Prevention, "Epidemiology of HIV Infection Through 2017," www.cdc.gov/hiv/pdf/library/slidesets/cdc-hiv-surveillance-epidemiology-2017.pdf, accessed September 9, 2019.
11. A. Garg, "Acquired and Inherited Lipodystrophies," *New England Journal of Medicine* 350 (2004): 1220.
12. B. Masquelier et al., "Prevalence of Transmitted HIV-1 Drug Resistance and the Role of Resistance Algorithms," *Journal of Acquired Immune Deficiency Syndrome* 40 (2005): 505–511.
13. U.S. Food and Drug Administration, "Antiretroviral Drugs Used in the Treatment of HIV Infection," April 12, 2018, www.fda.gov/patients/hiv-treatment/antiretroviral-drugs-used-treatment-hiv-infection, accessed September 9, 2019.
14. M. A. Kay and B. D. Walker, "Engineering Cellular Resistance to HIV," *New England Journal of Medicine*, 370 (2014): 968–969.
15. A. Falkenhagen and S. Joshi, "Genetic Strategies for HIV Treatment and Prevention," *Molecular Therapy: Nucleic Acids* (2018).
16. T. Rosenberg, "H.I.V. Drugs Cost $75 in Africa, $39,000 in the U.S. Does It Matter?," *The New York Times*, September 18, 2019.
17. L. A. Altman, "Rethinking Is Urged on a Vaccine for AIDS," *The New York Times*, March 26, 2008.
18. K. O. Kallings, "The First Postmodern Pandemic: 25 Years of HIV/AIDS," *Journal of Internal Medicine* 263 (2007): 218–243.
19. National Institutes of Health, "NIH and Partners to Launch HIV Vaccine Efficacy Trial in the Americas and Europe," July 15, 2019, www.nih.gov/news-events/news-releases/nih-partners-launch-hiv-vaccine-efficacy-trial-americas-europe, accessed September 5, 2019.
20. S. Hendrix, "A Mystery Illness Killed a Boy in 1969. Years Later, Doctors Learned What It Was: AIDS," *The Washington Post*, May 15, 2019.

21. L. Garrett, *The Coming Plague: Newly Emerging Diseases in a World Out of Balance* (New York: Farrar, Straus and Giroux, 1994).

22. T. Zhu, B. T. Korber, A. J. Nahmias, E. Hooper, P. M. Sharp, and D. D. Ho, "An African HIV Sequence from 1959 and Implications for the Origin of the Epidemic," *Nature* 391 (1998): 594–597.

23. B. Le Guenno, "Emerging Viruses," *Scientific American* (October 1995): 56–64.

24. Centers for Disease Control and Prevention, "Outbreaks Chronology: Ebola Virus Disease," June 19, 2019, www.cdc.gov/vhf/ebola/outbreaks/history /chronology.html, accessed September 9, 2019.

25. R. Preston, *The Hot Zone* (New York: Random House, 1994).

26. World Health Organization, "Ebola Virus Disease," May 30, 2019, www.who.int/en/news-room/fact-sheets/detail/ebola-virus-disease, accessed September 5, 2019.

27. G. Vogel, "Scientists Say Ebola Has Pushed Western Gorillas to the Brink," *Science* 317 (2007): 1484.

28. E. M. Leroy, P. Rouquet, P. Formenty, S. Souquière, A. Kilbourne, J. M. Froment, et al., "Multiple Ebola Virus Transmission Events and Rapid Decline of Central African Wildlife," *Science* 303 (2004): 387–390.

29. K. R. Victory, F. Coronado, S. O. Ifono, T. Soropogui, B. A. Dahl, and Centers for Disease Control and Prevention (CDC), "Ebola Transmission Linked to a Single Traditional Funeral Ceremony—Kissidougou, Guinea, December, 2014–January, 2015," *Morbidity and Mortality Weekly Report* 64 (2015): 386–388.

30. M. Fernandez and K. Sack, "Ebola Patient Sent Home, Despite Fever, Records Show," *The New York Times*, October 10, 2014.

31. K. Sack, "Downfall for Hospital Where Ebola Spread," *The New York Times*, October 15, 2014.

32. M. Wines, "New York Ebola Patient's Condition Improves, Officials Say," *The New York Times*, November 2, 2014.

33. D. Grady, "After Nearly Claiming His Life, Ebola Lurked in a Doctor's Eye," *The New York Times*, May 7, 2015.

34. D. G. McNeil Jr., "New Ebola Vaccine Gives 100 Percent Protection," *The New York Times*, December 22, 2016.

35. D. G. McNeil Jr., "A Cure for Ebola? Two New Treatments Prove Highly Effective in Congo," *The New York Times*, August 1, 2019.

36. A. Hartocollis, "Doctor Who Survived Ebola Says He Was Unfairly Cast as a Hazard and a Hero," *The New York Times*, February 25, 2015.

37. A. Hartocollis and E. G. Fitzsimmons, "Tested Negative for Ebola, Nurse Criticizes Her Quarantine," *The New York Times*, October 25, 2014.

38. L. Robbins, M. Barbaro, and M. Santora, "Unapologetic, Christie Frees Nurse from Ebola Quarantine," *The New York Times*, October 27, 2014.

39. A. Harticollis, "Notable Absence of New Quarantines at New York Area Airports," *The New York Times*, November 24, 2014.

40. K. D. Reed, J. W. Melski, M. B. Graham, R. L. Regnery, M. J. Sotir, M. V. Wegner, et al., "The Detection of Monkeypox in Humans in the Western Hemisphere," *New England Journal of Medicine* 350 (2004): 342–350.

41. Centers for Disease Control and Prevention, "Monkeypox," September 5, 2008, http://www.cdc .gov/ncidod/monkeypox/index.htm, accessed May 19, 2015.

42. Centers for Disease Control and Prevention, "Outbreak of Acute Illness—Southwestern United States, 1993," *Morbidity and Mortality Weekly Report* 42 (1993): 421–424.

43. Centers for Disease Control and Prevention, "Hantavirus Disease, by State of Reporting," January 2017, www.cdc.gov/hantavirus/surveillance/reporting -state.html, accessed September 6, 2019.

44. Centers for Disease Control and Prevention, "Hantavirus Pulmonary Syndrome—Northeastern United States, 1994," *Morbidity and Mortality Weekly Report* 43 (1994): 548–549, 555–556.

45. Centers for Disease Control and Prevention, "Dengue," www.cdc.gov/dengue/index.html, accessed September 6, 2019.

46. Centers for Disease Control and Prevention, "Outbreak of West Nile-Like Viral Encephalitis—New York, 1999," *Morbidity and Mortality Weekly Report* 48 (1999): 845–849.

47. Centers for Disease Control and Prevention, "Update: West Nile Virus Encephalitis—New York, 1999," *Morbidity and Mortality Weekly Report* 48 (1999): 944–946.

48. Centers for Disease Control and Prevention, "Summary of Notifiable Diseases—United States, 2006," *Morbidity and Mortality Weekly Report* 55 (2006): 8.

49. Centers for Disease Control and Prevention, "West Nile Virus Disease Cases and Presumptive Viremic Blood Donors by State—United States, 2019," www.cdc.gov/westnile/statsmaps/preliminary mapsdata2019/disease-cases-state-2019.html, accessed September 9, 2019.

50. R. Voelker, "Effects of West Nile Virus May Persist," *Journal of the American Medical Association* 299 (2008): 2135–2136.

51. Centers for Disease Control and Prevention, "West Nile Virus," www.cdc.gov/westnile/, accessed September 6, 2019.

52. A. Coelho and S. Crovella, "Microcephaly Prevalence in Infants Born to Zika Virus–Infected Women: A Systematic Review and Meta-analysis," *International Journal of Molecular Sciences* 18, no. 8 (2017).

53. P. Belluck, "A 500-Square-Foot Area in Miami Is Ground Zero for the Zika Virus," *The New York Times*, August 8, 2016.

54. J. M. Barry, *The Great Influenza: The Story of the Deadliest Pandemic in History* (London: Penguin Books, 2004).

55. Centers for Disease Control and Prevention, "Disease Burden of Influenza," February 19, 2019, www.cdc.gov/flu/about/burden/index.html, accessed September 9, 2019.

56. E. C. Holmes, "1918 and All That," *Science* 303 (2004): 1787–1788.

57. E. C. Claas, A. D. Osterhaus, R. van Beek, J. C. De Jong, G. F. Rimmelzwaan, D. A. Senne, et al., "Human Influenza A H5N1 Virus Related to a Highly Pathogenic Avian Influenza Virus," *The Lancet* 351 (1998): 472–477.

58. Centers for Disease Control and Prevention, "Avian Influenza Current Situation," March 17, 2015, www.cdc.gov/flu/avianflu/avian-flu-summary.htm, accessed September 9, 2019.

59. World Health Organization, "Human Infection with Avian Influenza A(H7N9) Virus—China," January 17, 2017, www.who.int/csr/don/17-january-2017-ah7n9-china/en/, accessed September 6, 2019.

60. D. G. McNeil Jr., "A Flu Epidemic That Threatens Birds, Not Humans," *The New York Times*, May 4, 2015.

61. D. G. McNeil Jr., "Over 80,000 Americans Died of Flu Last Winter, Highest Toll in Years," *The New York Times*, October 1, 2018.

62. D. Grady and W. J. Broad, "Seeing Terror Risk, U.S. Asks Journals to Cut Flu Study Facts," *The New York Times*, December 20, 2011.

63. D. Grady, "Despite Safety Worries, Work on Deadly Flu to Be Released, *The New York Times*, February 17, 2012.

64. F. S. Kantor, "Disarming Lyme Disease," *Scientific American* (September 1994): 34–39.

65. R. M. Krause, "The Origin of Plagues: Old and New," *Science* 257 (1992): 1073–1078.

66. R. K. Aziz and M. Kotb, "Rise and Persistence of Global M1T1 Clone of *Streptococcus pyogenes*," *Emerging Infectious Diseases* 14 (2008): 1511–1517.

67. D. L. Heymann, *Control of Communicable Diseases Manual* (Washington, DC: American Public Health Association, 2004), 160–161.

68. Centers for Disease Control and Prevention, "Public Health Dispatch: Outbreak of *Escherichia coli* O157:H7 and *Campylobacter* Among Attendees of the Washington County Fair—New York 1999," *Morbidity and Mortality Weekly Report* 48 (1999): 803.

69. Department of Agriculture, "Vilsack Issues Conditional License for Vaccine to Reduce *E. coli* in Feedlot Cattle," March 13, 2009, www/usda.gov/wps/portal/!ut/p/_s.7_0_A/7_0_1OB?content id=2009/03/0058.xml, accessed May 20, 2015.

70. W. Witte, "Medical Consequences of Antibiotic Use in Agriculture," *Science* 279 (1998): 996–997.

71. B. M. Kuehn, "Antibiotic-Resistant 'Superbugs' May Be Transmitted from Animals to Humans," *Journal of the American Medical Association* 298 (2007): 2125–2126.

72. "Editorial: Antibiotic Use, and Abuse, on the Farms," *The New York Times*, March 28, 2014.

73. Centers for Disease Control and Prevention, "*Salmonella*," www.cdc.gov/salmonella/, accessed September 6, 2019.

74. Centers for Disease Control and Prevention, "*Campylobacter* (Campylobacteriosis)," www.cdc.gov/campylobacter/index.html, accessed September 6, 2019.

75. S. L. Gorbach, "Antimicrobial Use in Animal Feed—Time to Stop," *New England Journal of Medicine* 345 (2001): 1202–1203.

76. P. Hudvinen, "Macrolide-Resistant Group A *Streptococcus*—Now in the United States," *New England Journal of Medicine* 346 (2002): 1243–1245.

77. Centers for Disease Control and Prevention, "What CDC Is Doing to Combat MRSA," February 1, 2019, www.cdc.gov/mrsa/tracking/index.html, accessed September 9, 2019.

78. Centers for Disease Control and Prevention, "Methicillin-Resistant *Staphylococcus aureus* (MRSA): Healthcare Settings," www.cdc.gov/mrsa/healthcare/index.html, accessed September 8, 2019.

79. K. S. Sack, "Hospital Infection Problem Persists," *The New York Times*, April 13, 2010.

80. World Health Organization, "Global Tuberculosis Report 2018," www.who.int/tb/publications/global_report/en/, accessed September 9, 2019.

81. D. M. Anderson, K. K. Charles, C. Las Heras Olivares, and D. I. Rees, "Was the First Public Health Campaign Successful?" *American Economic Journal: Applied Economics* 11 (2019): 143–175.

82. B. R. Bloom and C. J. L. Murray, "Tuberculosis: Commentary on a Reemergent Killer," *Science* 257 (1992): 1055–1064.

83. T. A. Kenyon, "Transmission of Multidrug-Resistant Mycobacterium Tuberculosis During a Long Airplane Flight," *New England Journal of Medicine* 334 (1996): 935–938.

84. S. E. Kline, L. L. Hedemark, and S. F. Davies, "Outbreak of Tuberculosis Among Regular Patrons of a Neighborhood Bar," *New England Journal of Medicine* 333 (1995): 222–227.

85. "California School Becomes Notorious for Epidemic of TB," *The New York Times*, July 18, 1994.

86. R. Ridzon, J. H. Kent, S. Valway, P. Weismuller, R. Maxwell, M. Elcock, et al., "Outbreak of Drug-Resistant Tuberculosis with Second-Generation Transmission in a High School in California," *Journal of Pediatrics* 131 (1997): 863–868.

87. T. R. Frieden, P. I. Fujiwara, R. M. Washko, and M. A. Hamburg, "Tuberculosis in New York City: Turning the Tide," *New England Journal of Medicine* 333 (1995): 229–233.

88. Centers for Disease Control and Prevention, "Trends in Tuberculosis, 2017," www.cdc.gov/tb/publications/factsheets/statistics/tbtrends.htm, accessed September 9, 2019.

89. Centers for Disease Control and Prevention, "Implementation of New TB Screening Requirements for U.S.-Bound Immigrants and Refugees," *Morbidity and Mortality Weekly Report* 63 (2014): 234–236.

90. Centers for Disease Control and Prevention, "Federal Air Travel Restrictions for Public Health Purposes—United States, June 2007–May 2008," *Morbidity and Mortality Weekly Report* 57 (2008): 1009–1012.

91. Centers for Disease Control and Prevention, "Tuberculosis Technical Instructions for Panel Physicians," www.cdc.gov/immigrantrefugeehealth/pdf/TB-panel-tech-instructions-h.pdf, accessed September 8, 2019.

92. N. S. Shah, R. Pratt, L. Armstrong, V. Robison, K. G. Castro, and J. P. Cegielski, "Extensively Drug-Resistant Tuberculosis in the United States, 1993–2007," *Journal of the American Medical Association* 300 (2008): 2153–2160.

93. D. G. McNeil Jr., "Scientists Discover New Cure for the Deadliest Strain of Tuberculosis," *The New York Times*, August 14, 2019.

94. Centers for Disease Control and Prevention, "Public Health Interventions Involving Travelers with Tuberculosis—U.S. Ports of Entry, 2007–2012," *Morbidity and Mortality Weekly Report* 61 (2012): 510–513.

95. Interagency Coordination Group on Antimicrobial Resistance, "No Time to Wait: Securing the Future from Drug-Resistant Infections," Report to the Secretary General of the United Nations, April 2019.

96. R. G. Will, J. W. Ironside, M. Zeidler, S. N. Cousens, K. Estibeiro, A. Alperovitch, et al., "A New Variant of Creutzfeldt–Jakob Disease in the U.K.," *The Lancet* 347 (1996): 921–925.

97. P. G. Smith and S. N. Cousens, "Is the New Variant of Creutzfeldt–Jakob Disease from Mad Cows?" *Science* 273 (1996): 748.

98. Centers for Disease Control and Prevention, "Variant Creutzfeldt–Jacob Disease (vCJD): Risk for Travelers," www.cdc.gov/prions/vcjd/risk-travelers.html, accessed September 9, 2019.

99. Centers for Disease Control and Prevention, "Variant Creutzfeldt–Jacob Disease (vCJD): vCJD Cases Reported in the US," October 9, 2018, www.cdc.gov/prions/vcjd/vcjd-reported.html, accessed September 9, 2019.

100. Centers for Disease Control and Prevention, "Variant Creutzfeldt–Jacob Disease (vCJD): Confirmed Variant Creutzfeldt-Jakob Disease (vCJD) Case in Texas," October 7, 2014, www.cdc.gov/prions/vcjd/news.html, accessed September 9, 2019.

101. Centers for Disease Control and Prevention, "Bovine Spongiform Encephalopathy (BSE), or Mad Cow Disease: About BSE," October 9, 2018, www.cdc.gov/prions/bse/about.html, accessed September 9, 2019.

102. Centers for Disease Control and Prevention, "Bovine Spongiform Encephalopathy (BSE), or Mad Cow Disease: BSE in North America," www.cdc.gov/prions/bse/bse-north-america.html, accessed September 9, 2019.

103. Centers for Disease Control and Prevention, "Prion Diseases," October 9, 2018, www.cdc.gov/prions/index.html, accessed September 9, 2019.

104. Centers for Disease Control and Prevention, "Chronic Wasting Disease (CWD)," February 5, 2019, www.cdc.gov/prions/cwd/index.html, accessed September 9, 2019.

105. R. Karlin, "New York State Acts to Prevent Chronic Wasting Disease in Deer," *Times Union*, August 15, 2019.

106. Institute of Medicine, *Achieving Sustainable Global Capacity for Surveillance and Response to Emerging Diseases of Zoonotic Origin: Workshop Report* (Washington, DC: National Academies Press, 2008).

107. Institute of Medicine, *Microbial Threats to Health: Emergence, Detection, and Response* (Washington, DC: National Academies Press, 2003).

108. C. J. Davis, "Nuclear Blindness: An Overview of the Biological Weapons Programs of the Former Soviet Union and Iraq," *Emerging Infectious Diseases* 5 (2000): 509–512.

109. K. B. Olson, "Aum Shinrikyo: Once and Future Threat?" *Emerging Infectious Diseases* 5 (2000): 513–516.

110. T. J. Torok, "A Large Community Outbreak of Salmonellosis Caused by Intentional Contamination of Restaurant Salad Bars," *Journal of the American Medical Association* 278 (1997): 389–395.

CHAPTER 11

Evolution of the Research Study

The Biomedical Basis of Chronic Diseases

KEY TERMS

Atherosclerosis
Cancer
Cardiovascular disease

Cholesterol
Diabetes
Hypertension

Mutation

The early successes of public health against infectious diseases led to a change in the major causes of illness and death beginning in the 1920s. Chronic degenerative diseases, especially heart disease and cancer, are now the leading causes of death in the United States. While they are primarily diseases of old age—when everyone must die of something—they also strike people in their prime, robbing them of productive years of life. Cancer is the leading cause of death among Americans aged 45 to 65, and cardiovascular disease runs a close second. Cardiovascular disease kills the most people overall. Other significant diseases of current public health concern include diabetes, arthritis, and Alzheimer's disease, which may not be as deadly in the short run but have severe impacts on the quality of life. It is the mission of public health to prevent such premature death and disability.

Prevention of disease usually requires some understanding of the cause, a requirement that is generally much more difficult to fulfill for chronic diseases than for infectious ones. No single pathogen causes cancer or heart disease, nor is a single agent responsible for arthritis, diabetes, or Alzheimer's disease. In most cases, chronic diseases have multiple causes, making it more difficult for scientists to recognize significant risk factors and establish preventive measures. Moreover, these diseases tend to develop over long periods of time, further complicating the task of pinning down their causes. In some cases, however, the gradual onset provides the advantage of early detection, permitting secondary prevention—interventions early in the disease process that can mitigate its impact.

As chronic degenerative diseases became a growing problem during the 20th century, scientists began to focus on efforts to understand their causes. The growth of the National Institutes of Health (NIH), which sponsors most biomedical research in the United States, has reflected the growth of concern about these diseases. In its early days as a one-room Laboratory of Hygiene that opened in 1887, the NIH conducted research primarily on infectious diseases. Congress created the National Cancer Institute in 1937 and the Heart Institute—now called the National Heart, Lung, and Blood Institute (NHLBI)—in 1948. Currently, there are 27 different institutes and centers within the NIH, each focused on a different organ or problem, mostly chronic diseases. One institute, for example, is concerned with arthritis, one with diabetes, and one with neurologic disorders and stroke.

Research into the causes of chronic disease, like research into the causes of infectious disease, relies on epidemiologic methods and laboratory research, which usually includes studies of animals as models, or stand-ins for human patients. The importance of research on animal models to the understanding of human disease cannot be overemphasized. Epidemiology is generally limited to observation and analysis of events that occur spontaneously. Ethical concerns severely limit the experiments that can be done on humans. By contrast, in experiments on laboratory animals, scientists can carefully control the conditions so that cause-and-effect relationships can be clearly proven. Mice and rats are the most commonly used laboratory animals; as mammals, they share the majority of biochemical and physiological processes with humans. Because of their short lifespans, the effects of various exposures and interventions can be studied over the lifetime of the animals. However, mammals can differ in unpredictable ways in their susceptibility to infectious or toxic agents. Different experimental animals have proven useful for studying different diseases, and extrapolation of results from any particular mammal to humans is not always valid.

The identification of an animal model can significantly improve progress toward understanding a disease. It is not always easy to find an experimental animal that is susceptible to the disease a researcher wishes to study. For instance, there is no good animal model for acquired immunodeficiency syndrome (AIDS), a fact that has hampered progress in developing drug therapies or vaccines. Asian macaque monkeys, which can be made sick by exposing them to simian immunodeficiency virus, a relative of human immunodeficiency virus (HIV), are the closest substitute. Only chimpanzees can be infected with HIV, and chimps are no longer used for research for ethical reasons and cost.[1] Animals also differ in how they metabolize some chemicals; a dose of dioxin that would kill a guinea pig has no effect on a mouse or rat, and it is difficult from this evidence to predict the chemical's toxicity to humans.

Scientists have been increasingly successful in devising methods of growing cells and tissues in laboratory glassware for studying biomedical processes. Such laboratory cultures are commonly used to investigate the cancer-causing potential of various chemicals. Much of the research on HIV has been done using cultured human cells, and a great deal has been learned from these investigations. However, such experiments provide oversimplified conditions that may lead to invalid conclusions about the complex interactions that occur in intact animals. In the case of HIV, for example, a number of drugs that appeared to inactivate the virus in test-tube experiments have proved ineffective in human patients.

Cardiovascular Disease

Cardiovascular disease encompasses two of the three leading causes of death in the United States: heart disease and stroke. The risk for dying from cardiovascular disease increases with age, is higher in men than in women, and is higher in blacks than in whites.

The causes of cardiovascular disease have been relatively well established through epidemiologic studies, including the Framingham Study, which identified high blood cholesterol, high blood pressure, and smoking as major risk factors. Animal experiments and examination of the bodies of people who have died of the disease have also contributed to an understanding of how it develops. Knowledge about cardiovascular disease has been facilitated by its high prevalence in the United States and the fact that it follows a similar progression in many patients. The important role of blood components in determining individual risk was readily established because blood is easy to study; it can be drawn from patients and experimental subjects without major discomfort or ethical objections.

It has been known for decades that **atherosclerosis**—hardening of the arteries—is part of the development of cardiovascular disease. Pathologists performing autopsies on people who died of heart attacks found, within the inner-wall lining of the deceased's arteries, a buildup of plaque composed of fat and cholesterol, blood cells, and clotting materials. The formation of plaque begins at an early age in the United States. Fatty streaks, the first stage in the development of plaque, have been found on autopsy in half the children aged 10 to 14 who died of accidental causes.[2] A classic study, published in 1955, examined the arteries of American soldiers killed in the Korean War and found that 77% of the men, whose average age was 22, showed some signs of atherosclerosis.[3] More recent studies have confirmed these findings and have shown that plaque is more likely to be found in individuals with risk factors such as smoking, hypertension, obesity, and high levels of low-density lipoprotein cholesterol.[4]

Animal studies showed that diet plays a role in the formation of plaque. Rabbits fed milk, meat, and eggs instead of their normal vegetarian diet were found to develop atherosclerotic plaque very similar to that observed in humans.[5] More recently, cohort studies of humans have shown directly that diets rich in fruits and vegetables reduce the risk of atherosclerosis and heart disease.[6] It is therefore easy to deduce that the typical American diet, which is heavy in animal products and light in plant-based produce, contributes significantly to the high rate of cardiovascular disease in the United States.

Experiments on rats, rabbits, and monkeys have clarified the process by which high cholesterol and fat in the blood interact with other risk factors such as smoking, high blood pressure, and diabetes to form plaque in the arteries. These factors cause chronic injury of the artery's inner wall, which the body attempts to repair, leading to a "healing" process that runs wild, becoming a disease in itself. The higher the levels of cholesterol and other fats in the blood, the more they are incorporated into the scab-like buildup, and the faster the plaque forms. A heart attack or stroke results when the plaque ruptures, releasing clots that may block an artery in the heart or brain, cutting off the blood supply.[7]

Recent evidence suggests that atherosclerosis may also have an infectious component, caused by bacteria that are often found in plaque.[8] The blood cells in plaque are characteristic of an immune response, and a number of chemicals in the blood suggest that atherosclerosis is an inflammatory condition like arthritis. These findings may lead to new approaches to prevention, diagnosis, and treatment of atherosclerosis.

With the major risk factors for cardiovascular disease well established, much of the recent epidemiologic and biomedical research has focused on trying to understand what determines the relative presence or absence of these risk factors. A great deal has been learned about the various lipids (fats) in the blood, each of which plays a distinct role in an individual's risk of cardiovascular disease, and how their concentrations may be increased or decreased. Factors that affect blood pressure have also been extensively studied. Diabetes, which has its own research institute at NIH, greatly increases the risk of cardiovascular disease (see the discussion of the biomedical basis of diabetes later in the chapter). All of these risk factors are determined in part by genetics, but they can be significantly modified by individual behavior and, therefore, are susceptible to public health intervention.

High blood **cholesterol** is a well-known risk factor for atherosclerosis and heart disease. Cholesterol levels of 200 mg/dL (milligrams per deciliter of blood) or less are considered desirable: Persons with that level of cholesterol have less than one-half the heart attack risk of those with levels greater than 240 mg/dL.[9] Most of the cholesterol in the blood is bound up with protein in various forms, and some forms are more harmful than others. For example, if a high percentage of a person's cholesterol is in the form of high-density lipoprotein (HDL), sometimes called "good cholesterol," the person's risk of heart disease is much lower than that of someone with a high percentage of cholesterol in the form of low-density lipoprotein (LDL), "bad cholesterol." Many current studies try to identify factors that affect not only total cholesterol, but also the relative concentrations of HDL and LDL.

Although previous expert advice called for people to limit their consumption of eggs and other cholesterol-containing foods, recent evidence suggests that cholesterol-containing foods are not the source of cholesterol in the blood. Instead, the greater concern is saturated fat and trans fat, as well as a deficiency of fruit and vegetables. In humans, as in rabbits, vegetarians have lower cholesterol levels than do meat eaters. Vigorous exercise lowers total cholesterol and increases HDL. Some other dietary substances, such as fish, olive oil, and whole grains, also appear to have favorable effects on blood lipids. Smoking lowers HDL levels. Genes play an important role in the HDL–LDL balance. Some people can eat lots of fat yet experience very few effects on their blood cholesterol, while others must work much harder to maintain favorable levels.

In the past few decades, the use of cholesterol-lowering drugs called statins has increased dramatically. The number of Americans who took these drugs grew from approximately 11 million in 1999 to 43 million in 2014.[10,11] Epidemiologic studies have clearly shown that statins can prevent heart attacks, even in people with cholesterol levels previously considered normal. For the most part, these agents appear to be safe for long-term use. However, from a public health perspective, the trend toward prescribing drugs for healthy people to take for the rest of their lives is troubling when lifestyle changes may sometimes accomplish the desired outcome. Moreover, certain statins can be expensive. As a spokesman for the American Heart Association noted, "If you're going to increase my health insurance because my next door neighbor has borderline high cholesterol, and if he's sitting around and watching TV and eating and getting fat, do you want me to pay for that?"[11]

Although the availability of statins appears to be good news for secondary prevention in people who already have atherosclerosis or who have risk factors that put them at high risk, the preferable public health approach to preventing heart disease is primary prevention. This means promoting healthy behavior, including exercise, not smoking, and eating a healthy diet. Unfortunately, eating a healthy diet is not always easy in American society.

High blood pressure—**hypertension**—is a major risk factor for cardiovascular disease, especially stroke, contributing to the injury in the artery walls that is part of atherosclerosis. It also increases the risk of kidney disease. While some medical conditions are known to cause high blood pressure, the exact cause in most cases is unknown; such individuals are said to have "essential hypertension." Factors that have been associated with essential hypertension include obesity, smoking, lack of exercise, excess dietary salt, and stress. In the United States, 140/90 mm Hg has long been considered the borderline level, above which blood pressure is considered too high. In this reading, 140 is the systolic pressure, the pressure exerted by the blood on the artery walls during the heart's contraction when the pressure is greatest. The diastolic pressure—90, in this case—occurs between contractions, when the heart is relaxed. New evidence prompted the

NHLBI to issue guidelines in 2003 that classified blood pressure as "normal" only if it is below 120/80 mm Hg. Pressures between this level and 140/90 mm Hg were to be classified as "prehypertension," meaning that individuals with these readings are at risk of developing hypertension.[12] A more recent cohort study of approximately 4500 participants found that over a 22-year period, the risk of cardiovascular events such as heart attack, stroke, or death was no higher in participants with systolic pressure between 120 mm Hg and 140 mm Hg than those whose pressure was below 120 mm Hg. The authors concluded that it is most important for people to keep their systolic pressure below 140 mm Hg.[13] Then, in 2015, the NHLBI announced that a new study of more than 9300 older men and women had been halted early because it clearly showed that 120 mm Hg was a safer upper limit for systolic pressure. The researchers found that risks of heart attack, heart failure, or stroke were reduced by one-third among subjects assigned to reach a pressure of 120 mm Hg or below compared with those assigned a target of 140 mm Hg or below. Risk of death was reduced by one-fourth at the lower limit.[14] Based on the emerging evidence, the American Heart Association issued new blood pressure guidelines in 2017, specifying levels between 120 and 129 mm Hg as "elevated," with a recommendation of lifestyle changes, and levels of 130 mm Hg and above as the new cutoff for high blood pressure, which requires treatment with lifestyle changes and oftentimes medication.[15]

The U.S. government launched a major blood pressure awareness program in 1972; since then, the annual rate of fatal strokes has been cut by more than half, to an age-standardized death rate from stroke of 73 per 100,000 people in 2015.[16] Many people can keep their blood pressure under control by eating a healthy diet, exercising, and abstaining from smoking—the same behaviors that promotes healthy cholesterol levels. Secondary prevention is also important: People should know their own blood pressure and take appropriate measures, including drugs, if it is too high.

Dietary salt (sodium chloride) is believed to be a factor in causing some cases of essential hypertension, but sensitivity to salt is variable and probably determined by genetics. Laboratory studies have found that some strains of rats get high blood pressure when fed large amounts of salt, whereas other strains of rats do not seem to react to salt. Rats of one sensitive strain tend to have strokes when subjected to salt and stress, while rats of some other strains are unaffected.[17] Nevertheless, the question of whether salt-restriction measures would reduce blood pressure in the average person is controversial. Some researchers have argued that high dietary salt damages the heart and kidneys even in people with normal blood pressure.[18] The Department of Health and Human Services recommends that individuals limit their salt intake to 2300 mg per day, or about one teaspoon, a level that most Americans exceed.[19]

At a population level, it is clear that hypertension has a higher prevalence in groups that consume greater amounts of sodium, and that sodium intake is higher in the United States than in many other countries. The prevalence of hypertension in the United States is high: One in three adults has high blood pressure, and approximately 65% of those age 60 or older have it.[20,21] In turn, public health experts have noted that reducing the amount of salt in the American diet would be expected to reduce the prevalence of hypertension. They estimate that, for example, if the average systolic blood pressure could be reduced by five points, mortality due to stroke would be reduced by 14%. Because Americans tend to get most of their salt from packaged foods and restaurant meals, the American Public Health Association, together with an interagency committee coordinated by NHLBI, recommended in 2003 that the food industry, including manufacturers and restaurants, reduce sodium in the food supply.[12] Since then, modest reductions in sodium intake have been observed among some groups of Americans.[22]

Smoking is believed to increase the risk of cardiovascular disease through the actions of two components of tobacco smoke: nicotine and carbon monoxide. Nicotine, the addictive component of tobacco, is a stimulant that raises blood pressure, increases the pulse rate, stimulates release of stress hormones, and increases irritability of the heart and blood vessels. Carbon monoxide, a poisonous gas, binds to hemoglobin in the blood, blocking the hemoglobin's ability to carry oxygen throughout the body. Both nicotine and carbon monoxide place stress on the heart and blood vessels, with the long-term effect of contributing to atherosclerosis. In the short term, nicotine and carbon monoxide can provoke irregularities in heartbeat, which may result in sudden death.

Tobacco is especially significant as a cause of heart attack in younger adults. Although heart attacks are relatively rare among people in their 30s and 40s, those that do occur are likely to be caused by smoking. One epidemiologic study found that smokers in this age group have a five times greater rate of heart attacks compared to nonsmokers.[23]

Cancer

Cancer has proved much more difficult to understand than cardiovascular disease, in part because it has so many different manifestations. It is sometimes said that cancer is not one disease, but rather 100 diseases. In many ways, breast cancer is different from lung cancer, which is different from leukemia. These diseases typically differ in terms of risk factors, appearance under a microscope, response to various forms of treatment, and so forth. For the biomedical scientist and the public health professional trying to understand the cause and prevention of cancer, each kind of cancer must be studied separately. What all cancers have in common is that they arise when the activities of a cell are transformed and the cell begins to grow out of control.

Understanding cancer, therefore, requires understanding normal cell function, so that it is possible to recognize what goes wrong in a cancer cell. In general, a normal cell turns cancerous through a **mutation** in the body's genetic material, DNA—usually a mutation in one of the genes that regulate cell growth and differentiation. When that cell divides, the mutation is transmitted to the daughter cells, which, because of the disruption in control caused by the mutation, tend to divide more rapidly than normal. As the cells continue to divide abnormally, errors tend to occur as the DNA is copied, leading to additional mutations and more abnormalities in the cells that are becoming a tumor.[24,25] Other changes that may accompany the formation of a tumor include the stimulation of the growth of blood vessels that feed the tumor and the tendency to metastasize—a process by which cancer cells detach from the main tumor and spread to distant parts of the body. Understanding the molecular mechanisms through which tumors form and grow can lead to the development of effective therapies, specific approaches to halting the process or killing the cancerous cells.

To achieve the public health goal of preventing disease, it is important to know what causes the mutations that initiate the cancer. It turns out that mutations in DNA can be caused by many different types of agents, including chemicals, viruses, and radiation. Other factors, such as hormones and diet, play a role in determining whether a mutation progresses to the development of a tumor. Hormones, which function in the body to either stimulate or inhibit cell growth, may have an enhanced effect on a mutated cell. The mechanisms by which dietary factors influence the development of cancer are less well understood—although some foods may contain carcinogens, or cancer-causing chemicals. Some evidence indicates that dietary fiber protects against some cancers, perhaps because it speeds the passage of possible carcinogens through the digestive tract, lessening the likelihood that they will be absorbed. High fat in the diet increases the risk of many forms of cancer, but it is not clear why. Conversely, diets high in fruits and vegetables seem to be protective against cancer.

Exposure to certain kinds of radiation has long been known to cause cancer in humans. Many of the early scientists who unsuspectingly worked with radioactive materials died of the disease, including Marie Curie, the Nobel Prize winner who discovered radium. Curie died of leukemia in 1934 at age 66.[26] Laboratory studies demonstrated clearly that ionizing radiation was capable of damaging DNA and causing mutations in all forms of life, from bacteria to plants to mammals. Later, exposure to certain chemicals was observed to cause some of the same kinds of genetic damage as did radiation, and many of these same chemicals could be demonstrated to cause cancer in laboratory animals.

Viruses have long been known to cause some cancers in plants and animals, but only recently have some human cancers, including liver cancer and cervical cancer, been shown to be of viral origin. Cancer viruses transform cells by integrating themselves into the host cell's DNA; the viral genes may override the host's genes, for example, by turning on inappropriate cell division. In fact, viruses that cause cancer in humans have been found to carry altered forms of human genes.

The knowledge gained by studying cancer viruses has helped scientists to understand more generally how mutation of the cell's own genes can turn a normal cell into a cancer cell by inappropriately turning on cell division. Some of the genes that, when mutated, lead to cancer—known as oncogenes—stimulate cell division; others, known as tumor suppressor genes, normally function to keep cell division turned off. The new genetic understanding of cancer causation also helps explain why some families are more susceptible to some kinds of cancer.

In most cases more than a single mutation is required before a cell is fully malignant, so a member of a family that carries one mutation in a gene might need only one additional event to develop a tumor.

The public health approach to primary prevention of cancer is to prevent human exposure to the agents that cause mutation. In the case of ionizing radiation, whose danger was recognized early, government standards have been developed to protect the population against exposure from various sources such as nuclear power plants, medical and dental x-rays, and radon gas. Sunlight, another proven cause of cancer, cannot be regulated: Education in the importance of applying sunscreen and wearing hats is the favored approach. Because viruses have only recently been recognized to cause cancer in humans, the public health response to these agents is evolving. Immunization is one approach: Hepatitis B vaccination is now recommended for all children, not only to prevent acute hepatitis infection but also because chronic infection with hepatitis B virus has been shown to lead to liver cancer. A vaccine against human papillomavirus (HPV) became available in 2006 and has been shown to be effective in preventing cervical cancer. Since its introduction, the rate of HPV infection among American young women has plummeted, falling by two-thirds for one primary strain of the virus and by one-third for the other primary strain.[27] The HPV vaccine is controversial, however, because it must be given to young girls and boys before they become sexually active.

The extent to which chemicals in the environment cause cancer is one of the most difficult and controversial questions in public health. The tars in tobacco smoke are clearly a major cause, and the American Cancer Society estimates that almost one-third of cancer deaths in the United States are due to tobacco use.[28] In addition to being the major cause of lung cancer, smoking increases the risk of cancer in many other organs, including the mouth, lips, nose and sinuses, larynx, pharynx, esophagus, stomach, pancreas, kidney, bladder, uterus, cervix, colon and rectum, and ovary, and some kinds of leukemia. Although Americans are greatly concerned about the possibility of cancer-causing chemicals in their food, water, or air, little is known about whether these sources contribute significantly to the number of cases diagnosed each year. Most industrial chemicals have not been tested for carcinogenicity. Chemicals added to food, however, must be tested.

The testing of chemicals for carcinogenicity in humans is fraught with difficulties. The standard, most definitive approach is a controlled experiment in which a large group of rats, mice, or guinea pigs is fed a diet containing the suspect chemical over their whole lifetime—about two years for these animals—and the incidence of tumors in this group is compared with that in an equivalent group of animals that did not receive the chemical. If the exposed animals have more tumors than the unexposed animals, the chemical is labeled a carcinogen. Aside from the potential frustration of the experiment by some unpredictable factor—for example, an outbreak of mouse flu that kills off all the animals after the first year, necessitating a new start—there are many reasons why this approach may not accurately predict carcinogenicity in humans. Differences in metabolism between mice and humans sometimes mean differences in carcinogenicity of a chemical in the two species; or the dose of the chemical necessary to produce a detectable increase in tumors may be so high that it disrupts the animals' metabolism, making the results meaningless.

Another approach to determining carcinogenicity—one that is much faster, simpler, and cheaper—is to test whether the chemical can cause mutations in a colony of cells growing in a laboratory dish. This test has its own drawbacks. While mutation is necessary for the development of cancer, not all chemicals that cause mutations are carcinogens. These test-tube experiments ignore the role of hormones and other secondary influences that determine whether a mutated cell will actually grow into a tumor.

Diabetes

The number of Americans diagnosed with diabetes has been rising rapidly, having increased from 1% in 1965 to 3% in 1995 to more than 7% today.[29] Officially, diabetes ranks seventh overall as a cause of death in the United States; it is fourth among American Indians and fifth among blacks, Hispanics, and Asians.[30] However, there are reasons to believe that diabetes contributes to premature death more often than is reported by death certificates. Examinations of death certificates of people known to have diabetes have found that only 35% to 40% of them had diabetes listed anywhere on the certificate. Many deaths listed as caused by heart disease may be linked with diabetes. Heart disease death rates are two to four times higher for people with diabetes than for those without it. Overall, the risk of death for people with diabetes is double the risk for people of the same age who do not have diabetes.[31]

Diabetes is a major cause of disability. Although it is usually treatable and can be controlled over long periods of time, public health has generally been able to do little to prevent the disease except make unpopular recommendations for changes in lifestyle. The Centers for Disease Control and Prevention has referred to the twin epidemics of diabetes and obesity: Obesity greatly increases the risk of diabetes, and the number of Americans who are obese has been increasing rapidly.[32]

Diabetes is a deficiency in the body's ability to metabolize sugar, a function that is normally controlled by the hormone insulin. There are two major forms of diabetes: type 1 and type 2. Type 1 diabetes, which usually has its onset in childhood, is caused by a failure of the insulin-producing cells of the pancreas. In contrast, type 2 diabetes, which is more common with increasing age, involves a more complex mix of impaired insulin production and resistance to the hormone's action. Both forms of diabetes are significantly affected by genetics. Research on the causes of diabetes has thus far yielded very little information on how type 1 diabetes could be prevented. Type 2 is closely correlated with obesity, and is largely preventable with proper diet and exercise. However, public health has not been very successful in persuading most people to adopt such healthy behaviors, which could prevent a number of other chronic diseases as well.

While public health practitioners may not be able to prevent diabetes, they are concerned with preventing the disability that inevitably occurs when the disease is not well controlled. An estimated one out of four people with diabetes are unaware of their disease.[26] This is a major public health problem because the high blood sugar that is typical of uncontrolled diabetes causes damage to blood vessels throughout the body, especially the eyes and kidneys. Complications of diabetes include blindness, kidney failure, cardiovascular disease, poor wound healing, and amputations of the extremities. Secondary prevention requires early diagnosis of the disease so that treatment can begin at an early stage. Lack of access to routine medical care—a common problem in the United States—contributes to the seriousness of diabetes as a public health problem. The necessary long-term monitoring and treatment required to manage a case of diabetes can be complicated and expensive, and those who need it the most may have the greatest difficulty in receiving care.

Other Chronic Diseases

There is much more to learn about other diseases that have a major impact on the health of the population. Mental illness is a major cause of disability in the United States, yet very little is known about its causes and prevention. Alzheimer's disease and other forms of dementia in older people cause anguish to their families and force affected people into nursing homes at a tremendous cost to society. The NIH and other funding sources are supporting a great deal of research on understanding genetic and other factors that affect people's risk of developing dementia as they age, but not much is known yet on how people can protect themselves. Arthritis, while not a major killer, can severely impact the quality of life for many older people, causing great pain and suffering in their last years.

Conclusion

Chronic diseases are the leading causes of death and disability in the United States, with cardiovascular diseases and cancer leading the list. Diabetes is becoming increasing prevalent and is a major cause of disability. Preventing these diseases—an important public health priority—requires understanding their causes. The success of biomedical science and epidemiology in revealing the causes of cardiovascular disease and ways to prevent or delay its onset serves as a model for what society would hope to achieve for all the diseases that cause premature death or disability. Progress in understanding the functioning of normal cells and what goes wrong when they turn malignant has given researchers hope that they will eventually learn to prevent many kinds of cancer.

Despite the tremendous progress made by biomedical science in the understanding of the bases of chronic diseases, a great deal is left to learn about what can go wrong with the human body and how to prevent it. People cannot expect to live forever, and perhaps would not wish to do so, but biomedical research holds the key to preventing many premature deaths, as well as much of the pain and anguish that many people suffer toward the end of their lives. Because it offers such hope, NIH's work is generally well supported by the U.S. Congress and the American people.

References

1. J. Cohen, "Monkey Puzzles," *Science* 296 (2002): 2325–2326.

2. R. Ross, "The Pathogenesis of Atherosclerosis: A Perspective for the 1990s," *Nature* 362 (1993): 801–809.

3. W. F. Enos Jr., J. C. Beyer, and R. H. Holmes, "Pathogenesis of Coronary Disease in American Soldiers Killed in Korea," *Journal of the American Medical Association* 158 (1955): 912–914.

4. National Institutes of Health, "Who Is at Risk for Atherosclerosis," https://www.nhlbi.nih.gov/health-topics/atherosclerosis, accessed September 5, 2019.

5. S. J. Dudrick, P. R. Adams, D. M. Englert, and A. S. Feste, "Experimental and Clinical Atherosclerosis: Their Experimental Reversal," *Transactions and Studies of the College of Physicians of Philadelphia* 10 (1988): 35–61.

6. X. Wang, Y. Ouyang, J. Liu, M. Zhu, G. Zhao, W. Bao, and F. B. Hu, "Fruit and Vegetable Consumption and Mortality from All Causes, Cardiovascular Disease, and Cancer: Systematic Review and Dose–Response Meta-Analysis of Prospective Cohort Studies," *British Medical Journal* 349 (2014): g4490.

7. D. J. Rader and A. Daugherty, "Translating Molecular Discoveries into New Therapies for Atherosclerosis," *Nature* 451 (2008): 904–913.

8. C. L. Alviar, J. G. Echeverri, N. I. Jaramillo, C. J. Figueroa, J. P. Cordova, A. Korniyenko, et al., "Infectious Atherosclerosis: Is the Hypothesis Still Alive? A Clinically Based Approach to the Dilemma," *Medical Hypotheses* 78 (2011): 517–521.

9. National Heart Lung and Blood Institute, "High Blood Cholesterol: What You Need to Know," June 2005, https://www.nhlbi.nih.gov/files/docs/public/heart/wyntk.pdf, accessed September 9, 2019.

10. E. J. Topol, "Intensive Statin Therapy: A Sea Change in Cardiovascular Prevention," *New England Journal of Medicine* 350 (2004): 1562–1564.

11. Centers for Disease Control and Prevention, "Half of Those Who Need Them Not Taking Cholesterol-Lowering Medications," https://www.cdc.gov/media/releases/2015/p1203-cholesterol-medicine.html, accessed September 5, 2019.

12. A. V. Chobanian, G. L. Bakris, H. R. Black, W. C. Cushman, L. A. Green, J. L. Izzo Jr, et al., "Seventh Report of the Joint Commission on Prevention, Detection, Evaluation, and Treatment of High Blood Pressure," *Hypertension* 42 (2003): 1206–1252.

13. C. J. Rodriguez, K. Swett, S. K. Agarwal, A. R. Folsom, E. R. Fox, L. R. Loehr, et al., "Systolic Blood Pressure Levels Among Adults with Hypertension and Incident Cardiovascular Events: The Atherosclerosis Risk in Communities Study," *Journal of the American Medical Association Internal Medicine* 174 (2014): 1252–1261.

14. Sprint Research Group, "A Randomized Trial of Intensive Versus Standard Blood-Pressure Control," *New England Journal of Medicine* 373 (2015): 2103–2116.

15. P. Whelton et al., "2017 ACC/AHA/AAPA/ABC/ACPM/AGS/APhA/ASH/ASPC/NMA/PCNA Guideline for the Prevention, Detection, Evaluation, and Management of High Blood Pressure in Adults: A Report of the American College of Cardiology/American Heart Association Task Force on Clinical Practice Guidelines," *Journal of the American College of Cardiology* 71, no. 19 (2018): e127–e248.

16. Q. Yang, X. Tong, L. Schieb, et al., "Vital Signs: Recent Trends in Stroke Death Rates—United States, 2000–2015," *Morbidity and Mortality Weekly Report* 66 (2017): 933–939.

17. J. J. Nora, K. Berg, and A. H. Nora, *Cardiovascular Diseases: Genetics, Epidemiology, and Prevention* (New York, NY: Oxford University Press, 1991).

18. E. D. Frohlich, "The Salt Conundrum: A Hypothesis," *Hypertension* 50 (2007): 161–166.

19. Centers for Disease Control and Prevention, "Get the Facts: Sodium and Dietary Guidelines," https://www.cdc.gov/salt/pdfs/sodium_dietary_guidelines.pdf, accessed September 5, 2019.

20. Y. S. Oh, L. S. Appel, Z. S. Galis, D. A. Hafler, J. He, A. L. Hernandez, et al., "National Heart, Lung, and Blood Institute Working Group Report on Salt in Human Health and Sickness: Building on the Current Scientific Evidence," *Hypertension* 68 (2016): 281–288.

21. Centers for Disease Control and Prevention, "Health, United States, 2017," Table 053, https://www.cdc.gov/nchs/data/hus/2017/053.pdf, accessed September 5, 2019.

22. Centers for Disease Control and Prevention, "Sodium Fact Sheet," https://www.cdc.gov/dhdsp/data_statistics/fact_sheets/fs_sodium.htm, accessed September 5, 2019.

23. S. Parish, R. Collins, R. Peto, L. Youngman, J. Barton, K. Jayne, et al., "Cigarette Smoking, Tar Yields, and Non-fatal Myocardial Infarction," *British Medical Journal* 311 (1995): 471–477.

24. W. K. Cavenee and R. L. White, "The Genetic Basis of Cancer," *Scientific American* (March 1995): 50–57.

25. H. J. Burstein and R. S. Schwartz, "Molecular Origins of Cancer," *New England Journal of Medicine* 358 (2008): 527.

26. *The New Encyclopedia Britannica*, Vol. 3 (Chicago, IL: Encyclopaedia Britannica, 1995), 799.

27. L. E. Markowitz, G. Liu, S. Hariri, M. Steinau, E. F. Dunne, and E. R. Unger, "Prevalence of HPV

After Introduction of the Vaccination Program in the United States," *Pediatrics* 137 (2016).

28. American Cancer Society, "Tobacco and Cancer," http://www.cancer.org/cancer/cancer-causes/tobacco-and-cancer.html, accessed September 9, 2019.

29. Centers for Disease Control and Prevention, "Long-Term Trends in Diabetes," April 2017, https://www.cdc.gov/diabetes/statistics/slides/long_term_trends.pdf, accessed September 5, 2019.

30. Centers for Disease Control and Prevention, "Deaths: Leading Causes for 2017," *National Vital Statistics Reports* 68 (June 24, 2019).

31. Centers for Disease Control and Prevention, "National Diabetes Fact Sheet, 2011," https://www.cdc.gov/diabetes/pubs/pdf/ndfs_2011.pdf, accessed September 9, 2019.

32. Centers for Disease Control and Prevention, "Maps of Trends in Diagnosed Diabetes and Obesity," April 2017, https://www.cdc.gov/diabetes/statistics/slides/maps_diabetesobesity_trends.pdf, accessed September 9, 2019.

CHAPTER 12

Dangerous Genes

Genetic Diseases and Other Inborn Errors

KEY TERMS

Autosomal dominant disorder
Autosomal recessive disorders
Carcinogens
Chromosomes

Genetic diseases
Genomics
Human Genome Project
Newborn screening

Prenatal testing
Teratogens
X-linked disorders

Congenital defects are a major cause of death and disability in infants and children. Approximately 3% of all newborns have a major abnormality apparent at birth.[1] Other problems show up later, with as many as 7.5% of children being diagnosed with a congenital defect in their first five years.[2] Such abnormalities may be inherited in the child's genes, or they may be caused by birth injury or by the mother's exposure to an infectious agent or toxic substance during pregnancy. Genes also play a role in many diseases of later life.

Because the birth of healthy children has traditionally been a high priority for public health, education and prenatal care for pregnant women have been encouraged. As more has been learned about how certain infectious agents, drugs, and chemicals can cause birth defects, greater public health efforts have been directed toward preventing women's exposure to these substances. Until the past few decades, little could be done to prevent genetic abnormalities. Now, however, technological developments have opened up vast possibilities in the detection of defective genes. These discoveries have had many clear benefits, but they have also raised many difficult ethical questions.

Environmental Teratogens

Birth defects may be caused by a variety of environmental agents, called **teratogens**, which include some bacteria and viruses, various drugs and chemicals, and radiation. Many teratogens are also **carcinogens**, capable of causing cancer. In some cases, the teratogenic effect, like the carcinogenic effect, is known to result from a mutation in the DNA. However, much less is known about the disruptions of fetal development that lead to birth defects than is known about carcinogenesis.

Infectious diseases known to damage the fetus include syphilis, rubella (German measles), and toxoplasmosis. Congenital syphilis, caused by bacteria passed from a mother to her fetus through the placenta, was a devastating disease of newborns before penicillin was discovered. This disease damaged the infants' nerves, bones, and skin and often resulted in blindness and mental retardation. Beginning in the 1930s, many states required blood tests for syphilis—the Wasserman test—for all couples about to be married in an effort to identify and treat infected people before they could transmit the disease to a child.[3] Most states have now discontinued that requirement.

Rubella, ordinarily a mild disease of childhood, causes profound deafness in children whose mothers were infected by the virus while pregnant. Routine vaccination of children against rubella accomplishes the longer-term purpose of immunizing childbearing women, and the incidence of congenital deafness has been dramatically reduced. Toxoplasmosis, a parasitic disease that may go unnoticed in adults, can cause major neurologic damage in the fetus. Since cats are a reservoir for the parasite and the route of transmission is most commonly through cat feces, toxoplasmosis is best prevented by education—specifically, by warning pregnant women about the risks of contracting the disease through gardening and contact with litter boxes.

A pregnant woman's exposure to teratogenic drugs and environmental chemicals can have very obvious results because the effects usually become apparent within nine months, dramatically altering a young life. One memorable tragedy occurred in the 1950s at Minamata, Japan, where a plastics factory contaminated the bay with high levels of mercury. A highly toxic form of the mercury accumulated in the fish, the staple of the community's diet. While adults were relatively unaffected, many children were born with severe neurologic deformities, including profound brain damage.[4] The tragedy of Minamata, captured by the famous photographs of W. Eugene Smith

and Aileen M. Smith, accessible on the Internet, alerted the world to the dangers of environmental pollution.[5] Laws controlling air and water pollution and disposal of toxic wastes have been effective in preventing such disasters in the United States, but they continue to occur in other parts of the world, including the former Soviet Union.

Another famous teratogenic event was the epidemic of limb deformities that occurred in Europe and Australia in the early 1960s and was caused by the sedative thalidomide. Women who took the drug to relieve morning sickness gave birth to babies whose arms and legs were drastically shortened into flipper-like appendages.[4] The United States escaped the epidemic because one skeptical Food and Drug Administration (FDA) official, Dr. Frances Kelsey, was suspicious of the drug and resisted great pressure from the manufacturer to approve thalidomide for marketing before the dangers became apparent. In 1998, in a controversial decision, thalidomide was approved by the FDA as an effective treatment for leprosy and some forms of cancer. However, it can be used only under very strict regulations that require women taking it to undergo monthly pregnancy tests and to use two forms of birth control.[6]

One of the FDA's most important missions is to protect American citizens against such tragic side effects of drugs by prohibiting them entirely if their value is not judged to be worth the associated risks or by mandating clear communications about risks when these agents also have clear benefits. The antibiotic tetracycline, the anti-epilepsy drug Dilantin, the hormone diethylstilbestrol (DES), and the acne medication Accutane are among the common prescription drugs that have been found by painful experience to cause birth defects. Pregnant women are now advised to refrain from taking any medication that is not absolutely necessary.

Alcohol was recognized to be a teratogen only in the 1970s. Although most cases of fetal alcohol syndrome have been identified in children of heavy drinkers, no level of alcohol has been judged safe for the fetus, and pregnant women are advised not to drink at all. Tobacco smoke increases the risk of premature birth and low birth weight, as well as sudden infant death syndrome. Cocaine and heroin use by pregnant women causes addiction in the fetus, bringing about painful withdrawal symptoms in the newborn and sometimes leaving permanent neurologic damage.

Genetic Diseases

Essentially all the information required for the development of a new human being is contained in the genetic material located in the fetus's 46 **chromosomes**, half of which come from the mother's egg and half of which come from the father's sperm. Mistakes are common in the reproductive process. The most visible are chromosomal abnormalities, which can be seen under a microscope. Such defects cause a variety of malformations in the developing fetus, many of which are incompatible with survival. More than half of pregnancies in healthy women end in spontaneous abortion, and chromosomal abnormalities are obvious in many of these aborted fetuses.[2] When the affected fetus does survive, the disability is usually profound, almost always including mental retardation and often leading to early death. Down syndrome, caused by an extra copy of chromosome 21, is the best-known disorder of this type, largely because its effects are less lethal than those of other chromosomal defects, so that most affected infants survive.

The majority of **genetic diseases** are caused by defects that are not visible under a microscope. Those that are best known and understood are caused by a defect in a single gene inherited more or less according to classical Mendelian genetics (**Figure 12-1**). The first part of Figure 12-1 shows the pattern of inheritance of a dominant gene. In this case, the father carries the gene for Huntington's disease on one of a pair of chromosomes; the mother

carries two normal genes. Half of the children will inherit the disease from the father. The second part of Figure 12-1 shows the pattern of inheritance of a recessive gene. Both parents carry one recessive gene, but neither parent has symptoms, and the parents may be unaware that they are carriers. One-fourth of the children will inherit two recessive genes and will have the disease. Half of the children will be carriers.

In sum, of the two copies of each gene that an individual inherits, one from each parent, the gene for a disease may be dominant or recessive. When the presence of a single copy is sufficient to cause the disease—an **autosomal dominant disorder**—the affected person will transmit that gene, on average, to half of his or her children. (Autosomal genes are found on a non-sex chromosome.) Examples of autosomal dominant disorders include Huntington's disease, a midlife deterioration of the brain whose best-known victim was the folk singer Woody Guthrie; achondroplasia, a type of dwarfism made famous by the French painter Toulouse-Lautrec; and Marfan syndrome, characterized by extreme height and cardiovascular abnormalities, which occasionally makes the news after the sudden death of an unsuspecting basketball player.[2]

Autosomal recessive disorders do not become obvious unless the individual inherits two copies of the gene. The disease may appear unexpectedly in a child of two parents who were unaware that they each carried one copy of the gene. The best-known autosomal recessive disorders tend to predominate in certain ethnic groups: Tay-Sachs disease in Jews of Eastern European descent, sickle-cell disease in Africans and African Americans, cystic fibrosis in people of northern European ancestry, and thalassemia in populations of Mediterranean or Asian descent.[2]

X-linked disorders, such as hemophilia and Duchenne's muscular dystrophy, are caused by a defective gene on the female sex chromosome, called the X chromosome. These diseases occur predominantly in males. Since

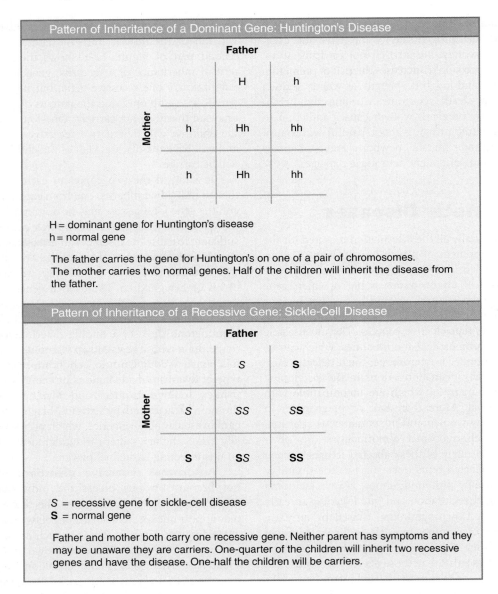

H = dominant gene for Huntington's disease
h = normal gene

The father carries the gene for Huntington's on one of a pair of chromosomes.
The mother carries two normal genes. Half of the children will inherit the disease from
the father.

S = recessive gene for sickle-cell disease
S = normal gene

Father and mother both carry one recessive gene. Neither parent has symptoms and they
may be unaware they are carriers. One-quarter of the children will inherit two recessive
genes and have the disease. One-half the children will be carriers.

Figure 12-1 Mendelian Genetics

females have two X chromosomes, inheritance of the defective gene has minimal impact on them because of the second, normal gene's presence. Males, who inherit an X chromosome from the mother and a Y chromosome from the father, can inherit the disease only from the mother.

While the patterns of inheritance are well established for many genetic diseases, new mutations may sometimes occur, affecting a child whose family has no history of the disease. Many autosomal dominant conditions cause such severe handicaps that the affected individuals are unable or unlikely to reproduce;

for these conditions, the majority of cases arise from mutations. With recessive and X-linked genetic defects, birth of an affected infant into a family that lacks a history of the condition may or may not indicate that a new mutation has occurred. A recessive gene would not be apparent unless someone who carried it had children with another carrier. X-linked genes might not appear for several generations in small families or those in which most of the children happened to be girls.

Some genetic conditions vary in their impact depending on environmental factors. For example, anencephaly—the absence of a brain—and the related spinal-cord defect, spina bifida, appear to be the result of a combination of genetic and environmental factors. The incidence of these disorders has been found to vary by geographic area, a hint that further research will provide evidence that environmental factors are involved. One important finding is that if a woman takes dietary supplements of folic acid before conception and during early pregnancy, her infant's risk of these devastating conditions is substantially reduced.

Genetic makeup also influences people's susceptibility to most of the common diseases of adulthood; most of these diseases involve complex interactions between genes and the environment. Genes for cholesterol and other blood lipids affect an individual's risk of cardiovascular disease. High blood pressure has a genetic component. A variety of genes affect people's risk for various forms of cancer, including breast cancer and colorectal cancer. Susceptibility to diabetes is strongly influenced by genes. Knowing individuals' family health history can help determine whether they need more intensive screening for these diseases.

Mental disorders including schizophrenia, manic depression, and Alzheimer's disease are also believed to be affected by genetics, although the evidence is fragmentary. While it is well known that people with high cholesterol can lower their risk of heart disease or diabetes by exercising, eating a healthier diet, and, if necessary, taking

appropriate medications, current knowledge offers little guidance about how to counteract a family history of Alzheimer's disease or other mental disorders. One can only hope that, with advances in biomedical research, prevention will someday be possible.

Genetic and Newborn Screening Programs

Short of performing surgery on the genetic material, the public health mandate of preventing death and disability from many genetic diseases can be fulfilled only by predicting and preventing the birth of affected children. This process involves various methods of prenatal diagnosis and, when an affected fetus is identified, termination of the pregnancy. One of the most common genetic abnormalities, Down syndrome, is caused by an extra copy of chromosome 21. Affected individuals have a distinctive appearance and are likely to have heart defects and mild to moderate mental retardation. The risk of bearing an infant with the syndrome is well known to increase with the mother's age. Thus, in the past, women age 35 and older were advised to undergo **prenatal testing** by amniocentesis, which involves using a needle to sample fetal cells from the uterus. With the option of abortion available, this practice reduced the number of Down syndrome births by approximately 33%.[7] However, even though younger women have a lower risk, the number of infants born to them is much higher overall, and they bear most of the affected infants. The American College of Obstetricians and Gynecologists currently recommends that all pregnant women be screened.[8] In the United States, nearly 67% of women who are found to be carrying an infant with Down syndrome choose to have an abortion.[9]

Public health has a more significant role in preventing disorders that are caused by recessive genes. When the gene is known, members of populations that have a high incidence of a disease, such as Jews of Eastern European descent, can be screened for carrier status, allowing young people to make informed decisions about marriage and childbearing. In the 1970s, after the gene for Tay-Sachs disease was identified, a major voluntary program offered screening to Jewish people. The response was enthusiastic because the horror of the disease was well known: Apparently healthy infants begin to deteriorate soon after birth, developing paralysis, dementia, and blindness, and they die by age 3 or 4. Couples who are both Tay-Sachs carriers can choose to undergo prenatal testing by amniocentesis, allowing for termination of an affected pregnancy.[10]

However, religious Jews are opposed to abortion. An alternative approach is offered by an organization called Dor Yeshorim, established in the 1980s by a rabbi who had lost four children to Tay-Sachs disease. The organization offers Jewish high school students in the United States, Israel, and other countries blood tests to determine if they are carriers. To maintain anonymity, and to avoid the stigma of being labeled a carrier, each student is given an identification number and a telephone number that couples can call to learn whether they are genetically "compatible." In ultra-orthodox communities that practice arranged marriage, a confidential registry was established that allows matchmakers to avoid arranging marriages between carriers of Tay-Sachs and several other debilitating or lethal genetic diseases.[11] As a result of the availability of screening, the incidence of Tay-Sachs has been reduced by more than 90% in the United States and Canada.[10]

Another public health approach to preventing the death and disability caused by genetic diseases is provided by **newborn screening** for metabolic disorders that can be treated if diagnosed soon after birth. An estimated 5000 of the 4.1 million infants born in the United States each year have a potentially severe or lethal condition for which screening and treatment could prevent many or all of the complications.[12] The first such condition to be recognized was phenylketonuria

(PKU), which was identified as the cause of mental retardation in a significant number of institutionalized adults. Biomedical scientists found that the problem was a genetic inability to metabolize the amino acid phenylalanine, which therefore accumulates in the blood with toxic effects on the brain. They recognized that if affected infants could be identified early, they could be put on a special low-phenylalanine diet, thereby preventing the damage.

Dr. Robert Guthrie, a pediatrician from Buffalo, New York, who is considered the "father of newborn screening," developed a simple, inexpensive test that could diagnose PKU from a drop of a baby's blood placed on a piece of filter paper. Routine newborn screening for PKU began in the 1960s and is now mandated in all states and most developed countries. Before each baby is discharged from the hospital, the blood sample is obtained by a prick of the baby's heel. Filter paper specimens bearing the dried blood spots are sent to state public health laboratories for testing.[13]

A number of other inborn metabolic errors can be identified from testing the same dried drop of blood, and tests for these conditions are mandated by various states depending on the characteristics of their populations. In addition to PKU, all states screen for congenital hypothyroidism, a deficiency of thyroid hormone leading to mental retardation and dwarfism that can be easily treated with regular doses of the hormone. All states now screen for sickle-cell disease, which is prevalent in African American populations, though this program raised ethical issues when first implemented, as discussed later in this chapter. The newborn blood samples are used in some states to identify infants who may have been exposed to the human immunodeficiency virus (HIV) prenatally.

Laboratory tests used for newborn screening have become increasingly more sophisticated. Starting in the 1990s, a method called tandem mass spectrometry was applied to search for more than 20 metabolic disorders in one process, using the dried blood-spot specimen.[14] However, the technical ability to detect these disorders has confronted states with dilemmas of how extensively to implement screening for them. Resources are needed to follow up on an abnormal test result, including further testing to confirm the presence of a disease and counseling of parents and pediatricians about a condition that may be extremely rare. Concerns have also been raised about who is responsible for treating a disease that has been identified through screening. For example, the special diet required for infants with PKU may be considered a food rather than a drug, so that it is not covered by a family's health insurance. For some conditions, no treatment exists. States differ not only on which conditions they screen for, but also on whether parental consent is required before screening, whether a fee is charged, and which services are provided for follow-up.[15]

The information gained from a genetic test or the screening of a newborn is not always so unambiguous as a fatal diagnosis of Tay-Sachs disease or a clear need for a special diet, as in PKU. With many conditions, uncertainties in the test results as well as in the prognosis complicate decision making. For example, cystic fibrosis (CF), which causes abnormal secretions of the lungs, pancreas, and sweat glands, is the among the most common lethal genetic diseases, affecting at least 30,000 Americans. The number of people in the United States living with the disease has been increasing, as their life expectancy has risen dramatically: Fifty years ago, affected children were not expected to live into adolescence, but today the median life expectancy exceeds 46 years.[16] About 1 in 25 Caucasian Americans, the group at highest risk, carries the recessive gene for CF, which has been identified. The screening test, which measures an enzyme in the blood, yields many false positives. Scientists learned that the accuracy of the diagnosis could be improved by following up the enzyme test with a DNA test. As scientists studied the gene, however, they found hundreds of different mutations that could cause CF, and

there seemed to be little correlation between the mutation and the symptoms. While many patients with CF die young of breathing problems associated with thick mucus in the lungs, some individuals identified by genetic tests have much milder symptoms. Although some questions arose about whether to include CF in newborn screening programs, a major clinical trial found that early identification of affected infants helped prevent some of the nutritional deficits and deterioration of lung function suffered by children who were identified only when they developed symptoms at an older age.[17] All states now screen for CF.[16,18]

The identification of the CF gene allows prospective parents to be tested for carrier status, as in Tay-Sachs disease. However, in the case of CF, the implications of the test results are not as clear-cut. Each of the many possible mutations must be tested for individually, and it is not feasible for laboratories to test for all of them. Currently, the accepted approach for white Americans is to test for the 23 most common mutations. Most carrier couples can be identified this way, but there is still a small risk that couples with a normal test result could bear a child with CF. The frequencies of mutations are lower in other ethnic groups, but identification of carriers is less reliable.[19] Scientists are learning more about the relationship between certain mutations and different symptoms, although affected individuals demonstrate significant variability in the severity of their symptoms.

In addition to the conditions that can be identified using the blood spot, the Centers for Disease Control and Prevention (CDC) recommends screening for hearing loss using computerized equipment now available in many hospitals, and 98% of newborns are now screened for such deficits. Congenital hearing loss is found to occur in 1.7 per 1000 births, with about one-third of these cases involving "severe" or "profound" permanent hearing loss in both ears. Approximately half of these cases are thought to be due to genetic mutations, with the other half being attributable to environmental factors, including prenatal drug exposures and infections such as rubella.[20,21]

Because of the state-to-state variations in the number of disorders included in newborn screening programs, a federal advisory committee was created in 2006 to recommend a panel of disorders that all states should include in their newborn screening programs.[18] By 2009, all states had implemented the full screening panel.[22] An additional six conditions have been added since then: severe combined immunodeficiency in 2010, critical congenital heart disease in 2011, Pompe disease in 2015, mucopolysaccharidosis type 1 and X-linked adrenoleukodystrophy in 2016, and spinal muscular atrophy in 2018.[23] **Table 12-1** lists the conditions for which the CDC recommends screening.

Table 12-1 Recommended Newborn Screening Panel and Estimated Number of U.S. Children Who Would Have Been Identified with Disorders in 2006

Disorder	Estimated Number of Cases in 2006
Amino acid disorders	
Classic phenylketonuria (PKU)	215
Maple syrup urine disease	26
Citrullinemia, type I	24
Homocystinuria	11
Argininosuccinic acidemia	7
Tyrosinemia, type I	–
Organic acid metabolism disorders	
3-Methylcrotonyl-CoA carboxylase deficiency	100
Methylmalonic acidemia (methylmalonyl-CoA mutase)	50
Glutaric acidemia type I	38
Isovaleric acidemia	32
Propionic acidemia	15
Methylmalonic acidemia (cobalamin disorders)	12
Beta-ketothiolase deficiency	7
Hydroxymethylglutaric aciduria	3
Multiple carboxylase deficiency	3
Hemoglobinopathies	
Hemoglobin SS (sickle cell anemia)	1,128
Hemoglobin SC (sickle C disease)	484
Hemoglobin S/beta thalassemia	163

Disorder	Estimated Number of Cases in 2006
Fatty acid oxidation disorders	
Medium-chain acyl-CoA dehydrogenase deficiency	239
Carnitine uptake defect	85
Very long-chain acyl-CoA dehydrogenase deficiency	69
Long-chain 3-hydroxyacyl-CoA dehydrogenase deficiency	13
Trifunctional protein deficiency	2
Other disorders	
Hearing loss (2009 data)	5,073
Primary congenital hypothyroidism	2,156
Cystic fibrosis	1,248
Classical galactosemia	224
Congenital adrenal hyperplasia	202
Biotinidase deficiency	62
Critical congenital heart disease	–
Glycogen Storage Disease Type II (Pompe)	–
Severe combined immunodeficiencies	–
Mucopolysaccharidosis Type 1	–
X-linked Adrenoleukodystrophy	–
Spinal Muscular Atrophy due to homozygous deletion of exon 7 in SMN1	–

Disorders listed in italics are those that were added since 2006.

Data from U.S. Department of Health and Human Services, "Recommended Uniform Screening Panel," www.hrsa.gov/advisory-committees/heritable-disorders /rusp/index.html, accessed September 6, 2019; and Centers for Disease Control and Prevention, *Morbidity and Mortality Weekly Report* 61 no. 21 (2012): 390–393.

Genomic Medicine

The science underlying human genetics has made great advances over the past two decades, with important early progress occurring through the federally sponsored **Human Genome Project**, which analyzed the whole of human DNA and mapped the most active parts of the human genome, including 92%

of the genome overall.[24] The successful identification of key genes has enabled many couples cursed with a family heritage of crippling disease to bear a healthy child. Most diseases that arise in later life are more complex, rather than single-gene defects, so the presence or absence of a specific gene does not provide any definite predictions. Nevertheless, an individual's risks of developing some cancers, heart disease, diabetes, Alzheimer's disease, and other major afflictions of adulthood are closely tied to his or her genetic makeup. Knowledge of the genes can potentially provide benefits in preventing the diseases as well as better treatments when the individual becomes sick with one of these diseases later in life. The study of how genes act in the body, and how they interact with environmental influences to cause disease, is called **genomics**, a science that promises to transform the prospects of medical practice and has major implications for public health.

Identifying genetic risks early in life can bring many potential benefits. For example, scientists are investigating ways to prevent the onset of type 1 diabetes in children whose genes put them at high risk for this disease. Antibodies detectable in the blood of these children attack and ultimately destroy the insulin-producing cells of the pancreas, but there is hope of disrupting this process with appropriate drugs or immune modifiers. If these experiments are successful, diabetes risk could be included in newborn screening programs, and treatment could avert the need for lifelong insulin therapy and lifestyle modifications.[25]

Genes have already been identified that significantly increase a woman's risk of breast cancer. The *BRCA1* and *BRCA2* genes can be screened for, but they account for a relatively small percentage of breast cancer cases; these genes also increase the risk of ovarian cancer. Genetic screening may benefit women who have a family history of breast cancer, especially when the cancer occurs at an early age, as tends to happen with inherited *BRCA* mutations. Women who inherit these mutations are advised to undergo more intensive and frequent breast exams than average and to begin this screening when they are younger. The most effective intervention currently available for *BRCA* carriers is the surgical removal of a woman's breasts and ovaries. The actresses Christina Applegate and Angelina Jolie, for example, had double mastectomies after testing

positive for the *BRCA1* gene.[26] Scientists hope that, in the future, a better understanding of the genes' actions may lead to less drastic therapy.[27]

Scientists have mapped hundreds of millions of places along the human genome where individuals or populations may differ in a base pair,[28] known as single-nucleotide polymorphisms (SNPs). Numerous studies are under way to find links between specific SNPs and risks of various diseases. In most cases, the difference in risk is relatively small—though this has not stopped companies from trying to patent and commercialize tests based on these SNPs. About a decade ago, several companies, such as 23andMe, started offering "gene profiles," promising that customers who sent a cheek swab and a fee would receive information on their risk of diseases such as diabetes, heart disease, and various forms of cancer. Since then, the FDA has imposed stricter regulation of these services, limiting the health information component, although other countries, including Canada and United Kingdom, now allow this reporting to consumers.

Most knowledgeable scientists believe that these promises are overblown, for several reasons.[29] First, because these tests are not regulated, their validity and accuracy are unreliable. Second, the science of predicting susceptibility to complex diseases based on the presence of specific genes is still at an early stage. The tests do a poor job of distinguishing people who will actually develop the disease from those who will not. Third, these tests raise the question of what can be done for a person who has been found at increased risk. Some sources argue that knowledge of an increased susceptibility to a disease might motivate people to practice a healthier lifestyle. For example, a person with a genetic susceptibility to lung cancer might be more likely to quit smoking, or individuals at risk of diabetes might increase their physical activity. However, little evidence supports that people really do respond in this way. Certainly, a concerned individual would be better off spending his money on a gym membership than on a genetic profile. From a public health perspective, it makes more sense to promote healthy behaviors for everyone.[30]

Findings from the Human Genome Project have had major implications for the use of drugs in the treatment of diseases. A great deal is being learned about how genes affect the metabolism of various drugs. For some time, researchers have known that different individuals may respond to some drugs in different ways. Medicines that are dramatically effective in some patients may be ineffective in others with the same disease and may cause major side effects in still others. It is becoming possible to predict which patients will respond to a drug and even to determine which patients may require higher or lower doses of the drug than others. Scientists are also able to design drugs for specific patients depending on their genetic makeup. Cancer therapy is especially suitable for targeted drug therapy: Already there have been successes in blocking tumor growth using specially designed drugs that attack cellular mechanisms specific to certain mutations. The lives of patients with leukemia, gastric cancer, melanoma, and colon cancer have been extended with such drugs.[31]

Even more promising are the possibilities of "genetic engineering"—that is, the prospect of "fixing" faulty genes, so that affected individuals can lead healthy lives. For example, researchers have been working to cure PKU, the genetic disorder that causes patients to be unable to break down a by-product of dietary protein called phenylalanine. The gene therapy approach of inserting working versions of the defective gene, called *PAH*, into patients' cells, has so far been unsuccessful. By comparison, a synthetic biology approach has shown more promise. Researchers have now bioengineered a harmless strain of *Escherichia coli* bacteria, which most people already have in their intestinal tract, by inserting new genes that allow the bacteria to break down phenylalanine. Patients drink a shake filled with these *E. coli*, which then take up residence in their gut and process the phenylalanine so that it washes away harmlessly in the patient's urine. This treatment has proved effective in mice with PKU, and in a 2018 trial was well tolerated in healthy human volunteers. Trials are now under way in humans with PKU and there are hopes for FDA approval in 2020 or 2021.[32]

Ethical Issues and Genetic Diseases

The potential uses of genetics and genomics in preventing and treating disease have generated great excitement in the medical community and among the public. However, the discoveries have opened a Pandora's box of ethical, legal, social, and scientific questions.

There are lessons to be learned from the mistakes made in early attempts to screen for sickle-cell disease, a disorder of hemoglobin, the oxygen-carrying protein in the blood. In this disease, painful crises of impaired blood circulation occur in individuals who have inherited two copies of the recessive gene, which was identified in the 1970s. However, well-meaning attempts to initiate screening programs for sickle-cell disease, inspired by the success of Tay-Sachs screening in Jews, caused widespread confusion and ill feeling among African Americans, the group at highest risk for carrying the sickle-cell gene. The meaning of the tests was not understood, and many people who were healthy carriers of one gene were discriminated against in school and in employment and were denied health insurance. Many African Americans became suspicious that the intent of the program was genocidal.[33] Considerable time, effort, and money were required to overcome the early mistakes. Now, most states include sickle-cell disease in their newborn screening programs. Although there is no cure for sickle-cell disease, infant and childhood mortality is reduced by prophylactic treatment with penicillin, which prevents infections associated with the crises.[34]

Difficult questions always arise when a serious disorder is diagnosed in a fetus or the genetic potential for such a problem is recognized in the parents. Aborting a fetus with a genetic or teratogenic abnormality is often the only alternative to the birth of a child with a handicap. Many Americans are uncomfortable with, if not morally opposed to, abortion. However, attitudes vary with the severity of the abnormality: Most people would support the parents' decision to abort a fetus with anencephaly (the absence of a brain), as this condition is rapidly and inevitably lethal. The acceptability of a child with Down syndrome varies significantly among prospective parents; some couples choose abortion, whereas others are happy to have the child.

Matters become even more complicated when the genes being identified are known to cause diseases of later life. One of the cruelest of these conditions is Huntington's disease, a single-gene defect in which symptoms first appear between the ages of 30 and 50. During the next 10 to 20 years, the disease progresses toward death, with symptoms that include extreme involuntary movements, intellectual deterioration, and psychiatric disturbances. Because Huntington's disease is inherited in an autosomal dominant fashion, each child of an affected individual has a 50% chance of developing the disease. Although a test is now available that allows individuals to learn whether they carry the gene and are destined to develop the symptoms, many people who are at risk have decided they would prefer not to know. The psychological impact of such knowledge can be devastating, and the potential for being denied insurance or employment is significant. Conversely, individuals with a family history of Huntington's disease may wish to know whether they carry the gene before deciding whether to beget children.[35]

There is a fine line between the worthy goal of preventing disease and disability and the use of genetic screening and abortion to select desirable traits and eliminate undesirable ones from the gene pool. The former is part of the mission of public health, but the latter comes dangerously close to the kind of eugenics practiced by Nazi Germany. The Human Genome Project set aside 3% to 5% of its funding to study the many social, ethical, and legal dilemmas that result from better understanding of human heredity. Since genetic screening first became possible in the 1960s, various groups have proposed guidelines for how screening should be done and who should be screened. Most of the principles are consistent with the recommendations proposed by an Institute of Medicine committee, which include the following:

- Newborn screening should be done only when there is a clear indication of benefit to the newborn, when a system is in place to confirm the diagnosis, and when treatment and follow-up are available for affected infants.
- Carrier identification programs should be voluntary and confidential, and they should include counseling about all choices available to the identified carriers.
- Prenatal diagnosis should include education and counseling before and after the test, informing the parents about risks and benefits of the testing procedure and the alternatives available to them.
- All tests should be of high quality, because life-and-death decisions are based on the results. New tests should be evaluated by the FDA, and there should be more government oversight of laboratory proficiency.
- There should be more education for the general public about genetics.[36]

With the increasing availability of genetic tests, there is great concern about how the information will be used. Such knowledge can help individuals and their doctors make informed decisions about their lifestyle and medical care. However, harmful consequences are also possible—for example, if insurance companies use the information to deny coverage or prospective employers deny employment to individuals who may be more vulnerable in the work environment or who may potentially be more expensive to insure. According to some estimates, every individual carries at least 5 to 10 genes that could make him or her sick under the wrong circumstances or could adversely affect his or her children.[9] All people have an interest in ensuring that any knowledge about their genetic makeup will be used to do them good and not harm. In 2008, Congress passed and President George W. Bush signed the Genetic Information Nondiscrimination Act, which prohibits discrimination by health insurers or employers on the basis of DNA. Part of the justification for this law was that some people might otherwise avoid getting genetic tests that could benefit their health. Another benefit is that the law encourages people to be more willing to participate in research studies without fear that their genetic information might be used against them.[37]

From a public health perspective, there is danger that the enthusiasm for genomics may deflect attention and resources from the important mission of preventing disease in the population. Although individuals differ in their genetic susceptibility to the most common diseases, these diseases are associated with well-known environmental and behavioral risks that are traditional targets of public health intervention. Smoking, for example, increases risks for heart disease, several kinds of cancer, and a number of other diseases. To reduce smoking in the whole population is a far more efficient and effective approach to improving the population's health than attempts to identify risk genes in individual smokers. There is certainly a place for genomics in understanding the biological basis of diseases that cannot be prevented with existing knowledge, such as breast cancer, type 1 diabetes, and Alzheimer's disease. However, many public health advocates believe that resources would be better spent on research and interventions aimed at modifying health-related behaviors, including smoking, diet and physical activity patterns, and sexual behavior.[38]

According to one skeptical epidemiologist, the benefits of genomics are likely to be greatest for treatment rather than prevention. Notably, "our resources allocated to treatment already massively outweigh those spent for disease prevention."[39]

Conclusion

People's health is determined significantly by their genes, and sometimes by prenatal exposure to infectious agents and toxic substances. Public health measures can sometimes prevent unfortunate health outcomes caused by genes or by exposures before birth.

A number of bacteria, viruses, and parasites are known to damage a developing fetus. Immunization of children against some of these infectious agents prevents infections from affecting future generations. Some chemical substances, including several well-known prescription drugs as well as alcohol and illegal drugs, can also cause birth defects. Public health efforts to prevent these exposures include environmental protection and regulation by the FDA.

With increasing knowledge about the genetic basis of some diseases, public health is able to take some actions to minimize their impact. Some conditions, such as Down syndrome, can be easily detected during pregnancy, permitting parents to choose whether to bear an affected child. For a few notorious diseases in children who receive a defective gene from each parent, such as Tay-Sachs disease and sickle-cell disease, prevention involves screening at-risk populations, allowing potential parents to choose whether to conceive an affected child. A major public health effort is focused on diagnosing severe metabolic disorders that can be treated if detected soon after birth. All states have newborn screening programs that test dried spots of blood taken from each infant soon after birth.

The increasing knowledge about the role of genetics in health and the growing capacity to test for individuals' genetic makeup raise many ethical issues concerning how the information should be used and whether application of this knowledge will divert resources from public health's mission of preventing disease in the whole population.

References

1. Centers for Disease Control and Prevention, "Data & Statistics on Birth Defects," https://www.cdc.gov/ncbddd/birthdefects/data.html, accessed September 5, 2019.

2. P. A. Baird and C. R. Scriver, "Genetics and the Public Health," in J. M. Last and R. B. Wallace, eds., *Maxcy-Rosenau Public Health and Preventive Medicine* (Norwalk, CT: Appleton and Lange, 1992), 983–994.

3. R. R. Faden et al., *AIDS, Women, and the Next Generation* (New York, NY: Oxford University Press, 1991), 62.

4. A. Nadakavukaren, *Our Global Environment: A Health Perspective*, 7th ed. (Long Grove, IL: Waveland Press, 2011).

5. W. E. Smith and A.M. Smith, "Minamata," http://aileenarchive.or.jp/minamata_en/slides/swf.html, accessed September 9, 2019.

6. U.S. National Library of Medicine, "Thalidomide," January 15, 2018, https://medlineplus.gov/druginfo/meds/a699032.html, accessed September 9, 2019.

7. Gert de Graaf, F. Buckley, and B. G. Skotko, "Estimates of the Live Births, Natural Losses, and Elective Terminations with Down Syndrome in the United States," *American Journal of Medical Genetics Part A* 167, no. 4 (2015): 756–767.

8. American College of Obstetricians and Gynecologists, "Ob-Gyns Release Revised Recommendations on Screening and Testing for Genetic Disorders," March 1, 2016. https://www.acog.org/About-ACOG/News-Room/News-Releases/2016/Ob-Gyns-Release-Revised-Recommendations-on-Screening-and-Testing-for-Genetic-Disorders?IsMobileSet=false, accessed September 9, 2019.

9. J. L. Natoli, D. L. Ackerman, S. McDermott, and J. G. Edwards, "Prenatal Diagnosis of Down Syndrome: A Systematic Review of Termination Rates (1995–2011)," *Prenatal Diagnosis* 32, no. 2 (2012): 142–153.

10. M. M. Kaback, "Population-Based Genetic Screening for Reproductive Counseling: The Tay-Sachs Model," *European Journal of Pediatrics* 159, suppl. 3 (2000): S102–S195.

11. A. George, "The Rabbi's Dilemma," *New Scientist*, February 14, 2004.

12. M. Mitka, "Newborn Screening Bill," *Journal of the American Medical Association* 299 (2008): 2141.

13. R. Guthrie, "Newborn Screening: Past, Present, and Future," in T. Carter and A. M. Willey, eds., *Genetic Disease Screening and Management* (New York, NY: Alan R. Liss, 1986), 318–339.

14. Centers for Disease Control and Prevention, "Using Tandem Mass Spectrometry for Metabolic Disease Screening Among Newborns," *Morbidity and Mortality Weekly Report* 50, no. RR03 (2001): 1–22.

15. American Academy of Pediatrics Newborn Screening Task Force, "Serving the Family from Birth to the Medical Home," *Pediatrics* 106 (2000): 389–422.

16. Cystic Fibrosis Foundation, "2017 Patient Registry Annual Data Report," August 2018, https://www.cff.org/Research/Researcher-Resources/Patient-Registry/2017-Patient-Registry-Annual-Data-Report.pdf, accessed September 6, 2019.

17. Centers for Disease Control and Prevention, "Newborn Screening for Cystic Fibrosis: Evaluation of Benefits and Risks and Recommendations for State Newborn Screening Programs," *Morbidity and Mortality Weekly Report* 53, no. RR-13 (2004).

18. Centers for Disease Control and Prevention, "Impact of Expanded Newborn Screening—United States, 2006," *Morbidity and Mortality Weekly Report* 57 (2008): 1012–1015.

19. Cystic Fibrosis Foundation, "Newborn Screening Clinical Care Guidelines," https://www.cff.org/Care/Clinical-Care-Guidelines/Diagnosis-Clinical-Care-Guidelines/Newborn-Screening-Clinical-Care-Guidelines/, accessed September 6, 2019.

20. Centers for Disease Control and Prevention, "Hearing Loss in Children," February 18, 2015, https://www.cdc.gov/ncbddd/hearingloss/facts.html, accessed September 6, 2019.

21. Centers for Disease Control and Prevention, "2016 Hearing Screening Summary," https://www.cdc.gov/ncbddd/hearingloss/2016-data/01-data-summary.html, accessed September 6, 2019.

22. Centers for Disease Control and Prevention, "CDC Grand Rounds: Newborn Screening and Improved

Outcomes," *Morbidity and Mortality Weekly Report* 61 (2012): 390–393.

23. U.S. Health Resources and Services Administration, "Summary of Nominated Conditions to the Recommended Uniform Screening Panel (RUSP)," July 2018, https://www.hrsa.gov/sites/default/files /hrsa/advisory-committees/heritable-disorders/rusp /previous-nominations/summary-of-nominated -conditions-to-RUSP-508c.pdf, accessed September 6, 2019.

24. J. Schmutz et al., "Quality Assessment of the Human Genome Sequence," *Nature* 429, no. 6990 (2004).

25. M. Iglesias et al. "Type-I Interferons Inhibit Interleukin-10 Signaling and Favor Type 1 Diabetes Development in NOD Mice," *Frontiers in Immunology* 9 (2018).

26. D. Grady et al., "Jolie's Disclosure of Preventive Mastectomy Highlights Dilemma," *The New York Times*, May 14, 2013.

27. J. Couzin, "Choices—and Uncertainties—for Women with BRCA Mutations," *Science* 302 (2003): 592.

28. 1000 Genomes Project Consortium, "A Global Reference for Human Genetic Variation," *Nature* 526, no. 7571 (2015).

29. E. Pennisi, "Breakthrough of the Year: Human Genetic Variation," *Science* 318 (2007): 1842–1843.

30. D. J. Hunter et al., "Letting the Genome Out of the Bottle—Will We Get Our Wish?" *New England Journal of Medicine* 358 (2008): 105–107.

31. A. Pollack, "Drugs May Turn Cancer into Manageable Disease," *The New York Times*, June 6, 2004.

32. C. Zimmer, "Scientists Are Retooling Bacteria to Cure Disease," *The New York Times*, September 4, 2018.

33. J. Rennie, "Grading the Gene Tests," *Scientific American* (June 1994): 89–97.

34. Centers for Disease Control and Prevention, "Mortality Among Children with Sickle Cell Disease Identified by Newborn Screening During 1990–1994—California, Illinois, and New York," *Morbidity and Mortality Weekly Report* 47 (1998): 169–172.

35. National Institute of Neurological of Neurological Disorders and Stroke, "Huntington's Disease: Hope Through Research," March 27, 2019, https:// www.ninds.nih.gov/disorders/huntington/detail_ huntington.htm, accessed September 9, 2019.

36. Institute of Medicine, Committee on Assessing Genetic Risks, *Assessing Genetic Risks: Implications for Health and Social Policy* (Washington, DC: National Academies Press, 1994).

37. National Institutes of Health, National Human Genome Research Institute, "Genetic Information Nondiscrimination Act of 2008," April 17, 2017, https://www.genome.gov/about-genomics/policy-issues/Genetic-Discrimination, accessed September 9, 2019.

38. K. R. Merikangas and N. Rich, "Genomic Priorities and Public Health," *Science* 302 (2003): 599–601.

39. W. C. Willett, "Balancing Life-Style and Genomics Research for Disease Prevention," *Science* 296 (2002): 695–598.

Social and Behavioral Factors in Health

© Vertismart/Shutterstock

CHAPTER 13

The Actual Causes of Death

Do People Choose Their Own Health?

KEY TERMS

Prohibition

Regulatory approach

Social norms approach

The early successes of public health, in its mission to prevent death and disability, often came from focusing on specific diseases or groups of diseases, seeking particular causes, and finding ways to interrupt the cause-and-effect relationships. This approach was validated during the 20th century by victories over infectious diseases. Public health professionals learned to break the chains of infection, most often by removing etiologic agents (bacteria, viruses, parasites) from the environment (water, food) or by developing vaccines to immunize potential hosts.

As infectious diseases were brought under control and chronic diseases became more significant as causes of death and disability, it became increasingly apparent that the challenges faced by public health regarding chronic diseases would be more complex. Consider the leading causes of death in the United States in 1900 (**Table 13-1**) versus those in 2017 (**Table 13-2**). The top three killers of 1900, which were of infectious origin, have moved down or disappeared from the 2017 list, while heart disease has moved

from fourth to first and cancer from eighth to second. The diseases at the top of the 2017 list have complex causes and most have no clear etiologic agent. Despite decades of biomedical research, there are no vaccines or environmental solutions to the problems of most cancers and heart disease.

In 1990, a group of public health experts from the Centers for Disease Control and Prevention (CDC) decided that they should look at the data in a different way. They observed that the leading causes were not, in fact, root causes but were merely the diagnoses identified at the time of death. These diseases result from a combination of inborn (largely genetic) and external factors. The panel of experts undertook to identify, where possible, the underlying causes of death from each of the leading diseases. They came up with a list of nongenetic factors that they called the leading actual causes of death.[1] While the mortality figures were only estimates, they were based on the best data available. These factors are highly significant for public health because they are

Table 13-1 Leading Causes of Death in the United States, 1900

Cause	Number of Deaths	Percentage of All Deaths
Pneumonia and influenza	40,362	11.8
Tuberculosis (all forms)	38,820	11.3
Diarrhea, enteritis, ulceration of intestines	28,491	8.3
Diseases of heart	27,427	8.0
Intracranial lesions of vascular origin	21,353	6.2
Nephritis	17,699	5.2
All accidents	14,429	4.2
Cancer and other malignant tumors	12,769	3.7
Senility	10,015	2.9
Diphtheria	8056	2.3

Data from National Center for Health Statistics, "Leading Causes of Death, 1900-1998," www.cdc.gov/nchs/data/dvs/lead1900_98.pdf, accessed September 21, 2019.

Table 13-2 Leading Causes of Death in the United States, 2017

Cause	Number of Deaths	Percentage of All Deaths
Diseases of heart	647,457	23.0
Malignant neoplasms (cancer)	599,108	21.3
Unintentional injuries	169,936	6.0
Chronic lower respiratory disease	160,201	5.7
Cerebrovascular disease	146,388	5.2
Alzheimer's disease	121,404	4.3
Diabetes	83,564	3.0
Influenza and pneumonia	55,672	2.0
Nephritis, nephrotic syndrome, and nephrosis	50,633	1.8
Suicide	47,173	1.7

Data from Centers for Disease Control and Prevention, "Deaths: Leading Causes for 2017," www.cdc.gov/nchs/data/nvsr/nvsr68/nvsr68_06-508.pdf, June 24, 2019, accessed September 21, 2019.

Table 13-3 Actual Causes of Death in the United States, 2000

Cause	Number of Deaths	Percentage of All Deaths
Tobacco	435,000	18.1
Poor diet and physical inactivity	365,000	15.2
Alcohol consumption*	85,000	3.5
Microbial agents	75,000	3.1
Toxic agents	55,000	2.3
Motor vehicles	43,000	1.8
Firearms	29,000	1.2
Sexual behavior	20,000	0.8
Illicit drug use	17,000	0.7

*16,653 deaths from alcohol-related crashes are included in both alcohol consumption and motor vehicle death categories.
Data from A. H. Mokdad and P. L. Remington, "Measuring Health Behaviors in Populations," July 2010, www.cdc.gov/pcd/issues/2010/jul/10_0010.htm, accessed September 21, 2019.

preventable causes of death and disability and because they provide targets for public health intervention. In 2000, CDC scientists repeated the analysis with new data and found some changes, although the order of importance is almost the same.[2] **Table 13-3** shows the leading actual causes of death in 2000, which are still reported on the CDC's website.[3]

Based on more recent studies, it seems likely that the combination of poor diet and physical activity has displaced tobacco as the leading actual cause of death, although tobacco was still the leading cause of disability-adjusted life years—a measure of the number of years lost due to poor health, disability, or early death—as of 2016.[4] Illicit drug use, especially opioid use, has increased significantly in importance, causing approximately 70,000 deaths in 2018.[5] While we can expect other modest changes in the numbers of deaths in Table 13-3, the general patterns continue to hold, with tobacco, poor diet, and physical inactivity remaining the leading actual causes of death.

As mentioned, tobacco was found to be the leading actual cause of death in the United States, and it remains the leading cause of disability-adjusted life years. According to the study, tobacco accounts for 30% of all cancer deaths and 21% of cardiovascular disease deaths. In addition, it causes chronic obstructive lung disease, infant deaths due to low birth weight, and burns due to accidental fires. Of the 435,000 deaths attributed to tobacco smoking, 35,000 were caused by second-hand smoke. (By 2014, these numbers had increased to more than 480,000 deaths, including 41,000 from second-hand smoke, with an even higher number of additional suspected cases included.[6])

Poor diet and physical inactivity are listed among the top two leading actual causes of death. These two factors are closely related to each other, with overeating and inactivity combining to produce obesity. Dietary fat, sedentary behavior, and obesity have all been associated with heart disease, stroke, several forms of cancer, and diabetes. The number of deaths attributed to this factor increased by 22% between the 1990 and 2000 estimates, and has continued to increase since then, with the estimated number of deaths from dietary factors in 2016 totaling 529,299, and 8.3% of deaths associated with inadequate physical activity.[4,7] The prevalence of overweight and obesity among Americans has increased dramatically since the 1990s and continues to increase.

In 2005, an analysis by scientists from the CDC and the National Cancer Institute found fault with the calculations of obesity as a leading cause of death.[8] The new calculations, using different statistical methods, led to the conclusion that being moderately overweight was actually protective, especially in older people, although obesity still caused premature deaths. The publication of this study prompted great glee among critics of the "health police" and libertarians who object to being told what to do by the government. It is not clear why this analysis produced such different conclusions from the previous ones. In fact, the authors, troubled by the contradictions, revisited the issue in 2010, investigating several possible systematic biases that might explain them. They concluded that the differences could not be explained by illness-induced weight loss or residual confounding by smoking, and they reaffirmed the findings of the 2005 study.[9] A 2013 review of existing research also supported the conclusion that being moderately overweight was not harmful, but that being obese was associated with higher mortality.[10] The evidence is still strong that obesity increases risks for heart disease, diabetes, high blood pressure, and some kinds of cancer. One possible explanation for the findings is that medical care has become increasingly effective in preventing deaths from these diseases. Despite the controversy, public health professionals continue to regard excess weight and obesity as major threats to people's health.

Misuse of alcohol was listed as the third actual cause of death, causing 35% to 40% of motor vehicle fatalities, as well as chronic liver disease and cirrhosis, home injuries, drowning, fire fatalities, job injuries, and 3% to 5% of cancer deaths.[2] Alcohol consumption by people younger than 21 years, the legal drinking age, is associated with many health and social problems, including alcohol-impaired driving, physical fighting, poor school performance, sexual activity, and smoking. Underage drinking to excess is responsible for more than 4300 deaths in the United States each year (and 119,000 emergency room visits by youth ages 12 to 21).[11]

Number four on the list—microbial agents—encompasses the top three killers of 1900. The fact that mortality from infectious diseases has become so much less significant is testimony to public health's successes. Nevertheless, infectious diseases have by no means been conquered, and they could move to a higher position on the list in the future.

The fact that toxic agents are listed fifth as an actual cause of death is evidence of successes in environmental health. The list's authors call this figure the most uncertain: Environmental threats may actually belong higher up in the list. Certainly, environmental pollution is much more significant as a cause of death in the countries of the former Soviet Union and in China, where environmental health has not been given the same priority as in the United States.

Firearms, sexual behavior, motor vehicles, and the illicit use of drugs round out the list. The authors, recognizing that some deaths may have multiple causes, chose what they believe to be the most significant. For example, they attributed most deaths from acquired immunodeficiency syndrome (AIDS) to sexual behavior or drug use, although they recognize that a microbial agent is involved. The number of deaths attributed to these actual causes has declined since 1990 because of improved treatments for human immunodeficiency virus (HIV). Deaths from alcohol-related motor vehicle crashes have also declined since

1990, largely due to better enforcement of drunk-driving laws.[2]

Perhaps the largest relative movement on the list of actual causes of death is illicit drug use—in particular, use of opioids, but also use of cocaine, methamphetamine, and other drugs. Deaths from overdoses have increased significantly since the data in Table 13-3 were tabulated, and accounted for 69,029 deaths for the 12 months ending February 2019.[12] The causes of this increase are complex and have roots in the economic and social changes that have occurred in the United States since the 1970s. The causes also involve the increasing availability of stronger and longer-acting painkillers since the 1990s.

These nine actual causes of death account for approximately 50% of all deaths in the United States. The causes of the remaining deaths include genetic factors, which were specifically excluded from the analysis, and other, less clearly identifiable causes. Lack of access to health care was cited as a significant factor. Over time, this problem may be largely alleviated by the Patient Protection and Affordable Care Act passed during the Barack Obama administration, assuming it survives the challenges from its many critics. Presumably, many deaths can legitimately be attributed to old age. The nine identified factors are of particular public health significance because they cause premature deaths, they are often preceded by impaired quality of life, and many could be prevented by public health measures.

In trying to prevent premature death and disability, public health must focus on these nine factors. Two of them—microbial agents and toxic agents—have traditionally been public health issues. The other seven are rooted in the behavioral choices made by individuals. Guiding these choices in a positive direction is the biggest challenge now faced by public health: How can people be persuaded to behave in healthier ways in a democratic society, where every step is fraught with political, economic, and moral controversy?

The government has traditionally taken two approaches to promote healthy behavior: education and regulation. Both of these approaches have had successes as well as failures. Both continue to be important components of public health's struggle to accomplish its mission.

Education

Most simply, education informs the public about healthy and unhealthy behavior. Many people who are concerned about their health and that of their families do, in fact, adjust their behavior in accordance with new information. For example, the 1964 Surgeon General's report called *Smoking and Health*,[13] the first authoritative statement from the federal government that smoking caused cancer and other life-threatening diseases, had a significant impact on the prevalence of smoking in the United States. Many people quit the habit after learning this information, and the prevalence of smoking began to decline for the first time after 1964.

Information on healthful eating habits has traditionally been provided by the federal government. In the early 20th century, concern focused on nutritional deficiencies, and the government conducted research on requirements for various vitamins and minerals, leading to listings of recommended dietary allowances or daily values. The educational process was furthered by Food and Drug Administration (FDA) requirements for labeling of prepared foods, which must accurately identify the percentage of the daily value provided by each serving.

While the prevention of nutritional deficiencies remains a valid concern, especially among the poor, the focus of government educational programs on nutrition has largely shifted to the prevention of the major killers of cancer, cardiovascular disease, and diabetes—all of which tend to be associated with nutritional excesses. Research over the past several decades has led to a greater understanding of the importance of overall dietary pattern in the onset of these diseases. The government's educational efforts have stressed the importance of avoiding saturated fat and too much salt, and consuming more fruits, vegetables, and whole grains. The FDA has revised its labeling requirements to provide consumers with the information that will allow them to follow its guidelines.

Results of efforts to modify dietary and smoking behaviors, while showing some success, also illustrate the limitations of the educational approach. The impact of both messages has been mixed. While the percentage of Americans who smoke has declined, 14% of adults maintains the habit despite widespread knowledge about the dangers of tobacco.[14] Particularly worrisome is the pattern that holdout smokers are concentrated among already disadvantaged groups: Approximately 30% of adults with a high school education or less smoke, compared to 7% with at least a college degree; 21% of adults living a household making less $35,000 per year smoke, compared to 8% who earn more than $100,000 per year; 25% of adults without health insurance or using Medicaid smoke, compared to 10% for those with private insurance or Medicare.[14] Evidence of dietary improvement is difficult to verify, as surveys of people's eating habits are notoriously unreliable. While the decline in heart disease is encouraging, the prevalence of obesity has increased, casting doubt on the extent to which Americans have really improved their eating habits.

To illustrate the limitations of the educational approach, consider that in 2008, New York City implemented a law requiring restaurant chains to label the calories for each food item on the menu. In 2009, the state of California followed suit. The 2010 passage of the Patient Protection and Affordable Care Act of 2010 (also known as Obamacare) extended this requirement to all restaurants in the United States with at least 20 locations. One

might have imagined customers being shocked by the 1220 calories in a Burger King Triple Whopper with Cheese or the 740 calories in the medium Oreo-flavored shake, but studies of these policies show that menu calorie postings have, at best, a small effect on consumers' menu choices.[15]

Educational efforts to modify health-related behavior can be controversial, even when the messages seem benign and obvious. For decades, the tobacco industry used all its political and economic power to dispute the evidence that smoking was harmful. Even the government's policy on diet has generated opposition, for example, from the meat industry, which has fought to delay the release of proposed recommendations that people should eat less meat and more fruits, vegetables, and grains—recommendations that, if widely followed, would financially harm the meat industry.[16] Similarly, the sugar industry has fought government recommendations that people should reduce the sugar intake in their diet.[17]

The educational messages most guaranteed to generate controversy, however, are those concerning sexual behavior. American attitudes about sex are notoriously ambivalent. Although movies and television shows frankly depict sexual activity, many people are puritanically reluctant to talk about how people can protect themselves against the natural consequences of that activity: unintended pregnancy and sexually transmitted diseases. For example, the tenure of Joycelyn Elders as President Bill Clinton's Surgeon General was extremely controversial because she spoke out openly on these issues, recommending condom use and masturbation, until she was forced by political pressures to resign her office.

Schools are naturally a prime site for health education programs. The goal is to teach children from an early age how to live healthy lives by providing information, for example, on diet, exercise, and the dangers of smoking, alcohol use, and drug abuse. Studies have shown that school education programs are effective in teaching children the facts about health and safety. It is less clear, however, that they actually influence young people to behave in healthier ways.

Sex education in the schools is highly controversial. Opponents have argued for years that teaching young people about sex encourages them to indulge in immoral behavior. When AIDS came along, the controversy became more intense because it meant that sexual behavior could be a matter of life and death. Many proponents of explicit education about safe sex argue that young people will have sex no matter what they are taught and that they should be informed about how to protect themselves. Opponents argue that condoms are only partially effective in preventing pregnancy and sexually transmitted diseases and that young people should be taught that they can protect themselves only by abstinence. This was the policy of the George W. Bush administration, which allocated hundreds of millions of dollars of federal funds for abstinence-only education. Many of these programs commonly contained multiple scientific and medical inaccuracies. According to Richard Daines, then the New York State Commissioner of Health, "the Bush administration's abstinence-only program is an example of a failed national health-care policy directive, based on ideology rather than on sound scientific evidence that must be the cornerstone of good public health-care policy."[18]

In fact, a number of studies have shown that students who have received comprehensive sex education in school delay initiation of sex, reduce the number of partners, and are more likely to use contraception when they do have sex. And while the use of condoms cannot guarantee protection against pregnancy and HIV transmission, condoms do reduce these risks. Nevertheless, the controversy continues in many communities. The decision on what students should be taught about sex is made by local school boards and depends on "community standards."

An extension of the educational approach to changing behavior is the use of advertising to reinforce the public health message. Most people are subjected to large doses of media messages promoting unhealthy behavior, including cigarette ads in magazines, beer commercials on television, and movie portrayals of unsafe sex. The occasional public service announcements meant to convey countervailing messages are feeble weapons in the battle for public health, although evidence shows that counter-advertising about the dangers of smoking helped reduce smoking rates in the 1960s. The "Just Say No" antidrug campaign during the Ronald Reagan administration was strong enough to make an impression; whether it persuaded people to change their behavior, however, is doubtful.

Another variation on health education that has become popular with college administrators to curb high-risk student drinking is the social norms approach. This approach is based on an influential study from the 1980s, which surveyed students about their perception of the frequency and amount of drinking among their peers. It turned out that students generally believed that other students drank more than they actually did. The remedy to the misperception that "everyone is doing it" is to advertise the actual norms on campus. Institutions could reduce high-risk drinking by as much as 20% over a relatively short period of time by conducting surveys on campus and advertising the results.[19] Although use of the social norms approach is in an early stage, its proponents believe that it can be used for a variety of other issues, such as tobacco prevention, seat belt use, and prevention of high-risk sexual activity.

Health education messages may also be delivered by a medical professional during an office visit. Doctors who care for people with chronic diseases such as diabetes and asthma know that they can keep their patients healthier if they include a health education component in their treatment plans. Studies have shown that, while patients do not always follow the doctor's orders, a physician's recommendation can increase the likelihood that people will change their behavior.[20]

Public health's mission is to prevent disease, whereas medicine traditionally focuses more on treatment and cure. However, the fact that the medical profession can—and often does—play an important role in communicating public health messages about healthy behavior means that public health has a role to play in educating medical providers about health risks and health-related behaviors.

Regulation

Governments have always regulated people's behavior by passing and enforcing laws. The **regulatory approach** is clearly warranted when its intent is to restrain people from harming others. Laws against murder and assault are, in effect, public health laws, and there is no question about their legitimacy. Traffic laws—also aimed at protecting public health—are clearly accepted as necessary. Though not scrupulously obedient, everyone recognizes the importance of stopping at red lights, keeping to the right side of the road (in the United States), and driving at speeds appropriate to the conditions.

Most states have laws concerning alcohol and tobacco use aimed at protecting the public's health. Laws against drunk driving are clearly justified as a means of protecting others. Laws that regulate smoking in indoor public places are also justified on the basis that smokers create a health hazard by polluting the air that others must breathe. Most adults agree with laws aimed at preventing children and teenagers from behaving in ways that may harm their health, such as restrictions on access to alcohol and tobacco. The greatest controversy about governmental attempts to regulate behavior arises when these efforts are perceived as interfering with a mature individual's freedom to take risks with his or her own health. The so-called individual mandate component of the Patient Protection and Affordable Care Act required most individuals in the United States to have a minimum level of health insurance or pay a fine. The requirement was controversial from the start, with some people preferring to take their chances that they would remain healthy. In 2017, the Donald Trump administration, with the help of the Republican-controlled Congress, effectively nullified the individual mandate.

Controversy over public health laws is not new. In the 19th century, major controversies raged in Britain and the United States over laws requiring immunization against smallpox. In the United States, the matter was decided in the 1905 Supreme Court decision *Jacobson v. Commonwealth of Massachusetts*, which upheld that state's right to require vaccination "for the common good."[21]

Another hot-button issue in the 19th century, both in Britain and in the United States, was the control of "venereal diseases" (sexually transmitted infections), a campaign fraught with moral and social implications that presaged more recent controversies over AIDS. In Britain, a series of Contagious Diseases Acts were passed in the 1860s and 1870s, providing for compulsory medical examinations of known and suspected prostitutes and detention of those found to carry disease. Such laws were justified by arguing that venereal diseases were a national defense issue: Military recruits affected by syphilis and gonorrhea would be unfit for service. Proponents also argued that irresponsible men, infected by prostitutes, carried diseases home to their innocent wives. It was especially urgent to prevent the spread of syphilis, which can be transmitted from an infected woman to her fetus during pregnancy, causing severe damage to the child. In the United States, most states adopted laws that required couples to be certified free of disease before they could obtain a marriage license.[22]

Many of the themes that occurred in the debates over venereal disease control have recurred in recent decades in debates about AIDS prevention. In fact, two states passed laws in the 1980s requiring premarital screening for HIV infection—similar to the old requirement for syphilis testing. However, these laws were soon repealed, as the syphilis laws have been.

Changes in social norms mean that premarital screening occurs too late to protect women—and men—against sexually transmitted diseases. The conflict between, on the one hand, the protection of the privacy and freedom of the infected individual and, on the other hand, the protection of the health of potential "innocent" victims is the same with AIDS as it was with syphilis. However, the political power of gay men, the group most affected by AIDS in the early days of the epidemic, was much stronger than was the power of prostitutes in the 19th century. The gay community fought against many proposals designed to prevent the spread of the virus. For example, legal battles were fought in San Francisco and New York over the closing of gay bathhouses, which were the site of many unsafe sexual practices. New York State's 1985 decision to close the bathhouses in New York City was upheld by the courts. In San Francisco, legal action by the gay community forced an overturn of the city's order to close the bathhouses. However, the court ordered bathhouse owners to hire monitors to prevent high-risk sexual activity.[23]

Does Prohibition Work?

The most ambitious attempt by the U.S. government to regulate the behavior of its citizens was **Prohibition**, a ban on alcohol manufacture, sale, and use passed by a constitutional amendment in 1919, only to be repealed 14 years later. Common wisdom holds that Prohibition was a failure, but today's society treats "recreational" drugs such as cocaine and hallucinogens in much the same way that the Eighteenth Amendment treated alcohol, and few public health leaders are willing to call for an end to these prohibitions. In fact, the Prohibition approach to regulating behavior appears to have mixed results, combining success and failure in a complex way.

The movement to legally ban alcohol became a moral crusade in the late 19th century, with prohibitionists blaming alcohol for all the ills of society. According to the rhetoric during that era, drinking drove men to violence, especially against their wives and children; drunkards were a threat to public safety; and drunkenness itself was looked on as a sin and a crime. In fact, public disapproval had convinced many people to cut down on or quit their use of alcohol, and consumption had declined even before the Eighteenth Amendment was approved.[24] During Prohibition, the rate of cirrhosis of the liver declined to half that of 1910. Despite the image of the Roaring Twenties—with speakeasies, flappers, and bathtub gin—consumption of alcohol fell by two-thirds over this period.[25] However, it was also true that flouting of the law became socially acceptable, and organized crime flourished as it sought to fulfill the ongoing demand for alcohol.

The debate about Prohibition resurfaces occasionally in the context of illegal drugs. In an exchange of letters published in the *Wall Street Journal* in 1989, two prominent conservatives debated whether the war on drugs was doing more harm than good.[26,27] The economist Milton Friedman argued that while drugs are "tearing asunder our social fabric, ruining the lives of many young people, and imposing heavy costs on some of the most disadvantaged among us," much of the harm, he suggested, results from the fact that the drugs are illegal.[26] The illegality drives up the price of the drugs, providing a financial incentive to drug dealers, causing desperate addicts to commit crimes to pay for their addiction, and corrupting law enforcement officials tempted by bribery. Removing the "obscene profits" from the drug market, Friedman wrote, would reduce the motivation of drug pushers to recruit future addicts among vulnerable young people.

Opposing this view was William Bennett, who was the leader of President George H. W. Bush's drug-control efforts. Bennett admitted that the war on drugs is costly, but argued that the cost of not enforcing laws against drugs would be higher. He claimed that after repeal of Prohibition, the consumption of alcohol soared by 350%; he then asked if the country could afford such a dramatic increase in drug use. Bennett blamed current levels of drug use for lost productivity, rising health insurance costs, flooding of hospitals with drug overdose emergencies, and drug-related accidents. He disputed the argument that addicts turn to crime to support their habit, claiming that many addicts were criminals before they turned to drugs.[27]

The argument has not been resolved. In 2001, the National Academy of Sciences published a report arguing that the Prohibition-like approach was not working. The report stated that, although the federal government spends some $17 billion each year on drug enforcement programs, there is little information on the effectiveness of these programs. The number of people arrested and incarcerated for drug offenses increased dramatically starting in the 1980s and has exceeded 2 million people since 1999 (about 2.2 million were incarcerated in 2017),[28] despite a lack of evidence that this approach helps deter illegal drug use. "It is unconscionable for the country to continue to carry out a public policy of this magnitude and cost without any way of knowing whether and to what extent it is having the desired effect," the report concluded.[29(p.279)]

Recent evidence on alternatives to the war on drugs was discussed by Nicholas Kristof in a 2019 *New York Times* column entitled "Seattle Has Figured Out How to Win the War on Drugs." Kristof notes that cities like Seattle and countries like Portugal that have decriminalized drug use have seen significant improvements in outcomes not only in terms of reducing both drug overdoses and recidivism to prison, but also in economic terms: The cost of treatment turns out to be far lower than the cost of incarceration. This approach quickly pays for itself by converting individuals with a drug addiction into more productive members of society. Unfortunately, there has been long-standing inaction on this issue in the United States at the federal level, so it has fallen on states and municipalities

to lead the way. Approaching three years into the Trump administration, a non-temporary administrator of the Drug Enforcement Agency has still not been appointed.[30]

Later in this text, we undertake a more theoretical discussion of what influences people to behave in the ways that they do. It is clear that, to be effective, public health must expand beyond the traditional approaches of education and regulation in its attempt to change people's unhealthy behaviors. Elsewhere, we discuss ways in which a combination of education and regulation is being used to change people's behavior in relation to the substance that tops the list of hazards to health: tobacco smoking.

Conclusion

As infectious diseases have become less predominant causes of death in the United States, a major focus of public health programs has shifted to people's behavior. An analysis conducted by a group of public health leaders concluded that the top three actual causes of death are smoking, poor diet and physical inactivity, and alcohol consumption. Other behavioral factors that are among the top nine causes of death are firearms, sexual behavior, motor vehicles, and the illicit use of drugs. For public health to significantly reduce the premature-death rates beyond what it can achieve in controlling infectious diseases, it must find ways to promote behavioral change.

Two approaches that government has traditionally taken to persuade people to change their behavior are education and regulation. Education about health includes simply informing people about risks, which can be an effective strategy when new knowledge becomes available, as occurred with the 1964 Surgeon General's report called *Smoking and Health*. Food labeling is also part of an educational effort to encourage Americans to eat a healthier diet. Regulation is another effective approach to promoting behavioral change, although it is often unpopular. Historically, the most ambitious attempt to regulate Americans' behavior was Prohibition, which did in fact improve their health by reducing the rate of cirrhosis of the liver. Whether the Prohibition-like approach currently used for control of illegal drugs provides real benefits has not been demonstrated, but the costs both financially and in terms of the long-term harm to incarcerated individuals has been enormous.

Research in the social and behavioral sciences has led to the development of theories of why people behave as they do and how they can be influenced to change their behavior. The evidence indicates that health promotion programs are most effective when they target individuals at many different levels of influence.

References

1. J. M. McGinnis and W. H. Foege, "Actual Causes of Death in the United States," *Journal of the American Medical Association* 270 (1993): 2207–2212.

2. A. H. Mokdad, J. S. Marks, D. F. Stroup, and J. L. Gerberding, "Actual Causes of Death in the United States, 2000," *Journal of the American Medical Association* 291 (2004): 1238–1245.

3. A. H. Mokdad and P. L. Remington, "Measuring Health Behaviors in Populations," July 2010. https://www.cdc.gov/pcd/issues/2010/jul/10_0010.htm, accessed September 21, 2019.

4. A. H. Mokdad, K. Ballestros, M. Echko, S. Glenn, H. E. Olsen, E. Mullany, et al., "The State of US Health, 1990–2016: Burden of Diseases, Injuries, and Risk Factors Among US States," *Journal of the American Medical Association* 319 (2018): 1444–1472.

5. Centers for Disease Control and Prevention, "Deaths: Final Data for 2017," *National Vital Statistics Report* 68 (June 24, 2019): Table 6, https://www.cdc.gov/nchs/data/nvsr/nvsr68/nvsr68_09-508.pdf, accessed September 16, 2019.

6. Centers for Disease Control and Prevention, "Smoking & Tobacco Use: Fast Facts," https:///www.cdc.gov/tobacco/data_statistics/fact_sheets/fast_facts/index.htm, accessed September 21, 2019.

7. S. A. Carlson, E. K. Adams, Z. Yang, and J. E. Fulton, "Percentage of Deaths Associated with Inadequate Physical Activity in the United States," in *Preventing Chronic Disease* (Atlanta, GA: Centers for Disease Control and Prevention, 2018), 15.

8. K. M. Flegal, B. I. Graubard, D. F. Williamson, and M. H. Gail, "Excess Deaths Associated with Underweight, Overweight, and Obesity," *Journal of the American Medical Association* 293 (2005): 1861–1867.

9. K. M. Flegal, "NCHS Health E-Stat: Supplemental Analyses for Excess Deaths Associated with Underweight, Overweight, and Obesity in the U.S. Population," January 7, 2010. https://www.cdc.gov/nchs/data/hestat/excess_deaths/excess_deaths.htm, accessed May 30, 2015.

10. K. M. Flegal, B. K. Kit, H. Orpana, and B. I. Graubard, "Association of All-Cause Mortality with Overweight and Obesity Using Standard Body Mass Index Categories: A Systematic Review and Meta-Analysis," *Journal of the American Medical Association* 309 (2013): 71–82.

11. Centers for Disease Control and Prevention, "Fact Sheets: Underage Drinking," August 2, 2018, https://www.cdc.gov/alcohol/fact-sheets/underage-drinking.htm, accessed September 21, 2019.

12. Centers for Disease Control and Prevention, "Provisional Drug Overdose Death Counts," Vital Statistics Rapid Release, https://www.cdc.gov/nchs/nvss/vsrr/drug-overdose-data.htm, accessed September 16, 2019.

13. Department of Health, Education and Welfare, *Smoking and Health: Report of the Advisory Committee to the Surgeon General of the Public Health Service* (Washington, DC: U.S. Department of Health, Education and Welfare, 1964).

14. Centers for Disease Control and Prevention, "Smoking & Tobacco Use: Fast Facts and Fact Sheets," https://www.cdc.gov/tobacco/data_statistics/fact_sheets/index.htm, accessed September 21, 2019.

15. M. W. Long, D. K. Tobias, A. L. Cradock, H. Batchelder, and S. L. Gortmaker, "Systematic Review and Meta-Analysis of the Impact of Restaurant Menu Calorie Labeling," *American Journal of Public Health* 105 (2015).

16. M. Nestle, *Food Politics* (Berkeley, CA: University of California Press, 2002).

17. "Editorial: The Food Pyramid Scheme," *The New York Times*, September 1, 2004.

18. T. Hampton, "Abstinence-Only Programs Under Fire," *Journal of the American Medical Association* 299 (2008): 2013–2015.

19. University of Virginia, National Social Norms Institute, "Social Norms Approach." http://www.socialnorms .org/social-norms-approach/, accessed May 30, 2015.

20. U.S. Public Health Service. *Healthy People 2000: National Health Promotion and Disease Prevention Objectives*, Publication No. (PHS) 91–50212 (Washington, DC: Department of Health and Human Services, 1990), 153–154.

21. T. Christoffel, *Health and the Law: A Handbook for Health Professionals* (New York, NY: Free Press, 1982).

22. H. M. Leichter, *Free to Be Foolish: Politics and Health Promotion in the United States and Great Britain* (Princeton, NJ: Princeton University Press, 1991).

23. R. Bayer, *Private Acts, Social Consequences: AIDS and the Politics of Public Health* (New York, NY: Free Press, 1989).

24. G. Pickett and J. J. Hanlon, *Public Health: Administration and Practice* (St. Louis, MO: Times Mirror/Mosby, 1990).

25. D. Beauchamp, *The Health of the Republic: Epidemics, Medicine, and Moralism as Challenges to Democracy* (Philadelphia, PA: Temple University Press, 1988).

26. M. Friedman, "An Open Letter to Bill Bennett," *The Wall Street Journal*, September 7, 1989: A14.

27. W. Bennett, "A Response to Milton Friedman," *The Wall Street Journal*, September 19, 1989: A30.

28. C. Robertson, "Crime Is Down, Yet U.S. Incarceration Rates Are Still Among the Highest in the World," *The New York Times*, April 25, 2019.

29. Committee on Data and Research for Policy on Illegal Drugs, *Informing America's Policy on Illegal Drugs: What We Don't Know Keeps Hurting Us* (Washington, DC: National Academies Press, 2001).

30. N. Kristof, "Seattle Has Figured Out How to End the War on Drugs," *The New York Times*, August 23, 2019.

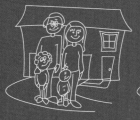
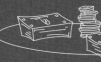

Healthy, Wealthy, and Wise

How Psychosocial Factors Affect Health Behavior

KEY TERMS

Ecological model
Health belief model
Self-efficacy

Social support
Socioeconomic status (SES)
Stress

Transtheoretical model

While individual behavior plays a major role in determining a person's health, many factors influence individual behavior. Humans are social creatures, and their behavior is strongly affected by their social environment. This accounts, at least in part, for the fact that diseases tend to be distributed in the population according to certain patterns: Certain groups have characteristic disease patterns that remain constant over time, even when individuals in the group change. Thus, from a public health perspective, it may be more efficient to try to change the social environment that influences people to behave in unhealthy ways than to try to change people's behavior one individual at a time.

Another reason to consider the social environment in studying health behavior is that when the focus is on the individual, the conclusion is likely to be that the person is to blame for his or her illness. Unhealthy

behaviors may be maintained and reinforced by aspects of the social environment that are beyond the individual's control. It may be more appropriate for public health intervention programs to focus on these social aspects or at least consider them in designing programs aimed at promoting healthy behavior.

Demographic factors—including race, gender, and marital status—are consistently found to influence health. Statistics show that most ethnic minorities in the United States have significantly higher mortality rates from most diseases than whites do. Males have higher mortality rates than females do at all ages, although females tend to suffer more from chronic illness. Married people are in general healthier than people who are not married, whether single, separated, widowed, or divorced. The reasons for these differences are believed to be primarily social.[1,2]

The most important predictor of health is **socioeconomic status (SES)**, a concept that includes income, education, and occupational status—factors that tend to be strongly associated with each other. SES accounts in part, though not entirely, for the health differences by race, sex, and marital status. For example, blacks tend to be less healthy than whites are, and they generally have lower SES than whites do. However, even wealthy, educated blacks have higher mortality rates than do whites of comparable SES.[3]

Groups with the lowest SES have the highest mortality rates, a relationship that holds in many different countries and has been true for centuries, for reasons known and unknown.[4] In London in 1665, the poor were more likely to die in the plague epidemic because of poor nutrition and sanitation and because they could not flee the city to escape infection as the wealthy did. In the United States today, the health of the poor is threatened by adverse environmental conditions, such as lead in paint and tap water, air pollution, and violence. Poor people also have poorer nutrition, less access to medical care, and more psychological stress.

It is not just the effects of poverty that account for socioeconomic variations in health, however. The association is seen at all levels of the socioeconomic scale, with the very rich being healthier than the rich, who are healthier than the middle class, and so on. In a study of British civil servants called the Whitehall Study, researchers compared mortality rates over a 10-year period across four employment grades. Top administrators were compared with executives and professionals, the clerical staff, and unskilled laborers.[5] As seen in **Figure 14-1**, higher employment status was associated with a lower risk of dying.

Part of the reason that people with higher SES are healthier seems to be that people with more education behave in healthier ways. For example, in 2017, 30% of Americans with a high school education or less smoked, while of those with at least a bachelor's degree, only 7% smoked.[6] Americans with more education were also more physically active.[7] Similarly, the Whitehall Study questioned U.K. subjects about their habits and found that those in higher employment grades were less likely to smoke, more likely to exercise, and more

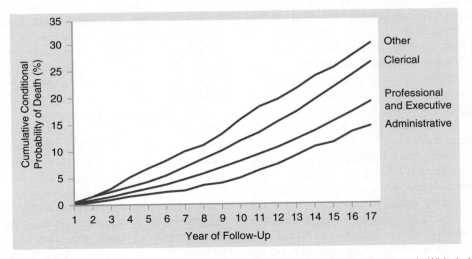

Figure 14-1 Mortality from All Causes by Year of Follow-Up and Grade of Employment, in Whitehall (U.K.) Male Civil Servants, Initially Aged 40–64

likely to eat a healthful diet that included whole grains and fresh fruits and vegetables.[5] Likewise, there is a strong link between socioeconomic status and drug abuse, both of illicit drugs and prescription drugs. The opioid crisis of the last decade is concentrated among Americans with less education, who are less likely to have ever been married, who have lower SES, and who are more likely to be out of the workforce.[8]

Variable access to medical care is another factor that has been blamed for some of the socioeconomic differences in health. In the United States, where 12.8% of adults—mostly those in low socioeconomic groups—lacked health insurance in 2017,[9,10] it was often argued that universal health insurance could reduce health inequalities. However, the SES differences in mortality are also seen in Britain, Scandinavian nations, and other countries that have national health programs. The British civil servants in the Whitehall Study all had the same medical coverage by the National Health Service, yet the mortality risks were still higher at lower employment grades, even when behavioral factors were taken into consideration.

Health of Minority Populations

Race and ethnicity have been seen to profoundly affect health in the United States. Most data on health status of different population groups show that the health of black Americans, the largest racial minority, constituting 13.4% of the population, is poorer than that of white Americans. Hispanics (classified as an ethnic group rather than a racial group by the U.S. Census) are a heterogeneous group, and their health status varies among different subgroups. American Indians generally have poorer health indicators than whites do, while Asian Americans have better health status.

While the overall health of the U.S. population has improved over the past decades, health disparities among racial and ethnic groups have persisted. Life expectancy at birth in 2017 was 78.8 years for whites and 75.3 years for blacks.[8] The infant mortality rate of blacks was almost double that for whites, and the rate for American Indians/Alaska Natives was 1.5 times higher than that of whites.[6] Mortality from diabetes is 27% higher for blacks compared to whites and 49% higher for American Indians compared to whites.[1] Black men die of prostate cancer at 2.2 times the rate of white men.[11] The death rate from human immunodeficiency virus (HIV)/acquired immunodeficiency syndrome (AIDS) is almost 6 times higher among black men than among white men, and 16 times higher for black women than for white women.[12]

The health disparities may be accounted for in part by the lower SES of blacks, who live in households with median incomes $21,181 less than the U.S. average. More than 20% of blacks were living in poverty in 2017, as compared with 8.1% of non-Hispanic whites.[13] Blacks have less education, on average, compared to whites, and they have higher unemployment rates. The reasons for the socioeconomic disparities are complex and somewhat inaccessible to public health interventions. Moreover, the relationship between socioeconomic status and health is not entirely understood. Nevertheless, public health must find ways to improve the health of groups that have historically been disadvantaged economically, educationally, and politically.

Public health interventions aimed at improving the health of minority groups include efforts to influence their health behaviors. These efforts begin with attempts to understand which factors influence health and health behavior, how these factors may affect people of various ethnic and racial groups differently, and which kinds of interventions can be effective in modifying these factors. This chapter examine how minority groups differs from the majority white population and how those differences may be related to the observed disparities in health.

Stress and Social Support

A number of psychological factors have been found to influence health, some of which may have a role in the health effects of SES. One of these factors is **stress**, which is due to the adverse physical and social conditions associated with lower SES. Stress may act both directly, by affecting physiological processes, and indirectly, by influencing individual behavior. Early evidence of the health effects of stress came from observations that widows and widowers seemed to have an unusually high risk of dying soon after the death of their spouses. Several studies in the 1960s and 1970s found that mortality rates of survivors are 40% to 50% higher during the six months after the death of a spouse compared to the mortality of married people of the same age. These studies were expanded to include the effects of other stressful life events such as death of other family members, divorce, and loss of a job, all of which were found to increase the risk of illness or death.[14]

Stress is well established as a contributor to heart disease, a relationship that has been demonstrated in a variety of epidemiologic studies. A particularly convincing example is a study of the male employees of two banks. At first, the two groups were similar, but one bank changed its management policies to become commercial. The employees of the commercial bank had to deal with considerable competition, risk, and responsibility for investing funds; employees of the other bank, a semipublic savings bank, had less competition and fewer responsibilities. Over a 10-year period, the employees of the commercial bank were found to have 50% higher rates of heart attacks and sudden death.[15]

Experiments on animals ranging from rats to baboons have found that various psychosocial stresses induce physiological changes such as decreased immune response and increased atherosclerosis. An experiment on humans demonstrated that stress suppresses the immune response in humans as well. In that experiment, investigators measured levels of psychological stress in 420 healthy volunteers, then administered nasal drops containing cold viruses to all but a small control group. They found that the subjects whose stress levels were higher were more likely to be infected with cold viruses and more likely to develop colds, with symptoms including sneezing, coughing, eye watering, nasal discharge, sore throat, and increased use of tissues.[16] A whole new field of research called psychoneuroimmunology has arisen to study the impact of stress on health.

Lower SES exposes people to greater life stress for many reasons. Daily hassles are greater at lower levels on the SES hierarchy: Cars break down, landlords complain about late rent checks, child care is unreliable, officials are rude. Members of racial and ethnic minorities may be exposed to incidents of racial prejudice. These minor but constant stresses may be as debilitating as such major life events as deaths in the family. By comparison, higher income and education provide resources that help buffer the impact of life's hassles, thereby protecting health.

A number of factors can help people cope with life's stresses. Money, of course, can solve a multitude of problems. Education is important because it provides the information and skills to solve problems. Family and friends can also help by providing both emotional and instrumental assistance. In fact, **social support** has proven to be surprisingly significant in determining an individual's health.

Early evidence for the influence of social support on health came from an epidemiologic cohort study conducted on residents of Alameda County in California. Persons aged 30 to 69 were surveyed in 1965 on their physical, mental, and social well-being as well as their health-related habits such as exercise and the use of cigarettes and alcohol. They were also asked about their social networks, such as marital status, number of close friends and relatives, church membership, and affiliation with other organizations. Death certificates were then monitored over the next 9 years to assess mortality rates and, in 1974, a follow-up survey was conducted on survivors to assess their health status.[17]

The study, as expected, found a strong association between certain unhealthy behaviors and higher mortality rates. More surprising, the study found that an individual's health status and risk of dying were strongly associated with the extent and nature of his or her social network. This was true for both men and women and for individuals of high SES and low SES. The association remained true even after unhealthy behaviors were taken into consideration. Across the socioeconomic spectrum, men and women with few social contacts had mortality rates two to three times higher than their counterparts with many social connections.

Many more recent studies have supported the conclusions of the Alameda County study. A review of 148 studies on the health effects of social relationships found much lower mortality rates for people with strong social connections. The association held regardless of age, gender, or the presence of preexisting conditions.[2] Why social support should have such a broad and consistent effect on health is not well understood, but it may act through one or more of the following channels. First, it may help buffer stress by way of emotional or other support from close social contacts, including hormonal responses to that support. Second, it may act through indirect channels such as having peers who model healthy behavior or, through belonging to a group, help establish norms for self-care. Third, social connections may help establish a better sense of purpose, well-being, and self-esteem.[2] A better understanding of the relationship between social support and health may come from research in the field of psychoneuroimmunology, which seeks to learn about the mind–body connection as it relates to the immune system.

Psychological Models of Health Behavior

While public health does not have much power to change people's SES, stressful life events, or social networks, it is hoped that understanding how these factors affect health may permit more effective interventions to promote healthier behavior. With this goal in mind, social and behavioral scientists have proposed various theories and models attempting to explain how psychosocial factors affect health-related behavior. Some of these theories focus on individual psychology, whereas others attempt to explain the effect of the social environment on individual behavior. The goal of these analyses is to understand the most effective ways to promote healthier behavior.

The classic frame of reference for understanding health behavior, and especially behavior change, is the **health belief model**. Assuming that people act in rational ways, the health belief model specifies several factors that determine whether a person is likely to change behavior when faced with a health threat: (1) the extent to which the individual feels vulnerable to the threat, (2) the perceived severity of the threat, (3) perceived barriers to taking action to reduce the risk, and (4) the perceived effectiveness of taking an action to prevent or minimize the problem.

Based on the health belief model, the public health approach to changing behavior would be to convince people that they are vulnerable, that the threat is severe, and that certain actions are effective preventive measures. For example, surveys of low-income minority women who had not had mammograms found that many had misperceptions about breast cancer. Some women underestimated their susceptibility to breast cancer (factor 1); others were embarrassed or afraid of the pain or radiation involved in a mammogram (factor 3); and others felt that cancer was not curable so there would be no point in diagnosing it early (factor 4). Screening rates among these women could be improved by counseling that included personally tailored messages that addressed the women's beliefs and concerns.[18]

Another important concept in understanding health behavior is **self-efficacy**, the sense of having control over one's life. People who are confident that they can control their lives are said to have high self-efficacy. Conversely, people who believe their lives are subject to chance or external forces are said to have low self-efficacy. Self-efficacy is often added as a fifth factor in the health belief model. People are more likely to adopt healthy behavior if they are confident that they have the ability to do so.[18]

A sense of control is beneficial for health in a number of ways. Clearly, it reduces stress. A number of studies in both humans and animals have shown that an individual's perception of the stressfulness of an adverse event can be reduced by two factors: knowledge of when the stressful event will occur and the ability to regulate the timing and intensity of the event. This knowledge and ability give the individual a sense of control, or self-efficacy. The lowest self-efficacy is seen in people (or animals) who have experience of being unable to avoid noxious events, especially if they have repeatedly tried and failed. They may develop a pattern of "learned helplessness"—a pattern described as a "numbed acceptance of a negative situation, so that an individual no longer tries to change that situation for the better because he or she does not expect those efforts to make any difference."[19(p.44)]

A number of studies have shown that people with high self-efficacy are more likely to engage in health-promoting behavior than are those with low self-efficacy. An attitude of learned helplessness is common in people who have repeatedly tried and failed to quit smoking or lose weight.

A great deal of research has been focused on how to increase people's self-efficacy, thereby motivating them to practice healthy behaviors. An individual's self-efficacy is increased by previous successful performance of the behavior in question. It may also be increased by seeing others successfully perform the behavior, especially if the observed behavior is performed by someone similar to themselves. For example, the most successful school drug prevention programs include role-modeling, small-group exercises, and skills practice to teach students how to identify and resist internal and external pressures to use drugs. These programs have been found to be much more effective in enhancing students' self-efficacy to resist drugs if they are led by older teens, with whom they can identify, rather than by adult health educators.[20]

A theory that has proved widely useful in health education is the **transtheoretical model**, which envisions change—for example, smoking cessation or adopting a healthy diet—as a process involving progress through a series of five stages: precontemplation, contemplation, preparation, action, and maintenance. People in the precontemplation stage have no intention to change their behavior; the first step in getting them to change involves consciousness-raising to increase their awareness that their behavior is unhealthy and should be changed. In the second, contemplation stage, the person is more aware of the benefits of change, but also very aware of the difficulties and barriers to change and still not ready to take action. The third step is preparation, when a person has decided to make the change and has planned concrete actions he or she could take, such as signing up for a class, discussing the plan with a physician, or buying a self-help book. The fourth step, action, requires that individuals actually modify their behavior by abstaining from smoking or adhering to a healthier diet. Finally, maintenance is the stage in which people have achieved the healthier behavior but must strive to prevent relapse.[21] Knowing which stage an individual has reached can help a physician or health educator move him or her along to the next stage.

The health belief model and the transtheoretical model are not contradictory; instead, they are alternative ways of looking at what may be the same psychological factors. Both models can be useful in designing public health messages aimed at changing behavior.

Ecological Model of Health Behavior

In accordance with the recognition that individual beliefs and behaviors occur in a social context and that health promotion may be more effectively achieved through changing the social environment, so-called ecological models have been proposed for understanding health behavior.[22] An **ecological model** looks at how the social environment, including interpersonal, organizational, community, and public policy factors, supports and maintains unhealthy behaviors. The model proposes that changes in these factors will produce changes in individual behavior.

The ecological model, illustrated in **Figure 14-2**, describes five levels of influence that determine health-related behaviors; each level is a potential target for health promotion intervention. The first level—*intrapersonal factors*—encompasses the knowledge, attitudes, and skills of the individual. This is the level that has been explored by the psychological theories discussed previously. The second through fifth levels—interpersonal relations, institutional factors, community factors, and public policy—all impact individual behavior both directly and indirectly, by interacting with the factors at other levels of influence.

The second level of influence, *interpersonal* relations—including family, friends, and coworkers—has very important effects on health-related behavior. Families, of course, are the origin of many health behaviors, especially habits learned early in life such as tooth brushing, exercising, and eating patterns. In the teen years, pressure from peers becomes more significant in influencing individual behaviors, such as smoking, using alcohol and drugs, and engaging in other risk-taking behavior. On the positive side, family and peer relationships provide the social support discussed earlier in this chapter.

Application of the ecological model at the interpersonal level would lead to different

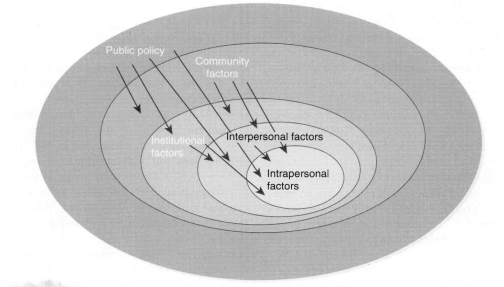

Figure 14-2 Ecological Model

strategies in a teen drug prevention program depending on the nature of the teens' social relationships. A teen who belongs to a dense, homogeneous network will be more influenced by the norms and values of that group than a teen who relates individually to a number of separate individuals. In the close-knit group, drug prevention programs would have to focus on changing the norms about drug use within the existing network. When social networks are more loosely organized, the program might focus on creating drug-free networks, encouraging teens to associate with those networks, and reducing the desirability of membership in drug-using networks.

The third level of influence is significant because people spend one-third to one-half of their waking lives in *institutional* settings, especially schools and workplaces, which may have profound effects on their health and health-related behavior. In the workplace, employees may encounter hazardous chemicals or risks from injuries and accidents. Stress may be a problem. Alternatively, organizations may provide a corporate culture that supports positive behavior change. Workplace or school cafeterias may provide health-conscious menus; exercise facilities may be available and their use encouraged; smoking restrictions may prevail. Schools and workplaces provide ideal settings for public health intervention.

The larger *community*—the fourth level—can be a significant influence on behavior. Organizations can work together in a community to jointly promote healthy goals. An understanding of community organizations and networks can offer insights into promising avenues for health promotion. For example, churches are the social centers for many black and rural communities and may provide a focal point for health-related interventions. Conversely, community factors may sabotage public health efforts to promote healthy behavior. In the South, where tobacco is a pillar of local economies, public health advocates may find it difficult to even raise the issue of the health consequences of smoking.

At the fifth level, *public policy* encompasses the regulations and limitations on behavior that have been discussed previously. These are the most explicit and controversial measures that local, state, and national governments take to promote healthy behaviors. Such measures include smoking restrictions, age limits on alcohol sales, seat belt laws, and so forth.

Health Promotion Programs

As social and behavioral scientists gain a better understanding of how people's behavior is affected by their own beliefs and by the various levels of influence in their social environment, theories such as the health belief model and the ecological model are being used to design more effective public health and disease prevention programs. A good example is provided by an AIDS prevention program targeted at gay men in San Francisco in the mid-1980s.[23] Prevention of infection through behavior change was, and still is, the most effective approach to AIDS control because there is as yet no biomedical solution to the problem—no vaccine and no proven cure.

In the 1980s, San Francisco was the city with the second-highest number of AIDS cases in the United States. Most of the cases occurred in gay men, and the primary means by which the virus was transmitted was by sexual intercourse between men. Almost as soon as this relationship was understood, the city health department launched a prevention campaign in collaboration with community-based AIDS organizations and a research group from the University of California. They mounted an intensive media effort to inform at-risk individuals about the practice of safer sex. However, researchers understood that merely providing knowledge was not sufficient to change people's behavior. By interviewing small groups of gay men, they identified key beliefs that must be addressed to convince the target population to act on the message.

This approach combines elements of three theories discussed earlier: the health belief model, self-efficacy, and the ecological model. The campaign's goals were to promote the following beliefs among high-risk individuals:

1. Belief in personal threat (i.e., "I am susceptible to infection").
2. Belief in response efficacy (i.e., "There is something I can do that will lessen the threat of infection").
3. Belief in personal efficacy (i.e., "I am capable of making these changes").
4. Belief that new behaviors are consistent with group norms (i.e., "My peers support new behaviors").[18]

The first belief was relatively easy to achieve because of the extensive publicity about AIDS in the general media. News and entertainment media aimed at gay men, including gay newspapers, comic books, and leaflets, as well as telephone hotlines could be used to focus more on the second and third beliefs. Gay-related organizations held small group training sessions to teach skills in the use of condoms as well as interpersonal communication skills such as the ability to negotiate safer sex practices with prospective sex partners; this helped to enhance perceptions of self-efficacy among those at risk. To achieve the fourth belief, messages sought to encourage the perception that low-risk behaviors could be pleasurable and satisfying.

The first three elements of the campaign focused on individual health beliefs and self-efficacy, whereas the fourth element addressed interpersonal and community influences. The campaign targeted community influences by providing educational programs for bartenders in establishments frequented by gay men. Condoms were made widely available in bars and small-group meetings and were distributed by volunteers on street corners. Through public policy, the government level of influence was addressed by the city's provision of free, confidential testing for the HIV antibody. Because public bathhouses were a frequent

site of high-risk behavior, the city government faced pressure to close them, as was done in New York City. However, the campaign as a whole was so successful in changing the behavior of gay men that business at the bathhouses fell off, and public health officers were satisfied with merely posting warnings to the clientele about safe sex.[24]

The San Francisco AIDS prevention program was highly successful. Surveys done between 1984 and 1988 found that gay men had dramatically reduced their high-risk sexual behaviors during that period. For example, the percentage of men who reported engaging in unprotected receptive anal intercourse—the behavior most likely to transmit HIV—fell from 44% to 3% over the four years of the study.[25]

The early success of AIDS prevention programs among gay men, in the rest of the United States as well as in San Francisco, was attributable largely to the fact that the gay community was in general well educated and politically astute. The epidemic's potential victims tended to be of high SES, motivated to preserve their health, and able to mobilize resources to cope with the impending threat. Thus, they were more receptive to the health promotion campaign than other groups at risk for HIV. Unfortunately, the initial success in reducing high-risk behavior has not been maintained over time. Ongoing studies of gay men in San Francisco found that the prevalence of unprotected anal intercourse had increased from 31% in 1998 to approximately 60% in 2014, and held steady at that level through 2018.[26–28] Nevertheless, the rate of new HIV cases among gay men fell every year between 2012 and 2018, from about 350 new cases in 2012 to about 150 new cases in 2018.[28]

Public health workers attribute the resurgence of high-risk sexual behaviors to the advent of highly active antiretroviral therapy in 1995. Because of the remarkable effectiveness of the new drug treatments, many younger gay men saw HIV infection as a less severe threat (a factor in the health belief model) than did older gay men. The total number of infected individuals continued to increase until 2014, but has held steady since then due to the balance between infected individuals now living longer because of therapy and the declining number of new infections.[28]

In other parts of the United States, different approaches may be necessary to reach high-risk groups. For example, among blacks—the population with the highest prevalence of HIV—men who have sex with men (MSM) often do not identify as gay. Thus prevention messages targeted at them might need to be different from those used in San Francisco.[29] A large number of studies have been done on behavioral interventions for HIV prevention and their effectiveness at reducing risky sexual behaviors. Evidence has shown the effectiveness of individual person-to-person counseling, group-level programs that include a skill-building component delivered by other MSM, and, to a lesser extent, community-level programs that can motivate and reinforce behavior change. There is little evidence, however, on how to reach minority MSM who do not regard themselves as part of the gay community. Other high-risk groups that need targeted programs include black women, who may be at risk of infection because of heterosexual intercourse with bisexual black men, and intravenous drug users.

Unfortunately, health promotion and disease prevention programs cannot be done once and for all. They must be repeated for every generation and every new at-risk group.

Changing the Environment

As more is learned about what influences people to behave the way they do, many advocates believe that public health programs, to be effective, must concentrate less on individual behavior and more on changing the environment—both the social environment and the physical environment—to make it easier for people to behave in healthy ways. For example, many fewer deaths occur from motor vehicle crashes now than took place

three decades ago. This public health success comes less from educational programs about safe driving than it does from safer design of highways and automobiles.

Similarly, the San Francisco HIV researchers suggested that social biases against homosexuality might contribute to the AIDS epidemic. They proposed that recognition of same-sex marriage might encourage more stable relationships among gays, reduce the number of sexual partners by each individual, and thereby reduce the individual's risk of being infected. Public policy affects risk of HIV infection among intravenous drug users by providing access to needle exchange programs, which are illegal in some communities.

Environmental factors influence people's diet and activity patterns, which are key factors in Americans' poor health. The government recommends that people eat five to nine servings daily of fresh fruit and vegetables, but educating people who live in poor areas will not help improve their diets if they do not have access to supermarkets or produce stands. Similarly, federal policies that since World War II have favored a suburban lifestyle must bear much of the blame for Americans' lack of exercise: People live in their cars because most places are not within walking distance.

The environmental perspective forces people to think of public health problems as social and political issues that require collective action. Instead of blaming smokers for lack of willpower, public opinion has shifted its focus to the tobacco industry and the enormous resources the industry had put into making its products attractive to young people, a way of thinking that has led to a remarkable change in public attitudes toward smoking. People are now taking action against the tobacco industry, as black activists did against the alcoholic beverage industry when it began aggressively marketing high-powered malt liquors to young black males.[30] This approach may lead to confrontations with very powerful economic interests, and it will not always be successful. However, having whole communities become involved has the potential of being the most effective way to bring about major changes in health and behavior.

Conclusion

Because health is so strongly affected by behavior, it is important for public health advocates to understand what influences people to behave in healthy versus unhealthy ways. The social and behavioral sciences offer insights into why people behave as they do, and they provide a basis for developing interventions aimed at persuading people to change their behavior.

Evidence suggests that factors such as race, gender, marital status, and especially SES influence health in various ways, and the reasons for these differences are likely to reflect differences in the social environment. Life expectancy, infant mortality, and mortality rates from a variety of diseases vary profoundly among different racial and ethnic groups. Stress, which may be brought on by social factors, has an adverse effect on health for a number of reasons. Social support has been found to have a positive effect on health, probably in part by providing a buffer against stress. The health of black Americans tends to be poorer than that of the white majority. Health data for populations are usually analyzed by race and ethnicity, and public health efforts focus on understanding the disparities and trying to eliminate them.

Theories of health behavior include the health belief model and the theory of self-efficacy. Both of these theories focus on individuals' attitudes and beliefs as determinants of their behavior. The transtheoretical model of stages of change can be used in health education programs to promote behavior change. A broader perspective is provided by the ecological model of health behavior. This model considers all the levels of influence that may affect the individual's attitudes and beliefs, including interpersonal relationships such as family and friends, institutional influences such as school and work, the larger community and its values and beliefs, and public policy including laws and regulations.

The most effective public health intervention programs influence people's beliefs at several levels with the goal of creating a social environment favorable to healthy behavior. The San Francisco AIDS prevention program is an example of an effective program that succeeded in significantly reducing the transmission of HIV early in the epidemic. Evidence shows, however, that to maintain the success of such a program, intensive public health efforts must be maintained, both to prevent relapses into unhealthy behavior and to educate new generations of at-risk people.

Increasingly, public health advocates realize that the most effective ways of improving the health-related behaviors of individuals will focus on involving whole communities in improving the social and physical environment to be more conducive to healthy behavior.

References

1. Centers for Disease Control and Prevention, "Deaths: Leading Causes for 2017," *National Vital Statistics Report* 68, no. 6 (June 24, 2019).
2. J. Holt-Lunstad, T. B. Smith, and J. B. Layton, "Social Relationships and Mortality Risk: A Meta-Analytic Review," *PLoS Medicine* 7, no. 7 (2010).
3. Centers for Disease Control and Prevention, National Center for Health Statistics, "Health, United States, 2011: With Special Feature on Socioeconomic Status and Health," May 2012.
4. N. Adler, T. Boyce, M. A. Chesney, S. Folkman, and S. L. Syme, "Socioeconomic Inequalities in Health: No

Easy Solution," *Journal of the American Medical Association* 269 (1993): 3140–3145.

5. M. G. Marmot et al., "Health Inequalities Among British Civil Servants: The Whitehall II Study," *Lancet* 337 (1991): 1387–1393.

6. Centers for Disease Control and Prevention, "Smoking & Tobacco Use: Fast Facts and Fact Sheets," https://www.cdc.gov/tobacco/data_statistics/fact _sheets/index.htm, accessed September 21, 2019.

7. National Center for Health Statistics, "Health, United States, 2014," May 2015, https://www.cdc.gov/nchs /data/hus/hus14.pdf, accessed September 21, 2019.

8. A. Case and A. Deaton, "Mortality and Morbidity in the 21st Century," *Brookings Papers on Economic Activity* 1 (2017).

9. Kaiser Family Foundation, "Health Coverage & Uninsured," https://www.kff.org/state-category/health -coverage-uninsured/, accessed September 21, 2019.

10. Centers for Disease Control and Prevention, "United States Life Tables, 2017," *National Statistics Vital Reports* 68, no. 7 (June 24, 2019), https://www.cdc .gov/nchs/data/nvsr/nvsr68/nvsr68_07-508.pdf, accessed September 14, 2019.

11. National Cancer Institute, "Cancer Stat Facts: Prostate Cancer," https://seer.cancer.gov/statfacts/html/prost .html, accessed September 21, 2019.

12. Centers for Disease Control and Prevention, "Atlas Plus: HIV Deaths," https://gis.cdc.gov/grasp/nchhst patlas/tables.html, accessed September 21, 2019.

13. J. Semega, M. Kollar, J. Creamer, and A. Mohanty, *Income and Poverty in the United States: 2018*, U.S. Census Bureau, Current Population Reports, P60-266 (Washington, DC: U.S. Government Printing Office, 2019).

14. K. J. Helsing and M. Szklo, "Mortality After Bereavement," *American Journal of Epidemiology* 114 (1981): 41–52.

15. F. Kittel, M. Kornitzer, and M. Dramaik, "Coronary Heart Disease and Job Stress in Two Cohorts of Bank Clerks," *Psychotherapy and Psychosomatics* 34 (1980): 110–123.

16. S. Cohen, D. A. J. Tyrrell, and A. P. Smith, "Psychological Stress and Susceptibility to the Common Cold," *New England Journal of Medicine* 325 (1991): 606–612.

17. L. F. Berkman and L. Breslow, *Health and Ways of Living: The Alameda County Study* (New York, NY: Oxford University Press, 1983), 31–54.

18. N. K. Janz, V. L. Champion, and V. J. Strecher, "The Health Belief Model," in K. Glanz, B. K. Rimer, and F. M. Lewis, eds., *Health Behavior and Health Education: Theory, Research, and Practice*, 3rd ed. (San Francisco, CA: Jossey-Bass, 2002), 45–66.

19. R. R. Lau, "Beliefs About Control and Health Behavior," in D. S. Gochman, ed., *Health Behavior: Emerging Research Perspectives* (New York, NY: Plenum Press, 1983), 43–63.

20. C. A. Marlatt, J. S. Baer, and L. A. Quigley, "Self-Efficacy and Addictive Behavior," in A. Bandura, ed., *Self Efficacy in Changing Societies* (Cambridge, UK: Cambridge University Press, 1995), 289–315.

21. J. O. Prochaska, "The Transtheoretical Model and Stages of Change," in K. Glanz, B. K. Rimer, and F. M. Lewis, eds., *Health Behavior and Health Education: Theory, Research, and Practice*, 3rd ed. (San Francisco, CA: Jossey-Bass, 2002), 99–120.

22. K. R. McLeroy, D. Bibeau, A. Steckler, and K. Glanz, "An Ecological Perspective on Health Promotion Programs," *Health Education Quarterly* 15 (1988): 351–377.

23. A. L. McAlister, P. Puska, M. Orlandi, L. L. Bye, and P. L. Zbylot, "Behaviour Modification: Principles and Illustrations," in W. Holland, R. Detels, and G. Knox, eds., *Oxford Textbook of Public Health*, 2nd ed., vol. 3. (Oxford, UK: Oxford University Press, 1991), 3–16.

24. R. Bayer, *Private Acts, Social Consequences: AIDS and the Politics of Public Health* (New York, NY: Free Press, 1989).

25. L. McKusick, T. J. Coates, S. F. Morin, L. Pollack, and C. Hoff, "Longitudinal Predictors of Reductions in Unprotected Anal Intercourse Among Gay Men in San Francisco: The AIDS Behavioral Research Project," *American Journal of Public Health* 80 (1990): 978–983.

26. S. Scheer, T. Kellogg, J. D. Klausner, S. Schwarcz, G. Colfax, K. Bernstein, et al., "HIV Is Hyperendemic Among Men Who Have Sex with Men in San Francisco: 10-Year Trends in HIV Incidence, HIV Prevalence, Sexually Transmitted Infections and Sexual Risk Behaviour," *Sexually Transmitted Infections* 84 (2008): 493–498.

27. J. M. Snowden, C. Wei, W. McFarland, and H.F. Raymond, "Prevalence, Correlates and Trends in Seroadaptive Behaviors Among Men Who Have Sex with Men from Serial Cross-Sectional Surveillance in San Francisco, 2004–2011," *Sexually Transmitted Infections* 90 (2014): 498–504.

28. San Francisco Department of Public Health, Public Health Division, "HIV Epidemiology Annual Report 2018," September 2019, https://www.sfdph.org/dph /files/reports/RptsHIVAIDS/HIV-Epidemiology-Annual -Report-2018.pdf, accessed September 21, 2019.

29. J. H. Herbst, C. Beeker, A. Mathew, T. McNally, W. F. Passin, L. S. Kay, et al., "The Effectiveness of Individual-, Group-, and Community-Level HIV Behavioral Risk-Reduction Interventions for Adult Men Who Have Sex with Men: A Systematic Review," *American Journal of Preventive Medicine* 32, suppl. 1 (2007): 38–67.

30. L. Wallack, L. Dorfman, D. Jernigan, and M. Themba, *Media Advocacy and Public Health: Power for Prevention* (Newbury Park, CA: Sage Publications, 1993).

CHAPTER 15

Deadly Habit

Public Health Enemy Number One: Tobacco

KEY TERMS

Carcinogenicity
Disability-adjusted life years

E-cigarettes
Menthol cigarettes

Second-hand smoke

Cigarette smoking—one of the two leading actual causes of death in the United States—is the nation's most significant public health issue: It is both the leading preventable cause of death and the leading cause of **disability-adjusted life years**, which is a measure of overall disease burden, capturing the number of years lost from poor health, disability, or premature death.[1,2] The problem of tobacco-caused disease embodies the complex interactions by which psychological, social, cultural, economic, and political factors influence individual behavior to cause more than 480,000 deaths each year, and perhaps as many as 575,000 deaths each year if additional suspected cases are included.[1,3] **Table 15-1** lists the major diseases thought to be caused by smoking, and provides estimates of the relative risk for each disease among current smokers age 55 and older relative to people who never smoked. The mortality rate among current smokers is 2.8 times higher than that for never-smokers,[3] and smokers, on average,

die 10 years younger than do nonsmokers.[4] **Table 15-2** lists the numbers of premature deaths caused by smoking in the United States over the 50-year period ending 2014 by major cause. An astounding 20,830,000 premature deaths have been attributed to smoking.[3]

The struggle to understand and deal with tobacco-caused illness involves all areas of public health. Epidemiology provided the first solid evidence that smoking caused cancer and heart disease and has continued to yield information on the health effects of this very human habit. Biomedical studies were slow to provide evidence because laboratory animals could not be persuaded or forced to smoke cigarettes, but eventually they yielded valuable information on the role of tobacco in the causation of cancer and heart disease. In more recent years, smoking has come to be seen as an environmental health threat, producing indoor air pollution that has been shown to cause adverse health effects in nonsmokers. Ultimately, however, smoking is a behavior,

Table 15-1 Relative Risk of Death from Smoking for Persons 55 Years of Age and Older by Cause and Gender

	Relative Risk for Current Smokers Compared to Never-Smokers	
	Women	Men
All causes	2.8	2.8
Cancers		
Acute myeloid leukemia	1.1	1.9
Breast cancer	1.3	–
Cancers of unknown site	2.7	3.2
Colorectal cancer	1.6	1.4
Esophogeal cancer	5.1	3.9
Kidney and renal pelvis cancer	1.2	1.8
Laryngeal cancer	103.8	13.9
Lip and oral cancer	5.6	5.7
Liver cancer	1.8	2.3
Lung cancer	22.9	25.3
Pancreatic cancer	1.9	1.6
Prostate cancer	—	1.4
Rare cancers	1.1	1.6
Stomach cancer	1.7	1.9
Urinary bladder cancer	3.9	3.9
Diseases of the heart		
Aortic aneurysm	10.1	7.5
Atherosclerosis	2.1	5.0
Essential hypertension and hypertensive renal disease	2.4	2.6
Hypertensive heart disease	1.9	2.9
Ischemic heart disease	3.0	2.6
Total stroke	2.1	1.9
Other arterial diseases	5.6	5.3
Other heart disease	1.9	2.0

	Relative Risk for Current Smokers Compared to Never-Smokers	
	Women	Men
Respiratory diseases and infections		
COPD	25.0	27.8
Pneumonia, influenza, and tuberculosis	1.9	2.0
Other infections	2.5	2.2
Other respiratory diseases	1.9	2.0
Other diseases		
Diabetes	1.5	1.6
Ischemic disorders of the intestines	6.1	5.6
Liver cirrhosis	2.6	3.6
Renal failure	1.9	2.1
Additional rare causes combined	2.0	1.9
Other digestive diseases	2.1	2.6
Unknown causes	2.2	1.9

Data from Table 2 of B.D. Carter et al., "Smoking and Mortality—Beyond Established Causes," *New England Journal of Medicine* 372 (2015): 631–640.

Table 15-2 **Premature Deaths Causes by Smoking and Exposure to Second-hand Smoke, 1965–2014**

Smoking-related cancers	6,587,000
Cardiovascular and metabolic diseases	7,787,000
Pulmonary diseases	3,804,000
Conditions related to pregnancy and birth	108,000
Residential fires	86,000
Lung cancers caused by exposure to second-hand smoke	263,000
Coronary heart disease caused by exposure to second-hand smoke	2,194,000
Total	20,830,000

Data from U.S. Department of Health and Human Services, "The Health Consequences of Smoking—50 Years of Progress: A Report of the Surgeon General, Executive Summary, Table 1, 2014," https://www.hhs.gov/sites/default/files/consequences-smoking-exec-summary.pdf, accessed September 22, 2019.

and it is the social and behavioral sciences that must provide insights into why people smoke and how they can be persuaded to quit.

Public health faces a fundamental dilemma in confronting the current epidemic of tobacco-caused disease: What should be the role of a democratic government in confronting a behavior that is practiced by nearly one in seven adults and will kill as many as half of them? Political and economic forces that favored tobacco have opposed strong government measures against cigarettes. Public health efforts involving education and health promotion campaigns have persuaded many people to stop smoking but seem to have reached the limit of their effectiveness in bringing smoking prevalence down to approximately 14% among U.S. adults.[5]

The 1990s saw a major shift in federal and state governments' attitudes toward smoking. Recognition that the nicotine in tobacco is addictive, together with evidence that cigarette companies have purposely manipulated nicotine levels in cigarettes to keep people hooked, has forced politicians to look with suspicion on what was previously considered a freely chosen behavior. Moreover, evidence of the high economic costs paid by government-financed programs, including Medicare and Medicaid, for the treatment of tobacco-caused disease has forced governments to question their previous assumptions about the economic advantages of supporting the tobacco industry.

Biomedical Basis of Smoking's Harmful Effects

The basic fact underlying the popular success of cigarettes is that they deliver nicotine, an addictive drug. Nicotine is absorbed by the linings of the mouth and the respiratory tract, from which it travels rapidly to the heart and then to the brain. The drug produces a sense of enhanced energy and alertness, while also having a calming effect on addicted smokers. When people try to quit smoking, they experience withdrawal reactions with unpleasant physical and psychological symptoms. In 2015, 68% of smokers reported wanting to quit smoking and 55% had tried in the past year to quit; only about 7% of them succeeded.[6]

In addition to nicotine, an important component of tobacco smoke is tar, the residue from burning tobacco that condenses in the lungs of smokers. Tars provide the flavor in cigarette smoke; they are also a major source of its **carcinogenicity**. As early as the 1930s, experiments were done in which these tars were painted on the ear linings of rabbits or the shaved backs of mice and found to cause tumors. Decades of studies by biomedical researchers—and clandestinely by tobacco companies, which did not wish to publicize their results—have confirmed the carcinogenicity of the tars as well as other ingredients of the smoke, including arsenic and benzene. When filters were added to cigarettes with the ostensible purpose of removing tars and other harmful ingredients, it turned out that they tended also to remove the taste and "satisfaction" from smoking. Thus filter cigarettes, to be acceptable to smokers, had to deliver significant levels of tar and nicotine, meaning that there were limits to how "safe" a cigarette could be.

Tars not only cause cancer but also contribute to other lung diseases by damaging cilia, the tiny hairs on the linings of the respiratory tract that sweep the lungs and bronchi clear of microbes, irritants, and toxic substances. Damage to cilia and irritation of respiratory tract linings by components of smoke increase susceptibility to infectious diseases such as bronchitis, influenza, and pneumonia as well as to diseases brought on by chronic irritation such as emphysema and asthma.

In contrast to the long-term processes leading to cancer and emphysema, smoking can have very rapid effects on the cardiovascular system. The nicotine in cigarette smoke raises blood pressure and heart rate. It may also cause spasms in the blood vessels of the heart, especially if damage already exists, increasing the risk of sudden cardiac death. Carbon monoxide in cigarette smoke interferes with the oxygen-carrying capacity of red blood cells, leading to oxygen shortages in the hearts of patients suffering from coronary artery disease. Smoking increases the risk of stroke and heart attacks by altering the clotting properties of blood. Components of cigarette smoke also have been shown to raise total blood cholesterol levels and reduce levels of high-density lipoprotein (HDL), the "good" cholesterol.

Historical Trends in Smoking and Health

Although it has been smoked and chewed for hundreds of years, tobacco was not used intensively enough to cause widespread illness until the 20th century. Before then, almost all tobacco was smoked in pipes and cigars or used as chewing tobacco and snuff. Cigarette rolling machines and safety matches were invented in the 1880s, but cigarette smoking began to increase dramatically only after 1913, when Camel, followed by other brands, began mass marketing campaigns.[7] The distribution of free cigarettes to soldiers during the two world wars further stimulated smoking among men. Smoking among women was frowned upon early in the century, but women began to take up the habit during and after World War II, and by 1960 approximately 34% of American women smoked.[8] While estimates of the percentages of men and women who smoked during the early part of the century are imprecise—they were developed before the Centers for Disease Control and Prevention (CDC) began systematic surveys of the population in 1965—a general idea of the trends in much of the century can be seen in **Figure 15-1**. The percentage of Americans who smoke has continued to decline since 1980. A better sense of the extent of smoking in this country, and the circumstances influencing it, comes from U.S. Department of Agriculture data on total manufactured cigarette consumption (**Figure 15-2**).

The first disease clearly linked to smoking was lung cancer, which is caused predominately by smoking and is relatively rare in nonsmokers. Lung cancer was virtually nonexistent in the United States and Britain in 1900. In the 1930s, the increase in deaths from lung cancer began to attract attention, and a link to cigarette smoking began to be suspected. Epidemiologic studies published in the 1950s eventually confirmed this link. Cigarette consumption dropped as a result of these reports (as shown in Figure 15-2), but began to climb again when tobacco companies promoted filter cigarettes as a safer alternative.

In 1964, the U.S. Surgeon General released the *Smoking and Health* report, a summary of the evidence to date, which resulted from an exhaustive deliberation by a panel of 10 renowned scientists.[9] The panel unanimously agreed that cigarette smoking caused lung cancer and chronic bronchitis and was strongly associated with cancer of the mouth and larynx. It also reported that smoking increased the risk of heart disease. The Surgeon General's report was very influential, convincing many smokers to quit and providing ammunition for advocates wishing to impose controls on the tobacco industry.

Women were hardly mentioned in the 1964 Surgeon General's report. Lung cancer was rare in women, and all the studies had been done on men. However, women soon began to catch up. In 1980, the Surgeon General issued another report that focused entirely on women. *Health Consequences of Smoking for Women* addressed "the fallacy of women's immunity."[10] The report points out that the first signs of an epidemic of smoking-related diseases among women were just beginning to appear, because women had begun smoking intensively nearly 25 years after men had. Indeed, lung cancer was about to surpass breast cancer and become the leading cause of cancer death in women,

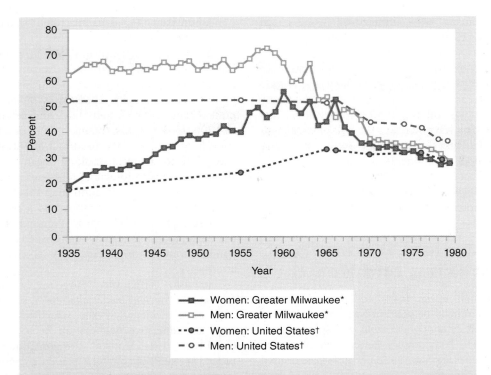

*Adapted from Howe 1984: *Milwaukee Journal*, Consumer analysis of the Greater Milwaukee market, 1924–1979. Before 1941, the wording of questions eliciting information on cigarette use and type of respondent are not recorded. In 1941–1954, men were asked, "Do you smoke cigarettes?" In 1955–1959, respondents were asked, "Do any men [women] in your household smoke cigarettes with [without] a filter tip?" In 1960–1965 and 1967, women and men were asked, "Have you bought, for your own use, cigarettes with [without] a filter tip in the past 30 days?" In 1966 and 1968–1979, women and men were asked, "Have you bought, for your own use, cigarettes with [without] a filter tip in the past 7 days?" Data since 1955 are based on the sum of the percentage of smokers who bought filter-tipped cigarettes and the percentage who bought nonfilter-tipped cigarettes in the past 30 days. Results overestimate smoking prevalence because respondents could answer "yes" to both questions. Data for women in 1976–1979 include only the percentage buying filter-tipped cigarettes; the question on the use of nonfilter-tipped cigarettes was dropped because of low response.

†Absence of data points from national surveys from 1935–1965 means these lines should not be interpreted as trends. The 1935 data are from the 1935 *Fortune* Survey III (*Fortune Magazine,* 1935), the 1955 data are from the 1955 Current Population Survey (Haenszel et al., 1956), and the 1965–1979 data are from the National Health Interview Survey (Giovino et al., 1994).

Figure 15-1 Prevalence of Current Smoking Among Adults Aged 18 Years or Older in the Greater Milwaukee Area and in the General U.S. Population, by Gender 1935–1979

Reproduced from Centers for Disease Control and Prevention, "Women and Smoking: A Report of the Surgeon General, 2001," Figure 2.1, http://www.ncbi.nlm.nih.gov/books/NBK44311/#A6558, accessed September 22, 2019.

as it remains today.[11] The 1980 report noted that, in addition to suffering the same ill health effects as men, female smokers are at increased risk for complications of pregnancy and infants of female smokers are more likely to be premature or lagging in physical growth.

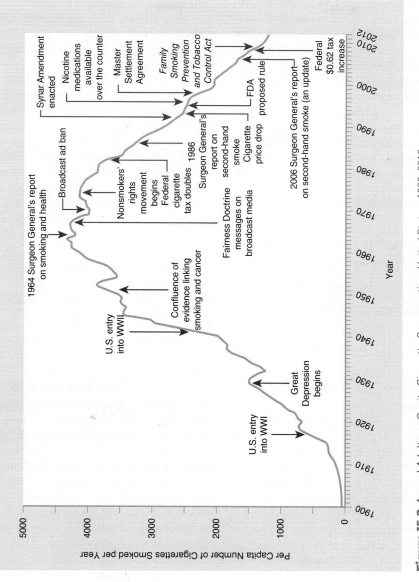

Figure 15-2 Annual Adult per Capita Cigarette Consumption, United States, 1900–2012

Historically, the prevalence of smoking among black men was higher than that among white men; accordingly, lung cancer mortality rates have been higher among black men. Rates of smoking among blacks have declined, however, and are now slightly lower than those among whites. American Indians and Alaskan Natives smoke at much higher rates than other ethnic groups, averaging 21% overall, while the rates for Hispanics and Asians are both less than 10%. Very large differences in smoking rates are seen among groups of different socioeconomic status, and there is a particularly strong association between smoking and lack of education. Prevalence of smoking is only about 7% among male and female college graduates, whereas nearly 30% of those with a high school education or less are smokers.[12]

Regulatory Restrictions on Smoking: New Focus on Environmental Tobacco Smoke

Public health efforts at discouraging smoking have had to contend with the enormous economic and political power of the tobacco industry. Congress, which until recently provided subsidies to tobacco growers, has been very reluctant to pass legislation opposed by the industry. However, the 1964 Surgeon General's report carried great credibility, and its publication led to a number of government actions aimed at restricting cigarette marketing. These included Federal Trade Commission requirements that cigarette packages contain warning labels and a Federal Communications Commission mandate in 1968 that radio and television advertisements for cigarettes be balanced by public service announcements about their harmful effects. The latter requirement, called the Fairness Doctrine, was so effective in countering the tobacco companies' ads, as seen in the drop

in cigarette consumption shown in Figure 15-2, that in 1971 the industry submitted to a total ban on cigarette advertising on radio and television. In return, the public service announcements ceased. The tobacco companies then shifted their advertising efforts to magazines, newspapers, billboards, product giveaways, and sponsorship of sporting and cultural events.[8]

Over the past four decades, new awareness of the harm caused by **second-hand smoke** has led to some of the most effective actions against smoking. Studies began to show that exposure to environmental tobacco smoke caused some of the same health problems as active smoking. For example, the nonsmoking spouses of smokers have an increased risk of lung cancer and heart disease, and children of parents who smoke are more likely to suffer from asthma, respiratory infections, and sudden infant death syndrome. In 1992, the Environmental Protection Agency issued a report that declared environmental tobacco smoke to be a carcinogen, causing 3000 lung cancer deaths per year.[13] Evidence of the harm caused by second-hand smoke inspired the nonsmokers' rights movement, which largely bypassed the U.S. Congress and focused political pressure on state and local governments.

In 1974, Connecticut became the first state to enact restrictions on smoking in restaurants. Minnesota passed a comprehensive statewide clean indoor air law in 1975. In 1983, San Francisco passed a restrictive law against smoking in the workplace, including private workplaces. The clean indoor air movement blossomed. At the state level, laws were passed that restricted smoking on public transit vehicles and in elevators, cultural and recreational facilities, schools, and libraries. Over the objections of the tobacco industry, Congress banned smoking on all domestic airline flights in 1989.[8] Restrictions on indoor smoking became more widespread in the 1990s. As of September 2019, 27 states and the District of Columbia had banned or severely restricted smoking in all public places, including work sites, restaurants, and most bars, and were given a rating of A or B by the American Lung Association for the strength of their smoke-free air laws. All other states had enacted some limitations on indoor smoking, although 10 states received an F rating from the American Lung Association for their laws: Alabama, Kentucky, Mississippi, Missouri, New Hampshire, North Carolina, South Carolina, Texas, Virginia, and Wyoming. It is probably not a coincidence that the leading tobacco-growing states are on this F-rating list. Many counties and municipalities have also passed legislation to promote clean indoor air.[14]

The effectiveness of the nonsmokers' rights movement stems from its success in transforming smoking into a socially unacceptable activity. Bans in so many public places force smokers to refrain for extended periods and to segregate themselves when they wish to smoke, often by going outdoors. By making smoking inconvenient, bans encourage people to quit. As Figure 15-2 shows, cigarette consumption has declined steadily since the nonsmokers' rights movement began.

Advertising: Emphasis on Youth

Although smoking rates among adults have fallen, public health advocates are especially concerned about smoking among youth. Teenagers tend to be less worried about their health in the distant future than they are with their image and social status among their peers. Tobacco companies exploit those concerns in their attempts to win over young people to smoking.

To maintain a constant number of customers over time, the tobacco industry must persuade around a million people to take up the habit each year to balance the number of smokers who die or quit. Cigarette and smokeless tobacco advertising and promotional expenditures amounted to $9.5 billion in 2016, or $29 for every person in the United States.[15]

Because the teen years are the critical period for smoking initiation—nearly all adult smokers started before age 18—tobacco companies have targeted their advertising toward children and young people.[8] For example, Joe Camel ads were strongly appealing to children. A 1991 study found that 91% of 6-year-olds recognized the cartoon character—the same percentage that recognized Disney's Mickey Mouse logo.[16] Between 1988, when the Joe Camel ad campaign was introduced, and 1990, it is estimated that Camel cigarette sales to minors rose from $6 million to $476 million.[8] In response to an outburst of negative publicity and public anger at the tobacco companies, Joe Camel was retired in 1997.

Tobacco companies also targeted youth with promotional items, such as T-shirts, caps, and sporting goods bearing a brand's logo. They managed to evade the ban on broadcast advertising by sponsoring sporting events, at which brand names were displayed in the background, ensuring that they would be visible on television throughout the event.

As part of the 1998 Master Settlement Agreement (MSA), discussed later in this chapter, major tobacco companies agreed to stop advertisements targeted at children, including some promotional activities. Although the most blatant appeals to youth have disappeared, the companies began running ads that, while ostensibly antitobacco public service ads, were actually more sophisticated messages designed to encourage youth smoking.[17] The messages stated that smoking is for adults only, and that parents should talk to their children about not smoking. Analyses of their impact on teens have shown that these ads were ineffective in discouraging young people from smoking and may have increased their intention to smoke. This may have been the intention when the ads were designed. While a combination of public health efforts, including the MSA, contributed to a decline in the number of teens who smoke for a period, the rate at which youths use tobacco products is again on the rise. Between 2011 and 2018, the percentage of high school students who used tobacco products increased from 24.2% to 27.1%; the smoking rates for middle school students were 7.5% in 2011 and 7.2% in 2018.[18] As discussed later in this chapter, electronic cigarettes (e-cigarettes) have fueled this increase.

All states have laws prohibiting the sale of tobacco to minors. In fact, as of September 2019, 18 states had increased the minimum age for purchasing tobacco products to 21. Nevertheless, enforcement of the laws varies.[19] The CDC's 2013 survey found that 18% of the student smokers bought cigarettes from a store or gas station.

As advertising to children and teens has become increasingly restricted, tobacco companies have focused their efforts on young adults, who are still receptive to social pressures, may smoke occasionally, and may be vulnerable to advertising. The companies use promotional activities, such as distributing free cigarette samples or brand-labeled articles of clothing, with the goal of turning occasional smokers into addicts. Indoor smoking bans, which have become widespread in recent decades, have blocked the effectiveness of this kind of marketing. Portrayal of smoking in movies and on television has been shown to exert a powerful influence in inspiring adolescents to smoke, and the Institute of Medicine has recommended that the movie rating system take this factor into consideration when assigning G, PG, PG-13, or R ratings.[20] However, the recommendation has had only limited effect.[21] Among the major movie studios in 2018, Fox and Comcast movies that were rated G, PG, or PG-13 had at least 35 tobacco-use incidents per movie, while Sony and Time Warner had fewer than 10, and Viacom and Disney movies had none.[22]

The tobacco industry has targeted advertising at both women and minorities—groups identified as promising sources of new smokers. Young women have been attracted by suggestions that smoking will help them lose weight, beginning with the Lucky Strike ads of the 1920s that advised, "Reach for a Lucky instead of a sweet." More recently, Virginia Slims ads have taken a similar approach. Shortly after the Virginia Slims advertising campaign began in the 1960s, the proportion of 14- to 17-year-old girls who started smoking nearly doubled.[8] Tobacco companies advertise to African American communities with campaigns that, for example, use urban culture and language to promote menthol cigarettes and offer tobacco-sponsored hip-hop bar nights. The companies also target Asian American communities by sponsoring events such as Chinese and Vietnamese New Year festivals.[15]

Taxes as a Public Health Measure

Antismoking activists, supported by economic research, have concluded that one of the most effective measures to discourage young people from smoking is to raise the tax on cigarettes. A pack of cigarettes represents a more significant proportion of a teenager's disposable income than it does for adults, and the higher price is likely to have more impact on someone who is not yet addicted. Low-income smokers are also sensitive to price.[23]

Research on teenage smoking suggests that teenagers are indeed sensitive to price. For example, after Philip Morris cut the price of Marlboro cigarettes, a brand favored by young people, by 40% in April 1993, the proportion of teenagers in 8th, 10th, and 12th grades who smoked rose from 23.5% to 28% in 1996. Other studies have shown that a 10% increase in price reduces the number of teenagers who smoke by approximately 7% to 12%.[24] "Raising tobacco taxes is our number one strategy to damage the tobacco industry," an American Cancer Society executive was quoted as saying. "The industry has found ways around everything else we have done, but they can't repeal the laws of economics."[24(p.293)]

Raising taxes on cigarettes is effective in reducing smoking among adults as well.

In 1989, California increased cigarette taxes from 10 cents to 35 cents per pack. The law specified that 20% of the proceeds were to be designated for programs designed to prevent and reduce tobacco use, especially among children. Surveys conducted before and after implementation of the tax increase found that the prevalence of cigarette smoking among adults in California was reduced from 22.7% in 1988 to 20.0% in 1992, then to 16.9% in 1995, and then to 13.3% in 2008.[25] It is difficult to determine the share of the decline that can be attributed to the price increase as compared with other antismoking measures, including indoor smoking bans and the antismoking campaign funded by the tax.

In recent years, state and local governments have found that raising taxes on cigarettes is a painless way of closing budget shortfalls, and many states have followed this policy.[26] In 2019, for example, Connecticut and New York had the highest cigarette tax rates, collecting a tax of $4.35 per pack. By contrast, tobacco-producing states have low cigarette taxes: Virginia's rate was 30 cents per pack, and Missouri's rate, the lowest, was 17 cents.[27] California, a leader in raising cigarette taxes for public health goals, had fallen to a rank of 32nd among states, with a tax of 87 cents per pack. In June 2012, California voters rejected a proposed $1 per pack increase, the proceeds of which would have been used to finance cancer research. The tobacco industry spent nearly $50 million to defeat the measure.[28] However, in 2016, the state was able to push through a $2 increase, bringing its current cigarette tax per pack to $2.87.[29] The federal tax on cigarettes, last raised in 2009, is $1.01 per pack.[27]

California's Tobacco Control Program

California's voter-initiated tobacco control program, which began in 1989 with a 25-cent tax increase on cigarettes, has proved successful in maintaining low smoking rates statewide, though the state no longer leads the nation in terms of tobacco control efforts. The initiative mandated mass-media antitobacco advertising as well as school and community education and intervention activities. It also mandated that the effectiveness of the program be evaluated after a decade. Thus, the California experience has provided evidence on which methods are effective in reducing smoking.

The tax increase itself contributed to the success of the program, as discussed in the previous section. Immediately after the increase was implemented, cigarette consumption declined significantly in California compared with the rest of the nation. In 1994, the California legislature passed a law prohibiting smoking statewide in all workplaces except bars, taverns, and casinos. The law has since been strengthened to include these workplaces as well. Overall, per capita cigarette consumption in California fell dramatically from 120 packs per capita annually in 1980 to 17 packs per capita in 2018. This reduction was achieved by a combination of a reduction in the number of smokers and a reduction of the number of cigarettes each smoker consumed per day.[28,29]

In 2017, the prevalence of smoking had declined to 11.1% in California, compared to 17.1% for the rest of the nation.[29] California's antitobacco campaign suffered budget cuts after the first few years, however, and tobacco companies stepped up their political efforts to oppose the state's control measures, as well as their advertising and promotion of cigarettes. Even so, the permanent changes in policy, as well as additional tax increases, have helped California maintain its lead over all other states except Utah in keeping smoking levels relatively low.[29]

California's campaign included an aggressive advertising component, which contributed significantly to its overall success. Studies of the effectiveness of antismoking messages have shown that some messages are much more effective than others. In fact, some programs sponsored by the tobacco industry, which are presented as smoking prevention efforts, have been shown to make smoking more attractive to youths. Examination of industry documents, discussed in the next section, has found that the industry has purposely used these "forbidden fruit" messages to generate good public relations and fight restrictive legislation without actually discouraging youth smoking.[30]

The evaluation component of California's media campaign identified which antismoking messages were most effective in reaching youth. Researchers found that the message most effective in reaching both youths and adults is that "Tobacco industry executives use deceitful, manipulative, dishonest practices to hook new users, sell more cigarettes and make more money."[31(p.774)] One successful ad based on this premise, called "Nicotine Soundbites," showed the actual footage of tobacco executives testifying before Congress, raising their right hands and swearing that nicotine is not addictive. Ads with this message made both adults and teenagers angry, because no one likes to learn that they are being manipulated. Another message found to be effective among both adults and teens emphasized that second-hand smoke harms others. One ad portrayed a boy smoking, sitting with his little sister watching television. The little girl begins coughing and smoke comes out of her mouth.

Researchers concluded that, to be effective, antitobacco advertisements need to be "ambitious, hard-hitting, explicit, and in-your-face."[31(p.776)] The industry recognized the effectiveness of the ads and worked hard to limit them. R. J. Reynolds threatened to sue the California Department of Health and the television stations that ran the Nicotine Soundbites ad; the lawsuit was not filed, but the ad was later dropped. During the state campaign, the tobacco industry tried to counter the antitobacco efforts by increasing spending in California on advertising, incentives to merchants, and promotional items. One study calculated that after 1993, the industry spent nearly $10 for every $1 spent by the state.[32]

The Master Settlement Agreement

The 1990s saw dramatic developments in the battle against smoking, and suddenly it seemed possible that effective tobacco control measures would be enacted at the federal level. The changes resulted from several separate political and legal events, as well as public revelations that have discredited the tobacco industry.

In February 1994, David Kessler, then Commissioner of the Food and Drug Administration (FDA), launched an offensive against the tobacco industry by asserting that his agency had the authority to regulate tobacco. Kessler, who was appointed by President George H. W. Bush but now had the support of an antismoking president, Bill Clinton, based his claim on thoroughly documented evidence that nicotine is an addictive drug and cigarettes are drug delivery systems. He proposed a series of measures aimed to protect children and teenagers against tobacco company efforts to get them hooked.

Coincidentally, in March 1994, a class-action lawsuit was filed against American tobacco companies in federal district court in Louisiana on behalf of "all nicotine-dependent persons in the U.S." and their families and heirs, seeking compensatory and punitive damages, attorneys' fees, an admission of wrongdoing, and other remedies. Although this suit was dismissed, it was followed by other major lawsuits, including one in May 1994 by Michael Moore, the attorney general of Mississippi, who sought to recover the medical costs that the state had incurred treating smoking-related illnesses. Attorneys general from most of the other states followed suit over the next three years.[33]

Also in 1994, an anonymous informant from the Brown & Williamson tobacco company, who called himself "Mr. Butts" after the *Doonesbury* comic strip character, sent a box of top-secret tobacco industry internal documents to Stanton Glantz, a professor of medicine at the University of California at San Francisco and a well-known critic of the tobacco industry. The papers provided a wealth of information on discrepancies between what the industry knew about the ill effects of tobacco and what they were telling the public. For example, a lawyer for Brown & Williamson had written in a 1963 internal memo, "Nicotine is addictive. We are, then, in the business of selling nicotine, an addictive drug effective in the release of stress mechanisms."[34(p.58)] Glantz, with the support of University of California lawyers and librarians, published the papers on the Internet.

The tobacco companies, of course, challenged the FDA's authority to regulate tobacco, and they vigorously defended themselves against the lawsuits by attorneys general and injured smokers. However, the documents released by Glantz, together with other internal industry documents that were leaked, seriously undermined the industry's ability to defend itself in court. In April 1997, a North Carolina court affirmed the FDA's authority over tobacco as a drug, although it struck down some of the advertising restrictions proposed by the agency. However, in August 1998, an appeals court ruled the other way, stating that only Congress has authority to regulate the tobacco industry. The U.S. Supreme Court agreed to take up the issue, and in 2000 it supported the appeals court decision that the FDA did not have the authority to regulate tobacco.[35]

In early 1997, when the tobacco industry was on the defensive, it began negotiations with the state attorneys general, hoping to reach a settlement that would protect tobacco companies against unlimited lawsuits and possible financial ruin. A historic settlement was announced in June 1997, in which the companies agreed to pay $368.5 billion over a 25-year period to compensate states for treating smoking-related illnesses and to set up a fund to pay damage claims for ill smokers, as well as for other purposes including financing

of nationwide antismoking programs. The industry also agreed to a number of restrictions on advertising and promotion and to allow the FDA to regulate the nicotine in cigarettes. However, the settlement required congressional approval, which did not materialize. In 1998, the tobacco industry reached a more limited settlement with the attorneys general, agreeing to pay 46 states $206 billion over 25 years and accepting some restrictions on advertising, including a ban on billboard ads. The settlement also provided $1.7 billion over a five-year period to create the American Legacy Foundation, which used the funds for public education and other tobacco control activities.[36]

The MSA has proved something of a disappointment for public health advocates. It was hoped that the states would use some of the settlement dollars for tobacco control programs. Smoking cessation programs that include counseling and nicotine-replacement therapy, such as nicotine gum or patches, can double or even triple a smoker's chance of quitting.[36] Telephone quit lines, sponsored by some states and sometimes by voluntary organizations, can be effective at motivating people to quit. However, most states have used few of the MSA funds for such programs, instead applying the windfall to close state budget gaps. For their part, tobacco companies have had to increase the price of cigarettes by 45 cents per pack to pay for the settlement. As discussed previously, higher prices discourage people from smoking, especially young people.

The American Legacy Foundation has used its part of the settlement to run aggressive ad campaigns against smoking targeted at youth, called the "truth" campaign. Drawing on findings from evaluations of the California and other tobacco control programs, the ads convey the message that tobacco companies manipulate the truth, deny adverse health effects and the addictive nature of tobacco, and try to make smoking appear attractive. The "truth" ads featured statements such as "In 1984, one tobacco company referred to new customers as 'replacement smokers" and "In 1990, tobacco companies put together a plan to stop coroners from listing tobacco as a cause of death on a death certificate." Another ad features a young man trying to ship a box of cigarettes at the post office, saying, "I'd like to ship this arsenic and cyanide spreading mechanism," insisting that his action is perfectly legal and being met with skepticism by the clerk.[37] The "truth" ads were placed in youth-oriented magazines and television programs. Two national youth surveys, used to evaluate the effect of the "truth" campaign, found that young people who had seen the ads were significantly more likely than those who had not seen them to hold negative attitudes toward tobacco.[38] The "truth" campaign and others like it, together with the increased tobacco prices, have contributed to reducing youth smoking to less than 10% in 2018.[8] Unfortunately, as discussed later in this chapter, e-cigarette use has skyrocketed among youths, reversing much of this progress—20.8% of high school students have reported using e-cigarettes in the last 30 days.[39]

Funding for the American Legacy Foundation (now called Truth Initiative) from the MSA expired in 2003. However, the foundation has succeeded in finding funds to continue the truth campaign and to launch the "EX" campaign, designed to help smokers quit by "re-learning to live their lives without cigarettes."[40] It also collaborates with the University of California at San Francisco in maintaining an online library of previously secret tobacco industry documents, which can be searched using a user-friendly interface. Ads for the "truth" campaign can be seen on the Foundation's website (www.thetruth.com); the digital library is found on the University of California's website.[41]

FDA Regulation

The original agreement negotiated by the state attorneys general and the tobacco companies contained a provision allowing the FDA to regulate tobacco. Because that agreement was not approved by Congress, the MSA did not contain such a provision. Assigning regulatory authority over tobacco to the FDA has many advantages from a health standpoint. Until 2009, there were no legal restrictions concerning ingredients in tobacco smoke or on labeling or advertising concerning health claims by the companies. Evidence indicates, for example, that companies manipulated nicotine levels in tobacco to promote addiction, and they added ammonia to increase the effect of the nicotine. Tobacco smoke contains toxic chemicals such as nitrosamines and arsenic in addition to the tars known to be carcinogenic.[34] It also contains radioactive polonium, which is not widely recognized.[42] In fact, the American Legacy Foundation has focused on some of these toxic ingredients in its antismoking ads.

Finally in 2009, after previous attempts had failed, Congress passed and President Barack Obama signed the Family Smoking Prevention and Tobacco Control Act.[43] This law gives the FDA authority to regulate tobacco products and to restrict advertising and promotion. It requires larger and more graphic warning labels on cigarette packages, and it forbids tobacco companies from sponsoring sporting events. The law requires the disclosure of ingredients of cigarettes, as is done with food. It gives the FDA authority to require the removal of harmful ingredients, and to regulate health-related claims made by the tobacco companies, insisting that such claims be proven. The truth-in-advertising provision makes it possible for cigarettes to be made safer, so that smokers who cannot or will not quit would suffer less harm. Unless the government has the authority to verify claims, tobacco companies could continue to label their products as "light" or "safer" even if they do not actually reduce the hazards of smoking. One proposed advantage of giving the FDA regulatory authority would be to allow the agency to gradually reduce the amount of nicotine allowed in cigarettes to make them less addictive and to taper smokers off the addictive drug.[20]

The new law bans candy-flavored cigarettes, designed to appeal to young people. However, menthol was not included in the banned flavorings. Menthol masks the harshness of inhaled smoke and appears to ease the initiation of smoking among youths. It is also popular among black smokers, three-fourths of whom smoke menthol cigarettes, while only 25% of white smokers choose the menthol flavoring.[1] In 2018, the FDA announced a move to ban **menthol cigarettes**, with the support of the NAACP, National Urban League, and the African American Tobacco Control Leadership Council.[44] The proposal, unsurprisingly, has proved controversial, and has stalled. A massive lobbying effort by the tobacco company Reynolds American, which enlisted the assistance of Al Sharpton and his group, the National Action Network, effectively tabled the motion in New York State. Sharpton has raised the concern that the ban would spur an underground market for menthol cigarettes that would disproportionally involve African Americans. At the same time, it was revealed that the National Action Network has taken financial contributions from cigarette makers for the last two decades. Sharpton has argued that his motives are pure.[45]

"The key to public health action on the tobacco front seems to lie in combining strategies to discourage children from smoking and in producing a safer and less addictive cigarette for those who cannot, or will not, resist the temptation to smoke," wrote the ethicist George Annas in January 1997,[46(p.307)] when the possibility of a negotiated settlement was first being considered. Whether Congress or the courts, or both, will finally make possible the demotion of tobacco as public health enemy number one remains to be seen.

Electronic Cigarettes

E-cigarettes (also known as nicotine vaping) are a recent addition to the repertoire of nicotine delivery systems. A CDC study found that between 2010 and 2013, awareness of e-cigarettes grew to 80% and use more than doubled among U.S. adults.[47] By 2017, 2.8% of U.S. adults regularly used e-cigarettes. Some of these adults are attempting to quit traditional combustible cigarettes, and some seek to reduce the amount of carcinogens and tar they are inhaling.[48] Although conventional cigarette advertising is banned from television, electronic cigarettes are heavily marketed on television. For example, the e-cigarette maker Juul launched a $10 million TV campaign called "Make the Switch" in 2019; the message is a subtle (or not-so-subtle) suggestion that e-cigarettes are less harmful than traditional cigarettes—a claim that is not legally allowed because the health benefits have not been proven to the FDA.[49] In fact, the FDA gained the authority to regulate e-cigarette makers in 2016, but besides attempting to block health claims (not always successfully), the FDA has not yet taken much concrete action other than issuing warning letters and levying a limited number of modest fines.

Perhaps the most concerning aspect of e-cigarettes is their appeal to youth. A survey funded by the National Institutes of Health (NIH) called Monitoring the Future found that the rate of smoking traditional cigarettes has fallen sharply—in 2018, 3.6% of high school seniors reported daily smoking, compared to 22.4% 20 years ago—but nicotine vaping appears to be taking its place. Among 12th graders, 11.0% reported nicotine vaping in the previous 30 days in 2017, 20.9% in 2018, and 25.4% in 2019. For 8th graders, the corresponding rates were 3.5%, 6.1%, and 9.0% for 2017, 2018, and 2019, respectively.[50] E-cigarette marketing helps explain this rise: In 2016, 78% of middle and high school students reported that they were "sometimes," "most of the time," or "always" exposed to e-cigarette advertising from certain sources including the Internet, television, and magazines.[51]

In the summer of 2019, the dominant e-cigarette maker Juul Labs was formally accused by the FDA of illegally marketing its products as a less harmful alternative to traditional cigarettes. It is not clear if significant enforcement action will result from this warning. Also worrisome is its recent tie-up with Altria, the parent company of Marlboro, which bought a 35% stake in Juul in December 2018 for almost $13 billion. With the ample resources and marketing and distribution experience from Altria, one of the largest cigarette companies in the world, Juul's presence is only likely to grow.[52]

Stricter regulation, however, does appear likely. In September 2019, the Donald Trump administration announced plans to ban flavored e-cigarettes, which are particularly appealing to youth. The states of Michigan and New York have already implemented this ban, and Walmart has announced that it will stop selling e-cigarettes.[53] The city of San Francisco has gone even further, banning e-cigarettes altogether, and becoming the first major American city to do so.[54] Major TV channels such as CNN, CBS, TNT, TBS, MTV, Nickelodeon, and BET have also announced that they will eliminate all e-cigarette advertisements on their shows.[55] In addition, the former mayor of New York City and one of the world's major philanthropists, Michael Bloomberg, recently announced that he will dedicate $160 million of his $1 billion antitobacco efforts toward banning flavored e-cigarettes.[56]

This push for regulation could not come soon enough. In the summer of 2019, an epidemic of lung illnesses tied to vaping broke out, causing 2291 hospitalizations for lung injury and 48 deaths as of December 2019 (these numbers are likely to rise).[57] Public health officials are rushing to determine the exact cause, but preliminary evidence indicates that most patients had combined nicotine with tetrahydrocannabinol (THC) or cannabidiol (CBD), the latter two substances usually being derived from marijuana. The New York State Department of Health has tentatively linked many cases to high levels of vitamin E acetate, a thickening agent sometimes added to liquid vaping products. However, a definitive explanation is not yet available.[54]

This regulatory pressure and the spate of vaping illnesses seemed to be having an effect on the dominant E-cigarette maker Juul. In late September 2019, the company announced it was suspending all advertising in the United States, would end its "Make the Switch" campaign, and would not lobby against the regulatory push to ban flavored e-cigarettes. At the same time, the CEO of Juul stepped down, to be replaced by an executive from Altria.[53] China has effectively blocked Juul's entry into the country, and India also announced that it would ban e-cigarettes.[53]

Electronic cigarettes have not been studied enough to determine the full extent of their potential risks. While some evidence indicates that they are safer than conventional cigarettes, recent usage trends suggest they may lead young people to try tobacco products and thus act as a gateway to nicotine addiction, and perhaps eventually traditional cigarette smoking itself.[58,59]

Conclusion

Cigarette smoking is one of the two leading actual causes of death in the United States and the leading cause of disability-adjusted life years. The fact that smoking causes lung cancer has been known since the 1950s, and this behavior has been responsible for an epidemic of lung cancer, now the leading cause of cancer death among both men and women. Smoking also causes cardiovascular disease, chronic lung disease, low birth weight in infants, and a number of other unhealthy conditions.

Since the Surgeon General's *Smoking and Health* report was published in 1964, summarizing the evidence about the harm caused by smoking, public health advocates have been attacking the habit in as many ways as possible. Cigarette consumption in the United States peaked in the early 1960s and has declined since then, confirming the significant success of the public health efforts. Currently 14% of the adult U.S. population smokes cigarettes, down from more than 42% in 1965.

Public health practitioners have fought the tobacco industry on many fronts. In the 1960s, Congress passed legislation that required cigarette ads on radio and television to be balanced by counter-advertising about the harmful effects of smoking. This publicity, together with warning labels on cigarette packages, helped persuade many people to quit. Tobacco companies have become increasingly sophisticated about marketing their products, especially to children, and public health agencies have had to work hard to oppose them. Since nicotine in tobacco is addictive, it has become clear that the most effective approach to reducing smoking is to prevent young people from taking up the habit.

Public health interventions that have demonstrated some success in preventing the onset of smoking and in reducing its prevalence include the enactment and enforcement of laws prohibiting the sale of tobacco to minors, restrictions on indoor smoking, and—most effectively—increases in cigarette prices through imposition of taxes. California was a leader among states in imposing a tax on cigarettes to be used for tobacco control programs. Evaluation of its mass-media advertising campaign has helped antismoking activists understand what messages are most effective in persuading youths not to smoke. California was also a leader in legislation to ban smoking in public places.

In the mid- and late 1990s, the Clinton administration and a number of states launched legal and regulatory attacks on the tobacco industry. The MSA between the attorneys general of 46 states and the tobacco industry contained restrictions on tobacco advertising aimed at young people and provided billions of dollars to the states to compensate them for medical costs they incurred for treating smoking-related illnesses. This agreement also provided funds to establish the American Legacy Foundation, which has run an effective media campaign to discourage young people from smoking.

In 2009, Congress passed and President Obama signed a law authorizing the FDA to regulate tobacco products. It is hoped that the agency will devise ways to wean tobacco users off their addiction to nicotine and reduce demand for tobacco products.

Electronic cigarettes are a recent addition to the repertoire of nicotine-delivery systems. They have not been studied enough yet to understand their potential risks, and the FDA, states, and municipalities are just starting to regulate electronic cigarettes, but that situation seems likely to change. In 2019, an epidemic of lung illnesses and fatalities were associated with vaping, the causes of which are still being studied.

The battle continues. It seems that progress is being made, yet prospects for victory in public health's battle against the powerful tobacco industry and the ongoing health disaster remain uncertain.

References

1. U.S. Department of Health and Human Services, "The Health Consequences of Smoking—50 Years of Progress: A Report of the Surgeon General," 2014, www.surgeongeneral.gov/library/reports/50-years-of-progress/full-report.pdf, accessed September 22, 2019.
2. A. H. Mokdad, K. Ballestros, M. Echko, S. Glenn, H. E. Olsen, E. Mullany, et al., "The State of US Health, 1990–2016: Burden of Diseases, Injuries, and Risk Factors Among US States," *Journal of the American Medical Association* 319 (2018): 1444–1472.
3. B. D. Carter, C. C. Abnet, D. Feskanich, N. D. Freedman, P. Hartge, C. E. Lewis, et al., "Smoking and Mortality: Beyond Established Causes," *New England Journal of Medicine* 372 (2015): 631–640.

4. P. Jha, C. Ramasundarahettige, V. Landsman, et al., "21st Century Hazards of Smoking and Benefits of Cessation in the United States," *New England Journal of Medicine* 368 (2013): 341–350.

5. T. W. Wang, K. Asman, A. S. Gentzke, et al., "Tobacco Product Use Among Adults—United States, 2017," *Morbidity and Mortality Weekly Report* 67 (2018): 1225–1232.

6. S. Babb, A. Malarcher, G. Schauer, K. Asman, and A. Jamal, "Quitting Smoking Among Adults—United States, 2000–2015," *Morbidity and Mortality Weekly Report* 65 (2017): 1457–1464.

7. Centers for Disease Control and Prevention, "Quitting Smoking Among Adults—United States, 2001–2010," *Morbidity and Mortality Weekly Report* 60 (2011): 1513–1519.

8. C. E. Bartecchi, T. D. MacKenzie, and R. W. Schrier, "The Global Tobacco Epidemic," *Scientific American* (May 1995): 44–51.

9. U.S. Public Health Service, *Smoking and Health: Report of the Advisory Committee to the Surgeon General* (Washington, DC: 1964).

10. U.S. Public Health Service, *Health Consequences of Smoking for Women: Report of the Surgeon General* (Rockville, MD: 1980).

11. American Cancer Society, "Cancer Facts & Figures, 2019," https://www.cancer.org/content/dam/cancer-org/research/cancer-facts-and-statistics/annual-cancer-facts-and-figures/2019/cancer-facts-and-figures-2019.pdf, accessed September 22, 2019.

12. Centers for Disease Control and Prevention, "Smoking & Tobacco Use: Fast Facts and Fact Sheets," https://www.cdc.gov/tobacco/data_statistics/fact_sheets/index.htm, accessed September 21, 2019.

13. U.S. Environmental Protection Agency, "EPA Designates Passive Smoking a 'Class A' or Known Human Carcinogen," January 7, 1993, https://archive.epa.gov/epa/aboutepa/epa-designates-passive-smoking-class-or-known-human-carcinogen.html, accessed September 25, 2019.

14. American Lung Association, "State of Tobacco Control, Smokefree Air Laws," https://www.lung.org/our-initiatives/tobacco/reports-resources/sotc/state-grades/state-rankings/smokefree-air-laws.html, accessed September 22, 2019.

15. Centers for Disease Control and Prevention, "Tobacco Industry Marketing," May 4, 2019, https://www.cdc.gov/tobacco/data_statistics/fact_sheets/tobacco_industry/marketing/index.htm, accessed September 22, 2019.

16. P. M. Fischer, M. P. Schwartz, J. W. Richards Jr., A. O. Goldstein, and T. H. Rojas, "Brand Logo Recognition by Children Aged 3 to 6 Years: Mickey Mouse and Old Joe the Camel," *Journal of the American Medical Association* 266 (1991): 3145–3148.

17. M. Wakefield et al., "Effect of Televised, Tobacco Company-Funded Smoking Prevention Advertising on Youth Smoking-Related Beliefs, Intentions, and Behavior," *American Journal of Public Health* 96 (2006): 2154–2160.

18. K. A. Cullen, B. K. Ambrose, A. S. Gentzke, B. J. Apelberg, A. Jamal, and B. A. King, "Notes from the Field: Use of Electronic Cigarettes and Any Tobacco Product Among Middle and High School Students—United States, 2011–2018," *Morbidity and Mortality Weekly Report* 67 (2018).

19. American Lung Association, "Tobacco 21 Laws: Tracking Progress Toward Raising the Minimum Sales Age for All Tobacco Products to 21," August 19, 2019, https://www.lung.org/our-initiatives/tobacco/cessation-and-prevention/tobacco-21-laws.html, accessed September 22, 2019.

20. Institute of Medicine, *Ending the Tobacco Problem: A Blueprint for the Nation* (Washington, DC: National Academies Press, 2007).

21. Centers for Disease Control and Prevention, "Smoking in the Movies," May 19, 2015, http://www.gov/cdc/tobacco/data_statistics/fact_sheets/youth_data/movies, accessed June 5, 2015.

22. Centers for Disease Control and Prevention, "Smoking in the Movies," April 22, 2019, https://www.cdc.gov/tobacco/data_statistics/fact_sheets/youth_data/movies/index.htm, accessed September 22, 2019.

23. Centers for Disease Control and Prevention, "Response to Increases in Cigarette Prices by Race/Ethnicity, Income, and Age Groups—United States, 1976–1993," *Morbidity and Mortality Weekly Report* 47 (1998): 605–609.

24. M. Grossman and F. J. Chaloupka, "Cigarette Taxes: The Straw to Break the Camel's Back," *Public Health Reports* 112 (1997): 291–297.

25. California Department of Public Health, "Adult Smoking Prevalence," https://data.chhs.ca.gov/dataset/adult-cigarette-and-tobacco-use-prevalence, accessed January 21, 2020.

26. S. Dewan, "States Look at Tobacco to Balance the Budget," *The New York Times*, March 20, 2009.

27. Centers for Disease Control and Prevention, "State Tobacco Activities Tracking and Evaluation (STATE) System," April 4, 2019, https://www.cdc.gov/statesystem/interactivemaps.html, accessed September 22, 2019.

28. I. Lovett, "California: Cigarette Tax Defeated," *The New York Times*, June 22, 2012.

29. California Department of Public Health, "California Tobacco Facts and Figures 2019," May 2019, https://www.cdph.ca.gov/Programs/CCDPHP/DCDIC/CTCB/CDPH%20Document%20Library/ResearchandEvaluation/FactsandFigures/CATobaccoFactsandFigures2019.pdf, accessed September 22, 2019.

30. A. Landman, P. M. Ling, and S. A. Glantz, "Tobacco Industry Youth Smoking Prevention Programs: Protecting the Industry and Hurting Tobacco Control," *American Journal of Public Health* 92 (2002): 917–930.

31. L. K. Goldman and S. A. Glantz, "Evaluation of Antismoking Advertising Campaigns," *Journal of the American Medical Association* 279 (1998): 772–777.

32. J. P. Pierce, E. A. Gilpin, S. L. Emery, M. M. White, B. Rosbrook, C. C. Berry, and A. J. Farkas, "Has the California Tobacco Control Program Reduced Smoking?" *Journal of the American Medical Association* 280 (1998): 893–899.

33. J. M. Broder, "Cigarette Makers in a $368 Billion Accord to Curb Lawsuits and Curtail Marketing," *The New York Times*, June 21, 1997.

34. S. A. Glantz et al., *The Cigarette Papers* (Berkeley, CA: University of California Press, 1996).

35. M. L. Myers, "Protecting the Public Health by Strengthening the Food and Drug Administration's Authority over Tobacco Products," *New England Journal of Medicine* 343 (2000): 1806–1809.

36. S. A. Schroeder, "Tobacco Control in the Wake of the 1998 Master Settlement Agreement," *New England Journal of Medicine* 350 (2004): 203–301.

37. American Legacy Foundation, "Truth," https://www.thetruth.com/, accessed June 8, 2015.

38. M. C. Farrelly et al., C. G. Healton, K. C. Davis, P. Messeri, J. C. Hersey, and M. L. Haviland, "Getting to the Truth: Evaluating National Tobacco Countermarketing Campaigns," *American Journal of Public Health* 92 (2002): 901–907.

39. Centers for Disease Control and Prevention, "Youth and Tobacco Use," February 28, 2019, https://www.cdc.gov/tobacco/data_statistics/fact_sheets/youth_data/tobacco_use/index.htm, accessed September 22, 2019.

40. American Legacy Foundation, "Truth Initiative," https://truthinitiative.org, accessed September 25, 2019.

41. University of California at San Francisco, "Truth Tobacco Industry Documents," https://industrydocuments.library.ucsf.edu/tobacco, accessed September 22, 2019.

42. M. E. Muggli, J. O. Ebbert, C. Robertson, and R. D. Hurt, "Waking a Sleeping Giant: The Tobacco Industry's Response to the Polonium-210 Issue," *American Journal of Public Health* 98 (2008): 1543–1650.

43. G. D. Curfman, S. Morrisey, and J. M. Drazen, "Tobacco, Public Health, and the FDA," *New England Journal of Medicine* 361 (2009): 402–403.

44. S. Kaplan and J. Hoffman, "F.D.A. Seeks Restrictions on Teens' Access to Flavored E-Cigarettes and a Ban on Menthol Cigarettes," *The New York Times*, November 15, 2018.

45. J. D. Goodman, "When Big Tobacco Invoked Eric Garner to Fight a Menthol Cigarette Ban," *The New York Times*, July 14, 2019.

46. G. Annas, "Tobacco Litigation as Cancer Prevention: Dealing with the Devil," *New England Journal of Medicine* 336 (1997): 304–308.

47. Centers for Disease Control and Prevention, "Electronic Cigarettes: Key Findings: Trends in Awareness and Use of Electronic Cigarettes among U.S. Adults, 2010–2013," September 23, 2014, http://www.cdc.gov/tobacco/basic_information/e-cigarettes/adult-trends/index.htm, accessed June 8, 2015.

48. T. W. Wang, K. Asman, A. S. Gentzke, et al., "Tobacco Product Use Among Adults — United States, 2017," *Morbidity and Mortality Weekly Report* 67 (2018): 1225–1232.

49. M. Andrews, "Cigarettes Can't Be Advertised on TV. Should Juul Ads Be Permitted?" National Public Radio, August 20, 2019, https://www.npr.org/sections/health-shots/2019/08/20/752553108/cigarettes-cant-be-advertised-on-tv-should-juul-ads-be-permitted?t=1569185671792, accessed September 22, 2019.

50. R. Miech, L. Johnston, P. M. O'Malley, J. G. Bachman, and M. E. Patrick, "Trends in Adolescent Vaping, 2017–2019," *New England Journal of Medicine* 381 (2019): 1490–1491.

51. K. Marynak, A. Gentzke, T. W. Wang, L. Neff, and B. A. King, "Exposure to Electronic Cigarette Advertising Among Middle and High School Students—United States, 2014–2016," *Morbidity and Mortality Weekly Report* 67 (2018): 294–299.

52. S. Kaplan and J. Hoffman, "Juul Illegally Marketed E-Cigarettes, F.D.A. Says," *The New York Times*, September 9, 2019.

53. S. Kaplan, M. J. de la Merced, and J. Creswell, "Juul Shake-Up: C.E.O. Steps Down," *The New York Times*, September 25, 2019.

54. J. McKinley and C. Goldbaum, "New York Moves to Ban Flavored E-Cigarettes by Emergency Order," *The New York Times*, September 15, 2019.

55. D. Yaffe-Bellany, "TV Networks Take Down Juul and Other E-Cigarette Ads," *The New York Times*, September 18, 2019.

56. V. Wang, "Bloomberg Takes on Vaping After Giving $1 Billion to Fight Tobacco," *The New York Times*, September 10, 2019.

57. Centers for Disease Control and Prevention, "Outbreak of Lung Injury Associated with E-Cigarette Use, or Vaping," December 6, 2019, https://www.cdc.gov/tobacco/basic_information/e-cigarettes/severe-lung-disease.html, accessed December 10, 2019.

58. B. Meier, "British Study Says Electronic Cigarettes Curb Smoking Risk," *The New York Times*, August 20, 2015.

59. J. Nocera, "Nicotine Without Death," *The New York Times*, November 29, 2014.

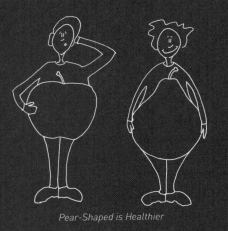
Pear-Shaped is Healthier

CHAPTER 16

Public Health Enemy Number Two—and Growing: Poor Diet and Physical Inactivity

KEY TERMS

Body mass index (BMI)
Calorie labeling
*Dietary Guidelines for
    Americans*

National Health and Nutrition
    Examination Survey
    (NHANES)
Obesity

Overweight
Sin tax
Sugar-sweetened beverage tax
Waist-to-hip ratio (WHR)

Throughout evolutionary history, humans had to exert a great deal of physical activity to obtain their food. Only over the past century has a substantial and increasing percentage of the population had access to an excess of food with no need to exercise. The consequence of this imbalance has been that Americans are becoming fatter—an exceedingly unhealthy trend. Today, poor diet and physical inactivity are ranked among the top two factors identified as leading actual causes of death in the United States.

Many studies have shown that weighing too much increases people's risk of cardiovascular disease, diabetes, most kinds of cancer, and a variety of other diseases. Thus, it is in the interest of public health to reduce the prevalence of overweight and obesity. In 2015 and 2016, 71.3% of the U.S. adult population was overweight, including 39.8% who were obese, and 7.7% who were severely obese.[1] The weight of a woman of average height (5 feet 4 inches) who is severely obese is at least 232 pounds; for a man of average height (5 feet 9 inches), it is at least 270 pounds.

Getting people to lose weight, however, seems to be even more difficult than getting them to quit smoking, although many of them want to be thinner. According to the 2013–2016 **National Health and Nutrition Examination Survey (NHANES)**, 56% of women and 42% of men are trying to lose weight, most of them unsuccessfully.[2] An Institute of Medicine report on the problem states, "It is paradoxical that obesity is increasing in the United States while more people are dieting than ever before, spending, by one estimate, more than $33 billion per year on weight-reduction products (including diet foods and soft drinks, artificial sweeteners, and diet books) and services (e.g., fitness clubs and weight-loss programs)."[3(p.27)]

The association of obesity with certain health risks is easy to measure, but the relationship may not be a simple one of cause and effect. **Obesity** is a complex condition, influenced by genes as well as by many individual and social factors that include eating and exercise patterns. While being overweight has a health impact in itself, a person's disease risk may also be affected independently by dietary patterns and the amount of physical activity, whether or not he or she is overweight. Public health advocates, therefore, seek to promote healthier eating patterns among Americans, to encourage them to exercise more, and to reduce the percentage of people who are overweight.

Epidemiology of Obesity

Obesity is, to an extent, in the eyes of the beholder—often the beholder who is looking in the mirror. From a public health perspective, obesity is usually defined more precisely in terms of **body mass index (BMI)**. BMI is calculated by dividing a person's weight in kilograms by the square of his or her height in meters. **Table 16-1** presents BMIs in terms of inches and pounds for a range that includes most Americans.

Most studies show that weight-associated health risks begin to appear at a BMI of about 25, and rise more significantly above 30, with the risks increasing in proportion to the severity of an individual's obesity. The National Institutes of Health and the Centers for Disease Control and Prevention (CDC) have agreed on a definition of **overweight** as a BMI between 25 and 29.9, obesity as a BMI of 30 or greater, and severe obesity as a BMI of 40 or higher.[4] Using this definition, 74.6% of men and 67.4% of women 20 years of age and older were found to be overweight or obese in the NHANES studies conducted between 2013 and 2016. The prevalence of obesity was 36.8% in men and 40.7% in women.[1] The prevalence of overweight and obesity has increased dramatically over recent decades, as shown in **Figure 16-1** and **Figure 16-2**.

There are significant racial differences in the prevalence of overweight among women: 80.6% of nonpregnant black women are overweight, compared with 64.6% of white women. Among men, the difference is reversed: 70.6% of black men compared with 75.2% of white men are overweight.[1] The health effects of overweight and obesity are also less marked among blacks. The optimal BMI has been calculated to be 23 to 25 for whites, but is 23 to 30 for blacks.[5] The risks of excess weight are known to be higher for Asian populations, so the BMI cutoffs recommended by the World Health Organization are lower for them.[6] Due to insufficient data, it has not been possible to calculate ideal weights in other ethnic groups, including Mexican Americans, in whom the prevalence of overweight and obesity is 82.9% among men and 84.5% in women. Overweight increases with age, as seen in Figures 16-1 and 16-2, but declines in the 75 years and older age group.[1]

Socioeconomic status has a significant influence on the prevalence of obesity. College graduates of both sexes are thinner than men and women with fewer years of education. The difference is especially significant among females: Those with less than 12 years of education are nearly twice as likely to be overweight as female college graduates. Among men, the relationship of obesity with education is less clear.[7]

The greater prevalence of obesity in black women compared to white women doubtless contributes to poorer health among blacks.

Table 16-1 Body Mass Index Table

BMI	19	20	21	22	23	24	25	26	27	28	29	30	31	32	33	34	35
Height (inches)							Body Weight (pounds)										
58	91	96	100	105	110	115	119	124	129	134	138	143	148	153	158	162	167
59	94	99	104	109	114	119	124	128	133	138	143	148	153	158	163	168	173
60	97	102	107	112	118	123	128	133	138	143	148	153	158	163	168	174	179
61	100	106	111	116	122	127	132	137	143	148	153	158	164	169	174	180	185
62	104	109	115	120	126	131	136	142	147	153	158	164	169	175	180	186	191
63	107	113	118	124	130	135	141	146	152	158	163	169	175	180	186	191	197
64	110	116	122	128	134	140	145	151	157	163	169	174	180	186	192	197	204
65	114	120	126	132	138	144	150	156	162	168	174	180	186	192	198	204	210
66	118	124	130	136	142	148	155	161	167	173	179	186	192	198	204	210	216
67	121	127	134	140	146	153	159	166	172	178	185	191	198	204	211	217	223
68	125	131	138	144	151	158	164	171	177	184	190	197	203	210	216	223	230
69	128	135	142	149	155	162	169	176	182	189	196	203	209	216	223	230	236
70	132	139	146	153	160	167	174	181	188	195	202	209	216	222	229	236	243
71	136	143	150	157	165	172	179	186	193	200	208	215	222	229	236	243	250
72	140	147	154	162	169	177	184	191	199	206	213	221	228	235	242	250	258
73	144	151	159	166	174	182	189	197	204	212	219	227	235	242	250	257	265
74	148	155	163	171	179	186	194	202	210	218	225	233	241	249	256	264	272
75	152	160	168	176	184	192	200	208	216	224	232	240	248	256	264	272	279
76	156	164	172	180	189	197	205	213	221	230	238	246	254	263	271	279	287

Data from National Heart, Lung, and Blood Institute, National Institutes of Health, "Body Mass Index Table," www.nhlbi.nih.gov/health/educational/lose_wt/BMI/bmi_tbl.htm, accessed September 23, 2019.

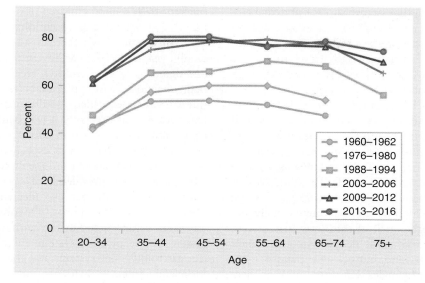

Figure 16-1 Percentage of Overweight Males, United States

Data from Centers for Disease Control and Prevention, "Health, United States, 2017," Table 58, 2018, www.cdc.gov/nchs/data/hus/hus17.pdf, accessed September 23, 2019.

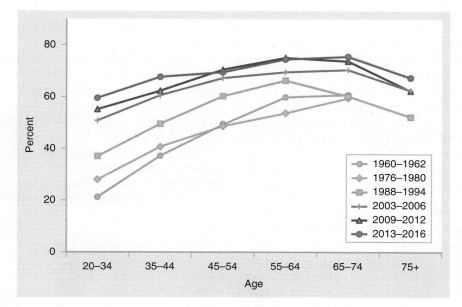

Figure 16-2 Percentage of Overweight Females, United States

Data from Centers for Disease Control and Prevention, "Health, United States, 2017," Table 58, 2018, www.cdc.gov/nchs/data/hus/hus17.pdf, accessed September 23, 2019.

Rates of cardiovascular disease and diabetes are higher in blacks than in whites, and an unhealthy diet is likely to be part of the problem. Many Hispanics and American Indians are also overweight, accounting for the high rates of diabetes found in these groups.

While being fat is bad for people's health, the distribution of fat on the body makes a difference in the health risks. Obesity researchers distinguish between apple-shaped people and pear-shaped people, and they have found health risks to be greater for those individuals shaped like apples. People who gain weight in the abdominal area, as men usually do, have a higher risk of cardiovascular disease and diabetes than do people who gain weight in the hips and buttocks—a pattern more common in females. Fat distribution is measured as a **waist-to-hip ratio (WHR)**, with the waist measured at the smallest point and the hips at the widest point around the buttocks. Health risks in men who have a WHR more than 1.0 and women whose WHR is more than 0.8 are greater than the risks due to excess weight alone.[3]

In an alarming trend, overweight among children has been increasing steadily since the 1960s. Definitions of overweight and obesity in children are complex calculations, based on growth curves of BMI for age. The CDC identifies children as overweight if they are at or above the 85th percentile on growth curves established before 1980 and as obese if they are above the 95th percentile.[8,9] The prevalence of obesity among children and adolescents 2 to 19 years old increased from less than 10.0% in the 1988–1994 NHANES to more than 17.8% in the 2013–2016 NHANES. Obesity is also more prevalent in some ethnic groups: Black and Hispanic teenage boys and girls are heavier than their white counterparts; Asian girls are especially unlikely to have a high BMI; and individuals of Hispanic or Latino origin have the highest rate of youth obesity.[1]

Children who are fat are likely to become fat adults and suffer the concomitant risks of chronic disease. For example, a study that tracked 679 school children for 16 years found that weight during childhood was a good predictor of whether an adult would exhibit risk factors for cardiovascular disease and diabetes.[10] Obese children are now often being diagnosed with type 2 diabetes—a condition sometimes called "adult-onset diabetes" because until recently it was believed to occur almost exclusively in adults.[11] A diagnosis of type 2 diabetes is especially likely to be made in American Indian adolescents, who have a high prevalence of obesity, but blacks and Hispanics are also affected. Complications of childhood obesity involve virtually every organ, including the cardiovascular system, the respiratory system, the kidneys, the gastrointestinal system, and the musculoskeletal system.[12] Evidence suggests that the harmful effects of excess weight increase with longer duration of obesity, implying that obese children are especially likely to suffer excess morbidity and mortality when they grow up.[5] One study found that the obese adolescent girls are two or three times as likely to die by middle age than are girls of normal weight.[12]

Obesity in children also tends to cause psychological problems such as depression, anxiety, social isolation, and low self-esteem. Children who are worried about their weight may adopt diets that affect their physical as well as their psychological health, and they are at increased risk for eating disorders such as anorexia and bulimia. Obese children are less likely than thinner ones to complete college and are more likely to live in poverty.[12]

Diet and Nutrition

Obesity is caused by unhealthy eating patterns combined with inadequate physical activity, with each being a significant factor that influences people's health whether or not they weigh too much. The public health aspects of physical activity are discussed later in this chapter. This section and the next explore the role of diet in the prevention of chronic diseases, including obesity, and describe public health efforts to encourage people to eat healthier diets.

Most analyses find that Americans eat too much protein and fat and too few fruits and vegetables. This pattern contributes to high levels of cholesterol and other blood lipids and to high blood pressure—all of which are risk factors for cardiovascular disease. The evidence is less clear on how the typical American diet increases cancer risk, but epidemiologic studies show that breast and colon cancer risks are greater in populations who eat diets high in meat and low in fruits and vegetables. Diet is a major factor in development of type 2 diabetes, which is often brought on by obesity and which can usually be controlled by careful eating. Osteoporosis, a debilitating disease of the elderly, especially white women, is likely to become increasingly common because young women are not getting enough calcium, best obtained in dairy products.

The federal government, in a number of reports produced over the years by various advisory committees, has developed recommendations on how Americans should eat to maintain health and prevent chronic disease. Since 1980, the U.S. Department of Agriculture and the U.S. Department of Health and Human Services have reviewed the recommendations every five years and have released reports called *Dietary Guidelines for Americans*.[13] Reaching agreement on these recommendations has often proved difficult, because the food industry tends to oppose any recommendation that calls for eating less of any food substance.[14] However, evidence clearly supports the recommendations included in the 2015–2020 guidelines that people's diets should emphasize fruits, vegetables, whole grains, and fat-free or low-fat milk and milk products; they should include lean meats, poultry, fish, beans, eggs, and nuts, but less saturated fats, trans fats, salt, and added sugar.[15] The image used to illustrate

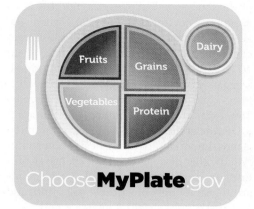

Figure 16-3 ChooseMyPlate.gov
U.S. Department of Agriculture, www.choosemyplate.gov, accessed December 11, 2019.

the recommendations is a place setting for a meal (**Figure 16-3**). ChooseMyPlate.gov recommends, for example, that half the plate should consist of fruits and vegetables, and at least half the grains should be whole grains. Its website includes an option for an individual to create a personal profile with a calorie limit, affected by his or her physical activity, and a recommended food plan.[16]

Dietary surveys conducted by the U.S. Department of Agriculture have shown that while the diet of Americans has improved over the past several decades, people fall far short of the federal recommendations. The diet of about three-fourths of the U.S. population is too low in vegetables, fruits, dairy, and healthy oils, and too high in added sugars, saturated fats, and sodium. Vegetables are the most commonly omitted item.[17]

Federal surveys suggest that one important cause of increasing obesity, especially in children, is increased intake of sweetened beverages. The proportion of calories that the average American obtained from soft drinks and fruit drinks more than doubled between 1977 and 2001 and remains high—for the period 2009–2016, NHANES shows that the average American consumed 154 calories per day from sugar-sweetened beverages, approximately 7%

of the total actual calories, though this is an improvement from 2003–2004, when the average American consumed 205 calories per day from sugar-sweetened beverages.[18–20] In 2011–2014, 63% of American youths drank a sugar-sweetened drink on any given day.[19] Meanwhile, consumption of milk decreased by 38% overall, including among children age 2 to 18, the group for whom milk consumption is most important for future health. Consumption of other beverages did not change significantly over the period studied. These trends are unhealthy, not only because soft drinks and sweetened juice drinks contain "empty calories" that contribute to weight gain, but also because consuming milk products appears to help people control their weight in addition to providing calcium for their bones. According to the researchers, reducing soft drink and fruit drink intake "would seem to be one of the simpler ways to reduce obesity in the United States."[18(p.209)]

Promoting Healthy Eating

It might seem that what each individual eats is under his or her individual control, but in reality many social, cultural, and economic factors contribute to dietary patterns. Eating habits and dietary preferences develop over a lifetime, and are influenced by family, ethnicity, the media, and other factors in the social environment. The high prevalence of overweight in the United States combined with the large numbers of people who are trying unsuccessfully to lose weight makes it clear that changing eating patterns is very difficult, even for highly motivated people. Studies of patients with a variety of medical conditions requiring special diets have found that even they have difficulty sticking to the prescribed diet. The rate of adherence to a diet by people with diabetes ranged from 20% to 53% to 73% in three different studies. People with kidney failure who were on dialysis were found to

have rates of adherence to the recommended diet of 39% and 42% in two separate studies. Another study found that only 30% of people with high cholesterol were able to successfully adhere to a low-cholesterol diet.[21]

Several major public health campaigns conducted in entire communities and aimed at reducing cardiovascular risks have found that obesity is the most difficult risk factor to control. The Stanford Three-Community Study, the Stanford Five-City Study, the Minnesota Heart Health Program, and the North Karelia (Finland) Project all had reasonable success in reducing risk factors such as smoking, hypertension, and blood cholesterol, but none of them interrupted the increase in the prevalence of obesity in the communities studied.[3]

Nevertheless, public health advocates have attempted to apply the ecological model of health behavior to create a social environment that favors healthier eating. For example, making nutritious foods more readily available—intervention at the community and institutional levels—should encourage people to choose their foods more wisely. The food industry is responding to many consumers' concerns about weight and health by providing a greater choice of low-calorie foods. Many restaurants offer "heart healthy" selections on the menu, with labels guiding customers to these choices. Worksite and school cafeterias may also provide healthy food choices, including salad bars. While such measures do not guarantee that people will eat a healthier diet, they remove barriers that make it more difficult for people to do so.

Enhancing self-efficacy and providing social support are ways of promoting healthy eating at the level of the individual and his or her family and friends.[21] Social support is provided when a whole family is willing to adopt a diet together, as well as by group programs such as Weight Watchers. Self-efficacy can be improved by "point of choice" postings of nutritional information, which can help shoppers who are concerned about the nutritional content of food but do not know how to make wise choices. Several major campaigns using point-of-choice postings have been conducted by supermarket chains in collaboration with health advocacy organizations such as the American Heart Association, but the results have been mixed. Other approaches to enhancing self-efficacy and adherence to diets include demonstrations of healthy cooking methods and practice in calculating portion sizes.

Public health advocates have looked at evidence from antismoking campaigns for ideas on how to improve the social environment to affect the American diet. The success of the public service announcements of the 1960s, together with later bans on cigarette advertising in the broadcast media, in reducing smoking prevalence inspired a number of media campaigns to promote more healthful eating. One such campaign was California's "5-A-Day" Campaign for Better Health, which attempted to increase fruit and vegetable consumption among state residents to five servings per day.[14] The assumption is that eating more fruits and vegetables leads to eating fewer non-nutritious foods. The program proved to be successful in increasing consumption of fruits and vegetables in the state. Later, the National Cancer Institute launched the program nationwide, although funding was never adequate to maintain the early successes of the California program. As in the case of antismoking campaigns, public health advocates must compete with well-financed advertising campaigns by food manufacturers that promote highly attractive but non-nutritious foods.

Another problem with the "5-A-Day" approach is that fresh fruits and vegetables are relatively expensive and are often unavailable in poor neighborhoods. Fast-food restaurants, by contrast, are inexpensive and are often concentrated in low-income neighborhoods. Moreover, U.S. government policy subsidizes industrial agriculture, which produces high-calorie commodities at the expense of more nutritious produce.[22] Food advertising focuses predominately on processed foods, which are more profitable for the industry.[3]

The food and beverage industries use some of the same approaches to increasing their sales as the tobacco companies have used. As documented in Marion Nestle's book *Food Politics: How the Food Industry Influences Nutrition and Health*,[14] food companies do everything they can to encourage Americans to eat more. For example, they process foods to make them taste good, which often means sweet, fatty, or salty. They push larger portions, often by promoting them as good buys—a large serving of fries might cost only pennies more than a small serving, yet have twice as many calories. Food companies also advertise extensively, especially to children. They take advantage of the fact that, with most women now working outside the home, convenience and efficiency are major factors in food choice and fewer family meals than in the past are home cooked. As Nestle describes, food companies "conduct systematic, pervasive, and unrelenting . . . campaigns to convince government officials, health organizations, and nutrition professionals that their products are healthful or harmless, to undermine any suggestion to the contrary, and to ensure that federal dietary guidelines and food guides will help promote sales."[14(p.26)] Like tobacco companies, food companies argue that diet is a matter of individual choice, and they use science to sow confusion about the harm their products can do.

The Institute of Medicine, after performing a thorough study aimed at developing criteria for evaluating the outcomes of programs to prevent and treat obesity, concluded in a report called *Weighing the Options* that prospects were dim for people seeking to lose weight. "The fact is that despite the billions of dollars spent, few people reduce their body weight to a desirable or healthy level and even fewer maintain the weight lost beyond two or three years."[3(p.158)] The report noted that for most people, weight is not lost once and for all, but rather its control demands continuing effort. Accordingly, the Institute of Medicine recommends thinking in terms of lifelong weight management, encouraging overweight people to try at least to avoid gaining additional weight. According to the report, even small weight losses can raise self-esteem and improve the health of people suffering from obesity-related chronic conditions.

Public health advocates believe that tackling the obesity epidemic will require community-based efforts to increase the availability of healthy foods, changes in national agricultural policy to encourage the availability of nutritious foods at a reasonable cost, and regulation of food industry advertising to promote ethical marketing standards.[23] A number of proposals have been made to tackle the obesity epidemic with tools similar to those that proved successful in the "tobacco wars." In addition to the educational campaigns such as the "5-A-Day" fruits and vegetables initiative, they include requirements for food labeling and advertising to carry information on calorie, fat, and sugar content and prohibitions on making misleading health claims. Fast-food restaurants would also be required to provide nutritional information on packages and wrappers. The nutritionist Nestle has proposed placing taxes on soft drinks and other junk foods to fund "eat less, move more" campaigns and perhaps to subsidize the costs of making fruits and vegetables more widely available.[14(p.367)]

Some of these proposals are beginning to be implemented. In May 2018, a provision of the Patient Protection and Affordable Care Act went into effect that requires restaurants in the United States with at least 20 locations to post calorie counts on their menus. That includes the calories in popcorn at movie theater chains and the calories in drinks at bar chains.[24] The effectiveness of providing this additional information may be relatively limited—but more study of these policies is needed and perhaps different implementations may prove effective. Unfortunately, the Donald Trump administration has been working against these policies. While the **calorie labeling** law went into

effect in 2018, that occurred only after the administration delayed the implementation at the behest of the restaurant lobby. As part of its renegotiation of the North American Free Trade Agreement (NAFTA), the Trump administration has also pushed to limit the ability of United States, Canada, and Mexico to include health warning labels on packaged foods that are high in sugar and fat.[24]

Taxing Sugar-Sweetened Beverages

Sugar-sweetened beverages are particularly unhealthy. They appear to cause more weight gain than equally sugary solid foods because liquid forms of sugar are less satiating and, therefore, do not reduce the amount of other foods being consumed. Experimental studies show that people tend to consume significantly more calories throughout the day when more of those calories come in liquid form. Experimental studies also show that youths given diet drinks instead of sugar-sweetened drinks over a 12- to 18-month period lose, on average, approximately 3 pounds.[20]

Notably, consumption of sugar-sweetened beverages significantly increases the risk of type 2 diabetes. Because the sugar in these drinks is more rapidly absorbed into the bloodstream compared to sugar in solid foods, they are particularly effective at promoting diabetes. A survey of research evidence shows that an additional serving of sugar-sweetened beverages per day increases the risk of getting type 2 diabetes by 13%. Moreover, sugary drinks significantly increase the risk of cardiovascular disease, with an additional serving per day increasing the risk of coronary heart disease by 17%.[20] These health burdens fall disproportionately on lower-income households. As **Figure 16-4** shows, there is a clear relationship between sugary drink consumption and income, with poorer households consuming about twice as many calories from sugary drinks compared to richer households.

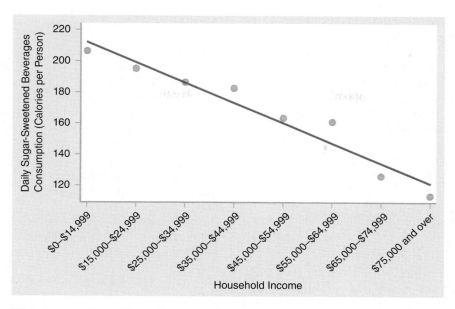

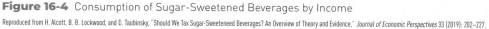

Figure 16-4 Consumption of Sugar-Sweetened Beverages by Income

Reproduced from H. Alcott, B. B. Lockwood, and D. Taubinsky, "Should We Tax Sugar-Sweeteneed Beverages? An Overview of Theory and Evidence," *Journal of Economic Perspectives* 33 (2019): 202–227.

The recognition of the important contribution of sugar-sweetened beverages to obesity, diabetes, and heart disease, and the relatively worse health effects of sugar in liquid form compared to solid form, have increased calls for a sugary drink tax. Although the Maine legislature passed a tax on sugar-sweetened drinks, the law was subsequently repealed by voters.[25] Chicago also passed a soda tax that was quickly repealed. However, in 2014, Berkeley, California, became the first U.S. city to pass a law taxing sugary drinks—and it has stuck. As of 2019, six additional U.S. cities—three in California, plus Boulder, Philadelphia, and Seattle—have implemented a **sugar-sweetened beverage tax**. Thirty-nine countries around the world also have such a tax. Moreover, 23 states and the District of Columbia do not charge sales taxes on groceries but exclude sugar-sweetened beverages in their definition of groceries, allowing these products to be taxed in stores.[20]

Like cigarette and alcohol taxes, soda taxes are a **sin tax**—a tax that raises the price of a product that is harmful to oneself and others—in an attempt to discourage consumption of that product. Excess sugary drink consumption not only harms the consumer, through the health consequences mentioned previously, but also others, through the large increase in healthcare costs that are shared across society through insurance programs such as Medicaid and Medicare.

Nevertheless, sugary drink taxes have proven controversial, most notably because of the relationship between consumption and income shown in Figure 16-4. This pattern has raised concerns about the regressivity of such a tax: If poor people consume more sugary drinks, then they would pay more of these taxes even though they are least able to afford it. This concern would indeed be well founded if poor people did not reduce their sugary drink consumption in response to the tax, but this is not the case. In fact, a large number of studies show that consumers, especially poor ones, are sensitive to the price of sugary drinks. These studies show that people will reduce their drink purchases, on average, by about 1.4% for every 1% increase in price. Thus, the large health benefits that result from drinking less sugary beverages easily outweigh the costs of the extra taxes they incur. Moreover, low-income people have systematically less knowledge about nutrition and the harm of sugary drinks, so this "paternalistic" intervention may be most helpful for this group.

In a wide-ranging 2019 analysis of sugar-sweetened beverage taxes, the authors Allcott, Lockwood, and Taubinsky put forward a set of principles for designing such taxes:[20]

1. Focus more on minimizing the harmful effects of sugary drinks, and less on minimizing sugary drink consumption itself. Many people enjoy unhealthy behaviors such as drinking soda or eating steak and dessert. The goal is not to deprive people of enjoyable activities, but instead to limit them to a level that balances the pleasure against the harm. This means a tax on soda may be more appropriate than, say, a ban.

2. Target the policies at the people who incur the most harm. For example, this may involve stronger policies related to sugary drink consumption by children.

3. Tax grams of sugar in these beverages rather than ounces of liquid. It is, after all, the sugar that is harmful. For example, Philadelphia's tax applies to regular and diet sodas equally, and excludes fruit juice, even though diet soda is far less harmful (or not harmful) and fruit juice is generally just as unhealthy as soda. In fact, there is little or no evidence that fruit juice is healthy—a common misconception among parents.[26]

4. Implement the taxes over as wide a geographic area as possible. Evidence indicates that taxes imposed at the city level cause some people to simply purchase their soda outside city lines. A state-level tax, for example, reduces this problems.

Youth Obesity

As mentioned earlier, there has been a sharp increase in overweight and obesity among American youth. Perhaps most alarming is the fact that very young children, those ages 2 to 5, are fully participating in this trend. The rate of obesity among 2- to 5-year-olds was already high in 2007–2008, at 10.1%, and increased to 13.9% as of 2015–2016.[27]

Many public health advocates believe that the best hope of preventing obesity in adulthood is to influence children's habits. Thus, they are devoting a great deal of attention to preventing overweight in children. It is also important to increase parents' awareness that their children are at risk and for children themselves to be aware of their weight status. In a follow-up to the 1988–1994 NHANES survey, after children were weighed and measured, mothers were asked whether their child was overweight, underweight, or about the right weight. Nearly one-third of mothers of overweight children ages 2 to 11 reported that their child was about the right weight.[28] In the 2007–2010 NHANES survey, parental perceptions were even less accurate. Among parents of overweight (but not obese) 8- to 15-year-olds, only 21% correctly identified their child's weight category.[29] The 2005–2012 NHANES survey asked 8- to 15-year-old children about their own weight. Among overweight boys, 81% said they were about the right weight, while 71% of overweight girls reported their weight was about right.[30]

Approximately half of all U.S. states have laws requiring schools to assess the BMI of their students, often requiring the schools to report the results to the students' parents. However, this practice is controversial because of concerns about stigma.[31] It is clear, though, that efforts to prevent and treat childhood obesity must involve parents. In 2015, the American Academy of Pediatrics issued new guidelines for pediatricians and parents on obesity prevention.

It recommends limiting sugar-sweetened beverages, high-calorie snacks, and sweets; making healthier options readily available and in plain sight for children—for example, on the kitchen counter; and encouraging children to eat fruits and vegetables.[32]

In 2005, the Institute of Medicine published a report called *Preventing Childhood Obesity: Health in the Balance*.[33] Calling childhood obesity a "critical public health threat,"[33(p.2)] the report recommends steps that federal, state, and local governments should take to make prevention of obesity in children and youth a national priority. These recommendations include developing guidelines for advertising and marketing of foods and beverages to children and giving the Federal Trade Commission authority and resources to monitor compliance. The report notes that "more than 50 percent of television advertisements directed at children promote foods and beverages such as candy, fast food, snack foods, soft drinks, and sweetened breakfast cereals that are high in calories and fat, low in fiber, and low in nutrient density."[33(p.172)] It also recommends that governments should develop and implement nutritional standards for all foods and beverages sold or served in schools. In recent years, food and beverage companies have invaded schools with vending machines selling unhealthy drinks and snacks, fast food in school cafeterias, and special educational programs and materials accompanied by advertisements for fast food and junk food.

As discussed later in this chapter, obesity and chronic disease are as much a result of lack of physical activity as they are of unhealthy diets. Weight-loss programs are most successful, in adults as well as in children, when they combine diet and exercise. "Exercise is today's best buy in public health," one commentator notes. "It is positive and acceptable, has insignificant side effects, and can be inexpensive."[34(p.252)]

Physical Activity and Health

Most studies on how to lose weight have found that the most effective approach combines dieting and physical activity. Dieters who are physically active are more likely to lose fat while preserving lean mass. This combination not only promotes a healthier distribution of body weight (a lower WHR), but also helps people avoid the weight-loss plateaus that can result from dieting. Because lean mass burns more calories than fat burns, a dieter who loses muscle mass will end up with a higher proportion of his or her weight consisting of fat; thus, the individual will need fewer calories to maintain the new weight, making it more difficult to lose additional pounds. Exercising when dieting helps ensure that the weight lost will consist of fat. Raising the amount of physical activity without reducing calorie intake, while a relatively inefficient way to lose pounds, is likely to reduce the WHR and, therefore, improve health.[35]

A number of epidemiologic studies have demonstrated that people who are more physically active live longer. For example, a study of almost 17,000 male Harvard alumni found that those who engaged in vigorous activities for 3 or more hours per week were less than half as likely to die within the 12- to 16-year follow-up period than those who had the lowest activity levels.[36] Among Harvard graduates who were sedentary at the beginning of the study, those who took up moderate sports activity at some time during the follow-up period had a 23% lower death rate than those who remained sedentary.[37]

Exercise clearly protects against cardiovascular disease, as demonstrated by both epidemiologic studies and biomedical evidence. The Framingham Study found, as early as the 1970s, that the risk for both men and women of dying from cardiovascular disease was highest among those individuals who were the least physically active and that more activity was associated with lower risk.[38] Exercise offers protection against both heart disease and stroke. Several studies have indicated that inactive men and women are more likely to develop high blood pressure than those who are active, and that moderate-intensity exercise may help reduce blood pressure in people whose pressure is elevated.[39]

Some biomedical evidence suggests how physical activity protects against cardiovascular disease. One major factor is the effect on blood cholesterol, especially the tendency for exercise training to increase levels of high-density lipoprotein (HDL), "the good cholesterol." Even a single episode of physical activity has been found to improve the balance of blood lipids, an effect persisting for several days.[40] By lowering cholesterol levels in the blood, exercise protects against atherosclerosis. Studies on monkeys have demonstrated that exercise has a protective effect even when the animals are fed a diet high in cholesterol and fats.[41] Other favorable effects of physical activity on the cardiovascular system include lowered blood pressure, increased circulation to the heart muscle, and a reduced tendency of blood to form clots. Moreover, physical activity reduces the risk of diabetes, which is an important risk factor for cardiovascular disease.

Type 2 ("adult-onset") diabetes is related to weight gain in adults, especially weight gain distributed in an "apple" shape, a consequence of insufficient physical activity. The high prevalence of obesity among Americans contributes to the ranking of diabetes as the seventh leading cause of death in the United States—though this is probably an underestimate because many cardiovascular deaths have diabetes as an underlying cause.

Early suspicions that physical inactivity contributed to diabetes were raised by observations that prevalence of the disease was higher in societies or groups that moved from a traditional lifestyle to a more technologically advanced environment. This transition has been extensively studied in certain American Indian and Pacific Islander communities. While the increased risk stems in part from changes in diet and increased prevalence of obesity, physical activity may be an independent risk factor.[42] The Nurses' Health Study and the Physicians' Health Study have both found that regular physical exercise reduces the incidence of type 2 diabetes.[43,44] The protective effect of exercise against the development of diabetes seems to work largely by increasing the sensitivity of muscle and other tissues to insulin.

Some evidence also shows that physical activity protects against cancer, especially colon cancer and breast cancer. Some studies suggest a protective effect against cancer of the lung, prostate, and uterine lining. Exercise also improves survival and quality of life among individuals who have been diagnosed with several kinds of cancer.[45]

How Much Exercise Is Enough, and How Much Do People Get?

In 2006, the Department of Health and Human Services decided that guidelines for physical activity should be developed, similar to the dietary guidelines. Together with the Institute of Medicine, it undertook a process similar to that used to develop the dietary guidelines. An advisory committee was appointed, which conducted an analysis of the scientific information, held a series of meetings, and released a report in 2008.[46] In 2018, the guidelines were revised based on the most recent scientific evidence and published as the second edition.[47]

Separate guidelines were developed for children and adolescents (60 minutes or more daily of physical activity) and adults (150 to 300 minutes per week of moderate-intensity activity or 75 to 150 minutes per week of vigorous-intensity aerobic activity). Adults gain increased benefits from exercising beyond 300 minutes of moderate-intensity activity or beyond 150 minutes of vigorous activity. Adults should also do muscle strengthening exercise at least two days a week. Older adults and people with disabilities or chronic medical conditions should do as much as they are able, in consultation with their doctor. **Table 16-2** provides examples of moderate- and vigorous-intensity activities.[47]

According to the National Health Interview Survey, only 26% of American men and 17% of American women met the aerobic nor the muscle-strengthening activity guidelines

in 2016.[47(Figure 1-1)] Lack of physical activity is a major factor in the trend toward increasing prevalence of obesity in children. The federal government recommends that children and adolescents should be physically active at least 60 minutes every day.[47] While most younger children report having engaged in exercise that makes them "sweat and breathe hard," surveys show that activity falls off dramatically during the high school years. Only 28% of high school boys and 10% of high school girls met the recommended physical activity and muscle-strengthening guidelines in 2011–2015.[47]

Evidence shows that television and computers may be important factors in children's physical inactivity. A number of studies have found that childhood obesity is positively associated with time spent watching TV.[48] The American Academy of Pediatrics issued new guidelines for children's media consumption in 2016, lowering the advised level. The group now recommends avoiding screen media altogether (except for video-chatting) for children younger than 18 months, and restricting media to high-quality programming, accompanied by an adult to help them understand what they are seeing, for children age 18 to 24 months. For children age 2 to 5 years, screen time should not exceed 1 hour per day and should be only high-quality programming. For children age 6 and older, parents should place consistent limits on screen time, and be sure to that such time does not displace adequate sleep, physical activity, and other healthy behaviors.[49] Surveys have found that American children age 8 to 18 devote, on average, 7.5 hours to screen time per day.[50] A trial conducted among third- and fourth-grade students in a California school found that reducing the hours they spent watching television by one-half to one-third over a period of 6 months reduced their BMI significantly compared with a control group.[51] A broad survey of research on this subject in 2019 found that children who had more than 2 hours per day

---

Table 16-2 **Examples of Different Aerobic Physical Activities and Intensities**

Moderate Intensity
- Walking briskly (2.5 miles per hour or faster)
- Recreational swimming
- Bicycling slower than 10 miles per hour on level terrain
- Tennis (doubles)
- Active forms of yoga (for example, Vinyasa or power yoga)
- Ballroom or line dancing
- General yard work and home repair work
- Exercise classes like water aerobics

Vigorous Intensity
- Jogging or running
- Swimming laps
- Tennis (singles)
- Vigorous dancing
- Bicycling faster than 10 miles per hour
- Jumping rope
- Heavy yard work (digging or shoveling, with heart rate increases)
- Hiking uphill or with a heavy backpack
- High-intensity interval training (HIIT)
- Exercise classes like vigorous step aerobics or kickboxing

Data from Office of Disease Prevention and Health Promotion, U.S. Department of Health and Human Services, "Physical Activity Guidelines for Americans," Second Edition, Table 4-1, https://health.gov/paguidelines /second-edition/pdf/Physical_Activity_Guidelines_2nd_edition.pdf, accessed September 25, 2019.

of screen time were significantly more likely to be overweight and obese compared to children who spent less time on such activities.[52]

Promoting Physical Activity

As with most attempts to change people's behavior, the most effective approach to promoting physical activity is likely to employ the ecological model, intervening at a number of levels of influence. Efforts to motivate individuals to be more active must be combined with interventions that make the physical and social environment more conducive to physical activity. In part because research on the effectiveness of these interventions is difficult to do, most studies have focused on short-term changes in exercise behavior. Very little evidence suggests that any program has had long-term success in increasing physical activity among significant numbers of people.

Many organizations and federal agencies recommend that healthcare providers counsel their patients about physical activity. However, the evidence is mixed as to whether such counseling actually motivates individuals to exercise more.[53] Studies of the effectiveness of counseling find that counseling practices of primary care physicians are highly variable, ranging from a brief recommendation to be more active to a referral for intensive counseling by health educators. Somewhat more effective are community-wide campaigns that include improving access to places for physical activity and using group settings to help people set individual goals, teaching skills for incorporating activity into daily routines, and providing social support to people trying to adopt healthier behaviors.[53]

The suburban lifestyle, which requires people to drive to wherever they want to go, is a major barrier to increasing physical activity that is very hard to overcome. As part of health promotion programs, some communities build walking trails or persuade shopping malls to open early for "mall walkers." Schools are a greatly underused resource for community recreation. Surveys of bicycle riders suggest that many more people would commute to work by bicycle if safe bike paths or bike lanes were available, and some communities have responded to this evidence by building such routes. Community trials designed to increase physical activity—usually as part of a "healthy heart" program—have incorporated such environmental modifications while also employing communications strategies ranging from public service announcements about physical activity to signs that provide cues to action. In one study, signs that said "Stay Healthy, Save Time, Use the Stairs" were placed next to an escalator. This measure increased the percentage of people who used the stairs from 8% to 17%.[35]

Pedometers are increasingly being used in campaigns to motivate people to increase their physical activity. Generally, it is recommended that healthy adults should walk about 10,000 steps per day, which is about 5 miles—a requirement that would more than fulfill the minimum federal recommendation of about 150 minutes of moderate-intensity physical activity per week. The recommendation for less active people is to measure their current number of steps and gradually increase the number until the goal is reached. A 2007 review of the effectiveness of pedometers in increasing physical activity found that people who wore the instruments did, in fact, increase the number of steps they took by an average of approximately 27%. Moreover, these individuals significantly reduced their BMI and blood pressure.[54] Other fitness tracking devices, such as the Fitbit and the Apple Watch, are available but comparatively expensive; they are more likely to appeal to people who are already motivated to exercise.

Many public health advocates believe that the best hope for increasing population-wide physical activity is to focus on developing good exercise habits in children and adolescents. Most young children engage in physical activity because they enjoy it. One strategy for promoting exercise is to encourage children to play outdoors.[55] Walking or biking to school is another straightforward way to increase children's physical activity. According to the CDC's 2014 School Health Policies and Practices Study, in 62% of schools, 10% or fewer students walked or biked to school; by comparison, in 23% of schools, 26% or more students walked or biked to school.[56] This is a large reduction from the 48% of children who walked or biked to school in 1960.[57] Today, the schools with higher rates of walking or biking are much more likely to have crossing guards, bicycle racks, and promotional material for parents about walking or biking to school. These associations suggest such simple and low-cost measures might boost the physical activity of students at schools with lower rates of walking or biking to schools.[56]

The CDC recommends that physical education classes teach school-age children about the health benefits of physical activity and help them develop skills that can be applied in lifelong physical fitness activities, such as jogging, tennis, and aerobic dance. These programs can be more effective if they are culturally appropriate for the targeted population. For example, one experimental program in a California middle school with predominantly black and Hispanic students was called "Dance for Health." Regular physical education classes were replaced with moderate- to high-intensity aerobic dance, accompanied by popular music recommended by the students themselves. At the end of the three-month program, participating students had lower BMIs and a more positive attitude toward physical activity compared to a control group. The program was especially popular and effective with girls.[58]

A youth development program focused on American Indian young people, who are particularly prone to obesity, type 2 diabetes, and suicide, is called Wings of America. Given that many American Indian communities include running in some of their celebrations,

Wings of America uses running as a catalyst for empowering youth to take pride in themselves and their culture. The organization sponsors cross-country teams, conducts youth development summer camps, and provides speakers and other assistance for wellness programs, conferences, clinics, and fairs.[59]

Despite such efforts, Americans' lack of exercise is one of the most intractable problems facing public health today. Very little is known about psychosocial, cultural, environmental, and public policy factors that may influence physical activity. The Surgeon General's *Physical Activity and Health* report called for more research on various interventions and their long-term effects.[35] Indeed, we have much to learn about how to motivate Americans to exercise adequately. In the words of one researcher, "The return of physical activity as the norm in everyone's everyday life—the 'restoration of biological normality'—will require cultural change on a scale similar to that which has occurred with smoking."[35(p.253)]

Confronting the Obesity Epidemic

The prevalence of overweight and obesity has increased so rapidly over recent decades (see Figures 16-1 and 16-2) that public health professionals have been calling it an epidemic. The health risks caused by overweight and obesity threaten to reverse many of the improvements in public health that were achieved in the 20th century. In fact, an analysis published in 2005 projected that the life expectancy of Americans will decline in the future due to obesity.[60] The authors predicted that if the present trends continued, the next generation will be the first to die younger and sicker than their parents. These predictions now seem prescient, as life expectancy did indeed fall over the five years ending in 2018. As discussed earlier in this text, rising obesity rates have likely contributed to the recent slowing in positive heart disease trends, a key factor in declining life expectancy (increased deaths of despair—drug overdoses, alcohol-associated deaths, and suicides—are the other major cause).[61]

Costs of treating the diseases caused by overweight and obesity are estimated to account for as much as 20.6% of total U.S. medical expenditures and may have reached as high as $190 billion annually from 2000 to 2005.[62] Approximately half of these costs are paid by Medicare and Medicaid (the government health insurance plans), and the other half by private health insurance and by individuals.

In 2000, then Surgeon General David Satcher organized a public "listening session" on this problem, which led to the publication of the *Surgeon General's Call to Action to Prevent and Decrease Overweight and Obesity*.[63] Its purpose was to develop a national plan and to forge coalitions of governments, organizations, and individuals to "promote healthy eating habits and adequate physical activity, beginning in childhood and continuing across the lifespan." As Dr. Satcher states in the report's foreword, "Many people believe that dealing with overweight and obesity is a personal responsibility. To some degree they are right, but it is also a community responsibility. When there are no safe, accessible places for children to play or adults to walk, jog, or ride a bike, that is a community responsibility. When school lunchrooms or office cafeterias do not provide healthy and appealing food choices, that is a community responsibility. When new or expectant mothers are not educated about the benefits of breastfeeding, that is a community responsibility. When we do not require daily physical education in our schools, that is also a community responsibility. There is much that we can and should do together."[63(p.xiii)]

The health consequences of obesity are serious, and the ineffectiveness of simply advising people to change their diet and exercise habits has led to the acceptance of more drastic measures. Bariatric surgery, which involves reducing the size of the stomach through implanting a gastric band or by surgically removing or bypassing part of the stomach, has been found effective in helping obese people to lose weight and to control diabetes. The National Institutes of Health suggests that bariatric surgery may be appropriate for obese people with a BMI of at least 40 and for people with a BMI of 35 together with serious coexisting medical conditions such as diabetes.[64] However, it warns that there are risks associated with the surgery and people must be prepared to change their habits afterward. Also, some people regain some of the lost weight.

An effective diet pill might be a less drastic approach than bariatric surgery in helping people to lose weight. In recent decades, the Food and Drug Administration (FDA) has been reluctant to approve weight-loss drugs because of fear of side effects. A drug combination called fen-phen introduced in the 1990s had to be removed from the market because it caused heart valve problems and pulmonary hypertension. More recently, the FDA has concluded that obesity has become such an important public health concern that pharmaceutical approaches to controlling it are badly needed and need not be risk-free. In turn, in 2012, it approved two new drugs:[65] Belviq works by activating a part of the brain that controls hunger; Qsymia is a combination of an appetite suppressant and a drug that was approved to treat epilepsy and migraines. An older drug, orlistat, works by inhibiting the absorption of dietary fats. The FDA approved it at a lower dose as the brand-name product Alli, for over-the-counter sales. Orlistat may have unpleasant gastrointestinal effects and on rare occasions has been reported to cause liver damage.[66]

Conclusion

Poor diet and physical inactivity are ranked among the top two behavioral factors identified as the leading actual causes of death in the United States. The combination of eating too much and exercising too little causes a very high prevalence of obesity among Americans. Obesity contributes to many health problems, including cardiovascular disease, diabetes, and most kinds of cancer. However, it is not just the extra pounds that adversely affect health, but how that weight is distributed. Extra weight in the hips and buttocks is less harmful to health than is extra weight in the midsection.

In general, Americans eat too much protein and fat and too few fruits and vegetables. This pattern of eating would be considered unhealthy even if it did not lead to obesity. Increases in the consumption of sweetened beverages and decreases in the consumption of milk over the past several decades, especially among children, have contributed to the obesity epidemic.

Recommendations for a healthy diet call for people to eat more vegetables, fruits, whole grains, and low-fat milk products. However, people have great difficulty in changing their eating patterns, as can be seen from the large number of individuals who are trying to lose weight, mostly without success. Public health programs to promote healthy eating employ the ecological model, trying to create a favorable social environment by conducting media campaigns, encouraging the ready availability of nutritious foods, and providing nutritional information so that people will choose their foods wisely. Taxing unhealthy products, notably sugar-sweetened beverages, can also play an important role.

Exercise helps protect against cardiovascular disease, diabetes, and some forms of cancer, in addition to helping to control weight. People who are physically active live longer than those who are inactive. Americans get far too little exercise—a factor that contributes to the high prevalence of obesity. Most public health interventions to promote physical activity apply the ecological model of behavior, using interpersonal and media messages to motivate people to exercise and removing environmental barriers that hinder such activity.

Because of the difficulty in changing diet and physical activity patterns of adults, the best hope of improving the population's behavior may be to focus on children. The prevalence of obesity in children is increasing in the United States. Some studies have shown that interventions that involve the whole family can be effective in reducing children's obesity. Encouraging children to play outside and to walk or bike to school can help increase their physical activity. In school, physical education classes that help children develop skills they can use later in life may encourage them to develop the habit of being physically active. One of the most important obstacles to the development of healthful diet and activity patterns in children is television watching and other types of screen time, which not only promote inactivity but also tempt children with advertisements for non-nutritious snacks.

References

1. Centers for Disease Control and Prevention, "Health, United States, 2017," Table 53, 2018, https://www.cdc.gov/nchs/data/hus/hus17.pdf, accessed September 23, 2019.

2. Centers for Disease Control and Prevention, "Attempts to Lose Weight Among Adults in the United States, 2013–2016," *NCHS Data Brief*, July 2018, https://www.cdc.gov/nchs/products/databriefs/db313.htm, accessed September 23, 2019.

3. U.S. Institute of Medicine, *Weighing the Options: Criteria for Evaluating Weight-Management Programs* (Washington, DC: National Academies Press, 1995).

4. Centers for Disease Control and Prevention, "Defining Adult Overweight and Obesity." https://www.cdc.gov/obesity/adult/defining.html, accessed September 23, 2019.

5. K. R. Fontaine et al., "Years of Life Lost Due to Obesity," *Journal of the American Medical Association* 289 (2003): 187–193.

6. World Health Organization Expert Consultation, "Appropriate Body-Mass Index for Asian Populations

and Its Implications for Policy and Intervention Strategies," *Lancet* 363 (2004): 157–163.

7. Centers for Disease Control and Prevention, "Health, United States, 2011," https://www.cdc.gov/nchs/data/hus/hus11.pdf, accessed December 11, 2019.

8. Centers for Disease Control and Prevention, "Basics About Childhood Obesity," September 11, 2018. https://www.cdc.gov/obesity/childhood/index.html, accessed December 11, 2019.

9. C. L. Ogden, M. D. Carroll, B. K. Kit, and K. M. Flegal, "Prevalence of Childhood and Adult Obesity in the United States, 2011–2012," *Journal of the American Medical Association* 311 (2014): 806–814.

10. A. Sinaiko, R. P. Donahue, D. R. Jacobs Jr, and R. J. Prineas, "Relation of Weight and Rate of Increase in Weight During Childhood and Adolescence to Body Size, Blood Pressure, Fasting Insulin, and Lipids in Young Adults: The Minneapolis Children's Blood Pressure Study," *Circulation* 99 (1999): 1471–1476.

11. A. Fagot-Campagna, D. J. Pettitt, M. M. Engelgau, N. R. Burrows, L. S. Geiss, R. Valdez, "Type 2 Diabetes Among North American Children and Adolescents: An Epidemiologic Review and a Public Health Perspective," *Journal of Pediatrics* 135 (2000): 664–672.

12. D. S. Ludwig, "Childhood Obesity: The Shape of Things to Come," *New England Journal of Medicine* 357 (2007): 2325–2527.

13. Office of Disease Prevention and Health Promotion, "Dietary Guidelines: Questions and Answers," https://health.gov/dietaryguidelines/2015/qanda.asp, accessed September 25, 2019.

14. M. Nestle, *Food Politics: How the Food Industry Influences Nutrition and Health* (Berkeley, CA: University of California Press, 2002).

15. Office of Disease Prevention and Health Promotion, "2015–2020 Dietary Guidelines for Americans," https://health.gov/dietaryguidelines/2015/, accessed September 30, 2019.

16. U.S. Department of Agriculture, "ChooseMyPlate," https://www.choosemyplate.gov, accessed September 30, 2019.

17. U.S. Department of Agriculture, "Dietary Guidelines 2015–2020: Shifts Needed to Align with Healthy Eating Patterns," https://health.gov/dietaryguidelines/2015/guidelines/chapter-2/current-eating-patterns-in-the-united-states/, accessed September 25, 2019.

18. S. J. Nielsen and B. M. Popkin, "Changes in Beverage Intake Between 1977 and 2001," *American Journal of Preventive Medicine* 27 (2004): 205–210.

19. Centers for Disease Control and Prevention, "Get the Facts: Sugar-Sweetened Beverages and Consumption," February 27, 2017. https://www.cdc.gov/nutrition/data-statistics/sugar-sweetened-beverages-intake.html, accessed September 25, 2019.

20. H. Allcott, B. B. Lockwood, and D. Taubinsky, "Should We Tax Sugar-Sweetened Beverages? An Overview of Theory and Evidence," *Journal of Economic Perspectives* 33 (2019): 202–227.

21. J. M. Chrisler, "Adherence to Weight Loss and Nutritional Regimens," in D. S. Gochman, ed., *Handbook of Health Behavior Research II: Provider Determinants* (New York, NY: Plenum Press, 1997), 323–333.

22. D. S. Ludwig and H. A. Pollack, "Obesity and the Economy: From Crisis to Opportunity," *Journal of the American Medical Association* 301 (2009): 532–535.

23. D. S. Ludwig and M. Nestle, "Can the Food Industry Play a Constructive Role in the Obesity Epidemic?" *Journal of the American Medical Association* 300 (2008): 1808–1811.

24. M. Fox, "Restaurant Menu Label Rules Go into Effect," *NBC News*, May 8, 2018, https://www.nbcnews.com/health/health-news/restaurant-menu-label-rules-go-effect-n872066, accessed September 25, 2019.

25. S. Chan, "A Tax on Many Soft Drinks Sets off a Spirited Debate," *The New York Times*, December 16, 2008.

26. E. R. Cheng, L. G. Fiechtner, and A. E. Carroll, "Seriously, Juice Is Not Healthy," *The New York Times*, July 7, 2018.

27. M. Richtel and A. Jacobs, "American Adults Just Keep Getting Fatter," *The New York Times*, March 23, 2018.

28. L. M. Maynard, D. A. Galuska, H. M. Blanck, and M. K. Serdula, "Maternal Perceptions of Weight Status of Children," *Pediatrics* 111 (2003): 1226–1231.

29. H. Y. Chen, S. C. Lemon, S. L. Pagoto, B. A. Barton, K. L. Lapane, and R. J. Goldberg, "Personal and Parental Weight Misperception and Self-Reported Attempted Weight Loss in US Children and Adolescents," *Preventing Chronic Disease* 11 (2014), https://www.cdc.gov/pcd/issues/2014/14_0123.htm, accessed September 30, 2019.

30. Centers for Disease Control and Prevention, "Perception of Weight Status in U.S. Children and Adolescents, Aged 8–15 Years, 2005–2012," *NCHS Data Brief*, no. 158 (July 23, 2014), https://www.cdc.gov/nchs/data/databriefs/db158.pdf, accessed September 30, 2019.

31. H. R. Thompson and K. A. Madsen, "The Report Card on BMI Report Cards," *Current Obesity Reports* 6, no. 2 (2017): 163–167.

32. S. R. Daniels and S. G. Hassink, "The Role of the Pediatrician in Primary Prevention of Obesity," *Pediatrics* 136 (2015): e275–e292.

33. Institute of Medicine, *Preventing Childhood Obesity: Health in the Balance* (Washington, DC: National Academies Press, 2005).

34. J. N. Morris, "Exercise Versus Heart Attack: History of a Hypothesis," in M. Marmot and P. Elliott, eds., *Coronary Heart Disease Epidemiology: From Aetiology to Public Health* (Oxford, UK: Oxford Medical Publications, 1992), 242–255.

35. U.S. Department of Health and Human Services, *Physical Activity and Health: A Report of the Surgeon*

General (Atlanta, GA: Centers for Disease Control and Prevention, National Center for Chronic Disease Prevention and Health Promotion, 1996).

36. R. S. Paffenbarger Jr., R. T. Hyde, A. L. Wing, C. C. Hsieh, "Physical Activity, All-Cause Mortality, and Longevity of College Alumni," *New England Journal of Medicine* 314 (1986): 605–613.

37. R. S. Paffenbarger Jr., R. T. Hyde, A. L. Wing, I. M. Lee, D. L. Jung, and J. B. Kampert, "The Association of Changes in Physical Activity Level and Other Lifestyle Characteristics with Mortality Among Men," *New England Journal of Medicine* 328 (1993): 538–545.

38. W. B. Kannel and P. Sorlie, "Some Health Benefits of Physical Activity: The Framingham Study," *Archives of Internal Medicine* 139 (1979): 857–861.

39. J. Boone-Heinonen, K. R. Evenson, D. R. Taber, and P. Gordon-Larsen, "Walking for Prevention of Cardiovascular Disease in Men and Women: A Systematic Review of Observational Studies," *Obesity Reviews* 10 (2009): 204–217.

40. A. D. Tsopanakis, E. P. Sgouraki, K. N. Pavlou, E. R. Nadel, and S. R. Bussolari, "Lipids and Lipoprotein Profiles in a 4-Hour Endurance Test on a Recumbent Cycloergometer," *American Journal of Clinical Nutrition* 49 (1989): 980–984.

41. D. M. Kramsch, A. J. Aspen, B. M. Abramowitz, T. Kreimendahl, and W. B. Hood, Jr., "Reduction of Coronary Atherosclerosis by Moderate Conditioning Exercise in Monkeys on an Atherogenic Diet," *New England Journal of Medicine* 305 (1981): 1483–1489.

42. T. J. Orchard et al., "Diabetes," in R. B. Wallace, ed., *Maxcy–Rosenau–Last Public Health and Preventive Medicine* (Stamford, CT: Appleton and Lange, 1998), 973.

43. J. E. Manson, E. B. Rimm, M. J. Stampfer, G. A. Colditz, W. C. Willett, A. S. Krolewski, "Physical Activity and Incidence of Non-Insulin-Dependent Diabetes Mellitus in Women," *Lancet* 338 (1991): 774–778.

44. J. E. Manson, D. M. Nathan, A. S. Krolewski, M. J. Stampfer, W. C. Willett, and C. H. Hennekens, "A Prospective Study of Exercise and Incidence of Diabetes Among U.S. Male Physicians," *Journal of the American Medical Association* 268 (1992): 63–67.

45. National Cancer Institute, Division of Cancer Epidemiology and Genetics, "Exploring the Link Between Leisure-Time Physical Activity, Sedentary Behavior, and Cancer," February 24, 2015, https://dceg.cancer.gov/news-events/news/2015/physical-activity-cancer, accessed September 30, 2019.

46. Office of Disease Prevention and Health Promotion, "2008 Physical Activity Guidelines for Americans," https://www.health.gov/paguidelines/guidelines/, accessed September 30, 2019.

47. U.S. Department of Health and Human Services, "Physical Activity Guidelines for Americans, 2nd edition," 2018, https://health.gov/paguidelines /second-edition/pdf/Physical_Activity_Guidelines _2nd_edition.pdf, accessed September 25, 2019.

48. U.S. Community Preventive Services Task Force, "Obesity Prevention and Control: Behavioral Interventions That Aim to Reduce Recreational Sedentary Screen Time Among Children," August 2014, www.thecommunityguide.org/findings/obesity -behavioral-interventions-aim-reduce-recreational -sedentary-screen-time-among, accessed September 30, 2019.

49. American Academy of Pediatrics, "American Academy of Pediatrics Announces New Recommendations for Children's Media Use," October 21, 2016, https://www.aap.org/en-us/about-the-aap/aap-press-room /Pages/American-Academy-of-Pediatrics-Announces -New-Recommendations-for-Childrens-Media-Use .aspx, accessed September 25, 2019.

50. Centers for Disease Control and Prevention, "Screen Time vs. Lean Time Infographic," https://www .cdc.gov/nccdphp/dnpao/multimedia/infographics /getmoving.html, accessed September 25, 2019.

51. T. N. Robinson, "Reducing Children's Television Viewing to Prevent Obesity," *Journal of the American Medical Association* 282 (1999): 1561–1567.

52. K. Fang, M. Mu, K. Liu, and Y. He, "Screen Time and Childhood Overweight/Obesity: A Systematic Review and Meta-Analysis," *Child: Care, Health, and Development* 45 (2019): 744–753.

53. U.S. Preventive Services Task Force, "Behavioral Counseling in Primary Care to Promote Physical Activity: Recommendations and Rationale," *American Family Physician* 66 (2002): 1731.

54. D. M. Bravata, C. Smith-Spangler, V. Sundaram, A. L. Gienger, N. Lin, R. Lewis, "Using Pedometers to Increase Physical Activity and Improve Health: A Systematic Review," *Journal of the American Medical Association* 298 (2007): 2296–2304.

55. R. C. Whitaker, "Obesity Prevention in Pediatric Primary Care: Four Behaviors to Target," *Archives of Pediatrics and Adolescent Medicine* 157 (2003): 725–727.

56. S. E. Jones and S. Sliwa, "School Factors Associated with the Percentage of Students Who Walk or Bike to School, School Health Policies and Practices Study, 2014," *Preventing Chronic Disease* 13 (2016): E63.

57. K. K. Davidson, J. L. Werder, and C. T. Lawson, "Children's Active Commuting to School: Current Knowledge and Future Directions," *Preventing Chronic Disease: Public Health Research, Practice, and Policy* 5 (July 2008): A100.

58. R. Flores, "Dance for Health: Improving Fitness in African American and Hispanic Adolescents," *Public Health Reports* 110 (1995): 189–193.

59. J. Spring, "Running from Despair: A Collection of American Indian Athletes Has Risen to Prominence," *The New York Times*, February 16, 2008.

60. S. J. Olshansky et al., "A Potential Decline in Life Expectancy in the United States in the 21st Century," *New England Journal of Medicine* 352 (2005): 1138–1145.

61. A. Case and A. Deaton, "Mortality and Morbidity in the 21st Century," *Brookings Papers on Economic Activity*, no. 1 (2017).

62. Institute of Medicine, *Accelerating Progress in Obesity Prevention: Solving the Weight of the Nation* (Washington, DC: National Academies Press, 2012).

63. U.S. Department of Health and Human Services, *Surgeon General's Call to Action to Prevent and Decrease Overweight and Obesity* (Rockville, MD: U.S. Government Printing Office, 2001).

64. National Institutes of Health, "Bariatric Surgery for Severe Obesity," June 2011, https://www.niddk.nih.gov/health-information/weight-management/bariatric-surgery/potential-candidates, accessed September 25, 2019.

65. U.S. Food and Drug Administration, "Medications Target Long-Term Weight Control," July 25, 2015, https://www.fda.gov/ForConsumers/ConsumerUpdates/ucm312380.htm, accessed November 19, 2015.

66. U.S. Food and Drug Administration, "Xenical (Orlistat) Capsules," 2010, https://www.accessdata.fda.gov/drugsatfda_docs/label/2010/020766s028lbl.pdf, accessed September 30, 2019.

CHAPTER 17

An Accident Waiting to Happen

Injuries Are Not Accidents

KEY TERMS

Consumer Product Safety
 Commission (CPSC)
Intentional injury
National Highway Traffic
 Safety Administration
 (NHTSA)

National Institute for
 Occupational Safety and
 Health (NIOSH)
Occupational Safety and Health
 Administration (OSHA)
Primary prevention

Secondary prevention
Tertiary prevention
"Three E's" of injury prevention
Unintentional injury
Years of potential life
 lost (YPLL)

Injuries are the third leading cause of death in the United States.[1] They are even more important than statistics suggest because injuries disproportionately affect young people and, therefore, cause many **years of potential life lost (YPLL)**. Injuries are the number one cause of death among people younger than age 50.[1] In addition to the people killed by injuries, almost as many survivors are left with permanent disabilities, representing a major economic and emotional drain on families and on society in general.

Traditionally, injuries have been thought of as "accidents," unavoidable random occurrences, or the results of antisocial or incautious behavior. It is only recently that public health practitioners have recognized that injuries can and should be treated as a public health problem, analyzable by epidemiologic methods and amenable to preventive interventions. While most injuries are caused to some extent by individual behavior, they are also influenced by the physical and social environment. Public health programs to prevent injury must find ways to change people's behavior by the classic methods of education and regulation—although for many types of injuries, prevention by changing the environment may be more effective.

Epidemiology of Injuries

Prevention of injury, like the prevention of most diseases, is based on epidemiology. Data are needed to answer the questions of *who, where, when*, and *how*, looking for patterns and connections that suggest where the greatest needs for prevention are as well as ways to intervene to prevent the injury. Fatal injuries are generally categorized as **unintentional injury** (sometimes referred to as "accidental") or **intentional injury** (homicide or suicide).

Injuries are an especially important cause of death in young people. In 2017, unintentional injuries caused 33% of deaths in children aged 1 to 4, 28% of deaths in children aged 5 to 14, and 42% of deaths in young people aged 15 to 24.[1] An additional 35% of deaths in the 15-to-24 age group were caused by suicide or homicide.

Both race and gender affect injury rates. Males are more likely to sustain injuries than are females, with a fatal injury rate 2.1 times higher than that of females for all age groups combined. Blacks have lower rates of injury mortality than whites do, including lower rates of alcohol- and drug-associated deaths, except for the high rates of homicide among black males, which is more than 11 times the rate for white males.[1]

Injury rates, like other indicators of poor health, are higher in groups of lower socioeconomic status. The death rate from unintentional injury is twice as high in low-income areas as in high-income areas. House fires, pedestrian fatalities, and homicides are all more common among the poor.[2] The poor are more likely to have high-risk jobs, low-quality housing, older, defective cars, and hazardous products such as space heaters, all of which contribute to higher injury risks.

Figure 17-1 shows the leading categories of injury deaths in the United States. Poisoning leads the list, followed by motor vehicle injuries, with firearms fatalities ranked third. As a result of the high priority that the federal government has placed on prevention of motor vehicle–related injuries, as described in a later section of this chapter, highway fatalities have declined over most of the past four decades—from a high of 54,589 such deaths

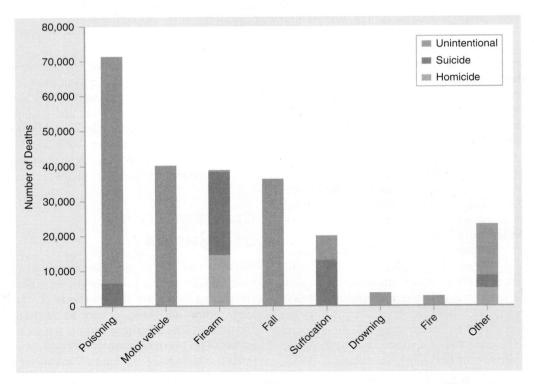

Figure 17-1 Leading Causes of Injury Death, 2017

Data from Centers for Disease Control and Prevention, "Deaths: Final Data for 2017," *National Vital Statistics Report,* Vol. 68, no. 9, ww.cdc.gov/nchs/data/nvsr/nvsr68/nvsr68_09-508.pdf, accessed September 16, 2019.

in 1972 to 40,231 deaths in 2017 (though the number hit a low of 35,303 deaths in between these years, in 2011). Firearm fatalities increased between 1968 and 1994, and the Centers for Disease Control and Prevention (CDC) predicted that if trends continued, the number of firearm-related deaths would surpass those related to motor vehicles by the year 2003.[3] The trend in firearm injuries held steady until 2014, at which time it increased from 10.5 age-adjusted deaths per 100,000 in 2014 to 12.2 age-adjusted deaths per 100,000 in 2017. In contrast, traffic fatalities have fallen modestly since the 2000s, so that the two causes are now about equal in the injury statistics, as shown in **Figure 17-2**).[4]

Death rates from poisoning overtook traffic fatalities in 2009, becoming the leading cause of injury death in the United States. Most poisonings are drug overdoses, including those caused by prescription painkillers, which increased five-fold between 1999 and 2017, and those caused by heroin and synthetic narcotics, which increased 16-fold over this period.[5] Other major causes of injury deaths that have drawn significant public health attention include falls, suffocation, drowning, and fires.

Many injuries are not fatal, of course, but fatal injuries are the ones that are most reliably reported. While data on nonfatal injuries are less complete, these injuries can have serious and even devastating effects. In 2017, for every fatal injury reported, more than 12 individuals were hospitalized for nonfatal injuries, and 187 were treated in the emergency department.[6] These numbers are illustrated in the "injury pyramid" shown in **Figure 17-3**, from which it is possible to estimate the impact of nonfatal injuries when data on fatal injuries are known.

Injuries that result in long-term disability, especially head and spinal cord injuries, are particularly costly to society. In 2014, for example, 2.9 million Americans sustained a traumatic brain injury (TBI).[7] Of these persons, approximately 56,800 died, and 288,000 were hospitalized and survived, often with lifelong disabling conditions. Many of these victims are young. Caring for these patients costs billions of dollars, much of it paid for with public funds.

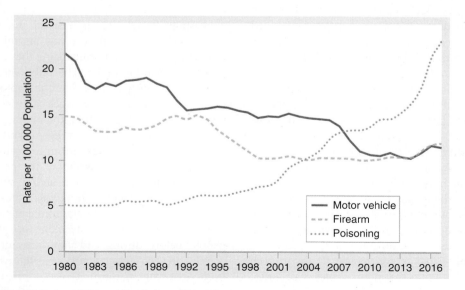

Figure 17-2 Age-Adjusted Death Rates for the Leading Causes of Injury, 1980–2017

Data from Centers for Disease Control and Prevention, CDC WONDER database, 1979-1998 data, http://wonder.cdc.gov/cmf-icd9.html; 1999-2017 data, http://wonder.cdc.gov/ucd-icd10.html, accessed September 28, 2019.

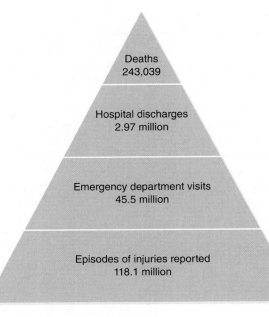

Figure 17-3 Injury Pyramid for 2016 (Deaths for 2017)

Data from Centers for Disease Control and Prevention, "All Injuries," www.cdc.gov/nchs/fastats/injury.htm, accessed September 28, 2019; discharge data: "National Hospital Ambulatory Medical Care Survey: 2016 Emergency Department Summary Tables, Table 24," https://www.cdc.gov/nchs/data/nhamcs/web_tables/2016_ed_web_tables.pdf, acceessed September 28, 2019.

Alcohol is a significant factor in a high percentage of injuries. An estimated 29% of traffic fatalities in 2017 involved alcohol.[8] Moreover, high alcohol levels were found in the blood of 32% of adult pedestrians killed by motor vehicles in that same year.[9] Many of those persons fatally injured in falls, drownings, fires, and suicides are under the influence of alcohol, as are many of the perpetrators and victims of homicides. Other drugs may play a role in injury, but because blood alcohol tests are much more commonly done than tests for other drugs, the role of alcohol in injury is better documented.

The importance of alcohol's contribution to injury accounts for its high placement on the list of "actual causes of death." To stress the importance of driving while intoxicated as a cause of death, the authors counted alcohol-related motor vehicle deaths in both the alcohol and the motor vehicle categories, making alcohol the third leading cause and motor vehicles the sixth leading cause.[10]

Analyzing Injuries

While injuries are generally brought on by human behavior, injury researchers have increasingly sought to understand the role of the environment in causing an injury-producing event and in influencing the severity of the resulting injury. The public health approach to injury control, like the approach to infectious diseases, analyzes injuries in terms of a chain of causation: the interactions over time between a host, an agent, and the environment. To analyze an injury-causing event requires information about the person (host) who initiates the event and/or suffers the injury, the agent (automobile, firearm, swimming pool), and the environment (road conditions, weather, involvement of other people) before, during, and after the event.

To prevent certain injury-causing events from occurring in the first place—**primary prevention**—analysts seek to understand the conditions prevailing before each such event.

For example, characteristics of the host (e.g., alcohol intoxication), the agent (e.g., defective brakes), and the environment (e.g., a dark and rainy night) are all relevant to whether a motor vehicle crash occurs. Conditions prevailing during the event affect the outcome of the crash. Thus, wearing a seat belt (host), equipping a car with an air bag (agent), and driving on a divided highway (environment) may allow the driver to avoid serious injury during a crash—**secondary prevention**. **Tertiary prevention** depends on conditions after the crash that determine whether the victim survives the injury and the extent of any resulting disability. The availability and quality of emergency care are major factors in tertiary prevention.

Because motor vehicle injuries cause so many deaths, they were the first category of injuries to be analyzed and subjected to systematic prevention efforts. Much data are available on conditions surrounding motor vehicle crashes, and methods for preventing motor vehicle injuries are highly developed. National highway safety programs were launched two decades before Congress identified injury as a general public health problem and established the National Center for Injury Prevention and Control at the CDC.

Injury-control efforts developed for motor vehicle injuries have served as a model for more embryonic efforts to control other categories of injury. Early prevention strategies focused on changing people's behavior by applying the classic public health methods of education and regulation. As with many public health issues related to behavior, regulation is usually more effective than education in getting people to change their behavior. In the earliest days of traffic safety efforts, for example, society learned that laws regarding speed limits and traffic lights were necessary to control the chaos on the roadways.

Modern injury control began with the recognition that engineering plays an important role in the causation of injuries and their severity. Sharp objects cause more damage

to the human body than do blunt ones; an impact distributed over a broad surface results in a less severe injury than an impact spread over a smaller surface; if deceleration can be controlled and made less sudden, the body can better withstand the force. In general, automatic protections are more effective than measures that require effort, and the more effort a measure requires, the less likely it is to be employed. Thus the **"three E's" of injury prevention** are education, enforcement, and engineering.

These insights, which were first applied in the auto industry, have also been applied to prevention of many other kinds of injury—especially childhood injuries—with considerable success. For example, when the New York City Health Department noted that a large number of children died from falls out of windows, it instituted the "Children Can't Fly" program, requiring landlords to install window guards. Subsequently, the number of fatal falls in the city was reduced by half.[11] The number of children who drown in swimming pools has been reduced by laws requiring pools to be fenced. Poisonings in children can be prevented by childproof caps on medicine containers and some household chemicals. The use of smoke detectors has reduced the number of deaths from fires. State and federal regulation of the flammability of fabrics has also saved lives, especially those of children—due to laws on children's sleepwear. As a result of these measures and others, fatal injury rates among small children have declined markedly in recent years.[1,12]

Motor Vehicle Injuries

Attention was focused on the problem of motor vehicle injuries by Ralph Nader's indictment of the automobile industry in his book, *Unsafe at Any Speed: The Designed-In Dangers of the American Automobile*, published in 1966. Congress responded by passing the National Traffic and Motor Vehicle

Safety Act of 1966, which established the **National Highway Traffic Safety Administration (NHTSA)** and empowered it to set safety standards for new cars, such as installation of seat belts, laminated windshields, collapsible steering assemblies, and dashboard padding. Prior to the implementation of such standards, hundreds of thousands of drivers had died from being impaled on unyielding steering columns. In addition, the heads and faces of front-seat passengers had been cut by sharp dashboard edges and by glass from broken windshields. The safer designs mandated by the 1966 legislation led to an enormous reduction in both injury and mortality.[11]

NHTSA was also required to collect data on motor vehicle–related deaths and to conduct research aimed at preventing motor vehicle collisions and ameliorating their effects. Among other activities, NHTSA has an ongoing program of crash-testing various vehicle models, seeking to understand how engineering-related changes could better protect occupants during a crash. These studies have led to further improvements in automobile design—including headrests that protect their occupants during rear-end collisions, strengthened side bars to protect occupants during side crashes, and air bags—that are now required by federal law.[13]

While requirements that vehicles more effectively protect their occupants during a crash are an important part of injury control (secondary prevention), preventing crashes from occurring in the first place (primary prevention) is the highest priority. Specific characteristics of vehicles, such as turn signals and brake lights, can help prevent crashes. State laws that require annual inspections of these devices, as well as of brakes and tires, are aimed at ensuring that defects in vehicles do not lead to injuries. Beginning with 2011 models, and with additions to the rating program in 2013, 2015, and 2016, the NHTSA has rated using a five-star safety rating system that includes crash avoidance technology such as electronic stability control, lane departure warnings, and forward collision warnings.[14]

Environmental features, especially improvements in highway design, have also been shown to prevent crashes. Divided highways, raised lane dividers embedded in road surfaces, rumble strips at road edges, and "wrong way" signs at off ramps can all help prevent mistakes by drivers.

Injury control methods that target the driver depend on both education and enforcement, and they exemplify the typical difficulties in getting people to practice healthier behaviors. Because alcohol plays such a major role in fatal crashes, laws against drinking and driving are virtually universal. Their effectiveness depends on how well they are enforced, however. The activism of volunteer groups such as Mothers Against Drunk Driving (MADD) has helped raise public consciousness about the extent of the problem, and tolerance for drinking and driving has declined in recent years. In addition to imposing severe penalties for being caught driving drunk, many states have expanded legislation to make establishments that serve alcohol liable for serving minors or persons who are already obviously intoxicated.

After alcohol, the second most important factor in fatal crashes is youth. In 2017, 8% of drivers in fatal crashes were between 15 and 20 years old, even though members of this age group made up only 5% of all drivers.[15] According to NHTSA, this disproportionate risk is believed to be due in part to inexperience: Driving is a complex task, and new drivers are more likely to make mistakes. Many of these crashes also involve risk-taking behavior and poor judgment.

Most states have now addressed the issue by implementing graduated driver-licensing systems, in which young drivers must pass through one or two preliminary stages of driver permits over a period of time before they are allowed a full license.[16] NHTSA has developed a model law that includes the following provisions:

- When a driver has a learner's permit, a licensed adult must be in the vehicle at all times; the young person must remain crash-free and conviction-free before being allowed to take a road test for a provisional license.
- Nighttime driving is restricted for those with a provisional license.
- Young drivers must remain crash-free and conviction-free for a year before moving to a full license.

As of 2008, all states had adopted some form of the graduated system, although states vary significantly in the restrictions they impose at different stages.[17] Graduated licensing has been successful in preventing traffic fatalities among young people: States that have adopted the system have experienced significant reductions in crashes by drivers younger than 20 years old.

In addition to being inexperienced, young drivers may be just starting to drink, and doing both together can be fatal. In 2017, 24% of drivers age 15 to 20 years who were killed in crashes had alcohol in their blood.[15] The federal government and many states have made concerted efforts to reduce drinking and driving among young people. One attempt to deal with this problem was a federal law requiring states to increase the drinking age to 21 to receive highway funds (the law became effective in 1988).[11] In 1995, a similar federal law required states to pass zero-tolerance laws for drivers younger than age 21. Since 1998, all states and the District of Columbia have had laws setting a limit of 0.02% blood-alcohol concentration or less for drivers, suspending driver's licenses for those found in violation. The evidence indicates that this is an effective approach to saving lives: The rate of teen drinking and driving has fallen steadily since the early 1990s.[18]

Speed limits are an important factor in highway injuries. In 1974, Congress imposed a national speed limit of 55 miles per hour to conserve fuel at the time of the Arab oil embargo. That law, which contributed to a 16% decline in traffic fatalities between 1973 and 1974, was revoked in 1995 as part of a larger deregulation trend.[11] Many states have since raised their speed limits, including 41 states that have limits of 70 miles per hour or higher on rural interstates.[19]

The use of seat belts has been shown to reduce fatalities by 40% to 50%. Child-safety seats can reduce the risk of a child being killed during a collision or sudden stop by 71%.[11] These engineering measures require people to use them correctly, however, and state laws requiring the use of seat belts and child-safety seats are widely ignored. In states that have primary seat belt laws—laws allowing police officers to pull over drivers and ticket them solely for not wearing a seat belt—the rate of seat belt use is higher than it is in states that have secondary laws—laws that permit police to issue tickets for seat belt violations only after stopping a driver for another reason. As of 2019, 34 states and the District of Columbia had primary seat belts laws, and 15 had secondary laws. New Hampshire has no seat belt law for adults. All states and the District of Columbia have child restraint laws, though the types of restraints required for children of various ages vary among the states.[20]

A relatively new issue that has come to the attention of traffic safety advocates is cell phone use while driving. The NHTSA collects data on distracted driving, which includes driving while using a cell phone, eating, reading, and using a navigational system, all of which degrade the driver's performance. According to NHTSA, 3166 people were killed in motor vehicle crashes involving distracted drivers in 2017.[21] As of 2019, 20 states and the District of Columbia had laws banning the use of handheld cell phones while driving, and 38 states and the District of Columbia ban their use by novice drivers.[22] No state has banned use of these devices altogether, although the evidence indicates that even hands-free phones can cause significant distraction to the driver.

Even more risky than talking on a cell phone is text messaging, which has become increasingly common, especially among younger drivers. One study that used video cameras installed in the cabs of long-haul trucks found that when drivers texted, their risk of a collision increased 23-fold.[23] Other studies suggest that the risk faced by drivers of passenger cars is similar. Forty-eight states and the District of Columbia completely ban text messaging while driving.[22]

In 1968, when implementation of federal traffic safety legislation began, almost 55,000 Americans died each year from motor vehicle–related injuries. The national effort to reduce this toll has had significant success. By 1993, the number had declined to a little more than 40,000 fatalities per year despite the fact that many more cars were on the roads and that the number of miles driven has more than doubled.[3] Subsequently, the downward trend halted for more than a decade, but then dropped dramatically to 32,479 fatalities in 2011. In the last several years, the number of motor vehicle–related fatalities has increased, reaching 37,133 deaths in 2017. The fatality rate per 100 million vehicle miles of travel, however, remained near its all-time low in 2017 due to the increase in miles traveled.[24]

Future progress in traffic safety could depend on factors such as the price of gasoline. High gas prices tend to lead people to drive less. They also encourage people to buy smaller cars. When gas prices are low, heavier vehicles such as minivans, pickup trucks, and sport-utility vehicles are popular, contributing to increases in traffic fatalities because crashes between vehicles of widely disparate size and weight cause high risk to the occupants of the smaller vehicle. Sport-utility vehicles, vans, and pickup trucks, with their higher center of gravity, are more likely to roll over in crashes than sedans, however, offsetting the advantage occupants get from their size.

Pedestrians, Motorcyclists, and Bicyclists

Approximately 16% of all people killed in motor vehicle crashes are pedestrians, so public health efforts are also directed at preventing these injuries.[24] Elderly people have the highest risk for being killed by a motor vehicle while walking. An estimated 19% of pedestrians killed by motor vehicles are age 65 or older.[25] Most of these injuries occur in urban areas.

When a 1985 study investigated reasons for the high fatality rate among older pedestrians along Queens Boulevard in a part of New York City inhabited by large numbers of senior citizens, the researchers found that elderly persons took an average of 50 seconds to cross the 150-foot wide boulevard, while the "walk" sign allowed only 35 seconds for navigation of this span. Moreover, because of the boulevard's width and because vision loss is common among the elderly, many pedestrians could not read the "walk/don't walk" signs, which were located on the far side of the boulevard. The traffic safety unit installed additional signs on the median strips so that they could be more easily seen, and they reset the signs to allow more time for crossing. After implementation of these and other measures, such as stricter enforcement of speed limits, the rate of death and severe injuries among pedestrians fell by 60%.[11]

Public health professionals viewed the Queens Boulevard story as a success, but residents of the neighborhood still call that stretch of roadway the "Boulevard of Death." The city's Department of Transportation has continued to make safety improvements, including more fences to curtail jaywalking, restricting vehicle U-turns and left turns, and posting safety signs to remind pedestrians about the danger.[26]

In 2017, 5172 motorcyclists and 777 bicyclists were killed in crashes.[24] Motorcycles are far more dangerous than cars, with the number of deaths per mile traveled being 28 times higher for motorcycles.[27] Children younger than 15 years of age account for 7% of all bicycle-related fatalities, making this one of the leading causes of injury-related death in children.[28] From 2004 to 2013, there was a steady increase in the average age of bicyclists killed or injured in crashes with motor vehicles, from 39 years to 44 years.[28] The most important protective measure for bicycle and motorcycle riders is wearing a helmet. At least 83% of bicyclists killed and 41% of fatally injured motorcyclists were not wearing helmets.[28,29] Head injuries from such crashes also cause profound, permanent disability in many survivors.

Public health advocates have devoted considerable efforts to promoting the use of bicycle and motorcycle helmets. As part of the 1966 National Highway Safety Act, Congress mandated that states pass laws requiring motorcyclists to wear helmets, leading to a dramatic decline in motorcycle fatalities. Because of vigorous objections to this mandate on grounds of personal liberty, however, the federal law was changed in 1976.[30] In response, 27 states repealed or weakened their laws, and by 1980 motorcycle fatalities had increased dramatically. As of 2019, 19 states and the District of Columbia required helmet use for all motorcycle operators and their passengers. In another 28 states, only operators younger than a certain age, usually 18, are required to wear helmets.[31] In states where only minors are required to wear helmets, laws are difficult to enforce. Data on crashes in these states show that, despite the laws, fewer than 48% of fatally injured riders were wearing helmets; by comparison, in states with universal laws, 97% of fatally injured riders were wearing helmets.[27] Only 21 states and the District of Columbia have laws requiring bicycle helmets, and these laws apply only to children, although some local governments have laws that apply to riders of all ages.[32] The public health effort regarding bicycle helmets typically focuses on community education programs.

Poisoning

During the last two decades, the number of poisonings has skyrocketed. In 2008, poisoning surpassed firearms as a cause of injury death (Figure 17-2). In fact, the rate of deaths from poisoning more than tripled between 1999 and 2017, although it appeared to have leveled off as of early 2019.[33,34]

In trying to understand the dramatic increase in poisoning fatalities, scientists at the CDC analyzed death certificates recorded at the National Center for Health Statistics. They found that the vast majority of them listed drugs—legal and illegal—as the cause of death.[35] Opioid pain medications were most commonly involved in the unintentional deaths, followed by cocaine and heroin. Suicide by poisoning most commonly involved psychoactive drugs, such as sedatives and antidepressants, followed by opiates and other prescription pain medications.

The CDC scientists noted that during the 1990s, pain specialists argued that opioid pain medications were being underprescribed because of fear of addiction, leading to suffering of patients who were being denied relief from chronic pain. In response, between 1990 and 2002 there was a dramatic increase in the number of prescriptions written for these drugs, including hydrocodone, oxycodone, and methadone. The increase in sales of methadone was explained by prescriptions filled at pharmacies for pain management rather than distribution of the drug through narcotics treatment programs. The scientists' conclusion was that the increase in unintentional poisoning deaths was largely a result of nonmedical, recreational use of prescription pain relievers. Further evidence for this explanation is the age and sex distribution of the individuals who died: They were primarily middle-aged and male, rather than the older females who typically suffer from chronic pain, and many of them had a history of drug abuse.[35]

The CDC analysis led to the conclusion that medically prescribed opioid painkillers were being diverted for illegitimate and dangerous uses. The authors noted that corrective actions might be necessary to reduce deaths without diminishing the quality of care for patients who need the drugs for pain relief. This may include better communication and education of healthcare providers to warn them about the risks and inform them how to recognize patients who may be prone to abuse. Stricter regulation of opiates by the Drug Enforcement Agency, which registers physicians and pharmacies that handle opiates and tracks the buying and selling of these drugs, may also be necessary.

The age group with the lowest poisoning mortality rate is children younger than age 15 years, in part due to public health measures designed to protect curious youngsters from ingesting toxic substances. Childproof caps on pharmaceuticals and cleaning products have helped keep poisons out of the hands and mouths of toddlers, and poison control centers staff emergency phone lines 24 hours per day. Nevertheless, parents are advised to stay alert to the risks of childhood poisonings.

Poisoning deaths from other substances of public health concern include alcohol poisoning as a result of binge drinking, which accounts for more than 2000 deaths per year.[36] Carbon monoxide poisoning, which is involved in a high number of suicides and many unintentional deaths, may result from breathing air containing motor vehicle exhaust or from malfunctioning stoves, furnaces, or other appliances.

Firearms Injuries

In 1994, firearms injuries surpassed motor vehicle injuries as the leading cause of injury-related death in eight states and the District of Columbia. It appeared at that time that firearm injuries would soon become the number one cause of such deaths nationwide (Figure 17-2). However, the number of homicides dropped dramatically in 1994 and 1995, and suicides and unintentional gun deaths fell slightly. The number of deaths caused by firearms continued to decline, falling from almost 40,000 in 1993 to fewer than 30,000 deaths in 2004. A number of reasons have been proposed for the decline, including tougher gun control laws, community policing, and demographic changes.[37] Since then, however, the number of firearms deaths has increased, once again approaching 40,000 fatalities in 2017.[1]

Violence is traditionally thought of as a criminal justice issue rather than a public health issue. Certainly no one is arguing that the criminal justice system should abandon its mission. But public health has a different mission: It focuses on prevention as opposed to punishment. The relative success of the public health approach against motor vehicle injuries has inspired calls for it to be applied against violence, especially against firearm violence, the behavior that has the most severe consequences for health.

Plenty of grim statistics show that America's permissive attitude toward guns is harmful to people's health. In 2017, firearms killed 39,773 Americans.[1] Of these deaths, 61% were suicides, 37% were homicides, and a little more than 1% were caused by unintentional shootings. Teenagers and young adults are especially at risk. Forty percent of people who die from firearms are between the ages of 15 and 34. Forty-one percent of these deaths among young people are suicides, and 58% are homicides. The death rate from firearms is six times higher for males than that for females. Young African American males are at increased risk relative to other groups, especially for homicide.[1]

In 2016, homicide rates in the United States were 5 to 20 times higher than those in other developed countries. For example, in the United States, 6.5 people per 100,000 died by homicide, compared to 1.3 in the United Kingdom, 0.7 in Spain and Germany, and 0.3 in Japan.[38] Although suicide rates among Americans are comparable to those in other developed countries, a high percentage of these acts are committed with firearms. The easy availability of guns in the United States is believed to be responsible for many of these deaths. Homicide and suicide are more likely to succeed if guns are used rather than less lethal weapons: In 2017, 50% of suicides and 74% of homicides were committed with guns.[1] Suicide among young people is especially tragic. While rates of suicide among people 15 to 24 years old have declined since 1990, suicide remains the second leading cause of death in this age group.[1] Almost half of these suicides are committed with firearms.[1]

A survey of U.S. households conducted in 2017 found that 41% of them possessed at least one firearm.[39] Although two-thirds of respondents said they owned a handgun to protect themselves, a number of case-control studies have shown that the opposite is true. One study found that the relative risk of death by an unintentional gunshot injury is 3.7 for people living in a home with at least one gun, compared to a home without guns.[40] Another study found that residents of a household with a gun present in the home are 3 times more likely to die in a homicide[41] and 5 times more likely to commit suicide[42] than when no gun is available. In another study, a gun kept at home was found to be 43 times more likely to kill its owner, a family member, or a friend than to be used to kill an intruder.[43] There is some controversy about these findings. An analysis by the National Academy of Sciences cast doubt on whether the association between gun ownership and homicide or suicide represents a cause-and-effect relationship. The report stated that the data were too unreliable to draw firm conclusions and noted that information such as that collected on guns traced to crimes by the Bureau of Alcohol, Tobacco, Firearms and Explosives is inaccessible to researchers.[44] Nevertheless, a number of published literature reviews have supported the findings that having a gun in the home increases risks to members of the household.[45]

The CDC had been collecting data on patterns of violence for almost two decades, and in the early 1990s the agency stepped up its efforts to identify and evaluate interventions to prevent and reduce the impact of violence. Politically, however, guns have proved a much more difficult issue to deal with than motor vehicles. Many conservative politicians, with the support of the National Rifle Association (NRA), regard any attempt to control access to firearms as an attack on the Second Amendment to the Constitution. Limits on the depiction of violence in the media are also vigorously opposed in the name of protecting freedoms, although some evidence indicates that viewing violent episodes on television or in the movies increases the cultural acceptance of violence and makes children and youths more likely to behave in aggressive ways.

Opponents of gun control have even gone so far as to try to prevent the CDC from conducting research on violence as a public health problem. In 1995 and 1996, conservative members of the U.S. House of Representatives, backed by the NRA, tried first to eliminate the CDC's National Center for Injury Prevention and Control and then to cut the center's budget by the exact amount—about $2.4 million—that it had proposed to spend on research on firearms injury.[46] President Bill Clinton supported the CDC's work, and attempts to cut the center's budget failed. However, the political opposition had an impact. Legislation passed in 1996 explicitly forbade the CDC from using any of its funding "to advocate or promote gun control."[47(p.190)]

Efforts to reduce firearms injuries are continuing nonetheless. The Harvard Injury Control Research Center, with funding from private foundations, developed a National Violent Injury Statistics System in 1999, modeled after the NHTSA's reporting system for motor vehicle injuries. This program became a pilot for what is now the National Violent Death Reporting System (NVDRS), established in 2002 by the CDC with support from a new Congress. The NVDRS is a state-based system that collects detailed data on homicides and suicides in an effort to better inform policy on violence and suicide.[48,49] As of 2019, the program operated in all 50 states, the District of Columbia, and Puerto Rico.

The successful passage of the Brady Handgun Violence Prevention Act and the federal assault weapons ban in 1994 showed that political support could be corralled to limit access to firearms even in an antiregulatory climate. However, the assault weapons ban expired in 2004, and the fact that it has not been renewed by Congress shows that the NRA still has clout in Washington. Some states and communities have similar bans, as well as violence prevention and youth development programs, including educational initiatives to promote nonviolent resolution of arguments. The economic cost of gun violence in terms of medical care—calculated at about $2.3 billion per year—has helped persuade some states to pass stricter gun control regulations. About half the medical costs of firearms injuries are borne by taxpayers.[50]

Public health advocates note that guns need not be banned to make them safer. The third "E" of injury prevention—engineering—has not been widely applied in the prevention of firearms injuries. Safety catches can be used to make guns childproof, for example, and there are even ways to personalize guns so that they can be used only by the owner. Safety features are required by law for many consumer products that are much less dangerous than guns. When the political climate is ready to support major efforts to prevent firearms-related injuries, the public health approach has much to offer.[51,52]

Occupational Injuries

Workplace injuries have been a significant public health problem since the Industrial Revolution, if not before. In 1907, more than 15,000 American workers were reported to have died on the job. Many states implemented occupational safety laws in the late 19th and early 20th centuries. In 1970, the Congress passed a federal law creating the **Occupational Safety and Health Administration (OSHA)**, which was empowered to set standards, inspect workplaces, and impose penalties for workplace hazards. The law also created the **National Institute for Occupational Safety and Health (NIOSH)** to conduct research, recommend standards, and conduct hazard evaluations.[11]

Workplaces are certainly safer now, with just 5147 fatal injuries reported by the Bureau of Labor Statistics in 2017, despite a large increase in the number of workers.[53] In part, this improvement reflects mandated safety measures and educational programs—but it also reflects an economy less dependent on heavy industry. However, in addition to the workplace-related deaths, almost 1 million American workers suffer an on-the-job injury each year that leads to lost workdays.[54]

Motor vehicles are the leading occupational cause of death, with highway crashes accounting for 40% of all worker deaths.[53] The second leading cause of injury mortality in 2017 was falls, which accounted for approximately 17% of deaths. Close behind falls were "violence and other injuries by persons and animals" and "contact with object or equipment," which includes being struck by falling objects and being caught in running equipment or machinery, accounting for 16% and 14% of workplace deaths, respectively. Not surprisingly, workers in some types of jobs have higher risks of occupational fatality than others. Logging and fishing are the most dangerous occupations, with the highest rate of deaths. Aircraft pilots/flight engineers and roofers, respectively, had the third- and fourth-highest fatality rates in 2017.[53] Other relatively risky professions include garbage collectors, iron and steel workers, and agricultural workers, who are at risk for amputations by machinery, electrocutions, and pesticide poisoning. The safest occupations are those that involve computers, mathematics, business, and finance.[53]

Injury from Domestic Violence

All too often, family conflict leads to violence against children or spouses. In 2012, an estimated 1640 children younger than age 18 died from child maltreatment; 70% of the deaths occurred in children younger than age 3. U.S. child protective services agencies estimated that 686,000 children were victims of maltreatment in 2012. More than 3 million reports of child abuse and neglect are received by state and local agencies annually.[55] Most often, the perpetrator is a parent.

Intimate-partner violence, including rape, physical violence, or stalking, is another serious problem in the United States, affecting more than 12 million women and men each year. In 2007, intimate-partner violence resulted in more than 2300 deaths. A number of surveys provide data on the extent of domestic violence in the United States. For example, in 1996, the CDC collaborated with the National Institute of Justice to sponsor the Violence Against Women Survey. In 2010, the two agencies, together with the Department of Defense, began conducting an ongoing National Intimate Partner and Sexual Violence Survey. The CDC's Behavioral Risk Factor Surveillance System includes questions about intimate-partner violence, and the Pregnancy Risk Assessment Monitoring System collects data about physical abuse during and after pregnancy.[56]

The risk factors for domestic violence victimization and perpetration are often the same. For example, childhood physical or sexual victimization is a risk factor for future victimization and perpetration. Other risk factors include low self-esteem, low income, young age, and heavy alcohol and drug use. The CDC puts a high priority on preventing domestic violence, but little is known about how to accomplish this goal. The agency conducts and supports research on ways to reduce or eliminate risk factors and increase protective factors.

Nonfatal Traumatic Brain Injuries

In addition to the more than 56,800 deaths from traumatic brain injuries (TBIs) each year, an estimated 2.9 million Americans are treated in hospital emergency departments for nonfatal TBIs, and uncounted others sustain such an injury but are treated elsewhere or do not seek care.[7] These data come from CDC surveys of general hospitals and children's hospitals, but do not include data from people treated in military hospitals or Veterans Administration hospitals. As members of the military are at high risk of TBIs, the CDC's data represent a significant underestimate of the prevalence of this condition.[57]

TBIs may be mild, moderate, or severe. A mild TBI, called a concussion, may cause only a brief change in consciousness or mental state. More severe TBIs can lead to changes in thinking, sensation, or language, and may cause permanent disability. They may also increase the risk later in life for Alzheimer's disease and other dementias and for Parkinson's disease. A well-known example of the latter is the boxer Mohammed Ali, who was diagnosed with Parkinson's syndrome at the age of 43 after years of enduring blows to the head.[58]

The age group at highest risk for hospitalization and death from TBIs is individuals 75 years and older, while the greatest number of emergency department visits for such injuries are by children age 4 and younger.[7] The leading causes of these injuries are falls, followed by being hit by an object and motor vehicle crashes; the last group includes injuries to drivers, passengers, pedestrians, motorcyclists, and bicyclists.

The **Consumer Product Safety Commission (CPSC)** administers another surveillance system that collects data from a nationally representative sample of 66 hospital emergency rooms. This system focuses on injuries associated with consumer products and identifies TBIs linked to products such as bicycles, swing sets, or inline skating equipment. Accordingly, the injuries identified through this system have different causes and affect younger individuals than those included in the CDC system. The group found at highest risk by the CPSC are aged 10 through 14 years, and the leading causes of the injury involve bicycles, football, playground activities, basketball, and riding all-terrain vehicles. Like the CDC system, the CPSC system has found that boys are much more likely than girls to suffer a TBI.[59]

The CDC recommends both primary and secondary prevention to minimize risks of suffering a TBI. Primary prevention calls for participants in dangerous activities to wear protective equipment such as helmets. Secondary prevention provides that anyone suspected of having a TBI should be removed from play and allowed to return only after being evaluated by a healthcare provider experienced in diagnosing and managing TBI.[59]

In recent years, attention has been drawn to the TBI risks from playing football, both professionally and as students. In October 2008, a 16-year-old high school football player in New Jersey died after suffering a brain hemorrhage during a game, the fourth high school player to die of a head injury in the United States that year.[60] The New Jersey student had had a concussion during a practice three weeks earlier, but had been cleared by a doctor to return to play. Young brains are especially vulnerable to repeat mild TBIs within a short period of time, and the question of how long young athletes need to recover from such an injury is controversial. Sports physicians note that athletes of all ages, eager to return to the game, tend to deny symptoms, and it is difficult for doctors to determine when it is safe for them to return.[61]

Similar issues have troubled the National Football League (NFL) in trying to develop a policy on when players may return to the game after a head injury. Several observations have suggested that professional football players may suffer a high rate of brain damage due to repeated head trauma. A study of retired players found a statistical link between multiple concussions and later-life depression. After evidence accumulated that retired football players had a higher than average risk of dementia, an NFL program to assist these retirees was launched, and dozens more candidates signed up than were expected. Another red flag was that when autopsies were done on five retired NFL players who had died before age 51, degenerative brain damage was found similar to that observed in boxers with dementia.

At a 2007 meeting of NFL officials, Troy Vincent, a former player who is currently executive vice president of football operations for the NFL, was quoted as saying that most players do not worry about concussions. Vincent himself had had six documented concussions, he said, but possibly dozens more. "Outside of me being knocked out, asleep, I went back in the game on all the other occasions. And 50 or 60 times, I'm in the huddle, I don't know where I'm at, don't know the call, and I've got a player holding me up. I'm not sure if athletes really know what a concussion is—get some smelling salts and back in the game."[62]

The issue of TBI in athletes is now being taken very seriously. The Boston University School of Medicine's Center for the Study of Traumatic Encephalopathy in 2008 established a Brain Bank to study the brains of deceased individuals who had suffered repeated blows to the head. The majority of the donated brains have come from the families of retired athletes who were exhibiting symptoms. A study of 85 of these brains found that 68 of them showed evidence of chronic traumatic encephalopathy. Fifty of them were former football players, of whom 33 played with the NFL, 9 were college football players, and 6 played football in high school.[63] Notable among the four hockey players was Derek Boogaard, who was known as an "enforcer" for the Minnesota Wild and the New York Rangers. His record after playing 255 games was 3 goals, 13 assists, and 589 minutes in the penalty box. Boogaard died at age 28 from an accidental overdose of alcohol and painkillers.[64]

In 2011, more than 4500 former football players filed a lawsuit against the NFL, claiming that the league had fraudulently concealed the dangers of repeated head trauma. The first evidence of a link between football and brain disease had appeared in the late 1990s. As the evidence grew, the NFL denied any connection. However, the league has been settling this and other lawsuits, and its payouts as of 2019 approached $1 billion. Negotiations are still ongoing: The number of retired players suing the NFL has increased, the number of ailments attributed to repeated TBI has grown, and concern has intensified about the risks to children of playing tackle football.[65–67]

Tertiary Prevention

For any kind of serious injury, the promptness and quality of emergency medical aid play a significant role in whether a victim survives as well as in the extent of permanent disability. Lack of prompt emergency care accounts for the fact that death rates from motor vehicle crashes are higher in rural areas than in more populated ones. The establishment of special trauma centers and the use of helicopters to transport injured patients over long distances have improved the prospects for survival in some locations, but many parts of the country still lack integrated trauma-care programs. Well-trained emergency medical technicians and well-equipped ambulances can make the difference between life and death. There is still a need for research to better understand the biomedical aspects of injury and to devise better treatments.

Conclusion

Injuries are a major cause of death and disability in the United States. They are of particular concern to public health because they disproportionately affect young people, and many injuries are preventable. Fatal injuries are categorized as unintentional—commonly called "accidents"—and intentional, a category that includes homicide and suicide. Poisoning surpassed motor vehicle crashes as the leading cause of injury deaths in 2009, and the number of such deaths continued to increase through 2017. As of February 2019, the rate appeared to have stopped increasing, but it remains at a very high level. Injuries caused by firearms are the third leading cause of injury deaths. Alcohol is a significant factor in a very high percentage of injuries. The number of deaths caused by injuries is just the tip of the injury pyramid: For every death, there are many injuries resulting in hospitalizations, many more injuries requiring treatment in emergency rooms and physicians' offices, and even more injuries treated at home.

Analysis of injuries provides guidelines for prevention. Such analysis involves considerations of the host, agent, and environment and how they may be altered to prevent an injury from occurring (primary prevention), to minimize the damage (secondary prevention), or to prevent resulting disability by providing prompt treatment (tertiary prevention). This kind of analysis was pioneered in the analysis of motor vehicle injuries, which focused not only on the driver (host) but also on making the vehicle (agent) safer and on developing safer highways (environment). Tertiary prevention included the provision of ambulances and trauma centers.

Prevention of motor vehicle injuries also includes campaigns to change people's behavior by persuading them, or requiring them by law, to wear seat belts when riding in motor vehicles and to wear helmets when riding on motorcycles. Bicycle helmets, which remain underutilized, are also an important safety measure.

The number of poisoning fatalities has increased dramatically over the last decade. Much of the increase is due to misuse of prescription drugs, especially painkillers. Regulatory approaches to reducing poisoning risks must be balanced against evidence that patients suffering from chronic disease have sometimes been denied the relief offered by appropriate medications.

Due to its large number of firearms injuries, the United States has higher rates of homicides and childhood suicides than other industrialized nations. The easy availability of guns in the United States contributes to the high death rate from firearms injuries. Some studies have suggested that the presence of a gun in the home increases the risk that a resident will be a victim of homicide or suicide. However, the data cited to support such studies are unreliable because of opposition by the gun lobby to the collection of such data.

Public health has made progress in preventing childhood injuries from falls, drowning, poisoning, and fires and burns. Much of this progress comes from laws requiring safety features such as window guards in apartment buildings, fencing around swimming pools, childproof caps on medicine containers, and fireproofing of children's sleepwear.

Workplace injuries have decreased since the late 19th and early 20th centuries. In part, this trend is due to the creation of the OSHA, which sets standards, inspects workplaces, and imposes penalties for workplace hazards, and NIOSH, which conducts research on the subject.

Domestic violence, including child abuse and intimate-partner violence, is a significant problem in the United States. Surveys sponsored by the CDC and other organizations provide evidence on the prevalence of these problems. The CDC has placed a high priority on prevention and sponsors and conducts research on how to reduce risk factors and enhance protective factors.

Because TBI, in addition to causing deaths, can have serious consequences, including lifelong disability, the federal government has surveillance systems in place to identify such injuries and their risk factors. Young people are especially vulnerable to TBI because their brains are more easily damaged and take longer to heal compared to adult brains. Recently, football-related brain injuries have drawn public health attention. There is evidence that professional football players may suffer degenerative changes to the brain because of repeated blows to the head, putting them at risk of depression and dementia. High school football players are even more vulnerable to serious consequences if they return to the playing field too soon after suffering a concussion.

References

1. Centers for Disease Control and Prevention, "Deaths: Final Data for 2017," *National Vital Statistics Report* 68, no. 9 (June 24, 2019), https://www.cdc.gov/nchs/data/nvsr/nvsr68/nvsr68_09-508.pdf, accessed September 16, 2019.

2. S. P. Baker, B. O'Neill, and R. S. Karpf, *The Injury Fact Book* (New York, NY: Oxford University Press, 1992).

3. Centers for Disease Control and Prevention, "Deaths Resulting from Firearm- and Motor-Vehicle-Related Injuries—United States, 1968–1991," *Morbidity and Mortality Weekly Report* 43 (1994): 37–42.

4. Centers for Disease Control and Prevention, "QuickStats: Death Rates for the Leading Causes of Injury Death—United States, 1979–2007," *Morbidity and Mortality Weekly Report* 59 (2010): 957.

5. National Center on Health Statistics, "Number of National Drug Overdose Deaths Involving Select Prescription and Illicit Drugs," CDC Wonder, National Institute on Drug Abuse, https://wonder.cdc.gov/mcd.html, accessed September 16, 2019.

6. Centers for Disease Control and Prevention, "FastStats: All Injuries," www.cdc.gov/nchs/faststats/injury.htm, accessed September 28, 2019.

7. Centers for Disease Control and Prevention, "TBI: Get the Facts," March 11, 2019, https://www.cdc.gov/traumaticbraininjury/get_the_facts.html, accessed September 28, 2019.

8. National Highway Traffic Safety Administration, "Traffic Safety Facts 2017 Data—Alcohol-Impaired Driving," November 2018, https://crashstats.nhtsa .dot.gov/Api/Public/ViewPublication/812630, accessed September 28, 2019.

9. National Highway Traffic Safety Administration, "Traffic Safety Facts, 2017 Data—Pedestrians," March 2019, https://crashstats.nhtsa.dot.gov/Api/Public/ ViewPublication/812681, accessed September 28, 2019.

10. A. H. Mokdad, J. S. Mark, D. F. Stroup, and J. L. Gerberding, "Actual Causes of Death in the United States, 2000," *Journal of the American Medical Association* 291 (2004): 1238–1245.

11. National Committee for Injury Prevention and Control, "Injury Prevention: Meeting the Challenge," *American Journal of Preventive Medicine* 5 (1989 suppl 3): 1–303.

12. Centers for Disease Control and Prevention, "Vital Signs: Unintentional Injury Deaths Among People Aged 0–19 Years—United States, 2000–2009," *Morbidity and Mortality Weekly Report* 61 (2012): 270–276.

13. National Highway Traffic Safety Administration, "Timeline of Federal Motor Vehicle Safety Standards," August 30, 2012, https://www.nhtsa.gov/staticfiles/pdf /Lives-Saved-Tech-Timeline.pdf, accessed September 28, 2019.

14. National Highway Traffic Safety Administration, "5-Star Safety Ratings Frequently Asked Questions," https://www.safercar.gov/Vehicle-Shoppers/5–Star -FAQ, accessed September 28, 2019.

15. National Highway Traffic Safety Administration, "Traffic Safety Facts: 2017 Data—Young Drivers," May 2019, https://crashstats.nhtsa.dot.gov/Api/Public /ViewPublication/812753, accessed September 28, 2019.

16. National Highway Traffic Safety Administration, "Teen Driving," https://www.nhtsa.gov/road-safety /teen-driving, accessed September 28, 2019.

17. Insurance Institute for Highway Safety, "Graduated Licensing Laws by State," https://www.iihs.org/topics /teenagers/graduated-licensing-laws-table, accessed September 28, 2019.

18. Centers for Disease Control and Prevention, "Teen Drinking and Driving," October 2012, https://www .cdc.gov/vitalsigns/teendrinkinganddriving/index .html, accessed September 28, 2019.

19. Insurance Institute for Highway Safety, "State Laws: Speed," July 2015, https://www.iihs.org/topics/speed/ speed-limit-laws, accessed September 28, 2019.

20. Insurance Institute for Highway Safety, "Seat Belts," May 2019, https://www.iihs.org/topics/seat-belts, accessed September 28, 2019.

21. National Highway Traffic Safety Administration, "Distracted Driving," https://www.nhtsa.gov/risky-driving/distracted-driving, accessed September 28, 2019.

22. Insurance Institute for Highway Safety, "Distracted Driving," https://www.iihs.org/topics/distracted-driving, accessed September 28, 2019.

23. M. Richtel, "In Study, Texting Lifts Crash Risk by Large Margin," *The New York Times*, July 28, 2009.

24. Insurance Institute for Highway Safety, "Fatality Facts 2017," December 2018, https://www.iihs.org/ topics/fatality-statistics/detail/yearly-snapshot, accessed September 28, 2019.

25. National Highway Traffic Safety Administration, "Traffic Safety Facts: 2013 Data—Pedestrians," February 2015, https://crashstats.nhtsa.dot .gov/Api/Public/ViewPublication/812124, accessed September 28, 2019.

26. J. Angelos, "On a 12-Lane Road Riders with an Agenda," *The New York Times*, November 28, 2008.

27. Insurance Institute for Highway Safety, "Motorcycles," May 2019, https://www.iihs.org/topics/motorcycles, accessed September 28, 2019.

28. National Highway Traffic Safety Administration, "Traffic Safety Facts: 2013 Data—Bicyclists and Other Cyclists," May 2015, https://crashstats.nhtsa.dot .gov/Api/Public/ViewPublication/812151, accessed September 28, 2019.

29. Insurance Institute for Highway Safety, "Fatality Facts 2017: Bicyclists," December 2018, https://www.iihs .org/topics/fatality-statistics/detail/bicyclists, accessed September 28, 2019.

30. G. S. Watson, P. L. Zador, and A. Wilks, "Helmet Use, Helmet Use Laws, and Motorcyclist Fatalities," *American Journal of Public Health* 71 (1981): 297–300.

31. Insurance Institute for Highway Safety, "State Laws: Motorcycle Helmet Use," May 2019, https://www .iihs.org/topics/motorcycles#helmet-laws, accessed December 11, 2019.

32. Insurance Institute for Highway Safety, "Pedestrians and Bicyclists," May 2019, https://www.iihs.org/topics /pedestrians-and-bicyclists, accessed September 28, 2019.

33. Centers for Disease Control and Prevention, "CDC Wonder: About Underlying Cause of Death, 1999–2017," https://http://wonder.cdc.gov/ucd-icd10.html, accessed September 28, 2019.

34. Centers for Disease Control and Prevention, "Provisional Drug Overdose Death Counts," Vital Statistics Rapid Release, https://www.cdc.gov /nchs/nvss/vsrr/drug-overdose-data.htm, accessed September 16, 2019.

35. L. J. Paulozzi, D. Budnitz, and Y. Xi, "Increasing Deaths from Opioid Analgesics in the United States," *Pharmacoepidemiology and Drug Safety* 15 (2006): 618–627.

36. Centers for Disease Control and Prevention, "Vital Signs: Alcohol Poisoning Deaths," January 2015, www.cdc.gov/vitalsigns/alcohol-poisoning-deaths/index.html, accessed September 28, 2019.

37. Associated Press, "Death Rate Up for Car Crashes, But Down for Shootings in 95," *The New York Times*, July 27, 1997.

38. World Health Organization, "Homicide Estimates by Country," 2016, http://apps.who.int/gho/data/view.main.VIOLENCEHOMICIDEv, accessed September 28, 2019.

39. Pew Research Center, "7 Facts About Guns in the U.S.," December 27, 2018, https://www.pewresearch.org/fact-tank/2018/12/27/facts-about-guns-in-united-states/, accessed September 28, 2019.

40. D. J. Wiebe, "Firearms in US Homes as a Risk Factor for Unintentional Gunshot Fatality," *Accident Analysis and Prevention* 35 (2003): 711–716.

41. A. L. Kellermann, F. P. Rivara, N. B. Rushforth, J. G. Banton, D. T. Reay, J. T. Francisco, "Gun Ownership as a Risk Factor for Homicide in the Home," *New England Journal of Medicine* 329 (1993): 1084–1091.

42. A. L. Kellermann, F. P. Rivara, G. Somes, D. T. Reay, J. Francisco, J. G. Banton, "Suicide in the Home in Relation to Gun Ownership," *New England Journal of Medicine* 237 (1992): 467–472.

43. A. L. Kellermann and D. T. Reay, "Protection or Peril? An Analysis of Firearm-Related Deaths in the Home," *New England Journal of Medicine* 314 (1986): 1557–1560.

44. National Research Council, *Firearms and Violence: A Critical Review* (Washington, DC: National Academies Press, 2005).

45. Harvard Injury Control Research Center, "Firearms Research," 2015, https://www.hsph.harvard.edu/hicrc/firearms-research/, accessed September 28, 2019.

46. N. A. Lewis, "N.R.A. Takes Aim at Study of Guns as Public Health Risk," *The New York Times*, August 26, 1995.

47. J. Rovner, "U.S. House Refuses Point-Blank to Restore CDC Gun-Research Funds," *Lancet* 348 (1996): 190.

48. Harvard Injury Control Research Center, "Death by Violent Means: Who's at Risk?" *Harvard Public Health Review*, Spring 2006.

49. Centers for Disease Control and Prevention, "National Violent Death Reporting System," January 22, 2019, https://www.cdc.gov/violenceprevention/datasources/nvdrs/index.html, accessed September 28, 2019.

50. P. J. Cook, B. A. Lawrence, J. Ludwig, and T. R. Miller, "Medical Costs of Gunshot Injuries in the United States," *Journal of the American Medical Association* 281 (1999): 447–454.

51. S. B. Sorenson, "Regulating Firearms as a Consumer Product," *Science* 286 (1999): 1481–1482.

52. N. Kristof, "Smart Guns Save Lives. So Where Are They?" *The New York Times*, January 18, 2015.

53. U.S. Bureau of Labor Statistics, "National Census of Fatal Occupational Injuries in 2017," December 18, 2018, https://www.bls.gov/news.release/pdf/cfoi.pdf, accessed September 28, 2019.

54. U.S. Bureau of Labor Statistics, "Employer-Reported Workplace Injury and Illnesses, 2017," November 8, 2018, https://www.bls.gov/news.release/osh.nr0.htm, accessed September 28, 2019.

55. Centers for Disease Control and Prevention, "Facts at a Glance: Child Maltreatment," 2014, https://www.cdc.gov/violenceprevention/pdf/childmaltreatment-facts-at-a-glance.pdf, accessed September 28, 2019.

56. Centers for Disease Control and Prevention, "Intimate Partner Violence Resources," October 23, 2018, https://www.cdc.gov/violenceprevention/intimatepartnerviolence/resources.html, accessed September 28, 2019.

57. Centers for Disease Control and Prevention, "Traumatic Brain Injury in the United States: Emergency Department Visits, Hospitalizations and Deaths, 2002–2006," March 2010, https://www.cdc.gov/traumaticbraininjury/pdf/blue_book.pdf, accessed September 28, 2019.

58. R. M. Thomas Jr., "Change in Drugs Help Ali Improve," *The New York Times*, September 9, 2004.

59. Centers for Disease Control and Prevention, "Nonfatal Traumatic Brain Injuries from Sports and Recreation Activities," *Morbidity and Mortality Weekly Report* 56 (2007): 733–737.

60. M. S. Schmidt and D. Caldwell, "High School Football Player Dies," *The New York Times*, October 16, 2008.

61. A. Schwarz, "New Guidelines on Young Athletes' Concussions Stir Controversy," *The New York Times*, June 7, 2009.

62. A. Schwarz, "Player Silence on Concussions May Block NFL Guidelines," *The New York Times*, June 20, 2007.

63. K. Nelson, "Study Bolsters Link Between Routine Hits and Brain Disease," *The New York Times*, December 3, 2012.

64. A. McLean, A. Tse, and J. Pennington, "Images of Brain Injuries in Athletes," *The New York Times*, December 3, 2012, https://www.nytimes.com/interactive/2012/12/03/sports/images-of-brain-injuries-in-athletes.html, accessed September 28, 2019.

65. Public Broadcasting System, "Frontline: League of Denial: The NFL's Concussion Crisis," October 8, 2013, https://www.pbs.org/wgbh/pages/frontline/sports/league-of-denial/timeline-the-nfls-concussion-crisis, accessed September 28, 2019.

66. B. Strauss, "Concussion Lawsuits Rankle School Groups," *The New York Times*, May 21, 2015.

67. K. Belson, "N.F.L. Says Fraud Plagues the Concussion Settlement," *The New York Times*, April 13, 2018.

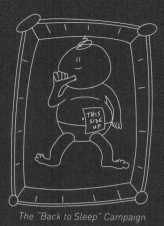

CHAPTER 18

The "Back to Sleep" Campaign

Maternal and Child Health as a Social Problem

KEY TERMS

Congenital anomalies
Contraception
Developmental disabilities
Family planning
Immunization
Infant mortality rate (IMR)
Maternal mortality rates

Prematurity
Prenatal care
Preterm birth
Special Supplemental Nutrition
Program for Women, Infants,
and Children (WIC)

Sudden infant death syndrome
(SIDS)
Supplemental Nutrition
Assistance Program (SNAP)
Teratogen

The health of pregnant women and children is traditionally one of the highest priorities of public health. In a society concerned with the welfare of its population, everyone should be guaranteed adequate conditions for the best possible start in life. The fetal and infant stages of development provide the foundations of good health throughout life. A growing body of evidence indicates that conditions in utero and during early life play a powerful role in increasing individuals' susceptibility to the chronic diseases that plague American adults, including high blood pressure, obesity, cardiovascular disease, and diabetes.[1] Moreover, because children are the most vulnerable segment of the population, like canaries in the coal mine, they are the first to suffer from any adverse conditions that affect human health in general.

Children's health first became a public concern in the United States at the end of the 19th century, prompted by alarm at the high infant and child death rates in the summer from diarrheal diseases.[2] Heat, poor sanitation, and lack of refrigeration contributed to heavy microbial contamination of milk, which was sickening poor children. In 1893, New York City established milk stations that provided safe milk; similar programs soon followed in other cities. The success of the milk programs in improving children's health inspired the formation of voluntary infant welfare societies with the mission of teaching poor and immigrant mothers about nutrition and hygiene. The federal government got involved in 1912 with the establishment of the Children's Bureau, which was mandated to "investigate and report on all matters affecting children and child life."[2(p.8)] In 1921, Congress first provided grants to states to develop health services for mothers and children. During the same period, advocates for child health and welfare were fighting to protect children from oppressive and exploitive labor, which was not regulated by the federal government until the 1930s.

Child health programs have, since the beginning, been plagued by a basic philosophical and political conflict: Society's responsibility for the well-being of infants and children was sometimes in conflict with the presumed right of parents to provide for, or neglect, their own children.[3] Until the 20th century, children were regarded as the property of their parents. Passage of the 1912 legislation establishing the Children's Bureau reflected a new view—that children were a national resource and that their health and vigor were important for the progress of society. In recent decades, children have increasingly been viewed as having rights on their own, independent of their parents or their prospective role in society. Current controversies concerning the role of government in the protection of children—issues that range from the removal of children from abusive parents to medical treatment for the children of Christian Scientists—are a continuation of a century-long tradition of conflict.

Table 18-1 Infant Deaths (per 1000 Live Births) in Organization for Economic Cooperation and Development (OECD) Countries, 2018

Japan	1.9	Hungary	3.5
Finland	2.0	Switzerland	3.5
Norway	2.3	Belgium	3.6
Sweden	2.3	Netherlands	3.6
Czech Republic	2.7	Denmark	3.8
Ireland	2.7	France	3.8
Italy	2.7	United Kingdom	3.9
Portugal	2.7	Poland	4.0
Spain	2.7	New Zealand	4.3
South Korea	2.8	Canada	4.5
Austria	2.9	Slovak Republic	4.5
Israel	3.1	United States	5.8
Australia	3.3	Chile	7.0
Germany	3.3	Turkey	9.2
Greece	3.5	Mexico	12.1

Data from Organisation for Economic Co-operation and Development (OECD), "Infant Mortality Rates," https://data.oecd.org/healthstat/infant-mortality-rates.htm, accessed September 29, 2019.

Maternal and Infant Mortality

The **infant mortality rate (IMR)** is a gauge of a society's attention to its children's health and is, in fact, an indicator of the health status of a population as a whole. This rate is a particular concern for American public health professionals because the IMR in this country is very high compared with that of other industrialized countries. As shown in (**Table 18-1**), the United States ranks 27th in terms of IMR, after many industrialized Asian and European countries. The infant mortality rate in the United States is two and half times higher than

the rates in most Scandinavian countries and three times higher than the rate in Japan.

The IMR, defined as the number of infant deaths within the first year of life for every 1000 live births, has been declining in the United States over the course of the last century (**Figure 18-1**)—from 100 in 1915 to 5.8 in 2018.[4] Reasons for this decline include improved socioeconomic status (SES), housing, and nutrition; immunization; clean water and pasteurized milk; antibiotics; and better prenatal care and delivery. The availability of **family planning** services and legalized abortion in the United States contributed to the lowering of IMR during the 1970s because wanted babies

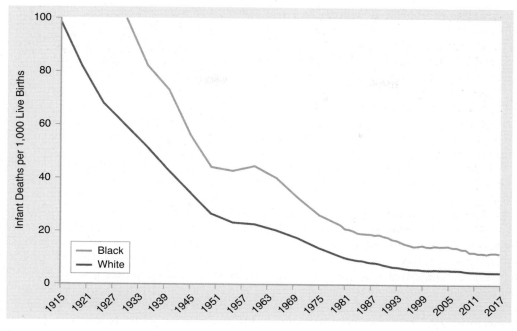

Figure 18-1 U.S. Infant Mortality Rates, 1915–2017
Note that data for black infants are available starting in 1930.

Data from B. Guyer et al., "Annual Summary of Vital Statistics: Trends in the Health of Americans During the 20th Century," *Pediatrics* 106 (2000): 1307–1317; Centers for Disease Control and Prevention, "Deaths: Final Data for 1998," *National Vital Statistics Report* 48 no. 11 (2000); "Deaths: Final Data for 2017, "*National Vital Statistics Report* 68 no. 9 (2019).

are more likely to thrive than are unwanted ones.[5] Progress in recent years is largely credited to technological advances in caring for premature infants and infants with low birth weight.

A very disturbing feature of the trends in infant mortality in the United States is the disparity according to race. The IMR for black Americans is more than double that for white Americans. While the high infant mortality among blacks accounts in part for this country's dismal showing on an international scale, the IMR for white Americans is worse than that of 25 other countries, as seen in Table 18-1. The IMR for Hispanics is nearly the same as that for whites.[4]

Maternal mortality rates also declined dramatically in the United States during the 20th century, so that today the death of a woman in childbirth is a very rare event. In 2015, 17.2 women died each year from causes related to childbirth for every 100,000 live births, as compared with 850 such deaths per 100,000 live births in 1900. Like IMRs, maternal mortality rates are significantly higher for black women than for white women—three to four times higher—although the mortality rates are nearly 15% lower for Hispanic women than for white women.[6,7]

Infant Mortality: Health Problem or Social Problem?

In the words of a former director-general of the World Health Association, "Infant mortality is not a health problem; it is a social problem with health consequences."[8(p.473)] In seeking reasons to explain the high IMR in the United States, epidemiologists find that the number one risk factor for infant mortality is poverty. The generally lower SES of African Americans in the United States accounts in large part (but not entirely) for their higher IMR. Poverty leads to high infant mortality for a variety of reasons—environmental, nutritional, behavioral, medical, and social. These same factors that raise the risk of infant death also have a more general harmful impact on the health of the children who survive, leading to increased rates of chronic illness and disability, both physical and mental.

An extreme example of an environmental cause of infant mortality is the epidemic of birth defects in Minamata, Japan, caused by mercury contamination of the bay from an industrial source. Poor families are more likely to live in such industrial areas, exposing pregnant women and their fetuses to the harmful effects of polluted air and water. Lead, which is highly toxic to the developing nervous system, is a common contaminant in the American inner city, both from deteriorating paint and from old plumbing. Other environmental chemicals known to harm the developing fetus include pesticides and organic solvents. More generally, to the extent that air or water pollution or substandard housing harm a mother's health, they harm her ability to give birth to a healthy infant. Subsequently, they may cause further harm to a sickly infant who is brought home to the unhealthy environment.

Poverty may interfere with a prospective mother's ability to consume an adequate diet for nourishing her fetus. Poor women may lack the knowledge, time, or energy to prepare nutritious meals for themselves and their children. They may live in rural or inner-city areas where fresh fruits and vegetables are not readily available or are too expensive. Ignorance or lack of financial resources may carry over to how a baby is fed. Breastfeeding, which provides the best nutrition for an infant, is less commonly practiced among poorly educated women than it is among those of higher SES.

Maternal behaviors that can harm the health of an infant include smoking, drinking alcohol, and the use of legal and illegal drugs. Women who smoke during pregnancy substantially increase their risk of giving birth to an infant of low birth weight. Moreover, infants are more likely to develop respiratory infections or die of sudden infant death syndrome when family members smoke in the home. Alcohol is a **teratogen**, an agent that can cause birth defects, and fetal alcohol syndrome is a risk for children of mothers who are problem drinkers. The use of illegal drugs by inner-city pregnant women, especially crack cocaine, became a major concern in the late 1980s and early 1990s. So-called "crack babies" were born addicted to the drug and suffered withdrawal symptoms after birth; some sustained permanent neurologic impairment. Unhealthy behaviors are not limited to poor women, of course; affluent women may smoke, drink alcohol, use drugs, and eat unhealthy diets while pregnant. However, these behaviors are more common among poor women.

Social factors that contribute to high-risk pregnancies include those common in poor neighborhoods: young maternal age and low maternal education, out-of-wedlock birth, and violence. Teenage mothers are more likely to deliver premature infants than older women of the same SES, apparently for biological reasons.[9] Poor women are more likely to be single mothers, who often lack social support. Infants and children of poor families are at greater risk from violence, both the impersonal violence of the neighborhood and child abuse by family members. Poor children are also more likely to die from unintentional injuries, including fires and falls.

Lack of prenatal care has been linked with a high risk of infant mortality. Poor women, who are more likely to lack access to medical care for financial and other reasons, are less likely to get prenatal care. However, it is not clear to what extent the lack of medical attention in itself contributes to the increased risk for poor women, as women who do not receive adequate prenatal care are likely to have other risk factors for infant mortality.[10]

Underlying and bound up with these factors that link poverty to infant mortality is the fact that poor women suffer higher levels of stress and have lower levels of social support than most women of higher SES. According to one definition, stress is "a state that occurs when persons perceive that demands exceed their ability to cope."[11(p.19)] Poor women may find that even such modest demands as paying the rent and the food bill, getting to work, or finding daycare services overwhelm them. Poor housing increases stress when residents must deal with leaky plumbing, malfunctioning appliances, and infestations of vermin. A mother's ability to cope with the needs of a sick child is limited when she has no health insurance, no transportation to a doctor's office, and no one to help her care for other children in the family. A poor, young, single mother may not have the coping skills that might come from experience, education, and the support of the child's father. To make matters worse, such a mother is more likely to seek stress relief through maladaptive behavior such as smoking, drug use, or entering into abusive relationships.

Preventing Infant Mortality

The United States has been successful in substantially reducing IMRs over the past several decades, as seen in Figure 18-1. However, much of this success is due to improved medical treatments for highly vulnerable infants after they are born.[12] The disadvantages of the technological approach are obvious: It disrupts normal bonding between parents and infants; it leaves a significant number of the survivors with long-term **developmental disabilities**, even severe handicaps; and it is very expensive. The countries that have better IMRs than the United States are generally much less dependent on neonatal intensive care for achieving their successes.

The public health approach to the prevention of infant mortality focuses on two groups: pregnant women in general, most of whom are highly motivated to bear a healthy child and are receptive to information on how to avoid risks; and high-risk women, including the poor, young, minority, unmarried women whose infants are most likely to suffer from their socioeconomic disadvantages. **Prenatal care** provides women with information on how to have a healthy pregnancy and bear a healthy child. Thus, prenatal care is the most public health–oriented kind of care that the medical profession provides. Prenatal visits also offer an opportunity for healthcare providers to diagnose problems that need medical intervention. For example, bacterial infections of the genital tract increase a mother's risk of giving birth prematurely, and treatment with antibiotics can reduce that risk. The Centers for Disease Control and Prevention (CDC) recommends that all pregnant women should be screened for common infections and treated if infected.[13] Beginning prenatal care as early as possible—preferably even before a woman conceives—greatly enhances a woman's prospects of bearing a healthy infant.

Prenatal care is especially important for the women with the lowest SES. Visits to a healthcare provider may be their only source of the education, services, and social support these women need. Most states recognize the importance of prenatal care and have tried to remove financial barriers by providing insurance or other sources of payment and by establishing prenatal clinics at health departments, hospital outpatient departments, and community health centers. In 2016, 77% of pregnant women in the United States received prenatal care in the first trimester of pregnancy.[14]

A number of barriers remain that discourage the women at highest risk from seeking prenatal care, including lack of information about available services, inconvenient hours of service, rudeness and long waits at the clinics, inadequate transportation, and lack of child care for older children. The percentage of black and Hispanic women who receive prenatal care in the first trimester is significantly lower than that for white women (67% for blacks and 72% for Hispanics in 2016, compared with 82% for whites). The percentage of women with less than a high school degree who receive such care is also significantly lower than that for women with at least a college degree (63% compared to 88%).[14] Reaching women who do not seek early prenatal care requires establishing active outreach programs including hotlines, community canvassing, and the provision of incentives to the expectant mother.[12] A new barrier arose with the wave of anti-immigrant sentiment and policies included in the 1996 federal welfare reform bill, which resulted in denial of prenatal care for immigrants in some states. From a public health perspective, this is a foolish and expensive policy, because the infants—U.S. citizens—born to these women will be more likely to be premature, unhealthy, and in need of neonatal intensive care. As of 2019, 16 states had passed legislation that provides prenatal care to undocumented immigrants using federal or state funds.[15]

To effectively reduce infant mortality, prenatal care for high-risk women should include a broad array of medical, educational, social, and nutritional services. Unfortunately, political realities too often mean that, although major efforts are made to increase the number of women who receive prenatal care, the clinics that provide it are understaffed, rushed, and not financed adequately to provide the services that could really make a difference in the health of the mother and infant.

Congenital Malformations

In the United States, the leading specific causes of infant mortality, according to the listings on death certificates, are the following: **congenital anomalies**, disorders related to preterm birth and low birth weight, maternal complications, sudden infant death

syndrome, and injuries such as suffocation. The birth of infants with congenital anomalies, which account for more than 20% of infant deaths, can be prevented in many cases.[16,17] Some disorders, such as Tay-Sachs disease, hemophilia, and Down syndrome, have a well-known genetic basis and can be identified through genetic screening and/or prenatal diagnosis. Newborn screening programs are designed to identify infants born with defects in body chemistry such as phenylketonuria and hypothyroidism that can be remedied by early diagnosis and treatment. Other congenital anomalies may be caused by known environmental exposures, such as tobacco smoke, viruses, heavy metals, or the use of legal or illegal drugs. Public health interventions include the Food and Drug Administration's (FDA) regulation of teratogenic drugs such as thalidomide and warnings to pregnant women such as those required on alcoholic beverage containers and on the packaging of legal teratogenic drugs such as the acne drug Accutane and the epilepsy drug Dilantin. Infection with the rubella virus (German measles), once a common cause of deafness and mental disability, can be prevented by immunization.

Despite these measures, the causes of more than 70% of birth defects remain unknown. It is believed that many defects are caused by a combination of genetic and environmental factors.

In an attempt to identify causes, the CDC is coordinating the National Birth Defects Prevention Study, a case-control study of babies born between 1997 and 2011.[18,19] Mothers of more than 30,000 infants with birth defects were interviewed about their own health, pregnancy history, diet, medication and substance use, work history, drinking water sources, and other questions thought to be relevant. They were also asked to provide DNA samples, which can help identify the role of genetics in their children's birth defects. The control group of 10,000 infants were chosen at random from birth certificates of live-born infants with no major birth defects, and their mothers were similarly interviewed and asked for DNA samples. Among the study's findings to date are that women who are obese are at much higher risk for bearing a child with a broad range of birth defects. Smoking during pregnancy increases the risk of premature birth and certain birth defects such as cleft lip and cleft palate. Drinking alcohol during pregnancy may cause fetal alcohol syndrome. Prescription pain medications increase the risk of congenital heart defects and neural tube defects, whereas most common antibiotics do not appear to increase risks of birth defects.

Nutritional factors are known to contribute to the risk of some defects. Two of the most severe are neural tube defects—anencephaly (a lethal condition in which all or most of an infant's brain is missing) and spina bifida (protrusion of the spinal cord from the spinal column accompanied by paralysis of the lower body)—which may be caused in part by a deficiency in folic acid, a B vitamin present in green leafy vegetables, dried beans, liver, orange juice, and grapefruit juice. The damage occurs early in the pregnancy, when the fetus's spinal column is being formed. Dietary supplementation with folic acid has been shown to reduce the incidence of these neural tube defects by 50% or more, but the supplementation must happen during the first month of pregnancy—even before the woman may recognize she is pregnant.[20] Public health campaigns to encourage all women of childbearing age to take folic acid supplements have had only modest success, and poor, high-risk women are probably the least likely to comply with the recommendation. To remedy the problem, the FDA decided to require that foods such as flour, cornmeal, pasta, and rice be fortified with folic acid, effective January 1, 1998. As a result of the fortification, the number of affected pregnancies in the United States declined by approximately 20% by 2000, though it has stabilized since then.[20]

The amount of folic acid used for fortification is not sufficient to provide a maximum protective effect, however, so young women are still advised to take supplements.

Preterm Birth

An analysis by CDC scientists, published in 2006, proposed that preterm birth is responsible for many more infant deaths than are indicated on the death certificates. The scientists noted that 6 of the 11 leading causes listed on the death certificates, including three separate diagnoses involving respiratory distress, are entirely attributable to **preterm birth**. When this information is taken into account, **prematurity**—disorders of short gestation and low birth weight—becomes the leading cause of infant death, causing more than one-third of these deaths. Thus reducing infant mortality rates in the United States will require "a comprehensive agenda to identify, to test, and to implement effective strategies for the prevention of premature births."[21(p.1573)]

The percentage of infants born prematurely amounted to 9.9% of all births in 2017—a rate essentially unchanged since 2010. Black infants are almost twice as likely to be born too small as are white and Hispanic infants. One factor contributing to the higher rate of small black infants is that the rate of births to black teenage girls is more than twice the rate in white teenagers. However, Hispanic teenage girls have babies at an even higher rate than blacks, and the rate of preterm births is much lower for this group than that for blacks.[22]

While the causes of premature labor and delivery are not well understood, many of the environmental, behavioral, nutritional, and social factors previously discussed can contribute to this phenomenon. In trying to understand how to reduce the mortality and disability caused by preterm births, scientists classify preventive measures as primary, secondary, or tertiary.[23] In the United States, most of the efforts have been focused on tertiary prevention, aimed at improving the outcomes for infants born prematurely, and requiring expensive use of neonatal intensive care. Secondary prevention seeks to identify women at risk of giving birth too early and reduce their risk. For example, maternal smoking causes a 25% increased risk of preterm birth; the CDC monitors the prevalence of smoking among pregnant women, which has declined significantly since 1990 but was still 7% in 2017.[22] In fact, a state-by-state survey found that 25% of pregnant women in West Virginia smoked in 2016.[24] Other risk factors include previous preterm births, carrying more than one fetus, obesity, diabetes, and bacterial infections of the genital tract. Recent evidence suggests that gum disease is associated with preterm births, such that periodontal treatment may reduce the risk.[25] Some of these factors can be helped by timely prenatal care. However, as many as half of preterm infants in the United States are born to women considered to be low risk.

Primary prevention of preterm birth is, from a public health perspective, the most desirable strategy. Many European countries accomplish this goal by providing social and financial support for low-risk pregnant women, but this approach might be politically difficult to implement in the United States.[23] Preterm birth, of the various causes of infant mortality, is clearly a social problem rather than a health problem, as discussed earlier in this chapter. The reason the United States has such a poor record in preventing infant mortality is that we have tried to approach it as a medical problem.

Sudden Infant Death Syndrome

Sudden infant death syndrome (SIDS) accounted for 1400 infant deaths in the United States in 2017, and is also not well understood.[17] Almost always, the death is unexpected; usually the infant appeared to be healthy before he or she died, and an autopsy fails to establish the cause of death. While SIDS is more common in infants of low birth weight and in infants of smokers or drug users, it is not limited to infants with these risk factors.[26] Until recently, because of the lack of understanding about the causes of SIDS, parents could do little to reduce the risk. Then, in the early 1990s, studies done in New Zealand, Australia, and the United Kingdom reported that SIDS occurred more frequently in infants who were sleeping on their stomachs. The American Academy of Pediatrics and the National Institute of Child Health and Human Development began a "Back to Sleep" campaign, now called the "Safe to Sleep" campaign, to educate maternity wards, doctors and nurses, and parents that infants should be put to sleep on their backs. Since the campaign was launched, the number of deaths from SIDS has declined dramatically: In 1990, 130 infants per 100,000 died from SIDs, but by 2017, this rate had fallen to 35. The SIDS death rate in 2017 for black infants was 74 per 100,000, while for white infants it was 39, and for Hispanic infants it was 21.[27]

There is still room for improvement: Surveys of infant sleeping positions have found that use of the back sleeping position varies widely and is least common among young women, black women, and women with less education and lower incomes.[28] The SIDS death rates for black and American Indian infants are about double the rate for white infants. Public health agencies and medical care providers are working with minority communities to educate them about the importance of putting infants to sleep on their backs. Other factors that increase the risk of SIDS include soft bedding, being overheated, and bed sharing.

SIDS is a diagnosis of exclusion, meaning that any unexplained death is thoroughly investigated and SIDS is listed as the cause of death only if no other explanation is found. Law enforcement officials participate in the investigation, which includes an autopsy as well as interviews with family members and other caregivers. The CDC publishes guidelines recommending how these investigations should be done, with the aim of better understanding causes and risk factors for SIDS.

Family Planning and Prevention of Adolescent Pregnancy

Because pregnancy is not good for the health of either a teenager or her infant, preventing adolescent pregnancy is a high public health priority. In addition to the health risks, pregnancy during the teen years has many harmful consequences, including interference with the young mother's education and career prospects, economic hardship, and interference with the formation of a strong family unit. Thus adolescent pregnancy, and all the accompanying socioeconomic consequences, increases the health risks to the child for all the reasons previously described as causes of infant mortality. Teenage mothers are less likely to seek prenatal care than are older women, and are more likely to have no care at all. They are also more likely to smoke and less likely to gain adequate weight during pregnancy. Infants of teenage mothers are at greatly increased risk of low birth weight, serious and long-term disability, and dying during the first year of life. These children are more likely to have lower school achievement, drop out of high school, be incarcerated, themselves become parents as teens, and face unemployment as young adults.[29]

Rates of adolescent pregnancy in the United States have declined since the 1950s, but in those days, social pressure forced marriage on many girls who became pregnant, producing a more stable economic and family environment for the young child. Today, most teenage mothers are unmarried, and a large increase in the number of adolescent births in the late 1980s alarmed public health advocates and policy makers.[30] However, after peaking in 1991, these rates declined steadily through 2017.[29] Birth rates have consistently been higher among black and Hispanic teenagers than among white teenagers, and rates have been lowest among Asian American and Pacific Islander teenagers. U.S. adolescent pregnancy rates are the highest in the industrialized world.

Unintended pregnancy in older women is also a matter of concern to public health because it is more likely to lead to poorer health outcomes for both mother and child. Some unintended pregnancies are merely mistimed, but many are unwanted, leading to some of the same risks as occur in teenage pregnancies. Surveys have shown that only half of all pregnancies among American women are planned. A frequent consequence of unintended pregnancy is induced abortion. In the United States in 2015, there was slightly less than one abortion for every five live births.[31] This represents a decrease from the ratio of more than one abortion for every three live births in the 1980s. From a public health perspective, every pregnancy should be an intended pregnancy.

Adequate access to **contraception** could go a long way toward reducing rates of unintended pregnancy and abortion. Americans' ambivalent feelings about sex probably contribute to the fact that many women lack access to comprehensive family planning services. Even private health insurance plans often do not provide coverage for contraception. Unmarried women, poor women, adolescents, and black women are especially likely to encounter difficulty in obtaining and paying for contraceptive services. President Barack Obama's Patient Protection and Affordable Care Act required all new health insurance plans to cover birth control without a deductible or copayment, a measure that would help prevent many unintended and unwanted pregnancies. Older plans are exempt from the requirement, however, as are plans offered by religious organizations. As of 2019, 29 states required insurance policies that cover prescription drugs to provide coverage for the full range of FDA-approved contraceptive drugs and devices.[32] In 2017, the Donald Trump administration issued new rules allowing insurers and employers to opt out of the contraception coverage mandate for religious or moral reasons; in 2019, this rollback of the mandate was blocked by a federal judge. The fate of the mandate remains to be seen.[33]

Female sterilization and vasectomy for men are the most effective methods of contraception and are commonly used in the United States, but they are permanent and therefore inappropriate for young people. Other highly effective methods—for women—include intrauterine devices (IUDs) and some hormonal implants and patches. These methods have a failure rate of less than 1 pregnancy per 100 women per year. Equally effective when used correctly are combination oral contraceptives—"the Pill"—and other hormonal contraceptives, such as Depo-Provera shots and the hormone-laden vaginal ring. Pills must be taken every day, however, and the other hormonal methods must be renewed at regular intervals. The effectiveness of hormonal methods may be reduced in women who are taking certain medications and supplements.[34]

All of these methods have drawbacks, although the general public tends to overestimate their health risks. Barrier methods, including the male and female condoms and the female diaphragm, can be fairly effective if used correctly (failure rates of 2 to 6 pregnancies per 100 women per year), and condoms have the added advantage of reducing the risk of sexually transmitted diseases. However, barrier methods are often used inconsistently and incorrectly. Spermicides used alone (foams, creams, and jellies) have failure rates of 15 pregnancies per 100 women per year for perfect use and much worse failure rates for typical use. The cervical cap has a failure rate of 14 pregnancies per 100 women who have

never been pregnant, but is much less effective in women who have given birth.[34]

The "morning-after pill," a form of emergency contraception, can be taken as long as five days after unprotected intercourse to prevent pregnancy. It works by preventing the release of a woman's egg for longer than usual and is at least 85% effective. Considerable controversy arose in the 2000s regarding whether these medications should be available without a prescription, especially to teenage girls, but now most brands are available over the counter.[34–36] In 2017, some universities began offering the morning-after pill in vending machines after students raised concerns about difficulty or confusion in obtaining the medication. Stanford University, the University of California, Davis, and the University of California, Santa Barbara, are among the schools that installed the option.[37] The availability of emergency contraception presumably has contributed to the reduction in the number of abortions in recent years. Insertion of an IUD within five days of unprotected intercourse is 99.9% effective as an emergency contraceptive. This device is relatively expensive and needs to be inserted by a healthcare provider, but it can be left in place for years to serve as ongoing birth control.

Public health programs specifically aimed at preventing teenage pregnancy include comprehensive sex education in the schools, which has been found to be effective in delaying young people's initiation of intercourse and increasing their use of contraception when they do have sex.[37] The exact message that should be conveyed in pregnancy prevention programs remains a topic of debate, however. The federal welfare reform bill implemented in 1998 included funding for programs that teach sexual abstinence only. Many states were reluctant to apply for this money because they believe such programs are much less effective than those that include education on contraception as well. A 2004 congressional review found that commonly used abstinence-only curricula contained "multiple scientific and medical inaccuracies."[37(p.2014)] For example, they teach that condoms are ineffective. Some of these programs encourage teenagers to sign virginity pledges; studies have shown that those who do sign may delay sex, but when they do initiate intercourse, they are less likely to use protection.[38]

Abstinence-only advocates took credit for the significant decline in adolescent pregnancy rates since 1991 described previously. However, despite hundreds of millions of dollars of federal funds spent on abstinence-only programs each year, studies have found no measurable impact on teen sexual behavior. An analysis of data from national surveys of young women ages 15 to 19 found that only 14% of the decline in pregnancy could be attributed to delayed initiation of sexual activity, while 86% of the decline was due to increased use of contraceptives.[38] The authors concluded that "abstinence promotion is a worthwhile goal, particularly among younger teenagers."[39(p.155)]—but it is insufficient to help adolescents prevent unintended pregnancies and sexually transmitted diseases. "Public policies and programs . . . should vigorously promote provision of accurate information on contraception and on sexual behavior and relationships, support increased availability and accessibility of contraceptive services and supplies for adolescents, and promote the value of responsible and protective behaviors, including condom and contraceptive use and pregnancy planning."[39(p.155)]

Nutrition of Women and Children

Since the establishment of milk stations in the 1890s, nutrition has been an important component of maternal and child health programs. At first, the emphasis was on breastfeeding and the safety of milk and baby foods. Public health is still concerned with promoting breastfeeding, which offers most

infants the healthiest start in life, reducing risks of infectious diseases, ear infections, respiratory infections, obesity, and chronic diseases such as asthma and allergies. Medical and public health organizations recommend that infants be exclusively breastfed for the first 6 months of their lives, and that breastfeeding should continue at least until their first birthday as new foods are introduced. The CDC tracks rates of breastfeeding at discharge from the hospital and at follow-up times through telephone surveys. The percentage of infants who were ever breastfed increased from 54% in 1986–1988 to 84% in 2016; in addition, in 2016, 57% of infants were still breastfed at 6 months and 36% were still breastfed at 12 months. However, these rates vary depending on the age and education of the mothers, from a rate of only 72% among women with a high school diploma or less, to a rate of 88% among women with at least a bachelor's degree. Approximately 69% of women younger than age 20 initiate breastfeeding. The rate of breastfeeding in 2016 for white mothers was 78%, compared to 60% for black mothers and 85% for Hispanic mothers.[40,41]

During the Great Depression of the 1930s, the federal government established several food assistance programs to ensure adequate nutrition for poor families. They formed the basis of current federal programs, run by the U.S. Department of Agriculture (USDA), which originated in the 1960s.[42] The **Special Supplemental Nutrition Program for Women, Infants, and Children (WIC)** provides vouchers for milk, fruit juice, eggs, cereals, and other nutritious foods for pregnant women, lactating mothers, infants, and children up to five years old. Nutrition education is also provided, and WIC centers often become a source of many support services for poor, young families. The USDA has evaluated the WIC program and found it to be effective in saving medical costs for the women and infants who participated.

The nutritional needs of older children are addressed through the School Meals Program. School lunches, which are provided at most schools, must meet certain nutritional standards, including offering a meat or meat alternative, fruit and/or vegetables, bread, and milk. Children from households with incomes at or below 185% of the poverty level receive the lunches for free or at reduced prices; children from families with higher incomes pay more. A more limited number of children receive free or reduced-price school breakfasts, and some schools offer after-school snacks. In addition, the Summer Food Service Program provides meals during school vacation periods.

A third federal program designed to help low-income families afford adequate food is the **Supplemental Nutrition Assistance Program (SNAP)**, formerly called the Food Stamp Program. Based on the household's size and income, families are issued an electronic benefits transfer card that can be used like a credit card to buy nutritious foods at grocery stores. The SNAP program, benefits of which cannot be used to purchase alcohol, tobacco, or nonfood items, has come under fire, in part because of some well-publicized abuses. Some limitations are also placed on immigrant families' eligibility to receive SNAP benefits.[43]

Despite food assistance programs, many children are at risk of going hungry in the United States. USDA surveys found that 11.1% of households were food insecure in 2018, meaning that they had limited or uncertain access to nutritionally adequate foods. Families headed by single women with children and black and Hispanic households are the most likely to experience food insecurity. Poor nutrition increases children's risks of stunting, inadequate cognitive stimulation, iodine deficiency, and iron deficiency anemia. It also increases the risk of overweight and obesity, in that high-calorie processed foods are often less expensive than fresh, perishable foods such as fruits, vegetables, and low-fat dairy products.[44,45]

While undernutrition is a real concern for the poorest American families, overeating is a more widespread problem, as discussed elsewhere in this text.

Children's Health and Safety

Deaths in childhood from infectious diseases have been vastly reduced because of widespread **immunization** programs. The vast majority of children are vaccinated against diphtheria, tetanus, pertussis (whooping cough), polio, measles, rubella (German measles), mumps, and hepatitis B before they enter school, because most of these immunizations are required by law. However, many preschool children are at risk because they do not receive immunizations at the recommended ages. Well-baby care is almost as important as prenatal care for child health, but children of poor families often miss out on these visits to the doctor for the same reasons that their mothers missed prenatal visits, including lack of affordable health care.

In 1993, the federal government launched a childhood immunization initiative aimed at increasing vaccination coverage among children ages 19 to 35 months. The federal government began to provide free vaccines for children who were uninsured or whose insurance did not cover vaccines. Public- and private-sector organizations and healthcare providers at the national, state, and local levels were enlisted to help meet the goals of the initiative, in the hope of virtually eliminating many of the traditional childhood diseases. In addition to the eight diseases mentioned previously, eight more recent vaccines are covered by the Vaccines for Children Program: *Haemophilus influenzae* type b (spinal meningitis), varicella (chickenpox), pneumococcal disease, hepatitis A, influenza, meningococcal disease, rotavirus, and human papillomavirus.[46]

The human papillomavirus (HPV) vaccine, which was approved by the FDA in 2008, has proved uniquely controversial. HPV comprises a group of sexually transmitted viruses that will, at some time in their lives, infect nearly half of all people who have ever had sex. Although some infections do not cause symptoms and are cleared by the immune system, others may lead to genital warts in men and women or cause cancers of the cervix or other genital organs. The HPV vaccine prevents infection with the types of the virus that cause most cervical cancers and genital warts, but is ineffective in people who are already infected. Thus vaccination is recommended for 11- and 12-year-old girls, with the aim of reaching them before they become sexually active, but is approved for women up to age 26. The vaccine is also recommended for boys, in whom the virus can cause cancers of the throat, penis, and anus. Vaccinated boys and men will be less likely to spread HPV to their current and future partners. The HPV vaccine is expensive, costing approximately $250 for each dose, and it is designed to be given as either two or three doses depending the person's age and dose spacing.[47] The Vaccines for Children Program will pay for poor and uninsured young people to be vaccinated.

The controversy about the HPV vaccine stems from several factors.[48] Some critics have questioned whether the expense is justified to prevent cervical cancer, a disease that is relatively rare in the United States. Because the vaccine prevents only 70% of cancer cases, women will continue to need regular Pap smears to screen for the disease. Moreover, it is unclear how long immunity persists, so individuals may eventually need booster shots. Some parents are reluctant for their daughters to be vaccinated because they fear it may encourage promiscuity. There is also concern about side effects of the vaccine. The greatest value of the vaccine would be in developing countries, where cervical cancer screening is rare and the death rate from this cancer is high, but the vaccine is too expensive to be used in such countries.

The CDC tracks all sorts of immunization rates. In 2017, more than 80% of children aged 19 to 35 months had received the recommended doses of the eight most highly recommended vaccines. More than 90% had received at least some doses of these vaccines. A little more than 1% had received no vaccinations. On balance, these rates have not improved over the last few years.[49] This may be due in part to an antivaccine movement that has arisen in some areas of the United States, as discussed in the chapter titled *The "Conquest" of Infectious Diseases*.

In some past years, there have been shortages of some vaccines. Many vaccine manufacturers have left the market or produced insufficient supplies because they concluded that profits were not high enough, and they feared lawsuits over possible side effects. That threat was removed by the National Childhood Vaccine Injury Act, passed by Congress in 1986, which provided that pharmaceutical companies cannot be sued over harm caused by a vaccine. As of September 2019, the CDC reported no shortages of the recommended pediatric vaccines.[50]

Other preventive services of concern to public health because they may be missed by children of low SES who do not get regular well-baby care include screening for tuberculosis, problems with vision and hearing, and scoliosis (curvature of the spine). Because recognizing these problems as early as possible is important for ensuring a child's future health and ability to learn, these services are usually provided in schools. Diagnosing a problem in a school screening program does not guarantee that the problem will be corrected, however. Children who are uninsured or underinsured may be unable to obtain treatment even after the problem is identified repeatedly.

Childhood asthma is a significant public health concern, affecting 8.4% of children. Its prevalence is higher among blacks (10.1%) than among whites (8.1%) and Hispanics (6.4%).[51] Asthma prevalence grew dramatically between 1980 and 1996 for reasons that are not well understood.[52] Since then, rates appear to have declined somewhat. Deaths from asthma are rare among children, but African American children have a risk of dying from the disease that is almost three times higher than the risk for white children.[53] Urban environmental factors are believed to be responsible, at least in part, for the increased asthma prevalence. Because asthma can generally be controlled by medication when patients and their parents are educated about self-management techniques, hospitalizations and deaths are thought to reflect a lack of access to regular, appropriate medical care.

Although fluoridation of community water supplies and other sources of fluoride have reduced tooth decay rates among children by more than 50% since the 1960s, some children still suffer from painful and debilitating tooth decay. Poor children are especially likely to experience dental decay when the water is not fluoridated, and communities vary in the extent to which they provide dental services through clinics or local health departments. The CDC has identified fluoridation of drinking water as one of the 10 great public health achievements of the 20th century. In 2014, 74.4% of the U.S. population served by public water systems received fluoridated water.[54]

The fact that most mothers now work outside the home—a major change from the norm in previous decades—means that young children are increasingly being cared for in daycare centers. Suddenly, the need for safe and affordable daycare programs has become a public health issue. Infectious diseases spread rapidly among young children, and adequate hygiene when caregivers change infants' diapers is especially important to ward off this risk. Daycare attendees also face risks of injury from an unsafe physical plant or play equipment, inadequate staffing, or unqualified caregivers. These risks can be reduced by state licensing of daycare centers, requiring them to meet basic health and safety standards.

Injuries constitute the main risk to the life and health of children once they pass their first year. Public health efforts to prevent childhood injury include education and regulations that encourage use of seat belts, child safety seats, and bicycle helmets. The U.S. Consumer Products Safety Commission monitors toys and children's furniture for safety hazards, issuing warnings and ordering recalls of products that are found to be dangerous to children.

While maternal and child health services, like public health in general, focus on prevention of death and disability, there is a long tradition of public concern about the care of children with handicaps. Since 1935, the federal government has funded state "crippled children's programs" that provide diagnosis, treatment, and rehabilitative services for children with special needs, many of whom are also eligible for support through Social Security.[2] In the past, many of these children might have been institutionalized, but current programs try as much as possible to keep them at home, supporting families and preparing disabled young people to live independent lives.

To better understand the various factors that influence children's health and development, Congress in 2000 authorized the National Institutes of Health (NIH), the CDC, and the Environmental Protection Agency to conduct the largest long-term study on children ever done in the United States. The National Children's Study was designed as a longitudinal cohort study, comparable to the Framingham Heart Study and the Nurses' Health Study. The plan was to follow 100,000 children from before birth to age 21, so as to better understand the link between children's genes; the physical, chemical, and psychosocial environments in which they are raised; and their physical and mental health and development. The first volunteers were recruited in January 2009. However, by December 2014, after more than $1 billion had been spent, only 5000 mother–infant pairs had been enrolled. Dr. Francis Collins, director of the NIH, announced the study was being terminated. An advisory panel had criticized the study for poor design, inadequate management, and failed oversight. Dr. Collins has said he intends to fund smaller studies that can answer some of the same questions.[55]

Conclusion

Maternal and child health is one of the highest priorities for public health. In the United States, city, state, and local governments have, for more than a century, conducted programs and enforced legislation aimed at protecting children and promoting their health.

Infant mortality is a gauge of society's attention to children's health and is often used as an indicator of the health status of a population as a whole. The United States compares poorly with other countries on infant mortality, ranking 27th overall. IMRs, along with other public health improvements, have greatly improved since the beginning of the 20th century. Like other indicators of health, infant mortality is higher among blacks than among whites and declines with increasing SES.

Leading causes of infant mortality include congenital anomalies, low birth weight, and SIDS. Public health programs to prevent infant mortality because of congenital anomalies, or birth defects, include prenatal and postnatal screening and diagnostic programs. They also include protection of pregnant women from exposure to environmental teratogens. Dietary supplementation with folic acid has been found to prevent some birth defects.

Low birth weight, caused by preterm birth, is closely linked to SES. Because pregnant adolescents are especially likely to give birth to infants of low birth weight, prevention of pregnancy in teenagers is a high priority for public health.

SIDS-related deaths declined dramatically during the 1990s after it was found that babies who were put to sleep on their stomachs were at increased risk of sudden death. An educational campaign about infant sleeping positions cut SIDS deaths by more than 50%.

Adequate family planning services are important for public health. Pregnancy in adolescence is risky for both mothers and infants. Comprehensive sex education is effective in preventing teen pregnancy. Political conservatives have promoted abstinence-only programs, which are less effective than programs that include information on contraception. Unintended pregnancy also increases health risks in older women and their infants. While a variety of effective contraceptive methods are available, many women do not have access to affordable family planning services. Nutrition is an important component of maternal and child health programs. Since the 1930s, the federal government supported a number of programs that provide supplemental foods for pregnant women, infants, and children.

Other public health initiatives that have a significant impact on children's health include immunization requirements, fluoridation of community water supplies, and injury-prevention measures. Regular access to medical care is important for the health of children, but many poor and minority children lack such access.

References

1. P. D. Gluckman, M. A. Hanson, C. Cooper, and K. L. Thornburg, "Effect of In Utero and Early-Life Conditions on Adult Health and Disease," *New England Journal of Medicine* 359 (2008): 61–73.
2. W. M. Schmidt and H. M. Wallace, "Development of Health Services for Mothers and Children in the United States," in H. M. Wallace, G. M. Ryan Jr., and A. C. Oglesby, eds., *Maternal and Child Health Practices* (Oakland, CA: Third Party Publishing, 1988), 3–21.
3. C. A. Miller, "Development of MCH Services and Policy in the United States," in H. M. Wallace, G. M. Ryan Jr., and A. C. Oglesby, eds., *Maternal and Child Health Practices* (Oakland, CA: Third Party Publishing Company, 1988), 39–45.

4. Centers for Disease Control and Prevention, "Deaths: Final Data for 2017," *National Vital Statistics Report* 68, no. 9 (2019).

5. W. S. Nersesian, "Infant Mortality in Socially Vulnerable Populations," *Annual Review of Public Health* 9 (1988): 361–377.

6. Centers for Disease Control and Prevention, "Pregnancy Mortality Surveillance System," June 4, 2019, https://www.cdc.gov/reproductivehealth /maternalinfanthealth/pregnancy-mortality-surveillance -system.htm, accessed September 29, 2019.

7. C. J. Berg et al., "Pregnancy-Related Mortality in the United States, 1998–2005," *Obstetrics and Gynecology* 116 (2010): 1302–1309.

8. M. G. Wagner, "Infant Mortality in Europe: Implications for the United States," *Journal of Public Health Policy* (Winter 1998): 473–484.

9. A. M. Fraser, J. E. Brockert, and R. H. Ward, "Association of Young Maternal Age with Adverse Reproductive Outcomes," *New England Journal of Medicine* 332 (1995): 1113–1117.

10. J. Huntington and F. A. Connell, "For Every Dollar Spent: The Cost-Savings Argument for Prenatal Care," *New England Journal of Medicine* 331 (1994): 1303–1307.

11. N. Adler et al., "Socioeconomic Status and Health: The Challenge of the Gradient," *American Psychologist* 49 (1994): 15–24.

12. S. S. Brown, "Preventing Low Birthweight," in H. M. Wallace, G. M. Ryan Jr., and A. C. Oglesby, eds., *Maternal and Child Health Practices* (Oakland, CA: Third Party Publishing, 1988), 307–324.

13. Centers for Disease Control and Prevention, "STDs During Pregnancy: CDC Fact Sheet," March 28, 2016, https://www.cdc.gov/std/pregnancy/stdfact-pregnancy .htm, accessed September 29, 2019.

14. Centers for Disease Control and Prevention, "Timing and Adequacy of Prenatal Care in the United States, 2016," May 30, 2018, https://www.cdc .gov/nchs/data/nvsr/nvsr67/nvsr67_03.pdf, accessed September 29, 2019.

15. Kaiser Family Foundation, "Health Coverage and Care of Undocumented Immigrants," July 15, 2019, https://www.kff.org/disparities-policy/issue -brief/health-coverage-and-care-of-undocumented -immigrants/, accessed September 29, 2019.

16. Centers for Disease Control and Prevention, "Infant Health," January 20, 2017, https://www .cdc.gov/nchs/fastats/infant-health.htm, accessed September 29, 2019.

17. Centers for Disease Control and Prevention, "Mortality in the United States, 2017," November 2018, *NCHS Data Brief* no. 328, https://www.cdc .gov/nchs/products/databriefs/db328.htm, accessed September 29, 2019.

18. P. W. Yoon, S. A. Rasmussen, M. C. Lynberg, C. A. Moore, M. Anderka, S. L. Carmichael, "The National Birth Defects Prevention Study," *Public Health Reports* 116 (2001 suppl 1): 32–40.

19. Centers for Disease Control and Prevention, "National Birth Defects Prevention Study (NBDPS)," November 1, 2018, https://www.cdc.gov/ncbddd /birthdefects/nbdps.html, accessed September 29, 2019.

20. Centers for Disease Control and Prevention, "Updated Estimates of Neural Tube Defects Prevented by Mandatory Folic Acid Fortification—United States, 1995–2011," *Morbidity and Mortality Weekly Report* 64 (2015): 1–5.

21. W. M. Callaghan, M. F. MacDorman, S. A. Rasmussen, C. Qin, and E. M. Lackritz, "The Contribution of Preterm Birth to Infant Mortality Rates in the United States," *Pediatrics* 118 (2006): 1566–1573.

22. Centers for Disease Control and Prevention, "Births: Final Data for 2017," *National Vital Statistics Report* 67, no. 8 (November 7, 2018), https://www .cdc.gov/nchs/data/nvsr/nvsr67/nvsr67_08-508.pdf, accessed September 29, 2019.

23. J. D. Iams, R. Romero, J. F. Culhane, and R. L. Goldenberg, "Primary, Secondary, and Tertiary Interventions to Reduce the Morbidity and Mortality of Preterm Births," *Lancet* 371 (2008): 164–175.

24. Centers for Disease Control and Prevention, "Cigarette Smoking During Pregnancy: United States, 2016," *NCHS Data Brief* no. 305, February 2018, https://www.cdc.gov/nchs/products/databriefs /db305.htm, accessed September 29, 2019.

25. N. P. Polyzos, I. P. Polyzos, D. Mauri, S. Tzioras, M. Tsappi, I. Cortinovis, and G. Casazza, "Effect of Periodontal Disease Treatment During Pregnancy on Preterm Birth Incidence: A Meta-Analysis of Randomized Trials," *American Journal of Obstetrics and Gynecology* 200 (2009): 225–232.

26. National Institute of Child Health and Human Development, "Safe to Sleep: Public Education Campaign," September 23, 2013, https://safetosleep .nichd.nih.gov, accessed September 29, 2019.

27. Centers for Disease Control and Prevention, "Sudden Unexpected Death and Sudden Infant Death Syndrome: Data and Statistics," September 13, 2019, https://www .cdc.gov/sids/data.htm, accessed September 29, 2019.

28. Centers for Disease Control and Prevention, "Surveillance for Disparities in Maternal Health-Related Behaviors—Selected States, Pregnancy Risk Assessment Monitoring System (PRAMS), 2000–2001," *Morbidity and Mortality Weekly Report* 53: SS-4 (2004).

29. Centers for Disease Control and Prevention, "About Teen Pregnancy," March 1, 2019, www .cdc.gov/teenpregnancy/about/index.htm, accessed September 29, 2019.

30. S. J. Ventura, S. C. Curtin, and T. J. Mathews, "Teenage Births in the United States: National and State Trends, 1990–96," *National Vital Statistics System* (Hyattsville, MD: National Center for Health Statistics, 1998).

31. Centers for Disease Control and Prevention, "Abortion Surveillance—United States, 2015," *Morbidity and Mortality Weekly Report* 67, no. 13 (November 23, 2018).

32. Guttmacher Institute, "Insurance Coverage of Contraceptives," https://www.guttmacher.org/state-policy/explore/insurance-coverage-contraceptives, accessed September 29, 2019.

33. M. Stevens, "Judge Blocks Trump's Attempt to Roll Back Birth Control Mandate," *The New York Times*, January 14, 2019.

34. Planned Parenthood, "Birth Control," 2014, https://www.plannedparenthood.org/learn/birth-control, accessed July 12, 2015.

35. F. Davidoff and J. Trussell, "Plan B and the Politics of Doubt," *Journal of the American Medical Association* 296 (2006): 1775–1778.

36. C. Caron, "Students Look to Vending Machines for Better Access to Morning-After Pill," The New York Times, September 28, 2017.

37. T. Hampton, "Abstinence-Only Programs Under Fire," *Journal of the American Medical Association* 299 (2008): 2013–2015.

38. H. Bruckner and P. S. Bearman, "After the Promise: The STD Consequences of Adolescent Virginity Pledges," *Journal of Adolescent Health* 36 (2005): 271–278.

39. J. S. Santelli, L. D. Lindberg, L. B. Finer, and S. Singh, "Explaining Recent Declines in Adolescent Pregnancy in the United States: The Contribution of Abstinence and Improved Contraceptive Use," *American Journal of Public Health* 97 (2007): 150–156.

40. Centers for Disease Control and Prevention, "Results: Breastfeeding Rates," August 1, 2019, https://www.cdc.gov/breastfeeding/data/nis_data/results.html, accessed September 29, 2019.

41. Centers for Disease Control and Prevention, "Health, United States, 2017," Table 9, https://www.cdc.gov/nchs/data/hus/2017/009.pdf, accessed September 29, 2019.

42. J. T. Dwyer and J. Freedland, "Nutrition Services," in H. M. Wallace, G. M. Ryan Jr., and A. C. Oglesby, eds., *Maternal and Child Health Practices* (Oakland, CA: Third Party Publishing, 1988), 261–282.

43. U.S. Department of Agriculture, "Food and Nutrition Services: FNS Nutrition Programs," https://www.fns.usda.gov/programs, accessed September 30, 2019.

44. T. Hampton, "Food Insecurity Harms Health, Well-Being of Millions in the United States," *Journal of the American Medical Association* 298 (2007): 1851–1853.

45. U.S. Department of Agriculture, "Household Food Security in the United States in 2018," September 2019, *Economic Research Report* no. ERR-270, https://www.ers.usda.gov/publications/pub-details/?pubid=94848, accessed September 29, 2019.

46. Centers for Disease Control and Prevention, "Vaccines for Children Program (VFC)," February 18, 2016, https://www.cdc.gov/vaccines/programs/vfc/about/index.html, accessed September 30, 2019.

47. Centers for Disease Control and Prevention, "Vaccine (Shot) for Human Papillomavirus," August 2, 2019, https://www.cdc.gov/vaccines/parents/diseases/hpv.html, accessed September 29, 2019.

48. E. Rosenthal, "Drug Makers' Push Leads to Cancer Vaccines' Rise," *The New York Times*, August 19, 2008.

49. Centers for Disease Control and Prevention, "Vaccination Coverage Among Children Aged 19–35 Months—United States, 2017," *Morbidity and Mortality Weekly Report* 67 (2018).

50. Centers for Disease Control and Prevention, "Current Vaccine Shortages & Delays," https://www.cdc.gov/vaccines/hcp/clinical-resources/shortages.html, accessed September 29, 2019.

51. Centers for Disease Control and Prevention, "Data, Statistics, and Surveillance," March 25, 2019, https://www.cdc.gov/asthma/asthmadata.htm, accessed September 29, 2019.

52. Centers for Disease Control and Prevention, "Summary Health Statistics for U.S. Children: National Health Interview Survey, 2012," December 2013, https://www.cdc.gov/nchs/data/series/sr_10/sr10_258.pdf, accessed September 30, 2019.

53. Centers for Disease Control and Prevention, "Most Recent National Asthma Data," May 2019, https://www.cdc.gov/asthma/most_recent_national_asthma_data.htm, accessed September 29, 2019.

54. Centers for Disease Control and Prevention, "Community Water Fluoridation: Water Fluoridation Data & Statistics," July 15, 2019, https://www.cdc.gov/fluoridation/statistics/index.htm, accessed September 29, 2019.

55. P. I. Landrigan and D. S. Baker, "The National Children's Study: End or New Beginning?" *New England Journal of Medicine* 372 (2015): 1486–1487.

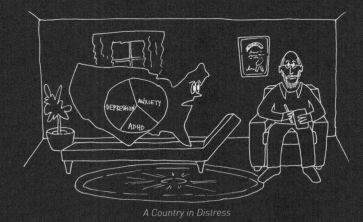

A Country in Distress

CHAPTER 19

Mental Health: Public Health Includes Healthy Minds

KEY TERMS

Anxiety
Community factor
Disturbances of mood
Eating disorders

Family factor
Individual factor
National Comorbidity Survey
(NCS)

National Survey on Drug Use
and Health (NSDUH)
Psychosis

According to the World Health Organization, mental illnesses account for more disability in developed countries than any other group of illnesses, including cancer and heart disease. In 2015, an estimated 17.9% of adults in the United States had a mental illness in the previous year. Nearly half of adult Americans will develop at least one mental illness during their lifetime.[1,2]

The most common mental illnesses in adults are anxiety and mood disorders. These disorders are often associated with chronic diseases, including cardiovascular disease, diabetes, asthma, epilepsy, and cancer. People with mental illness have an increased risk of injuries, both intentional and unintentional. They are also more likely than people without mental illness to use

tobacco products and to abuse alcohol and other drugs.

Major Categories of Mental Disorders

More than 200 types of mental illness are listed in the *Diagnostic and Statistical Manual of Mental Disorders* (*DSM*), the most authoritative compendium available, which attempts to standardize mental disorders into a common language for doctors, patients, researchers, health insurance companies, and others. The major categories of mental disorders listed in the 1999 Surgeon General's report *Mental Health*, which draws from the *DSM*, are anxiety, psychosis, disturbances of mood, and disturbances of cognition.[3] These categories are broad, heterogeneous, and somewhat overlapping. Any particular patient may manifest symptoms from more than one of these categories. Thus mental illnesses are sometimes hard to diagnose and, consequently, hard for epidemiologists to count.

Anxiety

Anxiety is a vitally important physiological response to dangerous situations that prepares one to either evade or confront a threat in the environment. However, inappropriate expressions of anxiety exist if the anxiety experienced is disproportionate to the circumstance or interferes with normal functioning. Examples include phobias, panic attacks, and generalized anxiety. Other manifestations of anxiety include obsessive–compulsive disorder and post-traumatic stress disorder (PTSD).

Psychosis

Disorders of perception and thought process are considered to be symptoms of **psychosis**. These disorders are most characteristically associated with schizophrenia, but psychotic symptoms can also occur in severe mood disorders. Among the most commonly observed psychotic symptoms are hallucinations (sensory impressions that have no basis in reality) and delusions (false beliefs held despite evidence to the contrary, such as paranoia).

Disturbances of Mood

Disturbances of mood characteristically manifest themselves as a sustained feeling of sadness or hopelessness (major depression) or extreme fluctuations of mood (bipolar disorder). Mood disturbances are also associated with symptoms such as disturbances in appetite, sleep patterns, energy level, concentration, and memory. Perhaps most alarming, major depression is often linked to thoughts of suicide.

Disturbances of Cognition

The ability to organize, process, and recall information, as well as to execute complex sequences of tasks, may be disturbed in a variety of disorders. Notably, Alzheimer's disease is a progressive deterioration of cognitive function, or dementia.

Epidemiology

A number of surveys of the U.S. population have yielded estimates of the prevalence of mental illness. One of the most comprehensive studies, the **National Comorbidity Survey (NCS)**, conducted from the fall of 1990 to spring of 1992, was sponsored by the National Institute of Mental Health, the National Institute of Drug Abuse, and the W. T. Grant Foundation. Researchers at Harvard Medical School interviewed 10,000 adults, asking questions designed to diagnose specific mental and substance use disorders.[4] The same respondents were reinterviewed in 2001–2002 to study patterns and predictors of the course of mental disorders and their relation to substance use. Another large survey, the **National Survey on Drug Use and Health (NSDUH)**, has been conducted by the U.S. government annually since 1971, with 67,500 interviews being performed each year.[2] The NCS and NSDUH are the sources of the commonly cited findings about the high incidence and prevalence of mental illness in the United States.

According to the NSDUH, the percentage of American adults with a mental disorder has not changed much since at least

2008. For 2015, it reported that 14.2% of adults had received mental health care in the past 12 months, and 83% of these individuals were treated with medication. Both of these percentages have increased slightly since 2002. Nearly 20% of individuals reporting a mental disorder also had a substance abuse disorder.[2]

Some of the surveys conducted by the Centers for Disease Control and Prevention (CDC) include questions on mental health. The Behavioral Risk Factor Surveillance System (BRFSS), a state-based telephone survey, conducts approximately 450,000 adult interviews each year. One question asked every year of all respondents is the number of mentally unhealthy days they experienced. Individual states may choose optional modules, including some that address other mental health issues in depth. For example, in 2006, 2008, and 2010, an optional module included one question on lifetime diagnosis of anxiety and one question on lifetime diagnosis of depression.[1]

Since 1997, the National Health Interview Survey, which conducts in-person interviews with carefully selected representative households, has asked a question designed to identify serious psychological distress in the past 30 days. In 2007, the survey included three questions on lifetime diagnoses: "Have you EVER been told by a doctor or other health professional that you had bipolar disorder? Schizophrenia? Mania or psychoses?"[1]

For the National Health and Nutrition Examination Survey, participants chosen from a carefully selected representative households are asked questions on the number of mentally unhealthy days, as well as questions designed to measure depression. A survey of women who have recently given birth, the Pregnancy Risk Assessment Monitoring System (PRAMS), asks questions about postpartum depression. Surveys on healthcare utilization gain information about mental health issues from data provided by hospitals, community health centers, office-based providers, and nursing homes.

The NCS provides data on the lifetime prevalence of mental disorders broken down by types of disorder—anxiety disorders, mood disorders, impulse-control disorders, and substance disorders—and the sex and age cohort of people suffering from each type. The total percentage of the population that has had an anxiety disorder is 31.2%; 21.4% have had a mood disorder; 25.0% have had an impulse-control disorder; and 35.3% have had a substance disorder. There is significant overlap among the specific disorders, with the total prevalence of any mental disorder amounting to 57.4%. **Table 19-1** shows details of the lifetime prevalence of various mental disorders by sex and age group.

When these data are broken down by sex, females report more anxiety disorders and mood disorders than males, while males have more impulse-control disorders and substance disorders. Notably, for all the disorders, younger cohorts have a higher prevalence than do cohorts older than age 60 years. In fact, the prevalence of anxiety disorders and mood disorders among those persons older than 60 is only about half of the prevalence among those age 18 to 59. Only nicotine dependence is comparable among older and younger groups.[1]

Two CDC surveys (BRFSS and PRAMS) collect data at the state or substate level, and the prevalence of some disorders varies substantially across regions of the country. The southeastern states generally have the highest prevalence of depression, serious psychological distress, and mean number of mentally unhealthy days. This finding likely reflects the association between mental illness and certain chronic diseases, such as obesity, diabetes, and cardiovascular disease, which are also more prevalent in the Southeast.

Table 19-1 Lifetime Prevalence (percent) of Mental Disorders by Sex and Cohort

	Total	Male	Female	18–29	30–44	45–59	60+
I. Anxiety Disorders							
Panic disorder	4.7	6.2	3.1	4.2	5.9	5.9	2.1
Agoraphobia without panic	1.3	1.6	1.1	1.2	1.4	1.8	0.9
Specific phobia	12.5	15.8	8.9	13	13.9	14.4	7.7
Social phobia	12.1	13	11.1	13.3	14.5	12.6	6.8
Generalized anxiety disorder	5.7	7.1	4.2	4.3	6.5	7.6	4
Post-traumatic stress disorder	6.8	9.7	3.6	6.3	8.1	9.2	2.8
Obsessive-compulsive disorder	2.3	3.1	1.6	3.1	3	2.4	0.6
Adult/Child separation anxiety disorder	9.2	10.8	7.4	12.4	11.1	9.2	3.1
Any anxiety disorder	31.2	36.4	25.4	32.9	37	34.2	17.8
II. Mood Disorders							
Major depressive disorder	16.9	20.2	13.2	16	19.3	20.1	10.7
Dysthymia	2.5	3.1	1.8	1.8	2.8	3.8	1.3
Bipolar I-II-sub-disorders	4.4	4.5	4.3	7	5.3	3.7	1.3
Any mood disorder	21.4	24.9	17.5	22.6	24.5	24.2	12.2
III. Impulse-Control Disorders							
Oppositional-defiant disorder	8.5	7.7	9.3	9.9	7.3	–	–
Conduct disorder	9.5	7.1	12	10.8	8.4	–	–
Attention-deficit/hyperactivity disorder	8.1	6.4	9.8	7.8	8.3	–	–
Intermittent explosive disorder	7.4	5.7	9.2	12.6	8.8	5.3	2.4
Any impulse-control disorder	25	21.6	28.6	27	23.4	–	–
IV. Substance Disorders							
Alcohol	13.2	7.5	19.6	14.5	16.4	14.1	6.3
Drug	8	4.8	11.6	11.1	12.1	6.8	0.3
Nicotine	29.6	26.5	33	26.5	29.4	34.3	27.3
Any	35.3	29.6	41.8	33.2	37.1	39.8	29.6
V. Any Disorders							
Any	57.4	56.5	58.4	58.7	63.7	60	44

This table includes updated data as of July 19, 2007. Updates reflect the latest diagnostic, demographic, and raw variable information.
Reproduced from R. C. Kessler, Harvard Medical School, *National Comorbidity Survey (NCS)*, (2005), www.hcp.med.harvard.edu/ncs/ftpdir/NCS-R_Lifetime _Prevalence_Estimates.pdf, accessed October 3, 2019.

Causes and Prevention

The precise causes of most mental disorders are not known, but much is known about the broad forces that shape them. The causes of mental disorders are viewed as a product of the interaction between biological, psychological, and sociocultural factors. Genetic factors are important in some mental disorders, including schizophrenia, bipolar disorder, autism, and attention-deficit/hyperactivity disorder. However, in the case of schizophrenia, studies of identical twins have found that when one twin has the disorder, in only half the cases does the second twin also have it, even though both twins have the same genes. This implies that environmental factors exert a significant role, so it may be possible to intervene to prevent the development of the disorder. Similarly, PTSD is clearly caused by exposure to an extremely stressful event, yet not everyone develops PTSD after such exposure. Again, appropriate treatment may prevent the disorder.[3]

Prevention of mental illness may depend on identification of risk factors that can be targeted, especially in children. Risk factors common to many disorders include individual factors, family factors, and community factors. **Individual factors** that may put a person at risk include neurophysiological deficits, difficult temperament, chronic physical illness, and below-average intelligence. **Family factors** that increase risk are severe marital discord, social disadvantage, overcrowding or large family size, paternal criminality, maternal mental disorder, and admission into foster care. **Community factors** such as living in an area with a high rate of disorganization and inadequate schools may also increase risk.[3]

Children

Both biological factors and adverse psychosocial experiences during childhood may influence the risk that a child will develop a mental disorder.

A risk factor may have no, little, or a profound impact depending on individual differences among children and the age at which the child is exposed to it, as well as whether it occurs alone or in association with other risk factors.

Biological risk factors that may lead to mental illness in children include intrauterine exposure to alcohol or cigarettes, environmental exposure to lead, malnutrition of pregnancy, birth trauma, and specific chromosomal syndromes. The quality of the relationship between infants or children and their primary caregivers is believed to be of primary importance to mental health across the lifespan. Maternal depression increases the risk of depressive and anxiety disorders, conduct disorder, and alcohol dependence in the child. Child abuse and neglect is a widespread problem in the United States, and is associated with depression, conduct disorder, delinquency, and impaired social functioning with peers.[3]

Autism is a severe, chronic developmental disorder characterized by a severely compromised ability to engage in, and lack of interest in, social interaction. Affected children may have a wide range of symptoms, skills, and levels of disability; thus they are referred to as "being on the autism spectrum." A 2014 CDC survey found that the rate of autism spectrum disorder was approximately 1 in 59 children. The prevalence in boys is about four times higher than in girls.[5]

The evidence for a genetic influence in autism development includes twin studies, which find that identical twins of autistic individuals will also have autism in 9 out of 10 cases. Researchers are starting to identify particular genes that may increase the risk of autism. Because autism results in significant lifelong disability, intensive special education programs in highly structured environments are recommended to help autistic children to acquire self-care, social, and job skills.

Mood disorders, including bipolar disorder, major depression, and suicide, are a matter of serious concern for anyone who cares about the mental health of children and adolescents. Mortality from suicide increases steadily through the teen years: Suicide is the second leading cause of death among young people age 15 to 24.[6] Boys are nearly four times as likely to commit suicide as are girls, whereas girls are more likely to report attempting suicide. Boys are more likely to use deadlier methods, such as firearms.[7]

Attention-deficit/hyperactivity disorder (ADHD) is the most commonly diagnosed behavior disorder of childhood, affecting approximately 5% of children in 2016. Boys are more than twice as likely to be diagnosed with ADHD than girls. ADHD tends to run in families, supporting the view that genes are important in this disorder. ADHD is often treated with psychoactive stimulants, but pharmaceutical treatment is more effective when accompanied by behavioral therapy aimed at helping a child organize tasks, follow directions, and monitor his or her own behavior.[8]

Concerns have been raised that children—especially active boys—are being overdiagnosed with ADHD and therefore receiving psychostimulants unnecessarily, in part because of the nation's push for greater academic achievement and school accountability.[9] This view is supported by the findings of one study that, although many children who do meet the full criteria for ADHD are not being treated, the majority of children and adolescents who are receiving stimulants do not fully meet the criteria. This reflects a failure of proper, comprehensive evaluation and diagnosis. The long-term safety of psychostimulant treatment has not been established.[3]

Disruptive disorders, such as oppositional defiant disorder and conduct disorder, are frequently found in children with ADHD. Other mental illnesses generally diagnosed in childhood include anxiety disorders, including separation anxiety, social phobia, eating disorders, and obsessive–compulsive disorder, which has a strong familial component.[3]

Several interventions that focus on enhancing mental health and preventing behavior problems have been found to be effective in enhancing children's success in the classroom and minimizing their involvement in the juvenile justice system—both of which are indicators of mental health. Project Head Start is probably the best-known prevention program in the United States. Although originally designed to improve the academic performance of economically disadvantaged preschool children, its advantages are mainly social in nature, including better peer relations, less truancy, and less antisocial behavior. A number of other early childhood programs for high-risk children, many of which involve home visits by nurses, are effective in part because they include a parental education component.[3]

Eating Disorders

Eating disorders typically appear during the teen years or young adulthood, but may also occur in older or younger individuals.[10] They are thought to be caused by a complex interaction of genetic, biological, behavioral, and psychological factors. Although they are clearly mental illnesses, these disorders may lead to serious physical problems.

With *anorexia nervosa*, a disorder more common in girls and women, the affected individual sees herself as overweight even when she is clearly underweight. She is obsessed with food, weight, and weight control, and typically eats only certain foods in very small portions. Anorexia may be life-threatening, as the person is starving herself to death. This disorder can cause heart damage, brain damage, and, eventually, multiple organ failure. People with anorexia are 18 times more likely to die young as are people in the general population of the same age.

People with *bulimia nervosa* are also obsessed with their weight, but they lack control over their eating. They binge on food and then try to compensate by engaging in purging behaviors such as self-induced vomiting or excessive use of laxatives, by fasting, or by performing excessive exercise. Bulimics tend to be of normal weight. They may develop symptoms such as chronic sore throat, tooth decay, various gastrointestinal problems, and electrolyte imbalance.

In *binge-eating disorder*, people lose control over their eating, but they do not purge. These individuals are often overweight or obese.

Eating disorders also affect males, but their preoccupation is often different from those of females. Unlike girls with eating disorders, who usually want to lose weight, boys often want to become more muscular. In consequence, they may use steroids or other dangerous drugs to "bulk up."

Treatment of eating disorders involves psychotherapy and family therapy. Patients with anorexia may need to be hospitalized for both mental health and medical treatment.

Mental Health in Adulthood

Mental health in adulthood is characterized by the successful performance of mental functions, enabling individuals to cope with adversity and to flourish in their education, vocation, and personal relationships. Traits or personal characteristics that contribute to mental health include self-esteem, optimism, and resilience traits that are needed to deal with stressful life events. Confidence in one's own abilities to cope with adversity is a major contributor to mental health in adulthood.[3]

The most common psychological and social stressors in adult life include breakup of intimate romantic relationships, death of a family member or friend, economic hardships, racism and discrimination, poor physical health, and accidental and intentional assaults on physical safety. Such events are more likely to cause mental disorders in people who are vulnerable biologically, socially, and/or psychologically.

Effective treatments for mental disorders are available, contrary to what many people think. A variety of psychotherapy approaches have been used successfully, from Freudian psychoanalysis to cognitive-behavioral therapy, which strives to alter faulty cognitions and replace them with thoughts that promote adaptive behavior. Drugs for the treatment of depression, anxiety, and schizophrenia have also been found effective in correcting the biochemical alterations that accompany these mental disorders.

Anxiety disorders are the most prevalent mental disorders in adults. They include panic disorders, agoraphobia (anxiety about being in situations from which escape might be difficult), generalized anxiety disorder, specific phobia, social phobia, obsessive–compulsive disorder, acute stress disorder, and PTSD. The prevalence of anxiety disorders among adults over their lifetime is approximately 31% (Table 19-1), and they significantly overlap with mood and substance abuse disorders. Females have a higher rate of most anxiety disorders compared to males. Some anxiety disorders, such as panic disorder, appear to have a strong genetic basis, whereas others are more rooted in stressful life events. Anxiety disorders are treated with some form of counseling or psychotherapy or drug treatment.[3,11]

Many veterans of the Iraq and Afghanistan wars suffer from post-traumatic stress disorder (PTSD). They may experience flashbacks to the traumatic events, have nightmares, or feel stressed and angry during the day, making it hard for them to do daily tasks, such as sleeping, eating, or concentrating. In August 2012, President Barack Obama signed an executive order that sought to strengthen access to mental health care for veterans, including suicide prevention efforts. The president also ordered the U.S. Department of Defense, the U.S. Department of Veterans Affairs, and the U.S.

Department of Health and Human Services to conduct research programs on how to better prevent, diagnose, and treat these disorders. Strategies for promoting evidence-based PTSD treatments are urgently needed.[9,12]

Two types of psychotherapies for PTSD are currently being evaluated: prolonged exposure (PE) therapy and cognitive processing therapy (CPT). PE involves helping people confront their fear and feelings about the trauma they experienced in a safe way through mental imagery, writing, or other ways. In CPT, the patient is asked to recount his or her traumatic experience, and a therapist helps him or her redirect inaccurate or destructive thoughts about the experience.[13]

Mood disorders, including major depression and bipolar disorder, are a major cause of disability. Bipolar disorder and major depression are more prevalent in women than in men. In 2015, 6.7% of adults had a major depressive disorder, defined as having a period of at least two weeks with a depressed mood or loss of interest or pleasure in daily activities, and at least some additional symptoms such as sleep or self-worth problems. This percentage has held steady since 2005.[2] The National Comorbidity Study found a lifetime prevalence of approximately 4% for bipolar disorder (Table 19-1). About half of those individuals with a primary diagnosis of major depression also have an anxiety disorder. Likewise, substance use disorders are common in individuals with mood disorders. The relative importance of biological and psychosocial factors varies across individuals and across different types of mood disorders. Genetic factors are strongly implicated in bipolar disorder.[14]

Several types of medications have been found effective in treatment of mood disorders, including four major classes of antidepressants and mood stabilizers such as lithium. Psychotherapy is often added to pharmaceutical treatment. Electroconvulsant shock therapy is sometimes used for severe depression.

Schizophrenia, which affects approximately 1% of the population, is characterized by profound disruption in cognition and emotion, affecting language, thought, perception, affect, and sense of self. Symptoms frequently include hearing internal voices (hallucinations) and holding fixed false personal beliefs (delusions). Onset generally occurs during young adulthood, although earlier and later onsets do occur. Twin and other family studies support the role of genetics in schizophrenia. Immediate biological relatives of people with the condition have about 10 times greater risk than that of the general population. Even so, only 40% to 65% of identical twins of someone diagnosed with schizophrenia have the disorder, indicating that environmental factors likely play a role as well.[3,15] Treatment of schizophrenia generally includes some form of antipsychotic medication, of which a variety of agents have been shown to be effective, combined with psychotherapy and family intervention programs.

Mental Health in Older Adults

A substantial proportion of the population age 55 and older experience specific mental disorders that are not part of "normal" aging. These include depression, Alzheimer's disease, alcohol and drug misuse and abuse, anxiety, late-life schizophrenia, and other conditions. Of all groups, older men have the highest rates of suicide, frequently as a consequence of depression.[6(Table 33)]

Risk factors for mental illness in the elderly include general medical conditions, admission to a nursing home, the high number of medications taken by many older individuals, and psychosocial stressors such as bereavement or isolation. Depression is particularly prevalent among older people, especially after loss of a spouse. Prevention through grief counseling or through participation in self-help groups is effective in improving social adjustment and reducing the use of alcohol and other drugs of abuse. Depression and suicide prevention strategies are also important for nursing home residents.

Anxiety symptoms not specific to any identified syndrome are prevalent in older adults, affecting approximately 18% of the elderly population (Table 19-1). Schizophrenia is commonly regarded as an illness of young adulthood, but it can both extend into and first appear in later life. Some younger patients who have received early intervention with antipsychotic medications demonstrate remarkable recovery after many years of chronic dysfunction. Symptoms of late-onset schizophrenia are similar to those in younger patients, and the risk factors are also similar.

Treatment of mental illness in older adults is similar to that in younger patients. However, physiological changes due to aging increase the risk of side effects from drug treatments. Interactions with medications used for other disorders of aging may also complicate effective treatment for mental illness, both by increasing side effects and by decreasing the efficacy of one or both drugs.

Treatment

A significant fraction of people with mental disorders do not seek treatment. In part, this reluctance may occur because they do not know that effective treatments are available. It may also reflect fear of the stigma of acknowledging the problem. Above all, the major deterrent is the cost of care. In general, insurance coverage of mental health care is inferior to coverage for physical health problems.

In the past, hospitalization was the norm for individuals with serious mental illness. People were sent to asylums, where they frequently endured poor and occasionally abusive conditions. In these settings, patients became excessively dependent and lost their connections to the community. More recently, inpatient units have been used for crisis care, focusing on reducing the risk of danger to self or others and ensuring the rapid return of patients to the community. Housing is often a major problem for people with severe mental illness, who often tend to be poor. It is estimated that as many as one in three individuals who experience homelessness has a mental illness.

Conclusion

Mental illnesses account for more disability in developed countries, including the United States, than any other group of illnesses. Nearly half of adult Americans will develop at least one mental illness during their lifetime. The most common mental illnesses in adults are anxiety and mood disorders. Schizophrenia, which occurs in about 1% of the population, is characterized by profound disruption in cognition and emotion and often includes hallucinations and delusions. Genetic factors are important in some mental disorders, including schizophrenia, autism, bipolar disorder, and ADHD. Most mental disorders are also influenced by environmental factors. PTSD is clearly caused by extremely stressful events. Eating disorders are caused by a complex interaction of genetic, biological, behavioral, and psychological factors. Most people with mental disorders do not seek treatment, although effective treatments do exist, including medications and psychotherapy.

References

1. Centers for Disease Control and Prevention, "Mental Illness Surveillance Among Adults in the United States," *Morbidity and Mortality Weekly Report*, 60 (2011 suppl 3): 1–32.

2. Center for Behavioral Health Statistics and Quality, "Key Substance Use and Mental Health Indicators in the United States: Results from the 2015 National Survey on Drug Use and Health," HHS Publication No. SMA 16-4984, NSDUH Series H-51, 2016, https://www.samhsa.gov/data/sites/default/files /NSDUH-FFR1-2015/NSDUH-FFR1-2015/NSDUH -FFR1-2015.pdf, accessed December 11, 2019.

3. U.S. Department of Health and Human Services, "Mental Health: A Report of the Surgeon General," 1999, https://www.psychosocial.com/policy/satcher .html, accessed October 3, 2019.

4. Harvard Medical School, "National Comorbidity Survey (NCS)," https://www.hcp.med.harvard.edu /ncs/, accessed October 3, 2019.

5. L. Wiggins, D. L. Christensen, et al., "Prevalence of Autism Spectrum Disorder Among Children Aged 8 Years—Autism and Developmental Disabilities Monitoring Network, 11 Sites, United States, 2014," *Morbidity and Mortality Weekly Report* 67, no. 6 (April 27, 2018).

6. Centers for Disease Control and Prevention, "Health, United States, 2014," May 2015, https://www .cdc.gov/nchs/data/hus/hus14.pdf, accessed October 3, 2019.

7. Stanford Children's Health, "Teen Suicide," https:// www.stanfordchildrens.org/en/topic/default?id=teen -suicide-90-P02584, accessed October 3, 2019.

8. Centers for Disease Control and Prevention, "Data and Statistics About ADHD," August 27, 2019, https://www.cdc.gov/ncbddd/adhd/data.html, accessed October 3, 2019.

9. S. P. Hinshaw and R. M. Scheffler, "Expand Pre-K, Not A.D.H.D.," *The New York Times*, February 23, 2014.

10. National Institute of Mental Health, "Eating Disorders," https://www.nimh.nih.gov/health/topics/eating-disorders/index.shtml, accessed October 3, 2019.

11. National Institute of Mental Health, "Any Anxiety Disorder Among Adults," https://www.nimh.nih .gov/health/statistics/prevalence/any-anxiety-disorder -among-adults.shtml, accessed October 3, 2019.

12. The White House, "Executive Order: Improving Access to Mental Health Services for Veterans, Service Members, and Military Families," August 31, 2012, https://obamawhitehouse.archives.gov/realitycheck /the-press-office/2012/08/31/executive-order -improving-access-mental-health-services-veterans -service, accessed October 3, 2019.

13. National Institute of Mental Health, "PTSD Treatment Efforts for Returning War Veterans to Be Evaluated," September 30, 2009, https://www.nimh.nih.gov /archive/news/2009/ptsd-treatment-efforts-for -returning-war-veterans-to-be-evaluated.shtml, accessed October 3, 2019.

14. National Institute of Mental Health, "Depression," https://www.nimh.nih.gov/health/topics/depression /index.shtml, accessed October 3, 2019.

15. National Institute of Mental Health, "Schizophrenia," https://www.nimh.nih.gov/health/topics/schizophrenia /index.shtml, accessed October 3, 2019.

PART V

Environmental Issues in Public Health

CHAPTER 20

An Environmental Hazard

A Clean Environment: The Basis of Public Health

KEY TERMS

Bisphenol A (BPA)
Consumer Product Safety
  Improvement Act
Environmental health

Environmental Protection
  Agency (EPA)
Factory farms
Polychlorinated biphenyls (PCBs)

Radiation
Radon gas

Humans are designed by eons of evolution to live on the earth: to breathe the earth's air, to drink the earth's water, to eat the plants and animals that grow on the earth's surface. People are adapted to the earth's environment. While that environment varies considerably in different parts of the planet, and while humans have found ways to live in many different climates and habitats, people's health depends on the presence of these basic ingredients of life—air, water, and food. Some natural phenomena in the environment can also harm human health: extremes of heat and cold, ultraviolet rays of the sun, toxic minerals and plants, and other living organisms, ranging from pathogenic bacteria to predatory mammals.

Human beings are social creatures, dependent upon other people to help them navigate the earth's environment. All humans in all parts of the world live in groups, from small bands of hunters and gatherers to the residents of teeming cities. When groups of people settle down to live together in one place, they change their shared environment: The larger the group, the greater the effect on the environment. Some of these changes may be made deliberately, to improve life for everyone; others are the inadvertent results of crowding, with harmful effects on people's well-being.

Archaeological evidence shows that the earliest cities were designed with consideration for the health of their inhabitants. As early as 2000 B.C., cities in India, Egypt, Greece, and South America had devised ways of providing clean water and draining wastes. These ancient systems of water supply, drains, and sewers are the first evidence of public health measures: organized community efforts to provide healthy conditions for the population.

Ensuring a clean water supply and the safe disposal of wastes—functions that fall into the category of **environmental health**—are still among the most important responsibilities of government. Other environmental health functions necessary in industrial countries are measures to ensure clean air and safe food. All of these concerns arise because of the human tendency to live in groups. Most people do not have the means or the desire to grow their own food, draw water from their own well, and dispose of wastes in their own yard. Instead, the majority of people live together in cities and suburbs, where they rely on others to provide their food and water and to dispose of their wastes. Because the earth is home to so many people today, and because of the prodigality of the modern lifestyle, the wastes that people produce have unprecedented potential to pollute the air and litter the earth.

Role of Government in Environmental Health

Environmental health is clearly the responsibility of government. Many environmental exposures, such as air pollution, are beyond the control of the individual. Others can be avoided only at significant trouble and expense—for example, if people grow their own vegetables, or buy them from farmers whose agricultural methods they have inspected themselves. Governments ensure a healthy environment by various means, sometimes providing services directly, in other cases by setting standards and regulating how the services should be provided.

Traditionally in the United States, local governments have provided water for their citizens. They are required by law to meet standards set by state and federal governments. Most local governments have also provided sewage systems to dispose of wastes from individual households and to handle runoff from the land.

In the 1960s, Americans became increasingly aware that the environment was deteriorating. Lakes and streams were choked with sewage and chemical wastes that killed fish and other wildlife. Cities were overhung with smog. Citizens were outraged by news stories of neighborhoods poisoned by long-dormant toxic waste dumps. State and federal governments were pressured to assume more responsibility for the environment. In the late 1960s and early 1970s, many new laws set standards for air, water, and waste disposal. The first Earth Day, celebrated in the United States on April 22, 1970, marked the beginning of the modern environmental movement, with advocates holding coast-to-coast rallies and teach-ins. That same year, the **Environmental Protection Agency (EPA)** was established to consolidate federal research, monitoring, standards-setting, and enforcement activities to achieve a cleaner, healthier environment in the United States.

Perhaps the most difficult environmental health issue people face today is the threat that human activities worldwide are changing the earth's climate. The biggest concern is the accumulation of "greenhouse gases" in the atmosphere. This problem, which may significantly affect human health, transcends national boundaries. Although the United Nations has sponsored international meetings on this issue and governments have signed treaties designed to bring the problem under control, there is no way of enforcing these agreements.

Identification of Hazards

A major role of the federal government in environmental health is to identify hazards in the environment and to set safety standards that must be met by industry and by state and local governments to protect people from these hazards. Both the identification of a substance as hazardous and the setting of standards are often difficult and controversial. The risks posed by most synthetic chemicals that are discharged into the environment by industrial processes or that are disposed of by consumers are unknown. Testing for potential harmful effects is expensive and time-consuming, and the choice of chemicals to test may be politically controversial. Even in cases where the health risk is obvious—such as the discharge of raw sewage into waterways or the air pollution caused by America's dependence on the private automobile—local governments, industry, and even the average citizen may resist requirements to meet standards because of the expense and inconvenience of cleaning up the environment.

Radiation is an environmental health hazard that people tend to worry about only when it is artificially produced. In reality, all people are exposed to cosmic radiation in varying amounts depending on where they live, and natural radioactive materials are found in soils and rocks in many parts of the world. **Radon gas**, produced by the natural radioactive decay of uranium, is present in many homes, a fact that was recognized only in the mid-1980s. Prolonged exposure to radon is potentially a cause of lung cancer, although the risks from radon in the home are not well understood. Ultraviolet radiation from the sun is a significant cause of skin cancer and melanoma. There is no way these exposures can be regulated by government, except for some testing requirements concerning radon.

In the mid-1890s, the discovery of x-rays, which could pass through flesh and reveal bones, aroused great public excitement and led to extensive human exposures before their dangers were recognized. During the early decades of the 20th century, x-ray treatments were popular as cure-alls for a variety of ailments, and radioactive ingredients were added to patent medicines. The first alarm was raised in the mid-1920s, following the deaths from kidney and bone disease of a number of

workers who painted watch dials with radium so they would glow in the dark. The workers had been touching the paintbrushes to their lips to sharpen the points, thereby ingesting toxic quantities of the chemical. Then in 1932, a rich, socially prominent businessman died in an agonizing manner from the same mysterious ailment, which was diagnosed on autopsy as radium poisoning. He had been dosing himself over a five-year period with hundreds of bottles of Radithor, a radium-containing patent medicine. The publicity surrounding the Radithor scandal led to strengthened Food and Drug Administration (FDA) powers to regulate patent medicines as well as specific limitations on radioactive pharmaceuticals.[1]

Evidence that chronic exposure to low levels of x-radiation caused cancer came from epidemiologic studies that began in the 1930s. One study compared death rates of radiologists with those of other medical specialists and found that the average age at death for radiologists was five years younger than that of other specialists.[2] Radiation's damaging health effects were confirmed by long-term follow-up studies of survivors of the atomic bombings of Hiroshima and Nagasaki, Japan, which ended World War II. The incidence of leukemia and other cancers was significantly increased among these people. Today, medical and dental x-rays constitute the largest source of nonbackground radiation exposure, although equipment has been continuously improved to reduce the hazard. As approximately one-third of the medical and dental x-rays that Americans receive are considered unnecessary, patients are advised to question whether each exposure is essential.

That some metals have harmful health effects has been common knowledge for decades or longer. For example, mercury was recognized in the 19th century as causing neurologic damage in workers who made felt hats—the origin of the expression "mad as a hatter" and the inspiration for the character the Mad Hatter in Lewis Carroll's *Alice in Wonderland*. The devastating effects of the mercury discharged by a plastics factory into

Japan's Minamata Bay in the 1950s caused some 700 deaths and varying degrees of paralysis and brain damage in 9000 other people. The mercury accumulated in fish, which were the staple of the community's diet. Another well-known episode of mercury poisoning occurred in Iraq in 1972, when the substance was used as a fungicide on seed grain. The contaminated wheat was turned into bread, which poisoned more than 6500 people, 459 of whom died.[3(Ch.7)]

In the United States, mercury enters the environment mainly by emissions from coal-burning power plants. The heavy metal falls to earth and becomes a hazard to humans mainly by getting into fish. Because the developing brain is most sensitive to the toxic effects of mercury, pregnant women and women who may become pregnant, as well as nursing mothers and young children, are advised to avoid eating fish species that have the highest average amounts of mercury in their flesh: bigeye tuna, king mackerel, marlin, shark, swordfish, and tilefish from the Gulf of Mexico. For other species of fish, there are limits on how many servings per week are considered safe.[4] Mercury is regulated under both the Clean Air Act and the Safe Drinking Water Act.

People may be exposed to mercury when the liquid metal is spilled, releasing toxic vapors—for example, after a glass thermometer breaks. Mercury may also be found in equipment used in school science labs, and exposure may occur if the equipment breaks or is mishandled. The EPA recommends that mercury-containing products be removed from homes and schools. The sale of mercury-containing fever thermometers is banned in many states; safer alternatives are now available. Cleanup of mercury spills requires great caution to prevent droplets of the metal from accumulating in small spaces and releasing vapors into the air. The EPA cautions against trying to clean up mercury with a vacuum cleaner or broom, or pouring it down a drain, because these methods are likely to put more of the toxic vapors into the air.[5]

Lead is another metal known to harm the brain and nervous system, especially in children. It also damages red blood cells and kidneys. Lead is believed to be the single most important environmental threat to the health of American children, who may be exposed to it from a variety of sources. Over the past three decades, evidence has accumulated that even low levels of lead can slow a child's development and can cause learning and behavior problems. The federal government recommends that all young children from families poor enough to be eligible for Medicaid be screened for lead in the blood, and some states have extended the mandate to children of all income levels. Permissible levels of lead have been steadily lowered from 60 micrograms per deciliter of blood in 1970 to 5 micrograms today.[6]

Lead has been used—and has been causing lead poisoning—since the time of the Roman Empire, when it was a component of wine casks, cooking pots, and water pipes. In fact, the Latin word for lead is "plumbum," the origin of the English word "plumbing." Even today, a major source of lead exposure for millions of Americans is water contaminated with lead from lead pipes or from lead solder used with copper pipes. The use of lead in pipes was phased out in the 1980s, and newer homes use plastic plumbing. Lead in public drinking water is also recognized as an increasingly common and serious problem. In recent years, one of the worst environmental crises was the discovery of lead in the municipal drinking water supply of Flint, Michigan, a city of more than 100,000 people, between 2014 and at least 2017. We cover the problem of lead in drinking water in more detail in the *Clean Water: A Limited Resource* chapter.

Until the 1980s, lead was a significant air pollutant, emitted from the tailpipes of motor vehicles that burned leaded gasoline. As a result of the phasing out of leaded gas, lead levels in the air have dropped to negligible amounts. Lead was also a component of paint, both interior and exterior, until its use was banned in 1977. Children—especially those who live in old, substandard housing—are still significantly exposed when they chew on chips of old peeling paint or when they put dirty hands in their mouths if the dirt is contaminated with dust from deteriorating paint. Attempts to remove old lead-containing paint can sometimes be even more hazardous if it turns to airborne dust as it is sanded or sandblasted off a surface and is inhaled.

New alarms about lead surfaced in 2007, when the Consumer Product Safety Commission (CPSC) recalled millions of wooden toys that had been painted with lead paint, including the popular Thomas the Tank Engine. The toys had been manufactured in China, which produces 70% to 80% of the toys sold in the United States.[7] Consumer advocates note that toy safety is largely the responsibility of the companies that import them. The CPSC suffered budgetary cuts during the George W. Bush administration and did not have the staff to monitor the safety of so many imports. Lead in toys is of special concern because young children often put them in their mouths. In 2008, Congress passed the **Consumer Product Safety Improvement Act**, which imposed regulations and testing requirements for toys and children's furniture on manufacturers, importers, distributors, and retailers. The law limited the amount of lead allowed in paint or any similar surface coating on these products.[8]

Arsenic, "the king of poisons," is well known as a means of committing homicide throughout the centuries. It was not recognized as an important environmental toxin until the United Nations Children's Fund inadvertently turned it into one in the 1970s in India and Bangladesh.[9] Concerned about epidemics of cholera, dysentery, and other waterborne diseases, the organization led a campaign to drill millions of wells so that the population would no longer need to drink contaminated surface water. Soon, however, people began to develop symptoms such as abdominal pain, vomiting, diarrhea, pain and swelling in the hands and feet, and skin eruptions. In some cases, symptoms progressed to progressive nervous system deterioration and death. Children with poor nutritional status proved to be especially susceptible to these problems. Subsequently, the well water, while free of disease-causing bacteria, was found to contain very high concentrations of arsenic. With 80% of Bangladeshis affected, the World Health Organization has labeled this "the worst mass poisoning in history."[9(p.A386)] Developing effective strategies for mitigating the effects of arsenic has been called one of the most important environmental health challenges of our time.

Studies have shown that, at somewhat lower concentrations, long-term exposure to arsenic in drinking water increases the risk of developing diabetes and cancer. In the United States, regulations call for public water systems to contain no more than 10 micrograms per liter of arsenic, a concentration significantly less than the levels known to cause harm. However, people in some parts of the country who have private wells may be drinking water that contains 50 to 90 micrograms per liter of arsenic. The risks from chronic exposure to these amounts are not known.[9]

Asbestos is a fibrous mineral valuable for a variety of uses because of its strength and fire resistance. The hazards of asbestos were first recognized in an occupational setting: Inhalation of high concentrations of asbestos dust caused stiffening and scarring of the lungs of miners and other asbestos workers, a condition known as asbestosis, which can be disabling and eventually fatal. Regulations limiting exposure were instituted, but as workers began to live longer, many of them developed cancer. They were especially likely to get lung cancer or mesothelioma, a rare cancer of the lining of the chest or abdominal cavity that seems to be caused exclusively by inhalation of asbestos. As a result of a succession of lawsuits brought by injured workers and their families in the 1960s and 1970s, the Manville Corporation—the largest asbestos company in the United States—filed for bankruptcy in 1982.[10] Once the dangers of asbestos were recognized, many uses of the material were banned, and standards for occupational exposure were tightened. However, asbestos can still be found in brake linings and a number of construction materials.[3(Ch.7)]

The general public is most likely to be exposed to asbestos fibers released into the air in the dust from crumbling walls and ceilings of old, deteriorating buildings. This possibility is a special concern in schools, because all schools built or renovated between 1940 and 1973 were required to install asbestos insulation as a fire safety measure. Children's exposure inspires special concern because they would live for many years with the fibers lodged in their lungs, and their likelihood of developing cancer would increase with time. In 1986, the Asbestos Hazard Emergency Response Act was passed. It required inspection of all primary and secondary schools; if loose asbestos was found, schools had to carry out plans for removing, enclosing, or encapsulating the material. Unfortunately, the removal was often done improperly, causing more asbestos to be released into the air than if the material had been left intact. Other schools, unable to afford the expense of asbestos removal, ignored the rulings.[3(Ch.7)] To date, no evidence shows that exposure to asbestos has been a significant cancer risk to the general population.

In contrast, the population of Libby, Montana, was clearly harmed by decades of exposure to asbestos. The vermiculite ore that had been mined in the Libby area since the 1920s was heavily contaminated with asbestos. A study by the National Institute of Occupational Safety and Health found that among 1675 Libby workers, 15 died of mesothelioma, a very rare disease, and the death rate from asbestosis was 165 times higher than expected. Death rates from asbestosis among residents of the area were approximately 40 times higher than those in the rest of Montana and 60 times higher than those in

the rest of the United States.[11] Follow-up studies found abnormalities in the chest x-rays of household contacts of asbestos workers, who presumably were exposed to asbestos dust brought home on the workers' clothes. Abnormalities were also found in the x-rays of children who had played in piles of vermiculite at the processing facilities.[12]

The fallout from the Libby crisis continues. A disease registry has been established to track individuals who were exposed, both to learn more about asbestos-related illnesses and to share information on new therapies and diagnostic tools. A community health center has been established with federal funds to provide medical services to affected individuals. In addition, Libby has been declared a Superfund site and is being cleaned up. In fact, in June 2009 the EPA declared a public health emergency under the Superfund law, the first time such an emergency had been declared.[13] W. R. Grace, the company that operated the mine, has been overwhelmed with lawsuits by injured residents, and the company filed for bankruptcy protection in 2001.[14] It was ordered to pay $250 million to the EPA for environmental cleanup. The EPA has warned that asbestos-containing vermiculite from Libby was used as insulation in millions of homes and businesses across the country and that asbestos fibers could pose a health threat if the insulation is disturbed.

Asbestos exposure concerns also arose as a result of the September 11, 2001, attacks on the World Trade Center. Beginning a few days after the collapse of the towers, the EPA and the New York City and New York State Health Departments monitored pollutants in the air, including asbestos. Concentrations near Ground Zero were quite high in the first few days and weeks after 9/11, but had decreased to background levels by January or February 2002.[15] These exposures were most likely to affect the thousands of rescue and recovery workers who labored at the site; they continue to be monitored for long-term health effects by the New York City Fire Department and the Centers for Disease Control and Prevention (CDC). One study of 12,781 firefighters and emergency medical workers who worked at the site found that they all exhibited significantly reduced lung function during the first year and the decline was persistent. A significant percentage were left with abnormal lung function.[16] Another study found a strong relationship between the rescue worker's arrival time at the World Trade Center after the September 11 attack and lung disease. Those arriving in the morning of September 11, who experienced the strongest exposure, suffered the worst symptoms; those arriving after noon on September 11 or on September 12 suffered less severe symptoms; and those arriving on September 13 or 14 experienced yet less severe symptoms.[17]

Pesticides and Industrial Chemicals

Rachel Carson's best-selling book *Silent Spring*, published in 1962, was a wake-up call to the American public, warning readers that chemicals in the environment cause harm. The publication of her book, more than any other single event, launched the environmental movement that led to sweeping legislation in the 1970s. *Silent Spring* called attention to the harmful effects of the virtually ubiquitous pesticide DDT, which at that time could be found in lakes and streams, plants, and insects. When eaten or drunk by fish and birds, it accumulated in their flesh; when these animals were eaten in turn by predators, the DDT became further concentrated in their own bodies. A worldwide survey measuring chemicals in the body fat of people on six continents found DDT in all of them.[18]

The use of DDT was banned in the United States in 1972. A number of other insecticides chemically related to DDT were also banned in the 1970s. These chemicals—including chlordane, aldrin, mirex, and Kepone—shared common features of solubility in fatty tissue and persistence in the environment: They break down very slowly, so they continue to cause harm long after their use is halted.

Studies looking for environmental pesticides discovered that a related group of chemicals, **polychlorinated biphenyls (PCBs)**, also turned up often. Unlike pesticides, these chemicals were used mainly in sealed systems—capacitors, transformers, and heat exchangers—but were still entering the environment in large quantities and getting into the food chain. PCBs frequently entered the environment through discharge of industrial wastes, a route similar to the mercury contamination of Minamata Bay. The contamination of New York's Hudson River with PCBs, discovered by environmentalists in 1975, was traced to two General Electric Company (GE) capacitor plants that had been discharging large volumes of PCBs into the river for more than 25 years.[19] Although the discharge was halted, the chemicals, unless cleaned up, would have persisted in the soil of the riverbed indefinitely. Even today, fish caught in the Hudson River contain PCBs at concentrations considered unsafe for women of childbearing age and children younger than 15 to eat at all, and for others to eat more than once a week.[20] The EPA developed a plan to clean the river by dredging the contaminated soil, a plan that generated controversy both because it would stir up the chemicals and cause more contamination of the river water in the short term, and because of vigorous objections by the communities proposed as disposal sites for the contaminated soil. After years of dispute, the dredging began in May 2009; the contaminated soil was to be transported by train to a hazardous waste landfill in Texas.[21] The dredging, paid for by GE, continued through 2016 over a 40-mile stretch of the river north of Albany.[22] Post-dredging data collected in 2016 show that PCB levels in the water, soil, and fish tissue were reduced by two-thirds or more through this cleanup effort. However, whether and when the PCB pollution can be considered effectively eliminated remains to be seen.[23]

Environmental scientists believe that PCBs are the most widespread chemical contaminants worldwide. Although production of these chemicals was halted in the United States in 1977, they and their chemical relatives, called persistent organic pollutants (POPs), are carried to remote regions of the globe, including the Arctic, by air, water, and migratory species. The effects on human health of exposure to these chemicals at the levels commonly found in the environment are still uncertain. However, people exposed to large doses of PCBs by a number of industrial accidents were made ill by the chemicals. In western Japan in 1968, a leak at a cooking oil factory contaminated a batch of the rice oil with heat exchanger fluids containing PCBs and related chemicals. Approximately 1800 people were sickened in what became known as the Yusho incident ("Yusho" means oil disease in Japanese).[24] Eleven years later, a similar accident occurred in Taiwan, affecting 2000 people with "Yu-cheng," which means oil disease in Chinese.[25] In the United States, two well-known incidents in the 1970s—a warehouse fire in Puerto Rico that caused PCB contamination of tuna meal used for animal and fish feeds, and a labeling mix-up in Michigan that contaminated cattle feed with polybrominated biphenyls, a chemical similar to PCBs—resulted in human exposure to this type of chemicals through the food supply.[26]

Victims of the Yusho, Yu-cheng, and other incidents have been the subjects of epidemiologic studies tracking the victims' health over the years since their exposure. The most conspicuous and consistent symptom is chloracne—severe skin rashes and discoloration that show up soon after exposure and may persist for years. Other effects include endocrine and immune system defects, fatigue, headaches, and aching joints. Many of these symptoms continue to affect victims more than 30 years after the original exposure.[27] An increased risk of some forms of cancer is now becoming apparent: According to the EPA,

PCBs are potentially carcinogenic in humans and have negative effects on the intellectual development of children and adults.[28] Infants born to Yusho and Yu-cheng mothers were small at birth and had dark discoloration of the skin (leading to the nickname "Coca-Cola babies"), which faded after a few months.[29] These infants suffered developmental delays and persistent cognitive deficits that were still apparent decades later.[30]

Some of the POPs, including dioxins and furans, are not manufactured intentionally but are by-products of some industrial processes. These contaminants of PCBs may have been responsible for some of the toxic effects observed in the Yusho and Yu-cheng incidents. Common pollutants of air and water, they are also produced by the burning of forests or household trash. They are highly toxic, and even relatively small exposures are thought to cause adverse effects on people's immune, endocrine, and neurologic systems. POPs are very stable, remaining in the fatty tissues of fish, animals, and humans indefinitely. Although levels of these chemicals are high in the blood and fatty tissues of people who eat fish from contaminated waters, in most Americans the levels appear to be declining.[31]

In 2001, the United States joined 90 other nations in signing the Stockholm Convention on Persistent Organic Pollutants, agreeing to reduce and/or eliminate the production, use, and release of 12 of the POPs of greatest concern. Since then, 16 new POPs have been added to the list.[32] The convention has been ratified or accepted by nearly all countries in the world except for the United States (Israel, Italy, and Malaysia are the other significant nonratifiers).[33,34]

Other chemicals that have stimulated concern in the last few years include **bisphenol A (BPA)** and phthalates. Both are components of the plastics commonly used in food and drink containers, capable of leaching into the containers' contents and being consumed. Traces of these chemicals are found in the blood of almost everyone in the United States.[35]

BPA is found in hard plastics used to make everything from compact discs to baby bottles and linings of soft drink and food cans.[36] Phthalates are used to produce soft and flexible materials such as vinyl flooring, shower curtains, and some water bottles; they are also used in personal-care products such as soaps, shampoos, hair sprays, and nail polishes.[37] Although government agencies have affirmed the safety of both chemicals at the low levels commonly found in humans, some evidence indicates that they may be especially harmful to infants and developing fetuses.

BPA and phthalates, as well as some POPs, have been shown to be endocrine disruptors in humans and wildlife, meaning that they interfere with normal hormone action in the body. BPA can mimic estrogen, causing early puberty in females and abnormalities in male and female sex organs. Phthalates interfere with testosterone synthesis in males, causing low sperm counts and abnormalities in the development of male sex organs. Some endocrine disruptors may interfere with the activities of the pancreas and thyroid glands, increasing the risk of obesity and diabetes.[35] A study using 1999–2002 data from the National Health and Nutrition Examination Survey found that concentrations of phthalates in the urine of adult American men were associated with increased waist circumference and insulin resistance. Although it does not prove cause and effect, the finding adds to the body of evidence suggesting that exposure to phthalates may contribute to the growing prevalence of obesity and diabetes.[38]

The Endocrine Society, the world's oldest and largest organization devoted to research on hormones and the clinical practice of endocrinology, has issued an "Introduction to Endocrine-Disrupting Chemicals" document that details the known evidence about the health effects of these substances; it strongly recommends that more research should be done to understand their role in the chronic diseases that are so common in the world today.[35] In contrast, the FDA's website in 2019

states: "FDA's current perspective, based on its most recent safety assessment, is that BPA is safe at the current levels occurring in foods. Based on FDA's ongoing safety review of scientific evidence, the available information continues to support the safety of BPA for the currently approved uses in food containers and packaging." Notably, the FDA and industry decided in 2012 and 2013 to ban BPA in baby bottles and sippy cups, and in coatings for packaging of infant formula.[39]

Occupational Exposures: Workers as Guinea Pigs

Workers are regularly exposed to larger amounts of toxic substances on the job than most of the population is ever likely to encounter. Consequently, workers tend to be the first and foremost victims who suffer from any harmful health effects caused by exposures to these chemicals. Many chemicals that all people encounter in everyday life may have unrecognized effects at low doses, causing unexplained cancer, neurologic disorders, and reproductive disorders in susceptible individuals. Workers, because they are often exposed to larger quantities, may inadvertently serve as the guinea pigs that call attention to the dangers.

That certain occupations are associated with an increased risk of certain kinds of cancer has long been known, and this information has been helpful in understanding some of the causes of cancer. The first environmentally caused cancer to be recognized came from an occupational exposure: Scrotal cancer was common in 19th-century English chimney sweeps. The soot to which they were exposed contained the same carcinogens found in tobacco smoke—chemicals that are now known to cause lung cancer. Few other cancers can be clearly linked to specific causative agents. Because most exposures are relatively low, and because the time lag between exposure and the development of cancer is long, cause and effect are difficult to establish. Workers are effective though unintentional guinea pigs because their exposure on the job is likely to be much higher than that in the general environment. An obvious increase in the rate of a specific cancer in a group of workers who have all been exposed to the same substance clearly throws suspicion on that substance as the cause.

Chemicals identified as carcinogens through occupational exposures include benzidine, which caused bladder cancer in dye factory workers; arsenic, which caused lung and lymphatic cancer in copper smelters; and vinyl chloride, used to make some plastics, which causes angiosarcoma, a rare cancer of the liver.[3(Ch.6)] Evidence that radiation exposure causes cancer came from the higher incidence of cancer among radiologists, as discussed earlier. Mesothelioma occurs almost exclusively in asbestos workers, who were also found to have high rates of lung cancer.

Neurotoxins, like carcinogens, may be hard to recognize because they act over a long period of time. In fact, nerve poisons may be even more insidious than carcinogens, because the damage they do—including deterioration of vision, muscle weakness, and failure of memory—may mimic common aspects of aging. Neurologic disorders that typically strike workers with specific exposures call attention to those chemicals as neurotoxins. In addition to mad hatter's disease caused by mercury, nerve damage was found in shoemakers exposed to hexane-containing solvents, dry cleaners exposed to trichloroethylene, pesticide applicators, and many other workers exposed to neurotoxins.[40]

Newer Source of Pollution: Factory Farms

Over the past few decades, there has been a revolution in farming that threatens to overwhelm the system for regulating environmental pollution. Thousands of hogs, cattle, and poultry are crowded into confined spaces where they can be fed and tended to by automated systems. The environmental problems caused by this approach to farming include the huge volumes of waste produced by these animals, which must be disposed of on a relatively limited amount of land. According to Farm Sanctuary, a farm animal rescue and protection organization, **factory farms**, also known as concentrated animal feeding operations (CAFOs), produce an estimated 1 million tons of manure every day, three times the total waste produced by the U.S. human population.[41] The farms deal with waste by creating "lagoons" in which the liquids are allowed to evaporate or from which they are sprayed on fields. Lagoons at many of these operations have broken, failed, or overflowed. They emit gases—including ammonia, hydrogen sulfide, and methane—that can be toxic to humans and contribute to global warming. People living near CAFOs suffer from symptoms caused by the lagoon gases: headaches, runny noses, sore throats, coughing, respiratory problems, nausea, diarrhea, dizziness, burning eyes, depression, and fatigue. Seepage from the lagoons pollutes groundwater that feeds wells used for drinking water. After heavy rains, lagoons may overflow or burst, spilling thousands of gallons of manure into rivers, lakes, streams, and estuaries; such spills have caused massive fish kills in at least 10 states. Water polluted by factory farms contains high levels of nitrate, which has been linked to spontaneous abortions and "blue-baby syndrome," which can kill infants.[42]

Most of these farms are owned by a very few major corporations, which have great economic and political power. In consequence, some state legislatures have passed laws protecting the industry from regulation. In addition, state universities may receive funding from the industry and may discourage research that makes the companies look bad.[43] Under the George W. Bush administration, the EPA and the U.S. Department of Agriculture

(USDA) halted enforcement investigations of the farms and suppressed research results unfavorable to the industry.[44] The farms should be regulated under the Clean Air Act, but the law was never enforced. The Clean Water Act requires large livestock operations to obtain permits, but this law has also been widely ignored.

Congress has repeatedly attempted to protect the corporations from enforcement of existing laws on clean air, clean water, and toxic chemicals. For example, the 2009 bill in the House of Representatives that appropriated funds for the EPA included provisions to block the agency from requiring factory farms to report greenhouse gas emissions.[45] Meanwhile, a number of environmental advocacy organizations, including the Sierra Club, the Environmental Integrity Project, and the Natural Resources Defense Council, sued the EPA in an attempt to force CAFOs to obey environmental laws. In 2010, the EPA agreed to strengthen the rules.[46,47] The Barack Obama administration strengthened these measures further in 2015 through the Waters of the United States rule, which placed stronger controls on the ability of farms to use fertilizers and other chemicals near water runoff areas. In 2019, the Donald Trump administration eliminated this rule, meaning that polluters will now be able to dump harmful substances into streams and wetlands with reduced oversight.[48]

Setting Standards: How Safe Is Safe?

Tens of thousands of synthetic chemicals have been manufactured since World War II and, in the United States alone, 3 to 4 billion pounds of these substances are released into the environment each year. Most have not been tested for the capacity to cause cancer, birth defects, neurologic damage, or other harmful effects on health. Because of the sheer number of chemicals, it is unrealistic to require testing them all.

The environmental legislation of the 1960s and 1970s tried to establish guidelines for identifying environmental hazards and required standards to be set that protected human health and the environment. Standards setting was required for air quality, water quality, radiation safety, food and drug safety, and the disposal of hazardous wastes. The Occupational Safety and Health Act of 1970 empowered the federal government to set standards for workers' exposure to toxic substances, and the Toxic Substances Control Act of 1976 allowed the government to require testing of potentially hazardous substances before they go on the market and to ban them in certain instances. The Federal Insecticide, Fungicide, and Rodenticide Act, originally passed in 1947 and amended several times since then, requires government approval of these substances before they can be used. Congress has also required a variety of federal agencies to set standards for exposure to toxic substances via various routes: The EPA, the FDA, the USDA, the U.S. Department of Transportation, the Nuclear Regulatory Commission, the CPSC, and the Occupational Safety and Health Administration (OSHA) are among the federal organizations responsible for various aspects of environmental health.[3]

Nevertheless, standards setting progressed very slowly after these laws were passed. For example, the Clean Air Act of 1970 required the EPA to develop a list of industrial pollutants that can cause serious health damage and set emission standards for them; as of 1993, only eight had been regulated.[3(Ch.13)] The Clean Air Act amendments of 1990 introduced measures designed to speed up the process.

Regulation tends to progress slowly for a number of reasons. One factor is the sheer volume of potentially toxic chemicals being manufactured in the United States. Today more than 80,000 chemicals are registered for use, with approximately 2000 new ones introduced each year.[49] Another problem is that toxicity testing on any single chemical can be expensive and time-consuming. The EPA has information suggesting that 10% to 15% of the newly introduced chemicals each year need more extensive toxicologic evaluation. The National Toxicology Program (NTP), an interagency program within the U.S. Department of Health and Human Services, can test only a few dozen agents each year, based on the extent of human exposure and/or suspicion of toxicity. One of the NTP's major goals for the 21st century is to develop and validate improved testing methods that will reduce the need for animal testing.

Another reason for the delays in standards setting is that each chemical must be regulated separately, each with the potential for controversy, legal challenge, and extensive litigation over each proposed regulation. Each standard is likely to have significant economic impact on some industry, whose members will naturally fight against the potential threat to their businesses and jobs. Emotions on the part of the public often run high because citizens believe that their health and the health of their children is endangered, yet their demands for safety may be perceived as unreasonable.

Risk–Benefit Analysis

The question "How safe is safe?" has been debated in connection with one potential health threat after another. Increasingly, policy analysts have come to agree that absolute safety is an impossible goal and that attempting to avoid risk of one sort may increase risks of other kinds. Furthermore, as one analyst asks and answers in the affirmative, "Does overregulation cause underregulation?"[50] He argues that too much effort is expended setting very strict standards for too few substances. In battling to achieve zero exposure to one carcinogen, for example, public health agencies may neglect to investigate other chemicals that are potentially more hazardous. Public health may be better served by aiming for looser, more easily achieved standards. This approach

would generate less controversy and opposition, allowing for a stepped-up pace of standards setting.

The argument is also made that prevention of risk must be balanced against other societal goals, including economic well-being. Until recently, the public health approach has ignored economic factors in seeking risk reduction. However, an increasing understanding of the fact that economic factors are significant to people's health and well-being has led to greater willingness on the part of public health advocates to consider costs as well as benefits in evaluating risks.

The Republican Congress elected in 1994 tried to roll back all kinds of regulations based on the argument that they were irrational and expensive, examples of government interference that had negative economic impacts on business. The fact that most of these initiatives failed demonstrated that most Americans want the government to protect their health and environment. At the same time, the initiatives made people ask how regulations could become more rational, less cumbersome, and more balanced. During the Bill Clinton administration, the political debate focused on how to achieve effective environmental protection while minimizing red tape and government intrusiveness. The George W. Bush administration was even more inclined to favor economic and business interests in policy making on environmental and public health issues.

President Obama placed a priority on many environmental issues, especially climate change. The Trump administration is rolling back environmental regulations at an unprecedented rate, seemingly attempting to reverse as many Obama-era regulations as possible. As of September 2019, the Trump administration has completed the rollback of 53 environmental regulations, and was in the process of rolling back 32 more.[51] Some examples of Trump-era rollbacks include ending enforcement of the ban on hydrofluo-rocarbons, a strong greenhouse gas used in air conditioners and refrigerators; weakening car fuel-efficiency standards; withdrawing from the Paris climate agreement; allowing more mercury to be emitted into the environment; allowing more natural gas drilling on public lands; changing the Endangered Species Act to make it more difficult to protect wildlife; rejecting a proposed ban on chlorpyrifos, a pesticide that can harm children; and allow-ing coal companies to dump more mining debris into local streams.[51]

Conclusion

Providing a clean environment, a necessity for human health, is one of the most important functions of government. When people began to live together in cities and towns, they became dependent on the government—traditionally the local government—to provide clean drink-ing water and safe disposal of wastes. As the American population grew, municipalities and industry discharged their wastes into the air, water, and land, and it became apparent that the environment was deteriorating. Pollution tends to spread beyond local areas, requiring state, federal, and international interventions to effectively deal with pollution-related issues. In the late 1960s and early 1970s, a number of significant federal laws were passed in the United States that set standards for air, water, and waste disposal aimed at protecting human health and cleaning up the environment.

Identification of hazards is an important first step in creating a safe environment. While environmental health has traditionally focused on microbial pathogens, many other phenom-ena can threaten human health. Radiation, both natural and human-made, can be highly dangerous to living organisms, something that was not recognized when x-rays were first discovered. Many metals and minerals, including lead, mercury, and asbestos, are toxic to humans. Pesticides and some indus-trial chemicals have been widely disseminated in the environment and have been absorbed into the fatty tissues of animals and humans, where they persist indefinitely, sometimes with harmful effects. Recently, concern has been raised about endocrine disruptors, including BPA and phthalates, common con-taminants of plastics, which are suspected to cause problems with development in fetuses and infants and to increase the risk of com-mon chronic diseases.

Sometimes hazards of environmental exposures are recognized first in workers who develop occupational illnesses after being exposed to chemicals on the job. The effects of a number of cancer-causing and neurotoxic substances have been recognized because workers have served as "guinea pigs," the first humans to test the safety of new chemicals.

In the United States, federal legislation in the 1960s and 1970s established a number of agencies charged with identifying environ-mental hazards and setting standards to pro-tect human health. These agencies include OSHA and the EPA. Standards setting was required for air quality, water quality, radia-tion safety, food and drug safety, the control of toxic substances, and the disposal of haz-ardous wastes. Many of these mandates have proved politically controversial, in that they have economic impact on various industries. Recent trends include greater willingness by public health advocates to weigh costs against benefits in evaluating risks.

Environmentalists have also recognized the hazards of animal wastes from factory farms. These wastes are collected in "lagoons" and may be sprayed on fields, causing air and water pollution. Nearby residents and communities are often powerless to object to the unpleasant odors and, sometimes, toxic fumes. Because of the economic power of agri-cultural companies, federal and state govern-ments have done little to regulate them.

References

1. R. M. Macklis, "The Great Radium Scandal," *Scientific American* (August 1993): 94–99.

2. R. Seltser and P. E. Sartwell, "The Influence of Occupational Exposure to Radiation on the Mortality of American Radiologists and Other Medical Specialists," *American Journal of Epidemiology* 81 (1965): 2–22.

3. A. Nadakavukaren, *Our Global Environment: A Health Perspective*, 7th ed. (Long Grove, IL: Waveland Press, 2011).

4. U.S. Food and Drug Administration, "Advice About Eating Fish," https://www.fda.gov/food/consumers/advice-about-eating-fish, accessed October 4, 2019.

5. U.S. Environmental Protection Agency, "Mercury Releases and Spills," https://www.epa.gov/mercury, accessed October 6, 2019.

6. Centers for Disease Control and Prevention, "Blood Lead Levels in Children" July 30, 2019, https://www.cdc.gov/nceh/lead/prevention/blood-lead-levels.htm, accessed October 4, 2019.

7. E. S. Lipton and D. Barboza, "As More Toys Are Recalled, Trail Ends in China," *The New York Times*, June 19, 2007.

8. U.S. Consumer Product Safety Commission, "Lead in Paint," https://www.cpsc.gov/Business--Manufacturing/Business-Education/Lead-in-Paint/, accessed October 6, 2019.

9. M. N. Mead, "Arsenic: In Search of an Antidote to a Global Poison," *Environmental Health Perspectives* 113 (2005): A379–A386.

10. P. Brodeur, *Outrageous Misconduct: The Asbestos Industry on Trial* (New York, NY: Pantheon Books, 1985).

11. National Institute for Occupational Safety and Health, "NIOSH Recommendations for Limiting Potential Exposures of Workers to Asbestos Associated with Vermiculite from Libby, Montana," October 7, 2014, https://www.cdc.gov/niosh/docs/2003-141/default.html, accessed October 6, 2019.

12. L. A. Peipins, M. Lewin, S. Campolucci, J. A. Lybarger, A. Miller, D. Middleton, et al., "Radiographic Abnormalities and Exposure to Asbestos-Contaminated Vermiculite in the Community of Libby, Montana, USA," *Environmental Health Perspectives* 111 (2003): 1753–1759.

13. C. Dean, "U.S. Cites Emergency in Asbestos-Poisoned Town," *The New York Times*, June 17, 2009.

14. J. M. Broder, "$250 Million Settlement over Asbestos Is Announced," *The New York Times*, March 12, 2008.

15. M. Lorber, H. Gibb, L. Grant, J. Pinto, J. Pleil, D. Cleverly, "Assessment of Inhalation Exposures and Potential Health Risks to the General Population That Resulted from the Collapse of the World Trade Center Towers," *Risk Analysis* 27 (2007): 1203–1221.

16. T. K. Aldrich, J. Gustave, C. B. Hall, H. W. Cohen, M. P. Webber, R. Zeig-Owens, et al., "Lung Function in Rescue Workers at the World Trade Center After 7 Years," *New England Journal of Medicine* 362 (2010): 1263–1272.

17. M. S. Glaser, M. P. Webber, R. Zeig-Owens, J. Weakley, X. Liu, F. Ye, et al., "Estimating the Time Interval Between Exposure to the World Trade Center Disaster and Incident Diagnoses of Obstructive Airway Disease," *American Journal of Epidemiology* 180 (2014): 272–279.

18. M. Wasserman, D. Wasserman, S. Cucos, and H. J. Miller, "World PCBs Map: Storage and Effects in Man and His Biologic Environment in the 1970s," *Annals of the New York Academy of Science* 320 (1979): 69–124.

19. E. G. Horn, L. J. Hetling, T. J. Tofflemire, "The Problem of PCBs in the Hudson River System," *Annals of the New York Academy of Science* 320 (1979): 591–609.

20. New York State Department of Health, "Hudson River: Health Advice on Eating Fish You Catch," March 2014, https://www.health.ny.gov/publications/2794.pdf, accessed October 6, 2019.

21. A. C. Revkin, "Dredging of Pollutants Begins in Hudson," *The New York Times*, May 15, 2009.

22. U.S. Environmental Protection Agency, "News Release: Sixth Season of Hudson River Dredging Begins," May 7, 2015, https://19january2017snapshot.epa.gov/newsreleases/sixth-season-hudson-river-dredging-begins-historic-dredging-project-draws-close-next_.html, accessed October 6, 2019.

23. U.S. Environmental Protection Agency, "Final Second Five-Year Review Report for the Hudson River PCBs Superfund Site," April 11, 2019, https://www.epa.gov/sites/production/files/2019-04/documents/hudson_final_second_five-year_review_report.pdf, accessed October 4, 2019.

24. Y. Masuda, "The Yusho Rice Oil Poisoning Incident," in A. Schecter, *Dioxins and Health* (New York, NY: Plenum Press, 1994), 633–659.

25. C. C. Hsu et al., "The Yu-Cheng Rice Oil Poisoning Incident," in A. Schecter, *Dioxins and Health* (New York, NY: Plenum Press, 1994), 661–684.

26. M. J. Schneider, *Persistent Poisons: Chemical Pollutants in the Environment* (New York, NY: New York Academy of Sciences, 1979).

27. Y. Kanagawa, S. Matsumoto, S. Koike, B. Tajima, N. Fukiwake, S. Shibata, et al., "Association of Clinical Findings in Yusho Patients with Serum Concentrations of Polychlorinated Biphenyls, Polychlorinated Quarterphenyls, and 2,3,4,7,8-Pentachlorodibenzofuran More Than Thirty Years After the Poisoning Event," *Environmental Health* 7 (2008): 47.

28. U.S. Environmental Protection Agency, "Polychlorinated Biphenyls (PCBs)," https://www.epa.gov/pcbs, accessed October 6, 2019.

29. F. Yamashita and M. Hayashi, "Fetal PCB Syndrome: Clinical Features, Intrauterine Growth Retardation and Possible Alteration in Calcium Metabolism," *Environmental Health Perspectives* 59 (1985): 41–45.

30. Y.-L. Guo, G. H. Lambert, and C. C. Hsu, "Growth Abnormalities in the Population Exposed In Utero and Early Postnatally to Polychlorinated Biphenyls and Dibenzofurans," *Environmental Health Perspectives* 103 (1995 suppl 6): 117–122.

31. U.S. Environmental Protection Agency, "Persistent Organic Pollutants: A Global Issue, a Global Response," December 2009, https://www2.epa.gov/international-cooperation/persistent-organic-pollutants-global-issue-global-response, accessed October 6, 2019.

32. Stockholm Convention on Persistent Organic Pollutants, "The 16 New POPs," http://chm.pops.int/TheConvention/ThePOPs/TheNewPOPs/tabid/2511/Default.aspx, accessed October 4, 2019.

33. E. Schor, "Obama Administration Steps up Pressure to Ratify Treaties on Toxics," *The New York Times*, September 24, 2010.

34. United Nations, "Status of Treaties, Stockholm Convention on Persistent Organic Pollutants," https://treaties.un.org/Pages/ViewDetails.aspx?src=IND&mtdsg_no=XXVII-15&chapter=27&clang=_en, accessed October 4, 2019.

35. Endocrine Society, "Introduction to Endocrine Disrupting Chemicals: A Guide for Public Interest Organizations and Policy-Makers," December 2014, https://www.endocrine.org/-/media/endosociety/files/advocacy-and-outreach/important-documents/introduction-to-endocrine-disrupting-chemicals.pdf?la=en, accessed October 4, 2019.

36. Centers for Disease Control and Prevention, "Bisphenol A (BPA) Factsheet," April 7, 2017, https://www.cdc.gov/biomonitoring/BisphenolA_FactSheet.html, accessed October 6, 2019.

37. Centers for Disease Control and Prevention, "Phthalates Factsheet," April 7, 2017, https://www.cdc.gov/biomonitoring/Phthalates_FactSheet.html, accessed October 6, 2019.

38. R. W. Stahlhut, E. van Wijngaarden, T. D. Dye, S. Cook, and S. H. Swan, "Concentrations of Urinary Phthalate Metabolites Are Associated with Increased Waist Circumference and Insulin Resistance in Adult U.S. Males," *Environmental Health Perspectives* 115 (2007): 876–882.

39. U.S. Food and Drug Administration, "Bisphenol A (BPA): Use in Food Contact Application," June 27, 2018, https://www.fda.gov/food/food-additives-petitions/bisphenol-bpa-use-food-contact-application, accessed October 4, 2019.

40. P. Spencer and H. H. Schaumburg, eds., *Experimental and Clinical Neurotoxicology* (Baltimore, MD: Williams & Wilkins, 1980).

41. Farm Sanctuary, "Factory Farming," https://www.farmsanctuary.org/learn/factory-farming/, accessed October 6, 2019.

42. Natural Resources Defense Council, "Livestock Production," https://www.nrdc.org/issues/livestock-production, accessed October 6, 2019.

43. S. Wing, "Social Responsibility and Research Ethics in Community-Driven Studies of Industrialized Hog Production," *Environmental Health Perspectives* 110 (2002): 437–444.

44. R. F. Kennedy Jr. and E. Schaeffer, "An Ill Wind from Factory Farms," *The New York Times*, September 20, 2003.

45. R. Bravender et al., "Farm Interests Use EPA Spending Bill to Fight Climate Regs," *The New York Times*, June 19, 2009.

46. S. N. Bhanoo, "Tougher E.P.A. Action on Factory Farms," *The New York Times*, May 28, 2010.

47. U.S. Environmental Protection Agency, "Proposed NPDES CAFO Reporting Rule," October 14, 2011, https://www3.epa.gov/npdes/pubs/2011_npdes_cafo_factsheet.pdf, accessed October 6, 2019.

48. L. Friedman and C. Davenport, "Trump Administration Rolls Back Clean Water Protections," *The New York Times*, September 19, 2019.

49. U.S. Department of Health and Human Services, National Toxicology Program, "About NTP," August 19, 2019, https://ntp.niehs.nih.gov/whoweare/about/index.html, accessed July 26, 2015.

50. J. Mendeloff, "Does Overregulation Cause Underregulation? The Case of Toxic Substances," *Regulation* (September–October 1981).

51. N. Popovich, L. Albeck-Ripka, and K. Pierre-Louis, "85 Environmental Rules Being Rolled Back Under Trump," *The New York Times*, September 12, 2019.

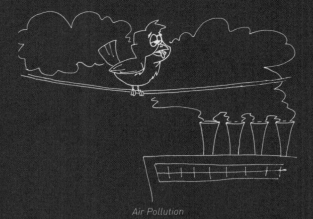

CHAPTER 21

Air Pollution

Clean Air: Is It Safe to Breathe?

KEY TERMS

Carbon dioxide
Chlorofluorocarbons (CFCs)
Clean Air Act
Criteria air pollutants

Emergency Planning and
Community Right-to-Know
Act (EPCRA)

Emissions standards
Greenhouse gases
Ozone layer

Air pollution caused by coal burning was a problem in London as early as the 17th century. With the advent of the Industrial Revolution in the 18th and 19th centuries, the air of many cities became blackened with smoke from industrial and household furnaces and railroad locomotives. In 1952, an unusual weather pattern caused a particularly severe air pollution crisis in London. A layer of cold, moist air hung motionless over the city for five days, and smoke, fumes, and motor vehicle exhaust accumulated. More than 4000 deaths from both respiratory and heart disease were attributed to the foul air. Britain's first clean air act was passed soon afterward.[1(Ch.13)]

In 1948, the United States had been shocked by a similar deadly air pollution crisis caused by a similar weather pattern. A five-day atmospheric inversion trapped smoke and fumes in a heavily industrialized Pennsylvania valley. In the small town of Donora, population 14,000, residents suffered eye, nose, and throat irritation and breathing difficulties resulting in 20 deaths.[1] The event drew national attention and helped raise awareness about the health consequences of air pollution. In 2008, on the 60th anniversary of this crisis, the town opened the Donora Smog Museum with the slogan "Clean Air Starts Here."[2]

For most cities, the effects of air pollution were not so dramatic, but air quality noticeably began deteriorating in the United States during the 1950s and 1960s. Increasingly, this trend was attributed to automobiles. Los Angeles became known for its photochemical smog, the yellowish-brown haze caused by intense sunlight acting on the complex mix of chemicals emitted in motor vehicle exhaust. The irritating effects of air pollution were obvious to everyone and were especially harmful to the health of children and people with heart and lung diseases.

Efforts by cities and states to regulate pollutant emissions proved unsuccessful, and the federal government began attacking the problem in the mid-1960s. The first emission standards for automobiles were passed in 1965, and took effect with 1968 model-year cars. The **Clean Air Act** established strict air quality standards, set limits on several major pollutants, and mandated reduction of automobile and factory emissions. Since then, improving air quality has been an almost constant political battle. Environmental and public health groups have pressed for compliance and ever stricter standards, while industries, supported by political conservatives, argue that the cost of pollution control is too high, hurting the nation's economy. Amendments to the Clean Air Act, strengthening some air quality regulations, were passed in 1977 and 1990. In general, the United States has cleaner air now than it did in 1970, but the battle is far from over.[1(Ch.13)]

Criteria Air Pollutants

The Clean Air Act and its amendments require monitoring and regulation of six common air pollutants, called **criteria air pollutants**, known to be harmful to health and the environment: particulates, sulfur dioxide, carbon monoxide, nitrogen oxides, ozone, and lead.[1(Ch.13)] All of these substances enter the air as a result of combustion—for energy in power plants or motor vehicles, or for solid waste disposal or industrial processes.

Particulate matter is the most visible form of air pollution—the smoke, soot, and ash that were so typical of the Industrial Revolution. Aesthetically, particulate matter is objectionable because it reduces visibility, forms layers of grime on buildings and streets, and corrodes metals. Epidemiologic studies have shown that particulates in the air also have harmful health effects. A groundbreaking cohort study conducted by Harvard epidemiologists compared the health of adults and children over the period 1975 to 1988 in six cities with markedly different amounts of particulate pollution in their air.[3] Residents of Steubenville, Ohio, the most polluted city in the study, were more likely to suffer from respiratory symptoms and had poorer lung function than residents of Portage, Wisconsin, the least polluted city. In addition, death rates in Steubenville were 26% higher than those in Portage. In a larger study of 151 cities, researchers found that death rates were increased by 15% in the cities with the dirtiest air.

Early air pollution regulation focused on limiting total particulate matter in the atmosphere. However, a number of studies, including the Harvard researchers' study of six cities, suggest that the smallest particles are the most dangerous because they can evade the body's natural defenses and penetrate deeply into the lungs, becoming a chronic source of irritation. In 1987, the Environmental Protection Agency (EPA) revised the air pollution standard to limit emissions of the smaller particles—those with a diameter less than 10 micrometers (PM10). In 1997, and again in 2006, the EPA focused on even smaller particles, issuing increasingly stringent limits for particles smaller than 2.5 micrometers (PM2.5). In 2012, the agency proposed a further strengthening of PM2.5. States have until 2020 to meet the new standards.[4]

Opponents of stricter regulations vigorously sought to discredit the six-city study and other data, but the evidence base has only grown stronger, showing increased hospitalizations and deaths associated with higher levels of the smallest particles. Opponents of the 1997 PM2.5 standard sued the EPA, demanding a cost–benefit analysis for implementing the new rules.[5] In 2001, the U.S. Supreme Court ruled unanimously that a cost–benefit analysis was not necessary and that the EPA must consider only public health and safety in setting the standards.[6] The importance of the PM2.5 level was affirmed in several other studies. In 2007, one large study, the Women's Health Initiative, found that every increase of 10 micrograms per cubic meter in PM2.5 almost doubled the risk of death from cardiovascular disease.[7] Another study examined the effect on infant health of the introduction of electronic toll collection technology (in this case, E-Z Pass) in New Jersey and Pennsylvania, which caused a sudden large reduction in air pollution near traffic toll plazas that had been caused by idling, decelerating, and accelerating traffic in these areas. Comparing mothers who lived less than 2 kilometers from toll plazas with mothers who lived 2 to 10 kilometers from toll plazas showed that preterm births decreased by about 7% and low birth weight decreased by about 10% for the less-than-2 kilometer mothers compared to the 2-to-10 kilometer mothers.[8]

Sulfur dioxide is produced by combustion of sulfur-containing fuels, especially coal. Although it irritates the respiratory tract, its most significant impact is as a precursor to acid rain, a major threat to the environment. Sulfur dioxide reacts with water vapor to form sulfuric acid; it also tends to stick to fine particulates in the air. Both of these mechanisms increase this pollutant's potential to cause respiratory damage.[1] Sulfur dioxide levels, which are highest in the vicinity of large industrial facilities, declined by 91% between 1980 and 2018.[9]

Carbon monoxide is a highly toxic gas, most of which is produced in motor vehicle exhaust. It interferes with the oxygen-carrying capacity of the blood and is therefore especially harmful to patients with cardiovascular disease, who are more likely to suffer heart attacks when exposed to higher concentrations of this pollutant. Carbon monoxide also affects the brain, causing headaches and impairing mental processes. Average carbon monoxide levels, which generally are highest in areas of high traffic congestion, decreased by 83% between 1980 and 2018.[9]

Nitrogen oxides are the chemicals responsible for the yellowish-brown appearance of smog. Like sulfur dioxide, nitrogen oxides are respiratory irritants that contribute to acid rain. They also contribute to the formation of ozone. The main sources of nitrogen oxides are on-road motor vehicle exhaust, off-road equipment, and power plant emissions. Nitrogen oxide levels declined by 65% between 1980 and 2018.[9]

Ozone, a highly reactive variant of oxygen, is produced by photochemical reactions in which sunlight acts on other air pollutants, including nitrogen oxides. This gas is very irritating to the eyes and to the respiratory system, and chronic exposure can cause permanent damage to the lungs. A study of 95 large urban communities in the United States, published in 2004, found that even short-term increases in ozone levels lead to increases in mortality from cardiovascular and respiratory diseases.[10]

Ozone levels in the air are an indicator of various other chemicals produced by motor vehicles, and they are often used as a general measure of air pollution. As discussed later, ozone is an important protective component of the upper atmosphere, but at low altitudes its effects are harmful. Although ozone levels tend to be high in many urban areas, many rural and wilderness areas may also be affected, as the wind can carry this pollutant hundreds of miles from its original source. Maximum ozone levels in the United States decreased 31% between 1980 and 2018.[9] However, in 2008, the National Parks Conservation Association and the Environmental Defense Fund filed suit to force the EPA to clean up emissions responsible for the haze that obscures the views in many national parks.[11] In 2015, the EPA strengthened the standards for ozone, though President Donald Trump's administration is attempting to roll back these regulations.[12,13]

Lead is a highly toxic metal that can damage the nervous system, blood, and kidneys; it poses a special risk to the development of children's intellectual abilities. In the past, the main source of lead as an air pollutant was the use of leaded gasoline, which was phased out in the United States by 1995.[1(Ch.13)] While environmental lead from other sources remains a threat to children, the amount of lead in the air has decreased dramatically, having dropped by 99% between 1980 and 2018.[9]

When an area does not meet the air quality standard for one of the criteria pollutants, the EPA may designate it as a nonattainment area and may impose measures designed to force the area to meet the standard. According to the EPA, 114 areas in 42 states, Puerto Rico, and the District of Columbia were classified as nonattainment areas for one or more criteria pollutants as of 2019.[14] Poor air quality due to excessive ozone levels is especially widespread, affecting broad areas in California, Texas, the East Coast from Boston to Atlanta, and parts of the Midwest. In 2018, 141 million people, representing 43% of the U.S. population, were exposed to polluted air, up from 124 million people in 2010.[15,16]

In addition to the criteria air pollutants, which are widespread, a large number of other toxic and carcinogenic chemicals are released into the air by local factories, waste disposal sites, and other sources. The Clean Air Act of 1970 directed the EPA to identify and set **emissions standards** for such hazards. In the years since this law's passage, the EPA has slowly added standards for new toxins, which now cover asbestos, mercury, beryllium, benzene, coke-oven emissions, and a host of others.[17] Legal battles over each standard have made progress on this front painfully slow.

The Clean Air Act amendments passed in 1990 contained a number of provisions designed to speed up this process. Congress identified 187 specific chemicals for the EPA to regulate. Rather than addressing each chemical individually, however, the agency was charged with identifying major sources that emit these pollutants and developing technical standards to reduce the emissions. Since then, the EPA has issued rules covering more than 80 categories of major industrial sources, including chemical plants, oil refineries, aerospace manufacturers, and steel mills, as well as categories of smaller sources such as dry cleaners.[17] It has also identified 30 toxic air pollutants that pose the greatest threats to public health in the largest number of urban areas and developed health risk assessments on them.[17]

Strategies for Meeting Standards

Motor vehicles are the primary source of air pollution in urban areas, and the number of motor vehicles is increasing far more rapidly than the population. The standard approach for limiting air pollution from motor vehicles has been to limit tailpipe emissions by mandating changes both in automobile engineering and in fuel. Significant improvement was achieved by the use of catalytic converters, devices that have been repeatedly improved to meet increasingly strict standards. The newest cars have reduced emissions of carbon monoxide and ozone-producing chemicals by approximately 90% and of nitrogen oxides by 70% below those of cars without emission controls.[1(Ch.13)] In addition, the ban on leaded gasoline has almost eliminated lead as an air pollutant.

Because of the continuing increase in the number of cars, however, and because older cars and poorly maintained vehicles continued to emit high levels of pollutants, a number of other requirements were included in the 1990 Clean Air Act amendments. Special attention was paid to geographic areas that failed to meet standards for one or more criteria pollutants. These requirements include installation of vapor recovery systems on gasoline pumps, and inspection and maintenance programs that require annual measurement of tailpipe emissions on each car, with mandatory remediation of cars that fail the test. Another mandate called for automakers to develop and market "zero-emission" vehicles—electric cars. This goal is beginning to be achieved, owing to the increasingly popular hybrid vehicles. Complicating efforts to reduce tailpipe emissions has been the increase in the number of pickup trucks and sport-utility vehicles (SUVs), to which the standards for passenger cars did not apply. In the 1990s, the rules were changed to require all new vehicles to meet the same standards by 2009, but vehicles manufactured under the old rules will still be on the road for many years.[1(Ch.13)]

In 2012, the Barack Obama administration established tighter rules requiring cars to have an average fuel efficiency of 54.5 miles per gallon for the 2025 model year. However, in 2018, the Trump administration announced that it would freeze this increase at 37 miles per gallon starting with the 2021 model year. This freeze has set up a major confrontation between the Trump administration and California and 19 other states (both Democratic- and Republican-leaning, including Colorado, Nevada, North Carolina, and Pennsylvania) that wish to set their own state-level fuel efficiency standards. Because these 20 states represent the majority of the U.S. car market, and because it is quite costly for car makers to make different variations of their cars, a large state like California or a coalition of states working together on a standard can exert great influence over car makers' emissions design decisions. The Trump administration is attempting to prevent these states from setting their own rules, and the legal battle is now working its way through the courts. It is expected to eventually be decided by the U.S. Supreme Court.[18,19]

Ideally, the number of cars on the road in highly populated areas should be reduced. Public transportation undoubtedly benefits air quality in New York City and Washington, D.C., but too many American cities—including Los Angeles—are not designed for efficient public systems. While Americans support most measures to ensure cleaner air, they consistently resist efforts to move them out of their private automobiles. Many urban areas have developed, with modest success, policies to encourage carpooling by providing high-occupancy vehicle lanes and by taxing parking spaces. Substantially higher taxes on gasoline, such as those in most European and Asian countries, would undoubtedly discourage unnecessary driving; however, raising gas taxes seems to be considered political suicide by most U.S. politicians. Developing efficient public transport systems will require public funds—and the accompanying dreaded increase in taxes. Spikes in gasoline prices in the early 21st century had some beneficial effects in encouraging people to buy smaller, more fuel-efficient, and less polluting vehicles. However when gasoline prices fell, the popularity of SUVs and vans surged again.

A variety of strategies have been effective in reducing industrial sources of pollution. Foremost among them have been installation of scrubbers on smokestacks and a move to less-polluting fuels, especially the transition away from high-sulfur coal. A new approach included in the 1990 Clean Air Act amendments is the creation of pollution allowances that can be bought and sold. Instead of requiring each factory or power plant to meet defined standards, an overall national or regional emissions goal is set, and that goal is moved lower each year. Each potential polluter is assigned a fraction of that amount as an allowance, which can be used or sold. Plants that choose to clean up their technology can recoup some of their investment by selling their allowances to plants that find such cleanup too expensive. This market approach was expected to achieve Clean Air Act goals with a maximum of flexibility and a minimum of political pain.[1(Ch.13)]

One provision of the 1977 Clean Air Act amendments that has generated a great deal of controversy is called "New Source Review." When the original Clean Air Act was passed in 1970, it set standards for newly built power plants but did not require changes to existing plants. Because this provision prompted companies to improve their existing facilities without cleaning up their emissions, the 1977 rules required that companies that substantially upgraded their old plants had to bring them into compliance with the standards. Many companies, however, ignored the rules. In the mid-1990s, after years of negotiations with the industry, the Bill Clinton administration sued seven electric utility companies in the Midwest and the South to force them to comply with the law and launched investigations of dozens of others.

When President George W. Bush took office in 2001, his administration responded to the complaints of the utilities by setting out to weaken the environmental laws. In 2002, the president proposed the "Clear Skies Initiative," which replaced the New Source Review requirement with a market-based trading system that clearly set weaker emissions standards than those required by the Clean Air Act. Congress did not act on the proposal, so the Bush administration began to administratively change the rules. It also dropped the investigations of noncompliant companies. In 2003, the attorneys general of 15 states, in cooperation with national environmental organizations, filed their own lawsuits against a number of the polluting power plants. Most of the states that sued were located in the Northeast, where the air is polluted by emissions blown in from the Midwest. The legal battles continued throughout Bush's term in office; by the end of his term, the New Source Review rule was still in place, but power plant emissions were still major sources of pollution.[20,21]

To address these shortcomings, in 2015, the Obama administration implemented the Clean Power Plan, which requires states to reduce carbon emissions by 2022, including closing heavily polluting coal-burning power plants and switching power generation to natural gas and renewable energy sources. The Clean Power Plan was expected to significantly reduce U.S. greenhouse gas emissions. In 2017, the Trump administration announced that it would roll back these coal plant restrictions. In response, a coalition of 29 states, led by California, filed a lawsuit to block this action. As with Trump's motor vehicle emissions rollback, the power plant lawsuit is expected to go all the way to the U.S. Supreme Court.[22]

The George W. Bush administration also issued rules on mercury pollution by coal-burning power plants that were later found by the courts to be inadequate and ineffective. The Bush rules used the same cap-and-trade system that has been effective for limiting air pollutants that disperse in the atmosphere; mercury, however, is heavy and tends to settle near the source of emission, causing local deposits that pollute soil and surface waters. Power plants, which produce more than 40% of mercury emissions, had lobbied heavily against strict rules requiring state-of-the-art technology at each site. The Obama administration promised to tighten the rules for mercury in accordance with the court order.[23] In turn, the EPA proposed stricter rules for emissions of mercury and other pollutants from coal-burning power plants in 2011.[24] The Trump administration is attempting to roll back these rules as well.[13]

One notable exception to Bush's attempts to weaken air quality rules occurred in May 2004, when the administration announced rules that would require vehicles using diesel fuel to meet stricter standards on emissions. Engine makers are required to install emission control systems, and refineries are required to produce cleaner-burning diesel fuel. These regulations, which took effect in 2012, apply to nonroad vehicles such as tractors, bulldozers, locomotives, and barges, as well as to buses and trucks. The change was expected to significantly cut emissions of particulate matter and, because diesel fuel contains high concentrations of sulfur, to decrease levels of sulfur dioxide in the air, helping to reduce acid rain.[1(Ch.13)] To date, this program has been something of a disappointment, because there are many more older, polluting diesel engines in use than newer, clean ones. In 2005, Congress authorized funding to retrofit old engines with a filter that reduces soot emissions. Due to budget-cutting fervor, however, the funding has not been sufficient to significantly reduce the health risks from diesel exhaust.[25]

A modest law that took effect in 1988, the **Emergency Planning and Community Right-to-Know Act (EPCRA)**, has had unexpectedly beneficial effects in prodding companies to voluntarily restrict their discharge of air pollutants. This law was passed in response to the infamous Bhopal disaster of 1984, in which a leak of isocyanate gas occurred at a Union Carbide pesticide factory in India, killing more than 10,000 people who lived nearby. EPCRA requires businesses to report the locations and quantities of chemicals stored at their sites. This information allows communities to better prepare for emergencies such as leaks and chemical spills. The law also requires that manufacturers disclose information on the kinds and amounts of toxic pollutants they discharge into the local environment each year.[26] Frequently, local communities, alarmed by this information, pressure the resident industries to cut back on their emissions. The program, known as the Toxics Release Inventory, is credited with reducing industrial releases of toxic chemicals in the United States by 54.5% between 1988 and 2001 and by another 33% between 2001 and 2013.[27,28]

Even before the terrorist attacks on September 11, 2001, some industries were pressuring the EPA to relax the EPCRA requirements, claiming, among other reasons, that publication of such information would increase communities' vulnerability to terrorism. Since September 11, the EPA has gone much further in trying to restrict public access to environmental information. Some critics claim that the terrorism argument is being used as a smokescreen to protect industry from lawsuits or bad publicity. As one of these critics noted, "What's tricky is finding the right balance between protection from terrorists on one hand and providing information for the neighbors so they can be safe."[29(p.107)]

The urban areas that are having the most difficulty meeting air quality standards by requiring controls on motor vehicles and factories must consider regulating sources of pollution that have thus far been left alone. For example, Los Angeles banned the use of charcoal lighter fluid for barbecues and regulates the exhaust of gas-powered lawnmowers. Dry cleaners, auto body shops, and furniture refinishers are also significant sources of toxic air pollutants that are regulated in the Los Angeles area.[30] In 2004, this region announced a program through which residents could turn in old gasoline lawnmowers in exchange for new, nonpolluting electric mowers.[31] California still struggles with pollution associated with its ports, caused by both cargo ships and the trucks that crowd the dock areas to move imported goods inland. The area's air pollution control agency in 2012 awarded $4.8 million to replace 163 older diesel trucks with newer, cleaner models.[32] In 2015, the agency announced the "Replace Your Ride" program, which provides up to $9500 to low-income residents for the replacement of their old vehicles with newer, less polluting ones.[33]

On a national scale, the Obama administration's 2009 program, nicknamed "Cash for Clunkers," provided rebates to people who turned in old vehicles for new, more fuel-efficient ones. It proved popular and helped to reduce pollution in areas with high emissions from motor vehicles.[34]

Overall, the United States has made substantial progress in fighting air pollution. As shown in **Figure 21-1**, emissions of most common pollutants have decreased significantly since 1970 despite significant increases in the nation's population and economic growth. In Los Angeles, concentrations of ozone—historically the most difficult pollutant to control—are now less than half of the mid-1970s levels; even so, ozone levels in Los Angeles air violated federal standards on 119 days per year, on average, between 2015 and 2017.[35]

Indoor Air Quality

While most public concern and political action have focused on outdoor air pollution, the 1980s saw increased attention paid to indoor air quality. In fact, most people spend more time indoors than outside, and concentrations

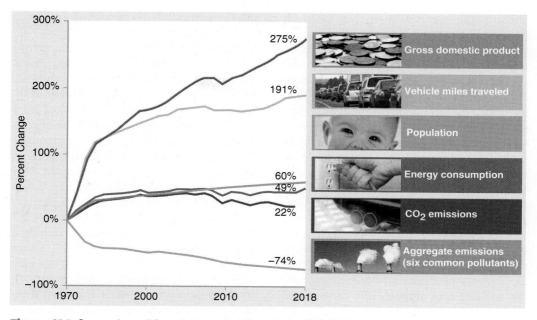

Figure 21-1 Comparison of Growth Areas and Emissions, 1970–2018

Reproduced from U.S. Environmental Protection Agency, https://gispub.epa.gov/air/trendsreport/2019/#growth_w_cleaner_air, accessed October 6, 2019.

of many pollutants trapped inside a building may exceed those outdoors in all but the most polluted cities. The problem is exacerbated by energy conservation measures that minimize the quantity of outdoor air allowed inside. In the extreme, a lack of sufficient ventilation may lead to "sick building syndrome," in which building occupants develop an array of symptoms that disappear when they go outdoors.

The most common indoor air pollutants are tobacco smoke, other products of combustion, radon gas, consumer products that release chemicals into the air, and biological pollutants, including bacteria, mold, dust mites, and animal dander. "Second-hand smoke" has become a political issue in recent years, and many states now ban smoking in various public places. In the homes of smokers— beyond the arm of laws and regulations— tobacco smoke may be the most significant air pollutant and the main source of particulate pollution for children. Smoking also increases levels of carbon monoxide in indoor air and

is a source of benzene, which is toxic and carcinogenic. Wood-burning stoves and fireplaces emit significant amounts of particulate matter and gases into the air. Gas ranges and furnaces burn more cleanly than wood stoves, but they produce carbon monoxide and nitrogen oxides.[1(Ch. 13)]

Radon is a radioactive gas emitted by the decay of radium and uranium. It has long been known to be a major health threat to uranium miners, who have a high risk of developing lung cancer. Then in 1984, a nuclear power plant worker set off radiation detection alarms on his way *into* the plant, near Philadelphia.[1(Ch. 13)] Investigation of his home found that radon gas levels there were 1000 times higher than normal. Since that discovery, elevated radon levels have been found in homes in most states; an estimated 1 of 15 homes in the United States has concentrations above the standard set by EPA.

The health threat from indoor radon pollution is not clear. The EPA and most other public health agencies assert that, based on extrapolation of the evidence obtained by studying uranium miners, radon in the home must be regarded as a serious cancer threat, causing an estimated 21,000 lung cancer deaths annually.[1(Ch.13)] Skeptics suggest that these estimates are too high, noting that miners' effective exposure is much greater than what is measured, because the radon adheres to dust particles that lodge in their lungs. In miners, smoking acts synergistically with radon to cause lung cancer, meaning that the risk to miners who smoke is many times greater than that of the average smoking non-miner or nonsmoking miner. By analogy, the danger of radon in homes would be greatly enhanced if the residents are smokers.

Radon enters homes by seeping up from the soil and rock through dirt floors, crawl spaces, cracks in cement floors and walls, and sump holes and floor drains. It may dissolve in well water and be released into the air during showers or baths. Measurement of radon is easily done with inexpensive kits and, in most homes where elevated levels are found, measures to seal cracks and openings are effective in reducing levels.

Other common indoor air pollutants include formaldehyde, a possibly carcinogenic gas that irritates the respiratory system and is contained in insulation, particleboard, plywood, some floor coverings and textiles, and tobacco smoke. In the past, elevated levels of formaldehyde were common in prefabricated and mobile homes. Although the U.S. Department of Housing and Urban Development requires that plywood and particleboard must conform to specified emissions limits, formaldehyde turned out to be a significant problem in mobile homes supplied by the Federal Emergency Management Agency (FEMA) to victims of the 2005 hurricanes Katrina and Rita. Since then, the Sierra Club and other organizations have noted that high levels of formaldehyde are more widespread in manufactured housing than previously thought,

and the Sierra Club has petitioned the EPA to tighten regulations.[36]

Drywall imported from China turned out to be a significant source of foul odors and health complaints in newly built houses, especially in those built in 2006 and 2007 during the housing boom that resulted from the hurricanes. The problem with the drywall appears to be emissions of sulfur compounds that also cause corrosion of metal objects in the homes. Thousands of lawsuits were filed as a result. The Consumer Product Safety Commission conducted an investigation, confirmed the problems, and recommended steps to be taken for remediation, including removing the problem drywall.[37-39] Other chemicals that may pollute indoor air and may have adverse health effects include pesticides, dry-cleaning solvents, paints and paint thinners, carpet glues, hair spray, and air fresheners. While most biological air pollutants, such as mold, house mites, and animal dander, are a problem only for people who are allergic to them, airborne microbes can pose serious health hazards: Witness Legionnaire's disease, an infection caused by bacteria vaporized from air-conditioning systems, and hantavirus released into the air from rodent urine or feces.

Global Effects of Air Pollution

Because air pollutants are the most mobile of all forms of pollution, their ill effects may spread far beyond the immediate area where they are released. In fact, a mounting body of evidence indicates that human activities are actually changing the composition of the atmosphere. The ultimate effects on public health from these changes remain a matter of speculation and controversy, but it has become clear that the effects may be quite harmful.

Acid rain is produced when two common air pollutants—sulfur dioxide and nitrogen dioxide—react with water to form sulfuric acid and nitric acid. In the United States, the industrial areas of the Midwest are a major source of the pollutants that acidify rainfall in the East, since prevailing winds blow from west to east. Acid rain in eastern Canada resulting from U.S. air pollution has been a cause of diplomatic tension between the two countries. The environment in Europe, the former Soviet Union, and southern China—everywhere that coal and oil are intensively used—is also seriously affected by acid rain.

Acid rain damages forests, reduces crop yields, and corrodes surfaces of buildings and statuary. It turns the water in lakes and rivers acidic, killing freshwater shrimp, wiping out bacteria on lake bottoms, and interfering with fish reproduction. Some lakes are so acidic that they can no longer support life: All fish species disappear in these bodies of water, as do most frogs, salamanders, and aquatic insects. Because many metals, such as aluminum, lead, copper, and mercury, are soluble in acid, the increasing acidity of water may lead to toxic levels of metals in drinking water supplies. Evidence indicates that regulations on industrial pollutants in the United States have helped decrease levels of sulfur dioxide and nitrogen oxides in the air and reduced the acidity of rainfall in the Northeast, but there is still wide geographic variation. EPA data show that 91% of monitoring sites in the Adirondack Mountains showed an improving acidification trend; 58% to 67% of sites in Maine, the Catskills region of New York, the North Appalachian Plateau of Pennsylvania, and Vermont showed improvement; but only 11% of sites in the Central Appalachians showed improvement.[40]

Depletion of the **ozone layer** is another manifestation of the global effects of certain air pollutants. Ozone, which is highly harmful to respiratory systems at ground level, is a natural component of the upper atmosphere that provides a layer of protection against ultraviolet radiation from the sun. The detection of **chlorofluorocarbons (CFCs)** in the ozone "hole" that opened over Antarctica in the early 1980s convinced scientists that these chemicals, which were used as refrigerants and spray-can propellants, were responsible for the breakdown of ozone. Because they are very stable, CFCs drift upward to the ozone layer, where they may cause damage for many decades. The increased ultraviolet radiation that reaches ground level through the thinner ozone layer is causing greatly increased rates of cataracts, already a major cause of blindness in the world, and skin cancer. It also has harmful effects on other organisms, including food crops, and could be a major threat to life on the planet.

This global problem clearly required international action. After several years of controversy and denial, diplomats from 29 nations met in Montreal, Canada, in 1987 to sign an agreement aimed at reducing the production and use of CFCs.[1(Ch.11)] As evidence of ozone depletion continued to mount, the Montreal Protocol was strengthened several times, and now calls for the elimination of chemicals that deplete ozone. The protocol has been signed by 197 nations, the first treaty in the history of the United Nations to achieve universal ratification.[41] The United States has ended production of CFCs and many other ozone-depleting substances, but millions of pounds of CFCs already in use will continue to be released into the atmosphere for years to come. The ozone layer appears to have stabilized, but there is still uncertainty about its prospects for the future.[42]

Carbon dioxide is not strictly an air pollutant—along with nitrogen, oxygen, and argon, it is one of the four major components of the atmosphere—but its increasing proportion in the air has ominous implications for the future of the earth's environment. Carbon dioxide levels have been rising since the beginning of the Industrial Revolution due to the burning of fossil fuels. They are now more than 45% higher than they were at the beginning of the Industrial Revolution, and are increasing rapidly.[43,44]

Atmospheric carbon dioxide acts like the glass of a greenhouse, allowing sunlight to enter but trapping the heat inside. The resulting "greenhouse effect" leads to warmer temperatures at the earth's surface. A growing body of evidence suggests that global warming is already under way. It has been hard to definitively prove that the average temperature of the earth's surface is increasing because of the normal fluctuations from year to year and even from one decade to another, but the evidence is now quite strong that the average temperature of the earth increased by about 1.6°F between 1880 and 2018.[43] The temperature is expected to continue increasing, with the extent of warming depending on how successful we are in curbing further emissions of **greenhouse gases**.

Conclusion

Air pollution, while a conspicuous problem in cities for more than two centuries, was recognized as a severe threat to health in the 1940s and 1950s. During this era, weather-related events together with smoke from the burning of fossil fuels in England and the United States caused local air pollution crises that led to deaths from respiratory and heart disease.

Because air pollution does not respect political boundaries, interventions, to be effective, must be implemented on a national and sometimes global scale. The United States began establishing regulations to control air pollution beginning in the 1960s. Regulations on both automobile and factory emissions have been repeatedly strengthened since the Clean Air Act of 1970. Each new standard has been highly controversial, opposed by industry, congressional conservatives, and some presidential administrations. For example, the Obama administration signaled an intention to support stricter rules against air pollution, but those efforts were later undone by the Trump administration.

The Clean Air Act identified six criteria air pollutants: particulate matter, sulfur dioxide, carbon monoxide, nitrogen oxides, ozone, and lead. These pollutants must be monitored by the EPA, and their levels in the air have fallen since 1970. A larger number of other chemicals have also been identified as toxic pollutants. The Clean Air Act amendments of 1990 required the EPA to identify major sources of these emissions and to set emission standards for the source categories rather than for individual pollutants.

Strategies for meeting air pollution standards include technological improvements in motor vehicles and factory smokestacks. Congress has encouraged a flexible approach by creating pollution allowances that can be bought and sold, permitting industries to cooperate in meeting the standards. Requirements that industries disclose information on their emissions often result in pressure on companies from local communities to reduce the pollution.

Indoor air may have even more significant effects on health than outdoor air does, since most people spend more time indoors than outside, and many indoor pollutants are trapped inside buildings at high concentrations. Common indoor air pollutants include tobacco smoke, radon gas, consumer products that release chemicals into the air, and biological pollutants such as bacteria and mold.

Air pollution can create acid rain, which profoundly affects the environment. Depletion of the ozone layer by CFCs increases the risk of skin cancer and cataracts and has harmful effects on other organisms. Increases in carbon dioxide concentrations in the air lead to the greenhouse effect, resulting in global warming.

References

1. A. Nadakavukaren, *Our Global Environment: A Health Perspective*, 7th ed. (Long Grove, IL: Waveland Press, 2011).

2. S. D. Hamill, "Unveiling a Museum, a Pennsylvania Town Remembers the Smog That Killed 20," *The New York Times*, November 2, 2008.

3. D. W. Dockery, C. A. Pope 3rd, X. Xu, J. D. Spengler, J. H. Ware, M. E. Fay, et al., "An Association Between Air Pollution and Mortality in Six U.S. Cities," *New England Journal of Medicine* 329 (1993): 1753–1759.

4. U.S. Environmental Protection Agency, "Table of Historical Particulate Matter (PM) National Ambient Air Quality Standards (NAAQS)," https://www.epa.gov/pm-pollution/table-historical-particulate-matter-pm-national-ambient-air-quality-standards-naaqs, accessed October 6, 2019.

5. J. H. Ware, "Editorial: Particulate Air Pollution and Mortality—Clearing the Air," *New England Journal of Medicine* 343 (2000): 1798–1799.

6. L. Greenhouse, "E.P.A.'s Right to Set Air Rules Wins Supreme Court Backing," *The New York Times*, February 28, 2001.

7. W. Dockery and P. H. Stone, "Cardiovascular Risks from Fine Particulate Air Pollution," *New England Journal of Medicine* 365 (2007): 511–513.

8. J. Currie and R. Walker, "Traffic Congestion and Infant Health: Evidence from E-Z Pass," *American Economic Journal: Applied Economics* 3 (January 2011): 65–90.

9. U.S. Environmental Protection Agency, "Air Quality: National Summary," July 8, 2019, https://www.epa.gov/air-trends/air-quality-national-summary, accessed October 6, 2019.

10. M. L. Bell, A. McDermott, S. L. Zeger, J. M. Samet, and F. Dominici, "Ozone and Short-Term Mortality in 95 U.S. Urban Communities, 1987–2000," *Journal of the American Medical Association* 292 (2004): 2372–2378.

11. Environment News Service, "EPA Sued for Allowing Haze to Obscure National Parks," October 23, 2008, https://www.nbcchicago.com/news/green/EPA_Sued_for_Allowing_Haze_to_Obscure_National_Parks.html, accessed October 6, 2019.

12. U.S. Environmental Protection Agency, "2015 National Ambient Air Quality Standards (NAAQS) for Ozone," July 20, 2018, https://www.epa.gov/ground-level-ozone-pollution/2015-national-ambient-air-quality-standards-naaqs-ozone, accessed October 6, 2019.

13. N. Popovich, L. Albeck-Ripka, and K. Pierre-Louis, "85 Environmental Rules Being Rolled Back Under Trump," *The New York Times*, September 12, 2019.

14. U.S. Environmental Protection Agency, "Criteria Pollutant Nonattainment Summary Report," September 30, 2019, https://www3.epa.gov/airquality/greenbook/ancl3.html, accessed October 6, 2019.

15. U.S. Environmental Protection Agency, "Our Nation's Air: Status and Trends Through 2018," https://gispub.epa.gov/air/trendsreport/2019/#home, accessed October 6, 2019.

16. U.S. Environmental Protection Agency, "National Emission Standards for Hazardous Air Pollutants (NESHAP)," August 29, 2019, https://www.epa.gov/stationary-sources-air-pollution/national-emission-standards-hazardous-air-pollutants-neshap-9, accessed October 6, 2019.

17. U.S. Environmental Protection Agency, "Urban Air Toxics," August 20, 2019, https://www.epa.gov/urban-air-toxics, accessed October 6, 2019.

18. C. Davenport, "Trump to Revoke California's Authority to Set Stricter Auto Emissions Rules," *The New York Times*, September 17, 2019.

19. C. Davenport, "California Sues the Trump Administration in Its Escalating War Over Auto Emissions," *The New York Times*, September 20, 2019.

20. B. Barcott, "Changing All the Rules," *The New York Times Magazine*, April 4, 2009.

21. J. M. Broder, A. C. Revkin, F. Barringer, and C. Dean, "Environmental Views, Past and Present," *The New York Times*, February 7, 2009.

22. L. Friedman, "States Sue Trump Administration Over Rollback of Obama-Era Climate Rule," *The New York Times*, August 13, 2019.

23. Editorial, "Mercury and Power Plants," *The New York Times*, July 24, 2009.

24. U.S. Environmental Protection Agency, "Fact Sheet: Overview of the Clean Power Plan," August 3, 2015, https://archive.epa.gov/epa/cleanpowerplan/fact-sheet-overview-clean-power-plan.html, accessed October 6, 2019.

25. J. P. Jacobs, "EPA Toxics Report Sparks Fight over Diesel Emissions," *The New York Times*, March 17, 2011.

26. G. E. R. Hook and G. W. Lucier, "The Right to Know Is for Everyone," *Environmental Health Perspectives* 108 (2000): A160–A162.

27. U.S. Environmental Protection Agency, "2001 Toxics Release Inventory (TRI): Public Data Release," July 2003, https://www.epa.gov/sites/production/files/documents/2001_national_analysis_executive_summary.pdf, accessed October 6, 2019.

28. U.S. Environmental Protection Agency, "2013 TRI National Analysis: Introduction," January 2015, https://19january2017snapshot.epa.gov/toxics-release-inventory-tri-program/2013-tri-national

-analysis-introduction.html, accessed October 6, 2019.

29. R. Dahl, "Does Secrecy Equal Security? Limiting Access to Environmental Information," *Environmental Health Perspectives* 112 (2004): A104–A107.

30. W. Boly, "Smog City Wants to Make This Perfectly Clear," Health (San Francisco, CA) 6, no. 2 (1992): 54.

31. B. Bergman, "To Cut Smog, Los Angeles Places a Bounty on Mowers," *The New York Times*, May 5, 2004.

32. South Coast Air Quality Management District, "SCAQMD Awards Nearly $5 Million to Replace Dirty Diesel Trucks Servicing Area Ports," July 2012, http://www.aqmd.gov/docs/default-source/publications/aqmd-advisor/july-2012-advisor.pdf, accessed October 6, 2019.

33. South Coast Air Quality Management District, "Need To Replace Your Ride?", http://www.aqmd.gov/docs/default-source/default-document-library/replace-your-ride/english.pdf?sfvrsn=7, accessed October 6, 2019.

34. M. L. Wald, "In Congress, a Jump Start for Clunkers," *The New York Times*, July 31, 2009.

35. American Lung Association, "State of the Air: California: Los Angeles," https://www.lung.org/our-initiatives/healthy-air/sota/city-rankings/states/california/los-angeles.html, accessed October 6, 2019.

36. B. M. Kuehn, "Stronger Formaldehyde Regulation Sought," *Journal of the American Medical Association* 299 (2008): 2015.

37. L. Wayne, "The Enemy at Home: Thousands in U.S. Attribute Ailments to Chinese Drywall," *The New York Times*, October 8, 2009.

38. U.S. Consumer Product Safety Commission, "Drywall Information Center," https://www.cpsc.gov/Safety-Education/Safety-Education-Centers/Drywall-Information-Center, accessed October 6, 2019.

39. U.S. Consumer Product Safety Commission, "Remediation Guidance for Homes with Corrosion from Problem Drywall as of March 15, 2013," https://www.cpsc.gov/s3fs-public/remediation031513.pdf, accessed October 6, 2019.

40. U.S. Environmental Protection Agency, "2015 Program Progress: Cross-State Air Pollution Rule and Acid Rain Program," August 14, 2018, https://www.epa.gov/sites/production/files/2018-08/documents/2015_full_report_0.pdf, accessed October 6, 2019.

41. United Nations Environment Programme, Ozone Secretariat, "Montreal Protocol on Substances That Deplete the Ozone Layer," https://www.state.gov/key-topics-office-of-environmental-quality-and-transboundary-issues/the-montreal-protocol-on-substances-that-deplete-the-ozone-layer/, accessed October 6, 2019.

42. National Oceanic and Atmospheric Administration, Earth System Research Laboratory, "Stratospheric Ozone Layer Depletion and Recovery," www.esrl.noaa.gov/research/themes/o3, accessed July 29, 2015.

43. National Oceanic and Atmospheric Administration, Earth System Research Laboratory, Global Monitoring Division, "Trends in Atmospheric Carbon Dioxide," https://www.esrl.noaa.gov/gmd/ccgg/trends/global.html, accessed October 6, 2019.

44. National Oceanic and Atmospheric Administration, Climate.gov, "Climate Change: Global Temperature," https://www.climate.gov/news-features/understanding-climate/climate-change-global-temperature, accessed October 6, 2019.

Water Pollution

Clean Water: A Limited Resource

KEY TERMS

Clean Water Act
Nonpoint-source pollution

Point-source pollution
Safe Drinking Water Act

The importance of safe drinking water to public health has been clear since John Snow identified polluted water as the source of London's cholera epidemic in 1855. Major epidemics of cholera and other waterborne diseases broke out periodically in the United States until the end of the 19th century. Ninety thousand people died of cholera in 1885 in Chicago—a toll that persuaded city officials to stop discharging the city's sewage into Lake Michigan, which was also the source of municipal drinking water.[1(Ch.16)] While contaminated water remains a major cause of disease and death in developing countries, Americans expect that their tap water will be safe to drink—and, for the most part, it is. Nevertheless, 647 outbreaks of waterborne diseases were documented by the Centers for Disease Control and Prevention (CDC) between 1971 and 1994, including the 1993 cryptosporidiosis outbreak in Milwaukee.[2] Each year between 1991 and 2010, the CDC and the Environmental Protection Agency (EPA) recorded an average of

16 outbreaks associated with contaminated drinking water.[3,4] Such outbreaks continue, as will be seen later in this chapter.

Common water pollutants include, in addition to microbial pathogens, a wide range of chemicals that may not only be toxic in drinking water, but also have harmful effects on fish and wildlife. Many chemicals have been discharged into waterways as industrial wastes, such as the mercury in Minamata Bay and the polychlorinated biphenyls (PCBs) in the Hudson River. People may then be poisoned by eating fish that have accumulated these toxins in their flesh. Other sources of water pollution include deposition of chemicals from the air, as in acid rain, and runoff from the land.

Until the early 1970s, individual states were responsible for the quality of their waterways and the purity of their drinking water. This arrangement did not control water pollution for the same reason that it could not control air pollution: The sources of pollution and the communities affected by that pollution may be under different political jurisdiction. For example, New Orleans draws its drinking water from the Mississippi River, yet it was helpless to stop cities upstream, located in other states, from discharging sewage and industrial wastes into the river.

A number of infamous pollution cases occurred in the United States in the 1960s and 1970s that inspired the passage of federal legislation to deal with this problem. The discovery of PCBs in the Hudson River led to a ban on commercial fishing there because the chemicals were so concentrated in the flesh of the fish. Residents of Duluth, Minnesota, were alarmed to learn that the Reserve Mining Company had been dumping asbestos-containing wastewater into Lake Superior, the source of municipal water, for more than 20 years.[5] While no one knew whether asbestos was as carcinogenic when drunk as it was when breathed, bottled water was distributed to the population for more than a year until a new water-filtration plant was completed. The James River was so badly polluted with the insecticide Kepone, discharged from a manufacturing plant in Hopewell, Virginia, between 1966 and 1975, that no practical way has ever been proposed to clean it up. The plant was eventually closed, not because of the environmental damage it caused, but because so many of its employees suffered neurologic, liver, and other damage from Kepone poisoning.[6] Perhaps the most dramatic call to action occurred in 1969, when the Cuyahoga River in Ohio caught fire because it had so much oil floating on its surface.[6]

The two goals of cleaning up lakes and rivers and ensuring safe drinking water are distinct but related, and Congress has addressed them in separate legislation: the Clean Water Act of 1972, amended in 1977 and several times since, and the Safe Drinking Water Act of 1974, which was rewritten in 1996.[1(Ch.15,16)] Given that half of the drinking water in the United States comes from lakes and rivers, success in meeting the goals of the Clean Water Act is obviously a help in achieving the goals of the Safe Drinking Water Act.

Clean Water Act

The **Clean Water Act** set national goals that lakes and rivers should be "fishable" and "swimmable" and that all pollutant discharges should be eliminated. The first attempts at cleaning up the nation's waterways focused on **point-source pollution**—well-defined locations that discharge pollutants into lakes and rivers. Most point-source pollution comes from municipal sewage and industrial discharges. The 1972 and 1977 legislation imposed strict controls on these sources; it also provided billions of dollars of funding to assist municipalities in building wastewater treatment facilities. With the success of these efforts, it became apparent that a great deal of pollution washed into waterways from the air and the land. Thus, the 1987 reauthorization of the Clean Water Act focused on cleaning up nonpoint-source pollution, which has proved a much more difficult task.[1(Ch.16)]

Laws governing point-source pollution set requirements for treating wastewater so that it can be discharged into waterways without causing human health problems or disrupting the aquatic environment. In the case of sewage treatment plants, achieving these goals requires several steps. The primary step is to remove suspended solids by screening them and then allowing them to settle out by gravity in settling tanks. The secondary step then breaks down the remaining organic material using biological processes: The wastewater is mixed with bacteria and plenty of oxygen, resulting in conversion of the organic wastes into carbon dioxide, water, and minerals. Finally, the wastewater is usually disinfected with chlorine before being discharged into the environment.[1(Ch.16)]

While the treatment process produces a liquid discharge that meets environmental safety standards, it also generates "sludge," the solid waste left behind on screens and at the bottom of settling tanks. Municipal sewage plants produce enormous amounts of sludge, creating a major disposal problem. In the past, sludge was often dumped in the ocean or incinerated, but these methods create other pollution problems. In 1992, Congress prohibited the ocean dumping of sludge. Some communities bury their sludge in landfills, but landfill space is running low. Since sludge is rich in nutrients, the EPA encourages the use of treated sludge as a fertilizer and soil conditioner to improve marginal lands and increase forest productivity. The EPA has developed strict regulations on sanitizing and removing hazardous contaminants from the sludge—called biosolids after treatment is complete—before it can be used on land. Recent analysis indicates that 55% of sewage sludge generated every year is used as fertilizer.[1(Ch.16)]

Approximately 70% of the U.S. population is served by sewage treatment plants. Most of the other 30% use on-site septic systems, which function as miniature sewage treatment plants, including the use of bacteria to break down organic wastes. Like the larger plants, septic systems produce sludge, which must be pumped out periodically. Improperly constructed and poorly maintained septic systems contribute to pollution of waterways and often result in public health problems.[1(Ch.16)]

Despite the laws and some occasional funding from the federal government, many cities have inadequate sewer systems that back up into basements or overflow and dump untreated sewage into waterways. In part, these problems are due to population growth, which has placed additional burden on aging systems, but they also occur because most systems combine rainwater runoff with sewage, which can overwhelm the system when it rains. According to an analysis of EPA data by *The New York Times*, sewage systems are the nation's most frequent violators of the Clean Water Act.[7] The American Society of Civil Engineers has estimated that $298 billion will be needed over the next 20 years to fix the nation's sewage infrastructure.[8]

Discharges from industrial sources are the second major category of point-source pollution, which is strictly regulated by the Clean Water Act. The EPA is required to develop standards for the release of various categories of pollutants into the environment. Industries that discharge substances directly into the nation's waterways are required to obtain a permit specifying allowable amounts and constituents of pollutants they may discharge. They must routinely monitor their discharges and report regularly to the EPA.[1(Ch.16)]

Industrial wastes may cause special problems if they are discharged into sewer systems and pass through a municipal sewage treatment plant, occasionally with disastrous consequences. In 1977, pesticide wastes illegally dumped into the sewers of Louisville, Kentucky, killed all the microbes responsible for the secondary treatment process, rendering the plant ineffective. For nearly two years while the plant was being cleaned up at a cost of millions of dollars, 100 million gallons of untreated sewage was discharged into the Ohio River every day. In 1981 in Cincinnati, a paint factory discharged hydrochloric acid into the city sewers, corroding the sewer pipe and causing it to collapse, leaving a hole in the street 24 feet in diameter.[9(Ch.15)]

To prevent such problems, the Clean Water Act requires pretreatment of industrial wastes before they are discharged into sewers. But standards have not been set for many smaller commercial establishments, including car washes and photo processing plants. Hazardous chemicals may also enter sewer systems from residences, when people dispose of bleaches, toilet bowl cleaners, paint thinners, and other household substances by flushing them down the drain.

As strict limits have been set on pollution from sewage systems and industry, **nonpoint-source pollution** has become an increasingly important threat to water quality. These contaminants come from stormwater runoff from farmland, construction sites, and urban streets. Agriculture is the leading source of water pollution in the United States, contributing soil, manure fertilizers, and pesticides that wash into streams and lakes.

Indeed, agricultural runoff is believed to have been the source of the Milwaukee cryptosporidiosis outbreak. Construction activities also contribute soil to runoff water, together with oil, tar, paint, and cleaning solvents. Contaminants contributed by urban street runoff include sand, dirt, road salt, oil, grease, heavy metal particles, pesticides and fertilizers from lawns, and animal and bird droppings.

A variety of approaches must be used to minimize pollution caused by stormwater runoff. These include preventing soil erosion by planting vegetation on exposed soil, incorporating more green space into urban areas, minimizing the use of chemical fertilizers and pesticides, and controlling litter.

Air pollution is also a source of water pollution. In addition to acid rain, a number of other chemicals are deposited into lakes, rivers, and oceans from the air—for example, lead, asbestos, PCBs, and various pesticides. In fact, the major portion of PCBs in the Great Lakes comes from the air. Industrial accidents and spills also contribute to pollution of waterways.[10]

To conform to the requirements of the Clean Water Act, the EPA regularly collects data from the states on water quality of rivers, lakes, and estuaries. The most recent reports available, which include data that are more or less up to date, depending on the state, showed that the nation still has a way to go to meet the fishable and swimmable requirements. Of the water bodies that were assessed, only 55% of river miles, 74% of lake acres, and 78% of bay and estuaries square miles were rated "good" for recreation (including fishing and swimming).[10]

Safe Drinking Water

Almost half of the drinking water in the United States comes from rivers and lakes. Thus, it is likely to be contaminated by the point-source and nonpoint-source pollutants just discussed. The other half of the nation's drinking water comes from underground aquifers; these are generally of better quality but are increasingly susceptible to contamination by leaching from landfills, leaky oil and gas storage tanks, and other sources of toxic chemicals. Improvements in surface-water quality brought about by the Clean Water Act make the job easier for community water systems, which must, however, meet much higher standards to produce potable water—water that is safe for human consumption.

All community systems need to treat their water so that, theoretically, all contaminants are removed. The steps needed to produce potable water vary depending on the source of the water and the type of contaminants. The basic steps common to most systems include sedimentation, coagulation, filtration, and disinfection. Incoming water is first allowed to sit quietly while suspended material settles out. Then alum is added, causing small particles to coagulate and settle out. Filtration through beds of sand or similar materials removes the smaller particles that do not settle, and chlorine is added to kill remaining pathogens. In areas of the country where water is "hard"—containing high concentrations of dissolved calcium or magnesium—or where it has objectionable tastes or odors due to dissolved iron or gases, additional treatments may be used. As a last step, fluoride is often added to protect community residents from tooth decay. **Figure 22-1** depicts a typical drinking-water purification plant.

To ensure that the treatment process is working effectively, regular laboratory tests are generally done on the final product. The traditional measures of water purity are turbidity and coliform levels. Turbidity indicates the presence of suspended particles, signifying a failure of the sedimentation and filtration steps. Suspended particles may interfere with the germicidal action of the chlorine. After the cryptosporidiosis outbreak, which accompanied an increase in the turbidity of Milwaukee's water, national turbidity standards were tightened. If coliform bacteria are

Typical municipal water treatment plant

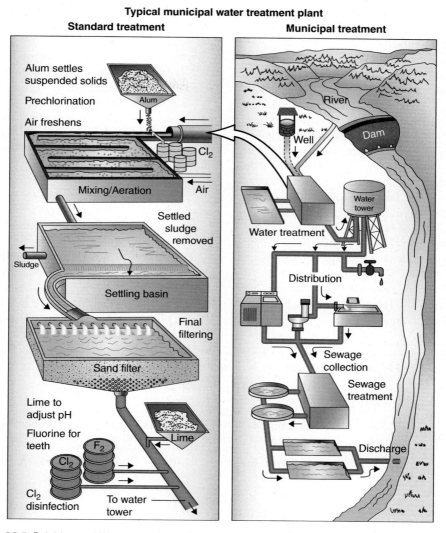

Figure 22-1 Drinking and Wastewater Treatment

Reproduced from U.S. Environmental Protection Agency, "The Water Sourcebook," September 11, 2013, p. 236.

detected, there has probably been a failure of disinfection. These bacteria are common inhabitants of the intestines of humans and other animals. Although they are rarely pathogenic themselves, their presence indicates that other, more harmful microorganisms may have survived the treatment process.[1(Ch.16)]

The general approach to water treatment described here is directed primarily against bacterial diseases, the most common and historically devastating type of waterborne disease. By contrast, it is not very effective against viruses and the parasites *Cryptosporidium* and *Giardia*, which are resistant to chlorine. Furthermore, it does nothing to address the problem of contamination with common chemical pollutants such as pesticides, herbicides, fertilizers, PCBs, lead, and other metals that may be harmful to health. Most community water systems are totally unprepared even to test for these pollutants.

The **Safe Drinking Water Act** of 1974 required the EPA to set standards for local water systems and mandated that states enforce these standards. Uniform guidelines were set for drinking-water treatment, and regular monitoring and testing were required, with the results to be reported to state governments. However, no deadlines were established for the standard setting, and state agencies were lax in enforcing the requirements that were in place. The 1986 reauthorization of the Safe Drinking Water Act specified 83 contaminants to be regulated by the EPA and set deadlines for action. In addition, it required water systems to take measures to prevent contamination with *Giardia* and *Cryptosporidia*.[9(Ch.16)] The EPA also stepped up the pace of regulation.

Currently, maximum contaminant levels have been set for 87 identified contaminants, including microorganisms, disinfectants, disinfection by-products, inorganic chemicals, organic chemicals, and radionuclides. A selected list of these contaminants is shown in **Table 22-1**). In addition, secondary standards have been set for 15 contaminants that do not cause health risks but that may affect taste, odor, or color, or that cause discoloration of skin or teeth.

In 1996, Congress again strengthened the Safe Drinking Water Act. New measures required that community water systems provide annual Consumer Confidence Reports to their customers on the source of the water, water contaminants, and the health effects of these contaminants.[11] The law also included requirements for source water protection, tightened standards for training and certification of operators, and provided funding

Table 22-1 EPA National Primary Drinking Water Regulations

Microorganisms		
Contaminant	**Potential Health Effects from Long-Term Exposure Above the MCL (Unless Specified as Short-Term)**	**Sources of Contaminant in Drinking Water**
Cryptosporidium	Gastrointestinal illness (e.g., diarrhea, vomiting, cramps)	Human and animal fecal waste
Giardia lamblia	Gastrointestinal illness (e.g., diarrhea, vomiting, cramps)	Human and animal fecal waste
Heterotrophic plate count (HPC)	HPC has no health effects; it is an analytic method used to measure the variety of bacteria that are common in water. The lower the concentration of bacteria in drinking water, the better maintained the water system is.	HPC measures a range of bacteria that are naturally present in the environment
Legionella	Legionnaire's disease, a type of pneumonia	Found naturally in water; multiplies in heating systems
Total coliforms (including fecal coliform and *Escherichia coli*)	Not a health threat in itself; used to indicate whether other potentially harmful bacteria may be present[5]	Coliforms are naturally present in the environment, as is feces; fecal coliforms and *E. coli* only come from human and animal fecal waste.

Microorganisms		
Contaminant	**Potential Health Effects from Long-Term Exposure Above the MCL (Unless Specified as Short-Term)**	**Sources of Contaminant in Drinking Water**
Turbidity	Turbidity is a measure of the cloudiness of water. It is used to indicate water quality and filtration effectiveness (e.g., whether disease-causing organisms are present). Higher turbidity levels are often associated with higher levels of disease-causing microorganisms such as viruses, parasites, and some bacteria. These organisms can cause symptoms such as nausea, cramps, diarrhea, and associated headaches.	Soil runoff
Viruses (enteric)	Gastrointestinal illness (e.g., diarrhea, vomiting, cramps)	Human and animal fecal waste
Disinfection By-Products		
Bromate	Increased risk of cancer	By-product of drinking water disinfection
Chlorite	Anemia; infants and young children: nervous system effects	By-product of drinking water disinfection
Haloacetic acids (HAA⁵)	Increased risk of cancer	By-product of drinking water disinfection
Total trihalo-methanes (TTHMs)	Liver, kidney or central nervous system problems; increased risk of cancer	By-product of drinking water disinfection
Disinfectants		
Chloramines (as Cl_2)	Eye/nose irritation; stomach discomfort, anemia	Water additive used to control microbes
Chlorine (as Cl_2)	Eye/nose irritation; stomach discomfort	Water additive used to control microbes
Chlorine dioxide (as ClO_2)	Anemia; infants and young children: nervous system effects	Water additive used to control microbes
Inorganic Chemicals		
Antimony	Increase in blood cholesterol; decrease in blood sugar	Discharge from petroleum refineries; fire retardants; ceramics; electronics; solder
Arsenic	Skin damage or problems with circulatory systems; may increase risk of getting cancer	Erosion of natural deposits; runoff from orchards, runoff from glass, electronics production wastes

(continues)

Table 22-1 **EPA National Primary Drinking Water Regulations (*Continued*)**

Inorganic Chemicals		
Asbestos (fiber > 10 micrometers)	Increased risk of developing benign intestinal polyps	Decay of asbestos cement in water mains; erosion of natural deposits
Barium	Increase in blood pressure	Discharge of drilling wastes; discharge from metal refineries; erosion of natural deposits
Beryllium	Intestinal lesions	Discharge from metal refineries and coal-burning factories; discharge from electrical, aerospace, and defense industries
Cadmium	Kidney damage	Corrosion of galvanized pipes; erosion of natural deposits; discharge from metal refineries; runoff from waste batteries and paints
Chromium (total)	Allergic dermatitis	Discharge from steel and pulp mills; erosion of natural deposits
Copper	Short-term exposure: gastrointestinal distress Long-term exposure: liver or kidney damage People with Wilson's disease should consult their personal doctor if the amount of copper in their water exceeds the action level	Corrosion of household plumbing systems; erosion of natural deposits
Cyanide (as free cyanide)	Nerve damage or thyroid problems	Discharge from steel/metal factories; discharge from plastic and fertilizer factories
Fluoride	Bone disease (pain and tenderness of the bones); children may get mottled teeth	Water additive that promotes strong teeth; erosion of natural deposits; discharge from fertilizer and aluminum factories
Lead	Infants and children: delays in physical or mental development; children could show slight deficits in attention span and learning abilities Adults: kidney problems; high blood pressure	Corrosion of household plumbing systems; erosion of natural deposits
Mercury (inorganic)	Kidney damage	Erosion of natural deposits; discharge from refineries and factories; runoff from landfills and croplands

Inorganic Chemicals		
Nitrate (measured as nitrogen)	Infants < 6 months who drink water containing nitrate in excess of the MCL could become seriously ill and, if untreated, may die. Symptoms include shortness of breath and blue-baby syndrome.	Runoff from fertilizer use; leaking from septic tanks, sewage; erosion of natural deposits
Nitrite (measured as nitrogen)	Infants < 6 months who drink water containing nitrite in excess of the MCL could become seriously ill and, if untreated, may die. Symptoms include shortness of breath and blue-baby syndrome.	Runoff from fertilizer use; leaking from septic tanks, sewage; erosion of natural deposits
Selenium	Hair or fingernail loss; numbness in fingers or toes; circulatory problems	Discharge from petroleum refineries; erosion of natural deposits; discharge from mines
Thallium	Hair loss; changes in blood; kidney, intestine, or liver problems	Leaching from ore-processing sites; discharge from electronics, glass, and drug factories
Organic Chemicals		
Acrylamide	Nervous system or blood problems; increased risk of cancer	Added to water during sewage/wastewater treatment
Alachlor	Eye, liver, kidney, or spleen problems; anemia; increased risk of cancer	Runoff from herbicide used on row crops
Atrazine	Cardiovascular system or reproductive problems	Runoff from herbicide used on row crops
Benzene	Anemia; decrease in blood platelets; increased risk of cancer	Discharge from factories; leaching from gas storage tanks and landfills
Benzo(a) pyrene (PAHs)	Reproductive difficulties; increased risk of cancer	Leaching from linings of water storage tanks and distribution lines
Carbofuran	Problems with blood, nervous system, or reproductive system	Leaching of soil fumigant used on rice and alfalfa
Carbon tetrachloride	Liver problems; increased risk of cancer	Discharge from chemical plants and other industrial activities
Chlordane	Liver or nervous system problems; increased risk of cancer	Residue of banned termiticide
Chlorobenzene	Liver or kidney problems	Discharge from chemical and agricultural chemical factories

(continues)

Table 22-1 EPA National Primary Drinking Water Regulations (*Continued*)

Organic Chemicals		
Dalapon	Minor kidney changes	Runoff from herbicide used on rights of way
1,2-Dibromo-3-chloropropane (DBCP)	Reproductive difficulties; increased risk of cancer	Runoff/leaching from soil fumigant used on soybeans, cotton, pineapples, and orchards
o-Dichlorobenzene	Liver, kidney, or circulatory system problems	Discharge from industrial chemical factories
p-Dichlorobenzene	Anemia; liver, kidney, or spleen damage; changes in blood	Discharge from industrial chemical factories
1,2-Dichloro-ethane	Increased risk of cancer	Discharge from industrial chemical factories
1,1-Dichloro-ethylene	Liver problems	Discharge from industrial chemical factories
cis-1,2-Dichloro-ethylene	Liver problems	Discharge from industrial chemical factories
trans-1,2-Dichloro-ethylene	Liver problems	Discharge from industrial chemical factories
Dichloro-methane	Liver problems; increased risk of cancer	Discharge from drug and chemical factories
2,4-Dichlorophenoxyacetic acid (2,4-D)	Kidney, liver, or adrenal gland problems	Runoff from herbicide used on row crops
1,2-Dichloro-propane	Increased risk of cancer	Discharge from industrial chemical factories
Di(2-ethylhexyl) adipate	Weight loss, liver problems, or possible reproductive difficulties.	Discharge from chemical factories
Di(2-ethylhexyl) phthalate	Reproductive difficulties; liver problems; increased risk of cancer	Discharge from rubber and chemical factories
Dinoseb	Reproductive difficulties	Runoff from herbicide used on soybeans and vegetables
Dioxin (2,3,7,8-TCDD)	Reproductive difficulties; increased risk of cancer	Emissions from waste incineration and other combustion; discharge from chemical factories
Diquat	Cataracts	Runoff from herbicide use
Endothall	Stomach and intestinal problems	Runoff from herbicide use
Endrin	Liver problems	Residue of banned insecticide

Organic Chemicals		
Epichlorhydrin	Increased cancer risk and, over a long period of time, stomach problems	Discharge from industrial chemical factories; an impurity of some water treatment chemicals
Ethylbenzene	Liver or kidney problems	Discharge from petroleum refineries
Ethylene dibromide	Problems with liver, stomach, reproductive system, or kidneys; increased risk of cancer	Discharge from petroleum refineries
Glyphosate	Kidney problems; reproductive difficulties	Runoff from herbicide use
Heptachlor	Liver damage; increased risk of cancer	Residue of banned termiticide
Heptachlor epoxide	Liver damage; increased risk of cancer	Breakdown of heptachlor
Hexachloro-benzene	Liver or kidney problems; reproductive difficulties; increased risk of cancer	Discharge from metal refineries and agricultural chemical factories
Hexachlorocycl-opentadiene	Kidney or stomach problems	Discharge from chemical factories
Lindane	Liver or kidney problems	Runoff/leaching from insecticide used on cattle, lumber, gardens
Methoxychlor	Reproductive difficulties	Runoff/leaching from insecticide used on fruits, vegetables, alfalfa, livestock
Oxamyl (Vydate)	Slight nervous system effects	Runoff/leaching from insecticide used on apples, potatoes, and tomatoes
Polychlorinated biphenyls (PCBs)	Skin changes; thymus gland problems; immune deficiencies; reproductive or nervous system difficulties; increased risk of cancer	Runoff from landfills; discharge of waste chemicals
Pentachlorophenol	Liver or kidney problems; increased cancer risk	Discharge from wood preserving factories
Picloram	Liver problems	Herbicide runoff
Simazine	Problems with blood	Herbicide runoff
Styrene	Liver, kidney, or circulatory system problems	Discharge from rubber and plastic factories; leaching from landfills
Tetrachloroethylene	Liver problems; increased risk of cancer	Discharge from factories and dry cleaners

(continues)

Table 22-1 EPA National Primary Drinking Water Regulations (*Continued*)

Organic Chemicals		
Toluene	Nervous system, kidney, or liver problems	Discharge from petroleum factories
Toxaphene	Kidney, liver, or thyroid problems; increased risk of cancer	Runoff/leaching from insecticide used on cotton and cattle
1,2,4-Trichloro-benzene	Changes in adrenal glands	Discharge from textile finishing factories
1,1,1-Trichloro-ethane	Liver, nervous system, or circulatory problems	Discharge from metal degreasing sites and other factories
1,1,2-Trichloro-ethane	Liver, kidney, or immune system problems	Discharge from industrial chemical factories
Trichloroethylene	Liver problems; increased risk of cancer	Discharge from metal degreasing sites and other factories
2,4,5-Trichlorophenoxy (2,4,5-TP; Silvex)	Liver problems	Residue of banned herbicide
Vinyl chloride	Increased risk of cancer	Leaching from polyvinyl chloride (PVC) pipes; discharge from plastic factories
Xylenes (total)	Nervous system damage	Discharge from petroleum factories; discharge from chemical factories
Radionuclides		
Alpha particles	Increased risk of cancer	Erosion of natural deposits of certain minerals that are radioactive and may emit alpha radiation
Beta particles and photon emitters	Increased risk of cancer	Decay of natural and human-made deposits of certain minerals that are radioactive and may emit forms of radiation in the form of photons and beta radiation
Radium-226 and radium-228 (combined)	Increased risk of cancer	Erosion of natural deposits
Uranium	Increased risk of cancer, kidney toxicity	Erosion of natural deposits

Data from U.S. Environmental Protection Agency, "Ground Water and Drinking Water: National Primary Drinking Water Regulations," September 17, 2019, www.epa.gov/ground-water-and-drinking-water/national-primary-drinking-water-regulations, accessed October 7, 2019.

to help localities improve their systems. The "right-to-know" measure was expected to evoke public pressure that would result in better compliance with standards.

A number of amendments to the Safe Drinking Water Act have occurred in more recent years. In 2005, a carve-out was created to allow energy companies to inject chemicals and fluids deep into the ground for hydraulic fracturing to obtain natural gas (a process commonly called "fracking"). A 2011 amendment was aimed at reducing lead in drinking water. Amendments in 2015, 2016, and 2018 helped fill in other gaps and provide additional resources that were missing in the existing law.

Ongoing surveillance for waterborne disease by the CDC provides data useful for evaluating the adequacy of existing water treatment technologies and the effectiveness of drinking water regulations. The CDC publishes its findings every two years, analyzing the outbreaks by causative agent, type of water system, type of deficiency in the system, and source of water. These data probably understate the incidence of waterborne diseases, because most cases go unrecognized or unreported.

The most recent CDC report found 42 outbreaks in the two-year period 2013–2014, affecting 1006 people and causing 13 deaths. Twenty-four of these outbreaks and all of the deaths were caused by *Legionella* bacteria, which caused respiratory disease. Many of these events occurred in hospitals, nursing homes, or other healthcare settings. Eight of the outbreaks were caused by *Cryptosporidium* or *Giardia*, parasites that cause acute gastrointestinal symptoms. Chemicals or toxins were responsible for an additional four outbreaks, and viruses or other bacteria caused another five outbreaks.[12]

A 2018 study examining trends in Safe Drinking Water Act violations over the period 1982–2015 found that in each of these years, between 9 million and 45 million people, or between 4% and 28% of the U.S. population, were affected by a violation. In 2015, 9% of community water systems, serving 21 million people, violated health-based water quality standards. Over the 34-year period, violations involving coliforms, which include *E. coli* and related bacteria that cause gastrointestinal illness, were the most common, representing 37% of total violations. Violations of water treatment rules and those involving nitrates (e.g., from farming fertilizer) accounted for 21% of violations. Violations involving arsenic, lead, and copper represented an additional 7% of violations. The states with the largest number of violations are Oklahoma (43% of community water systems in the state), Nebraska (35%), and Idaho (33%). Private water-treatment plants performed better than public ones, perhaps because private plants were at risk of lawsuits and public takeover should they fail to deliver quality drinking water. Rural areas, areas with larger minority populations, and areas with lower income had higher numbers of violations.[13]

In 1978, CDC's surveillance for waterborne disease outbreaks expanded to include outbreaks associated with recreational water, such as swimming pools, water parks, and beaches. These sources now account for more outbreaks than drinking water sources. In 2013–2014, there were 87 such outbreaks, affecting 3543 people and causing 4 deaths. Most of the illnesses were gastrointestinal in nature, caused by infectious agents or chemicals, but a significant number of cases involved respiratory or skin illnesses or symptoms.[14]

Private wells are not regulated under the Safe Drinking Water Act, although the EPA issues recommendations for ensuring that these wells are safe. Approximately 43 million Americans get their drinking water from private wells and, according to a study by the U.S. Geological Survey, more than one in five of these wells contains at least one contaminant at a concentration high enough to be a health concern. Different contaminants are more common in different regions of the country. The study authors note that these findings underscore a continuing need for public education and for testing of domestic wells.[15]

Many Americans choose to drink bottled water, believing that it is purer and tastes better than tap water. However, in a study published in 1999 by the Natural Resources Defense Council, many of the 103 brands tested contained chemical or biological contaminants, albeit not in concentrations high enough to cause health problems.[1] According to CDC data, every year or two, an illness outbreak occurs in the United States due to bottled water.[12,16] Bottled water is regulated by the U.S. Food and Drug Administration (FDA), which requires it to meet EPA's drinking water standards. Enforcement is not strict, however. Many, but not all, states impose additional regulations. An estimated 44% of bottled water sold in the United States is obtained directly from municipal water supplies.[1(Ch.16)]

Water Crisis in Flint, Michigan

Lead is toxic. Children who are exposed to lead have an elevated risk for serious neurologic problems including learning disabilities, attention-deficit/hyperactivity disorder (ADHD), and impulse control, which in turn have implications for society as a whole. For example, a reduction in lead exposure may help explain the sharp drop in crime in the 1990s: Studies show that when lead was removed from gasoline in the United States in 1974, ambient lead levels declined significantly and subsequent cohorts of children avoided the toxin; their exposure to lead may have caused children born before then to exhibit maladjusted behavior, including a propensity to commit crimes. Lead pipes were banned in the United States in 1986, but millions of homes, schools, and other types of structures were built before the newer codes, and are still inhabited today. Other studies have shown that, even after carefully controlling for a city's socioeconomic characteristics, cities whose drinking water is carried through lead pipes and whose natural water source is more acidic in nature, which causes more lead corrosion, have dramatically higher rates of violent crime compared to cities that have non-lead pipes or lead pipes but less acidic water.[17]

A large number of cities have experienced serious lead problems, often with only limited publicity. For example, widespread lead-contaminated drinking water was discovered in Washington, D.C., over the period 2000 to 2004; Columbia, South Carolina, in 2005; Durham and Greenville, North Carolina, in 2006; Sebring, Ohio, and Jackson, Mississippi, in 2016; New York City public schools in 2017; and Newark, New Jersey, from 2017 to 2019.[18,19] Nevertheless, it took the lead crisis in Flint, Michigan, to shine a needed spotlight on this issue.

Between 2011 and 2015, the city of Flint was in state receivership, which meant that, due to its financial troubles, the city's financial decisions were made by the state. To save money, in April 2014, the city's state-appointed emergency manager switched the source of drinking water away from Detroit's system, which the city had used for years without problem, to the Flint River. Almost immediately, city residents noticed their new water was discolored and smelled and tasted bad. By September, it had become clear that the Flint River's more acidic water was corroding the lead pipes that carried water to the city, causing lead levels in the public water supply to spike. The following month, the city switched back to using Detroit's water, but the crisis had already been set in motion.[20] Despite the return to less acidic water, the pipes now had a corrosion problem and continued to leach lead into the water supply. The solution was simple and cheap: add readily available anticorrosion chemicals to the water at a cost of a mere $200 per day. But city administrators inexplicably overlooked this basic action. By June 2015, the EPA had learned of this failure, but it was not until seven months later, in January 2016, that the EPA issued an emergency order to address the water crisis.[21] Compounding the problem, a Legionnaire's disease outbreak occurred at the same time that killed 12 people in the city. It is believed that the corroded pipes allowed the *Legionella* bacteria to multiply in the water supply during periods of warmer weather.

Since then, the EPA's Office of Inspector General has reported that management failures at the EPA delayed stronger intervention even as it became clear that state regulators had badly bungled the situation. Under the authority of the Safe Drinking Water Act, the Inspector General's report called for more aggressive federal intervention in states and municipalities when problems appear. Unfortunately, an increase in federal control is at odds with the mantra of the Republican party and Donald Trump's administration, which insists that federal authority should be scaled back. This tension will surely resurface in the future in relation to environmental issues.[22]

In 2017, criminal charges were filed against 15 state and local officials in the Flint case, including the former director of the Michigan Department of Health and Human Services, who was charged with involuntary manslaughter for the Legionnaire's disease–related deaths; a state epidemiologist; and the state-appointed emergency managers who were overseeing the city. In 2019, after political control of the state changed hands, the charges were abruptly dropped.[23,24]

In 2019, California implemented a novel policy to address drinking water problems that may represent a model for other locations. The plan is called the Safe and Affordable Drinking Water Fund. It involves charging modest fees to dairy producers and fertilizer manufacturers, who are responsible for nitrate and other water contamination, combined with a $0.95-per-month voluntary contribution by residential water customers that is collected through their water bills. Water customers can freely opt out of the small monthly contribution, but a survey of Californians showed that 70% were willing to pay this amount to improve water quality in needier communities. The

plan was signed into law by California Governor Gavin Newsom in June 2019 and is expected to raise $1.4 billion over 10 years for updating water systems in poorer communities.[25]

Dilemmas in Compliance

A dilemma recently faced by New York City illustrates why it is so difficult to ensure safe drinking water for many Americans. New York gets most of its tap water from six reservoirs in the Catskill Mountains built in the 1950s and 1960s. For many years, the city was justly proud of the purity and taste of its water. However, the population in the watershed region has grown, and the quality of the water began to suffer in the 1970s and 1980s. More than 100 community sewage treatment plants discharged their flows into the watershed area, many in violation of discharge permit standards. Substandard septic tanks also contributed to the problem. Dairy farms contributed tons of manure to the watershed. The amount of coliform bacteria measured in New York's water frequently violated EPA standards, and the amount of chlorine added to control bacteria increased to the level that it affected the water's taste. *Cryptosporidium* bacteria were also found in the city's water. The EPA ordered New York to clean up the pollution or to build a filtration plant for the water from upstate reservoirs, setting a deadline of December 1996 for achievement of this goal.[26]

New York City did not filter the water from its upstate reservoirs, and the cost of constructing a filtration plant was estimated at as much as $8 billion, a painful price for the city. As an alternative, the city proposed a plan to protect the watershed by helping communities to upgrade their sewage plants, buying sensitive land near the reservoirs, and making changes in the way farmers dispose of manure. The upstate communities, already angry at the city for taking so much of their land for the reservoirs, were concerned that New York's plan would further harm the region's economy by discouraging development. While most experts believe that all water systems should include filtration, they agree that watershed protection is also important. Milwaukee's cryptosporidiosis outbreak occurred despite the fact that this city's system filters the water. In early 1997, New York City reached an agreement with the upstate region to implement the watershed protection plan.[27,28] After years of further negotiation, the city reached an agreement in 2007 with the EPA and the upstate counties for a 10-year Filtration Avoidance Determination.[29] The city has continued to buy land in the watershed region, which can be used for recreational purposes such as hunting, fishing, and hiking, but cannot be developed. The agreement also calls for New York City to work with communities to upgrade wastewater treatment plants and septic systems. It is also working with agricultural groups to develop pollution prevention programs for farmers. As an added protection, the city has built an ultraviolet disinfection facility in Westchester County designed to kill *Cryptosporidium* and *Giardia* microorganisms.[29]

Meanwhile, New York City was under a court order to build a filtration plant for the older, more polluted reservoirs in the Croton system, located in suburban areas close to the city, which supplied as much as 10% of its water.[29] That highly controversial plant was built underground in the Bronx and was finally completed in 2015 at a cost of $3.2 billion.[30]

The cost of ensuring safe drinking water is a major obstacle for many communities, both large and small. While the federal government has provided some funds to assist states and localities in regulatory and remediation activities required by the Safe Drinking Water Act, the amount provided is never sufficient. In a report called *Drinking Water Infrastructure Needs Survey and Assessment*, the EPA has shown that spending on water and sewage systems is inadequate to cope with such problems as leaks in aging water pipelines and

failures in aging urban sewage systems.[31] The EPA estimates that addressing these needs will cost $384.2 billion over the next two decades. In the absence of adequate funding, attempts to upgrade water supplies always involve disputes over who should pay for improvements.

Another dilemma concerning drinking water is that the very chemicals used to kill microbes in water may themselves be harmful to health. Chlorine, the most common disinfectant, reacts with organic matter to form by-products that, some evidence shows, may be carcinogenic. Other, more expensive disinfection methods include bubbling ozone through the water, but these treatments tend to form other by-products that may be equally harmful to health. There is no simple solution to this problem—even bottled water is required to meet only the same standards of purity as tap water, as discussed earlier in this chapter. General steps to prevent water pollution through eliminating both point- and non-point-source pollution are helpful, however, since cleaner water sources require less treatment to meet drinking water standards.

A recent concern, the severity of which remains unknown, is the discovery in drinking water of trace amounts of a wide variety of hormones, pharmaceuticals, and household chemicals, most of which no one had thought to look for previously. Many of them probably get into wastewater when they are excreted by humans or animals and are not removed by sewage treatment systems. Some of the most frequently detected contaminants include steroids, insect repellants, antibiotics, and nonprescription drugs including caffeine and metabolites of nicotine. The health effects on humans of long-term exposure to low concentrations of these chemicals are not known, but evidence suggests that they have ecological effects on fish and other aquatic species. For example, female hormones in very small concentrations have been found to cause feminization of male fish. Some concern has been voiced that human fetuses might similarly be affected, although a more recent analysis concluded that the concentrations of estrogen in drinking water are too small to pose a significant risk to humans.[32,33] It is not clear that this kind of contamination can be prevented, but it may be reduced by employing more care in disposal of medications and other chemicals, which should never be flushed down the drain.

Is the Water Supply Running Out?

Although water covers 71% of the earth's surface, most of it is in the form of salt water or ice in glaciers or polar ice caps. Less than 1% of the total amount consists of fresh water, potentially suitable for drinking, cooking, bathing, farming, and other human needs.[1(Ch.15)] In many parts of the world, the supply of fresh water is inadequate to meet the demands of the local population. Already, political disputes are occurring in the United States over water shortages. Some heavily populated areas, including parts of Texas and New Mexico, are depleting finite underground water sources. In California, large quantities of water are transported to the central part of the state from the mountains for irrigation use, while cities in the south complain of shortages. Recent drought conditions in the western United States have exacerbated the problem. Water conservation measures of various kinds have been instituted throughout the United States, including legally mandated low-volume toilets and showerheads and limits on car washing and lawn watering in some areas during dry seasons.

As it becomes increasingly clear that pure water is a limited resource, it is also apparent that pure water is essential to public health.

Conclusion

Although Americans take it for granted that their tap water is safe to drink, outbreaks of waterborne illness are not uncommon in the United States; the 1993 cryptosporidiosis outbreak in Milwaukee is the most dramatic example. Two federal laws focus on keeping the water supply clean and safe.

The Clean Water Act specifies that lakes and rivers should be fishable and swimmable. It imposes controls on point-source pollution, mainly discharges from municipal sewage systems and from industry, and non-point-source pollution, which is washed into waterways from the air and the land. Laws governing point-source pollution set requirements for treating wastewater before it can be discharged. Nonpoint-source pollution is more difficult to control.

The Safe Drinking Water Act requires the EPA to set standards for local drinking water systems and requires states to enforce these standards. However, the EPA was lax in setting the regulations, and states have been equally lax in enforcing them. Legislation passed in 1996 requires that community water systems provide annual reports to their customers on water contaminants, in hopes that public pressure will force better compliance with the standards.

Complying with federal drinking water standards is expensive, and many communities do not do so—including New York City, which spent years trying to find a way to clean up its reservoirs without building a multibillion-dollar filtration plant. In a 2007 agreement with the EPA, the city agreed to work with upstate counties where its main reservoirs lie to protect the watershed. The city has also built a filtration plant in the Bronx to filter water from the more polluted reservoirs in areas closer to the city and an ultraviolet disinfection facility in Westchester County. Another dilemma concerning drinking water is that chlorine, the most common disinfectant used to kill microbes in the water, may itself cause harmful health effects. A recently discovered problem is that drinking water often contains pharmaceuticals and other household chemicals in low concentrations, the health effects of which are not well understood.

Lead-contaminated drinking water is a recurring problem in municipalities across the United States, but it took a major crisis in Flint, Michigan, to bring much needed attention to this issue. In 2019, California implemented a novel plan to help poorer communities upgrade their water supplies, which could provide a model for other areas.

The supply of fresh water on earth is finite, and many areas of the world, including parts of the United States, suffer from shortages.

References

1. A. Nadakavukaren, *Our Global Environment: A Health Perspective*, 7th ed. (Prospect Heights, IL: Waveland Press, 2011).

2. Centers for Disease Control and Prevention, "Surveillance for Waterborne-Disease Outbreaks—United States, 1993–1994," *Morbidity and Mortality Weekly Report* 45 (1996): SS-1.

3. G. F. Craun et al., "Waterborne Outbreaks Reported in the United States," *Journal of Water and Health* 4 (2006 suppl 2): 19–30.

4. Centers for Disease Control and Prevention, "Surveillance Reports for Drinking Water-Associated Disease and Outbreaks," June 2, 2015, https://www.cdc.gov/healthywater/surveillance/drinking-surveillance-reports.html, accessed August 1, 2015.

5. D. Zwick and M. Benstock, *Water Wasteland: Ralph Nader's Study Group Report on Water Pollution* (New York, NY: Grossman Publishers, 1971).

6. W. J. Hayes Jr., *Pesticides Studied in Man* (Baltimore, MD: Williams & Wilkins, 1982).

7. C. Duhigg, "Sewers at Capacity, Waste Poisons Waterways," *The New York Times*, November 23, 2009.

8. American Academy of Sewage Engineers, "2017 Infrastructure Report Card," 2019, https://www.infrastructurereportcard.org/cat-item/wastewater/, accessed December 20, 2019.

9. A. Nadakavukaren, *Our Global Environment: A Health Perspective*, 5th ed. (Prospect Heights, IL: Waveland Press, 2000).

10. U.S. Environmental Protection Agency, "Summary of Water Quality Assessments for Each Waterbody Type," https://ofmpub.epa.gov/waters10/attains_nation_cy.control#total_assessed_waters, accessed October 7, 2019.

11. U.S. Environmental Protection Agency, "Water on Tap: What You Need to Know," December 2009, https://nepis.epa.gov/Exe/ZyPURL.cgi?Dockey=P1008ZP0.TXT, accessed December 20, 2019.

12. Centers for Disease Control and Prevention, "Surveillance for Waterborne Disease Outbreaks Associated with Drinking Water—United States, 2013–2014," *Morbidity and Mortality Weekly Report* 66, no. 44 (November 2017): 1216–1221.

13. M. Allaire, H. Wu, and U. Lall, "National Trends in Drinking Water Quality Violations," *Proceedings of the National Academy of Sciences USA* 115 (2018): 2078–2083.

14. Centers for Disease Control and Prevention, "2013–2014 Recreational Water–Associated Outbreak Surveillance Report Supplemental Tables," https://www.cdc.gov/healthywater/surveillance/recreational/2013-2014-tables.html, accessed October 7, 2019.

15. L. A. DeSimone, P. A. Hamilton, and R. J. Gilliom, "Quality of Ground Water from Private Domestic Wells," *Water Well Journal* 63 (2009): 33–37.

16. Centers for Disease Control and Prevention, "Drinking Water: Commercially Bottled Water," July 7, 2014, https://www.cdc.gov/healthywater/drinking/bottled/index.html, accessed December 20, 2019.

17. J. Doleac, "New Evidence That Lead Exposure Increases Crime," *Brookings Up Front*, June 1, 2017.

18. M. Wines and J. Schwartz, "Regulatory Gaps Leave Unsafe Lead Levels in Water Nationwide," *The New York Times*, February 8, 2016.

19. K. Taylor, "Most New York City Schools Had High Lead Levels, Retests Find," *The New York Times*, April 28, 2017.

20. S. Atkinson, A. Haimerl, and R. Perez-Pena, "Anger and Scrutiny Grow Over Poisoned Water in Michigan City," *The New York Times*, January 15, 2016.

21. J. Bosman, "EPA Waited Too Long to Warn of Flint Water Danger, Report Says," *The New York Times*, October 20, 2016.

22. M. Smith and L. Friedman, "After Flint, Watchdog Urges EPA to Monitor Drinking Water More Closely," *The New York Times*, July 19, 2018.

23. S. Atkinson and M. Davey, "5 Charged with Involuntary Manslaughter in Flint Water Crisis," *The New York Times*, June 14, 2017.

24. M. Smith, "Flint Water Prosecutors Drop Criminal Charges, with Plans to Keep Investigating," *The New York Times*, June 13, 2019.

25. L. Firestone and S. De Anda, "Safe Drinking Water for All," *The New York Times*, August 21, 2018.

26. A. Finder, "Delay Sought on Approving Watershed Plans," *The New York Times*, April 7, 1995.

27. A. Revkin, "New York Begins Spending to Save City's Reservoirs," *The New York Times*, January 22, 1997.

28. A. Revkin, "Billion-Dollar Plan to Clean New York City Water at Its Source," *The New York Times*, August 31, 1997.

29. New York City Department of Environmental Protection, "New York City 2014 Drinking Water Supply and Quality Report," http://www.nyc.gov/html/dep/pdf/wsstate14.pdf, accessed August 2, 2015.

30. D. W. Dunlap, "As a Plant Nears Completion, Croton Water Flows Again to New York City," *The New York Times*, May 8, 2015.

31. U.S. Environmental Protection Agency, "Drinking Water Infrastructure Needs Survey and Assessment," April 2013, https://www.epa.gov/sites/production/files/2018-10/documents/corrected_sixth_drinking_water_infrastructure_needs_survey_and_assessment.pdf, accessed December 20, 2019.

32. B. M. Kuehn, "Traces of Drugs Found in Drinking Water," *Journal of the American Medical Association* 299 (2008): 2011–2013.

33. D. J. Caldwell, F. Mastrocco, E. Nowak, J. Johnston, H. Yekel, D. Pfeiffer, et al., "An Assessment of Potential Exposure and Risk from Estrogen in Drinking Water," *Environmental Health Perspectives* 118 (2010): 338–344.

CHAPTER 23

Not in My Backyard

Solid and Hazardous Wastes: What to Do with the Garbage?

KEY TERMS

Comprehensive Environmental
 Response, Compensation,
 and Liability Act
Municipal solid waste

Recycling
Resource Conservation and
 Recovery Act (RCRA)

Sanitary landfills
Superfund

In the spring and summer of 1987, the problem of solid waste disposal was brought to national attention by the plight of the "garbage barge" that could not find a place to unload its cargo. Carrying more than 3000 tons of commercial trash banned from the local landfill in Islip, New York, the barge's vain search for a disposal site somewhere along the Atlantic or Gulf coasts, Belize or the Bahamas, made national news over a five-month period. Finally, the barge returned to New York, and the trash was incinerated.[1(Ch.16)]

Americans dispose of about 260 million tons of municipal solid waste each year.[2] In 2015, this amounted to 4.48 pounds per person per day. **Municipal solid waste** includes durable goods, nondurable goods, containers and packaging, food scraps, yard trimmings, and miscellaneous inorganic wastes from residential, commercial, institutional, and industrial sources. It does not include construction and demolition debris, automobile bodies, municipal sludges, and industrial process wastes, all of which must also be disposed of in some way. **Figure 23-1** gives a breakdown of the composition of municipal solid wastes. The greatest portion of it is paper; much of it is packaging.

Garbage collection has been an important responsibility of local governments since the late 19th century. At that time, it was recognized that rats, flies, and other vermin attracted by garbage carry diseases such as plague and typhus. Even earlier, enlightened cities—including ancient Athens—required that wastes be disposed of outside the city walls.

Until the 1970s, little attention was paid to what was done with the garbage after it was

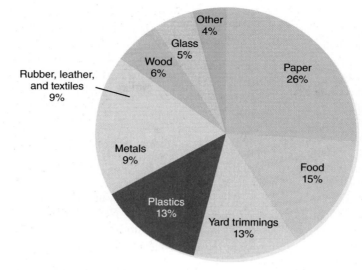

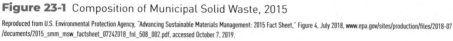

Figure 23-1 Composition of Municipal Solid Waste, 2015

taken away from residential neighborhoods. Most often, it was disposed of in open dumps. Sometimes it was burned, either in incinerators or out in the open, at the dump. Another approach was to pour it into nearby rivers, lakes, or oceans. The drawbacks of these methods became obvious as the volume of garbage increased. Garbage washed up on beaches and contaminated drinking water. Incinerators emitted foul odors, noxious fumes, and black smoke. Dumps, in addition to supporting large populations of vermin, produced toxic leachates that seeped through the soil and contaminated groundwater.

Environmental protection laws banned these methods of waste disposal, which merely transferred garbage from one part of the environment to another. The Clean Air Act made most incinerators illegal; the Clean Water Act outlawed dumping into rivers and lakes; and the Marine Protection, Research, and Sanctuaries Act of 1972, with later amendments, prohibited most ocean dumping. Open dumps were outlawed by many states and then by the federal government in 1976 with the

Resource Conservation and Recovery Act (RCRA). RCRA (colloquially known as "rickra") also set standards for sanitary landfills, which have replaced dumps as the most common method of municipal waste disposal.[3(Ch.17)]

Sanitary Landfills

Current standards for **sanitary landfills** require wastes to be confined in a sealed area. A properly designed landfill starts with an appropriate site, which should be dry and consist of impervious clay soil. A large hole is dug and lined with plastic. Refuse is spread in thin layers, compacted by bulldozers, and covered each day with a thin layer of soil. Since decomposing organic matter produces liquids, which may dissolve metals and other toxins, and potentially explosive gases, vents and drains must be constructed to control these hazards. In recent decades, some landfills have collected the gases and used them directly as an alternative fuel or burned them to produce renewable energy in the form of electricity.[2] When the landfill reaches its capacity, it is covered with a 2-foot layer of soil. The surface can then be used for a park, golf course, or other recreational facility.

The biggest drawback of sanitary landfills as a method of waste disposal is that they take up a lot of space. In many parts of the country, this commodity is readily available—but some urban areas are running out of land. It is expensive to transport garbage from crowded areas to disposal sites with plenty of free space. A measure of the availability of landfill space is the "tipping fee," the cost for disposing of a ton of municipal solid waste. In 2017, the average tipping fee in the United States for burial in a landfill was $50.30 per ton. The Northeast generally has the highest tipping fees, averaging $74.75; and western United States has lower fees, averaging $35.69.[4] Complicating the problem for cities is the phenomenon known as "NIMBY," meaning "not in my backyard." Simply put, people do not want a landfill in their neighborhood. Even people in areas of the country that have plenty of open space resist the idea of having to accept garbage sent from faraway cities.

The problem is epitomized by the garbage crisis in New York City, which was brought to a head by residents' complaints about the Fresh Kills landfill on Staten Island, a relatively rural borough located within city limits. Fresh Kills began taking garbage in 1948, and by 1996 it was accepting approximately 13,000 tons per day. It never met even minimal environmental standards, and in 1996 the U.S. Environmental Protection Agency (EPA) ordered it to cut down on emissions of noxious gases.[5] Meanwhile, the city's Department of Sanitation proposed to conduct regular tours of the site—"the world's largest dump"—a proposal that horrified city authorities and was promptly squelched.[6] Mayor Rudolph Giuliani then proposed to close it down. Fresh Kills was closed, with much fanfare, in March 2001. Except for its use to dispose of World Trade Center debris after the September 11 attacks, the site has remained closed. Since then, New York City has struggled with the difficulties of

sending its wastes to landfills in other states, mostly Pennsylvania and Virginia. City sanitation trucks took the 12,000 tons of residential wastes per day to transfer stations in the five boroughs and New Jersey, where it was loaded onto tractor trailers for the trip. Roughly the same amount of commercial waste is managed by private carting companies, but it ends up in the same place. The total cost to the city of disposing of a ton of trash in 2004 had risen to $75—40% more than it cost in 1997—and there was concern about the willingness of Pennsylvania and Virginia to continue accepting New York's garbage.[7] In 2006, the city published a comprehensive solid-waste management plan, designed to address environmental issues, to increase reliability, and to reduce costs. The plan, which is now being implemented despite many controversies, includes an increase in recycling, a shift from reliance on trucks to trains and barges for carrying trash out of the city (to reduce pollution and fuel costs), and an attempt to find landfill space within New York State.[8]

Meanwhile, Fresh Kills is being turned into a park. The mountains of garbage need to settle and then will be capped with more than 2 feet of soil. Work is under way to turn the former landfill into acres of marshes and streams full of wildlife, as well as paths for hikers, bikers, horses, and cross-country skiers. The park currently holds occasional events and tours. It will be opened in phases through 2036.[9,10]

Alternatives to Landfills

Currently, approximately 53% of municipal solid waste, as well as wastes from other sources, is disposed of in landfills.[2] It is obvious that the garbage crisis could be eased if the volume that goes to landfills could be reduced. The only way to make landfills last longer is to apply the "three R's": reduce, reuse, and recycle.

Prevention of a disposal problem by reducing waste materials at the source is obviously the most efficient approach. Consumer behavior holds the key to successfully reducing waste by this approach. The reduction strategy requires people to buy only the amount of a product that will be used, to choose items without excessive packaging, and to use reusable napkins, towels, diapers, dishes, and cups rather than the disposable variety. The popularity of yard sales is a favorable trend toward achieving reduction of waste through reuse. Although governmental action to encourage the reduction of wastes is still not widespread, some communities have taken concrete steps to incentivize the desired consumer behavior. For example, some residential garbage-pickup services charge by the bag, encouraging residents to cut down on volume. Some states impose taxes on hard-to-dispose-of items such as tires, batteries, and motor oil.

Recycling, technically called resource recovery, is rapidly growing as a method of reducing the amount of waste that must be put in landfills. In 2015, 35% of municipal solid waste was recycled or composted nationwide.[2] Providing curbside collection of separated recyclables is one way that communities encourage recycling. Having refundable deposits on bottles and cans is another very effective way to encourage recycling. As of 2019, 10 states required such deposits; recycling rates ranged from 70% to 90% in these states, about 2.5 times the rate in states without bottle bills. Michigan, which raised its deposit to 10 cents per bottle, the highest in the nation, has a recycling rate of 95%.[11]

The greatest obstacle to the growth of recycling is a lack of a market for used glass, metal, plastic, and paper. Paper is a special problem: It constitutes such a large proportion of trash, yet cannot be recycled indefinitely because the fibers break down. Some states require that newspapers contain a specified minimum percentage of recycled fiber. Since governments use large quantities of paper, they can make a significant impact on the recycled paper market. Some states and cities have passed laws requiring recycling of paper or use of recycled paper. Approximately 67% of paper and paperboard is currently recycled. Because a healthy market for recyclables depends on their use for new products, economic downturns, such as the great recession in 2008 and 2009, have a negative impact on the market for all recycled materials. Recycling will remain cost-effective, however, as long as the price of placing trash in landfills remains high.[1(Ch.17),12]

Composting is a form of recycling that allows natural decay processes to convert yard and food wastes to mulch, which is useful in gardening. Composting may be done on an individual or municipal level. Some communities mix their compost with sewage sludge to produce a rich fertilizer for agricultural uses.

Another approach to useful disposal of solid waste is waste-to-energy incineration, which both reduces solid waste and produces heat and energy. Special incinerators for this purpose have been designed to minimize the emission of air pollutants. However, the possibility still exists that they may emit toxic gases, including dioxins and furans from the burning of plastics, lead, cadmium, and mercury vapors from batteries mixed in with municipal wastes. Incinerator ash must be disposed of as a hazardous waste, because it frequently contains dangerous levels of heavy metals. NIMBY opposition tends to make finding a site for a waste-to-energy incinerator politically difficult, and building and operating one is expensive because of all the safety features required. Approximately 13% of municipal solid waste is disposed of by incineration.[2]

Hazardous Wastes

A small but significant percentage of solid waste consists of hazardous waste. These materials are toxic to humans, plants, or animals; are likely to explode; or are corrosive and thus likely to burn through containers or human skin. Two special categories of hazardous wastes that are regulated under separate laws are radioactive wastes and infectious medical wastes.

The problem of hazardous waste disposal first came to public attention in 1978 when Love Canal made the news. Residents of a 20-year-old housing development in the town of Niagara Falls, New York, had been noticing some alarming phenomena. After a season of heavy rains and snowfalls, noxious chemicals had begun to bubble up in backyards and seep into basements. Chemical odors were prevalent. Children developed rashes and watering eyes after playing outdoors. Heavy rains washed away soil to reveal buried metal drums, which were corroded and leaking. Reports began to circulate of cancer, birth defects, miscarriages, and other health problems among residents of the area. The alarmed citizens demanded that something be done.[1(Ch.17)]

The New York State Health Department and the EPA began to investigate. Analyses of soil samples from backyards, air samples in the basements of homes, and water samples in sump pumps and storm sewers revealed contamination by more than 200 different chemicals, including benzene, dioxin, pesticides, and a number of other known carcinogens and teratogens. In August 1978, President Jimmy Carter declared Love Canal a federal disaster area. Over the next several years, hundreds of Love Canal families were evacuated from their homes.[1(Ch.17)]

The source of the problem was an abandoned industrial dump, a trench originally intended to be a canal but never finished, which was used by a chemical company for disposal of its wastes over a 10-year period. In 1952, the trench was declared full and covered with soil. The city took over the property to build a school. By the time home building began in the neighborhood several years later, most people had forgotten about the former activities at the site, and it did not occur to anyone that the area might be hazardous.

Over much of the same period that the Love Canal problems were taking place, another hazardous waste drama was playing out in Missouri. The first act consisted of several episodes in 1971, when waste oil was sprayed on the floors of several horse arenas around the state, a practice used to keep the dust down. After the spraying, a wave of mysterious illnesses began affecting animals and people who came in contact with the dirt. Several children were sickened, some with chloracne, and some had to be hospitalized with severe flu-like symptoms. Horses were badly affected, and many died. Hundreds of dead birds were found in the area. The waste oil was suspected, but the hauler claimed there was nothing unusual about the oil. Investigators from the Missouri Department of Health and the Centers for Disease Control and Prevention (CDC) could find nothing unusual in the soil samples or in the blood of the victims. Meanwhile, the same hauler had been hired to spray oil on 23 miles of dirt roads in Times Beach, a community of about 2000 people near St. Louis, during the summer of 1972 and during each of the next four summers.[13]

CDC scientists continued to run tests on the soil from the horse arenas, and in 1974 they identified concentrations of dioxin as high as 31,000 parts per billion (ppb). This was more than high enough to cause human illnesses and the deaths of animals. Further investigation revealed that the oil hauler had been hired by a chemical company to dispose of wastes from the manufacture of Agent Orange, an herbicide used in the Vietnam War. The hauler was mixing this waste oil with used crankcase oil and using it for his spraying operations. The CDC was able to trace the hauler's activities and discovered Times Beach, among other places, where no problems had been suspected. That revelation came in 1982, at just about the time when the community was inundated by a flood, which, it was feared, spread the dioxin throughout the town. Tests found dioxin levels on the order of 100 ppb on roads and in yards. Residents panicked.[13]

In the end, Times Beach, like Love Canal, was evacuated. In retrospect, this decision has been widely criticized as an overreaction. The levels of dioxin in Times Beach were much lower than those in the horse arenas, and more modest remediation would probably have sufficed. However, little was known at that time about the toxicity and carcinogenicity of dioxin in humans. The effects on animals were certainly a cause of concern.

Love Canal residents have been carefully tracked for health outcomes that might be associated with the exposures. The New York State Department of Health interviewed more than 6000 former residents between 1978 and 1982, and in 1996 it began searching records of births and deaths and state registries of cancer diagnoses and congenital malformations for evidence of health problems. In a report of the study published in 2008, researchers identified clear evidence of adverse reproductive outcomes, including low birth weight and preterm birth, among women who had lived at Love Canal. Especially notable was the finding that women who had been exposed to waste at Love Canal as children were twice as likely to give birth to infants with congenital malformations than were comparable women who had grown up elsewhere. There were also indications of an increased risk of some forms of cancer, especially lung cancer.[14] The follow-up of these residents will be continued.

RCRA, the federal legislation first enacted in 1976 to deal with solid waste disposal, included special regulations on handling of wastes that potentially posed a hazard to health and the environment. These regulations, which were strengthened by amendments to RCRA in 1984 and 1992, can prevent future Love Canals and Times Beaches. They require that all hazardous wastes be accounted for "from cradle to grave," and impose criminal penalties for businesses and individuals who violate the laws. However, legal disposal of hazardous wastes is expensive, and no one knows how much illegal "midnight dumping" may actually go on today.[1(Ch.17)]

RCRA lists many specific wastes that are regulated under the law, including wastes from petroleum refining, pesticide manufacturing, and some pharmaceutical products. Wastes are also considered hazardous if they are ignitable, corrosive, reactive, or toxic. Stricter regulations apply to large-quantity generators, defined as facilities that generate more than 2200 pounds per month, than to small-quantity generators, defined as facilities that generate between 220 and 2200 pounds per month. Facilities that generate the smallest amounts of waste are subject to only minimal requirements. The RCRA regulations have two key elements: tracking and permitting. The tracking requirement, illustrated in **Figure 23-2**, mandates that paperwork document the progress of hazardous waste from its site of generation through treatment, storage, and disposal. Permitting means that any facility that treats, stores, or disposes of hazardous waste must be issued a permit from the EPA or the state; the permit prescribes standards for management of the waste. Transportation of hazardous waste, which must be clearly labeled, is regulated by the U.S. Department of Transportation.[15]

According to the EPA, more than 40 million tons of hazardous waste are managed annually under the RCRA regulations.[16] Like municipal solid waste, hazardous waste is managed by practicing the three R's: reduce, reuse, and recycle. One way of reducing this kind of waste is by treating it to make it less hazardous; this can be done, for example, by biological or chemical treatment, by burning the waste at high temperatures, and by separating solids from wastewater to reduce the volume of waste subject to disposal. A common method of disposing of liquid hazardous waste is to inject it under pressure into underground wells encased with steel and concrete. Specially designed landfills are also used for disposing of hazardous waste. Efforts to reduce the generation of hazardous wastes have paid off, however, and the volume that needs to be disposed of is much reduced from previous decades.[17]

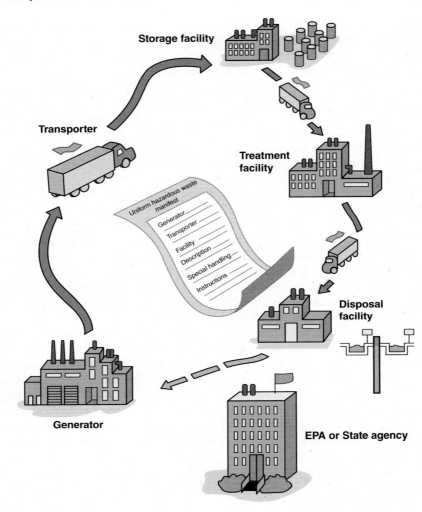

Figure 23-2 Tracking of Hazardous Wastes

Reproduced from U.S. Environmental Protection Agency, "RCRA: Reducing Risk From Waste," p. 18, September 1997, https://archive.epa.gov/epawaste/inforesources/web/pdf/risk-1.pdf, accessed October 6, 2019.

While RCRA was meant to control hazardous wastes as they are generated, it was inadequate to deal with the old waste sites that kept turning up in the news after public consciousness had been raised about these issues. In response, in 1980 Congress passed the **Comprehensive Environmental Response, Compensation, and Liability Act**, commonly known as "**Superfund**." That law required the EPA to compile a priority list of waste sites that threatened the public health or environmental quality, and it authorized $1.6 billion over a five-year period for emergency cleanup of these sites. The cleanup was paid for by a tax on industry, which created the trust fund that gave the program its name. Superfund was reauthorized in 1986 and 1990, allocating additional billions of dollars for cleanup.[3(Ch.17)]

The Superfund program has been mired in controversy from the beginning. The pace of the cleanup has been slow, and the cost has been very high. New sites are being added to the priority list more rapidly than old sites are being cleaned up and removed. As of October 2019, there were 1176 sites on the list and 45 sites had been proposed for addition. Cleanup had been completed on 407 sites, which had been deleted from the list.[18] Because the legislation calls for polluters to pay for the cleanup, a great deal of effort has been devoted to trying to establish who is liable. Congress did not reauthorize the corporate taxes that paid into the trust fund when the tax expired in 1995, and the fund has been exhausted. Although cleanup of many sites continues to move forward and is being paid for by the polluters—for example, General Electric Company is paying for the dredging of the Hudson River—cleanup of "orphan" sites, for which the responsible company could not be identified or could not pay, is now being funded by taxpayer dollars. The 2009 American Recovery and Reinvestment Act allocated $600 million to facilitate further cleanup of Superfund sites, giving hope that the most contaminated sites can be addressed.[3(Ch. 17)]

Another problem faced by the Superfund program is the shortage of cleanup options—that is, the question of what to do with the toxic materials removed from a site. To prevent the mere shifting of toxic materials from one place to another, Congress specified that cleanup actions should permanently and significantly reduce the volume, toxicity, or mobility of hazardous substances. Creative solutions are urgently needed. There are also disagreements over how clean is clean enough. The EPA's "Brownfields" initiative sets lower standards for sites designated for industrial use, an approach that makes cleanup easier but is less acceptable to some communities.[1(Ch.17)]

Americans have been very concerned about hazardous waste disposal and cleanup, especially when it affects their neighborhoods. Some critics believe that the degree of concern is out of proportion to the actual risk to public health. While the release of toxic gases into the air and the leaching of toxic liquids into water supplies are important public health risks because many humans are likely to be exposed to these hazards, the risks from toxic substances buried in the ground are much less certain. At times, nearly one-fourth of the EPA's entire budget has been allocated to the Superfund program, and additional funds are contributed by industry. At present, it is not clear whether this is a rational allocation of our spending on the environment. Methods of analyzing risk and understanding the balance between benefits and costs can help make such decisions.

Coal Ash

A previously obscure category of waste hit the news just before Christmas 2008, when a dam on the banks of a Tennessee River tributary broke, spilling a billion gallons of toxic sludge across 300 acres of East Tennessee. The earthen dam was holding back millions of cubic yards of wet coal ash, waste from a Tennessee Valley Authority power plant that burned 14,000 tons of coal per day and supplied enough electricity for 670,000 households. In addition to destroying and damaging homes in the area, the spill polluted the river water with thousands of pounds of arsenic, lead, and other toxic and carcinogenic metals.[19]

It turns out that coal ash was not regulated by the EPA, which had been studying the issue for more than 28 years amid controversy about whether to consider this material hazardous or nonhazardous waste. Meanwhile, the volume of ash produced grew from less than 90 million tons in 1990 to 121 million tons in 2007. Most of the waste is stored in more than 1300 open dumps around the country, where heavy metal contaminants have been leached into water in at least 26 states. The results have been decimated fish, bird, and frog populations and contaminated drinking water for an unknown number of people. Coal ash has also been used for construction landfill, mine reclamation, and "improvement" of soil for agricultural and golf courses.[20] The Barack Obama administration finally announced new regulations on coal ash in December 2014.[21] In 2018, the Donald Trump administration began rolling back these regulations, potentially leaving communities and wildlife exposed to these hazards once again.[22]

Conclusion

As concern about environmental pollution has grown, the problem of disposing of solid wastes has become more difficult to resolve. Traditional solutions, such as dumping garbage into waterways or incinerating it, can no longer be used because they increase water and air pollution. Old-fashioned open dumps cause noxious odors and attract vermin.

Solid-waste disposal is now confined to sanitary landfills, which must meet federal standards. But in many parts of the country, there is a shortage of space available for landfills. Communities typically resist having sanitary landfills sited near them—the NIMBY phenomenon.

The problem of finding space for garbage could be eased if the volume of garbage could be reduced—for example, by eliminating excessive packaging and charging consumers for disposal by volume. Recycling and use of reusable—as opposed to disposable—products also help reduce the volume of garbage.

Hazardous wastes present an especially difficult disposal problem. Several environmental scandals in the 1970s and early 1980s, including the Love Canal crisis in New York and the Times Beach incident in Missouri, brought national attention to the need for regulation of hazardous waste disposal. Federal legislation known as RCRA requires that all hazardous wastes be accounted for "from cradle to grave." Superfund legislation provides for identification and cleanup of hazardous-waste sites dating from before RCRA. Although both programs have shortcomings, they have contributed—along with federal laws on air and water pollution—to a significant improvement in the environment. Congress has not reauthorized the corporate taxes to support cleanup under Superfund, but the program continues, paid for by polluters and taxpayers.

An environmental problem that has emerged recently is coal ash, waste from coal-burning power plants, which had not been regulated by law. Recent spills from coal ash dumps into rivers and other bodies of water have called attention to the toxic contaminants contained in the ash, poisoning wildlife and threatening human health.

References

1. A. Nadakavukaren, *Our Global Environment: A Health Perspective*, 5th ed. (Prospect Heights, IL: Waveland Press, 2000).

2. U.S. Environmental Protection Agency, "Advancing Sustainable Materials Management: 2015 Fact Sheet," July 2018, https://www.epa.gov/sites/production/files /2018-07/documents/2015_smm_msw_factsheet _07242018_fnl_508_002.pdf, accessed October 7, 2019.

3. A. Nadakavukaren, *Our Global Environment: A Health Perspective*, 7th ed. (Prospect Heights, IL: Waveland Press, 2011).

4. "No End in Sight to US Landfill Cost Increases: Pacific Region to Experience Highest Growth," *Waste Business Journal*, June 13, 2018, http://www .wasteinfo.com/news/wbj20180613A.htm, accessed October 6, 2019.

5. I. Fisher, "EPA Tells Landfills to Curb Gas Emissions," *The New York Times*, March 3, 1996.

6. B. Weber, "Broadway, Statue of Liberty and Fresh Kills? World's Biggest Garbage Dump Hopes to Draw Tourists as Well as Gulls," *The New York Times*, March 27, 1996.

7. W. C. Thompson Jr., City of New York, Office of the Comptroller, "No Room to Move: New York City's Impending Solid Waste Crisis," October 2004, https://comptroller.nyc.gov/wp-content/uploads/documents/Oct06-04_No-room-to-move.pdf, accessed October 6, 2019.

8. S. Chan, "Gansevoort Deal Ends Impasse Over Waste," June 25, 2008, https://cityroom.blogs.nytimes.com/2008/06/25/gansevoort-deal-ends-impasse-over-waste, accessed October 6, 2019.

9. J. S. Russell, "Garbage Mountains Slowly Morph into $160 Million New York Park," *The New York Times*, September 23, 2010.

10. New York City Department of Parks and Recreation, "Freshkills Park," https://www.nycgovparks.org/park-features/freshkills-park, accessed October 6, 2019.

11. Container Recycling Institute, "Bottle Bill Resource Guide," http://www.bottlebill.org, accessed October 6, 2019.

12. M. Richtel and K. Galbraith, "Back at Junk Value, Recyclables Are Piling Up," *The New York Times*, December 8, 2008.

13. M. J. Schneider, *Persistent Poisons: Chemical Pollutants in the Environment* (New York, NY: New York Academy of Sciences, 1979).

14. New York State Department of Health, "Love Canal Follow-up Health Study," October 2008, https://www.health.state.ny.us/environmental/investigations/love_canal/docs/report_public_comment_final.pdf, accessed October 6, 2019.

15. U.S. Environmental Protection Agency, "RCRA: Reducing Risk from Waste," https://archive.epa.gov/epawaste/inforesources/web/pdf/risk-1.pdf, accessed October 6, 2019.

16. U.S. Environmental Protection Agency, "Hazardous Waste," July 11, 2019, https://www.epa.gov/hw, accessed October 6, 2019.

17. U.S. Environmental Protection Agency, "Analyzing Generation and Management of Priority Chemicals 2005–2007: The National Priority Chemicals Trends Report," February 8, 2013, https://archive.epa.gov/epawaste/hazard/wastemin/web/pdf/toc.pdf, accessed October 6, 2019.

18. U.S. Environmental Protection Agency, "Superfund: National Priorities List (NPL)," October 1, 2019, https://www.epa.gov/superfund/superfund-national-priorities-list-npl, accessed October 6, 2019.

19. S. Dewan, "At Plant in Coal Ash Spill, Toxic Deposits by the Ton," *The New York Times*, December 30, 2008.

20. S. Dewan, "Hundreds of Coal Ash Dumps Lack Significant Regulation," *The New York Times*, January 7, 2009.

21. U.S. Environmental Protection Agency, "Final Rule: Disposal of Coal Combustion Residuals from Electric Utilities," July 15, 2015, https://www.epa.gov/sites/production/files/2014-12/documents/factsheet_ccrfinal_2.pdf, accessed October 6, 2019.

22. N. Popovich, L. Albeck-Ripka, and K. Pierre-Louis, "85 Environmental Rules Being Rolled Back Under Trump," *The New York Times*, September 12, 2019.

CHAPTER 24

Meat Inspection

Safe Food and Drugs: An Ongoing Regulatory Battle

KEY TERMS

Clinical trials
Dietary Supplement Health
and Education Act
Foodborne diseases

FoodNet
Hazard analysis critical control
point (HACCP)

PulseNet
Toxins

Americans are very concerned about the safety of their food. Although Americans used to think of their food supply as the safest in the world, this confidence has been shaken in recent decades by widely publicized outbreaks of illnesses caused by foods ranging from bagged spinach to peanut butter.

Only the most serious cases of foodborne disease are reported, so the true extent of this problem is unclear. The Centers for Disease Control and Prevention (CDC) has estimated that 48 million people contract foodborne diseases each year, 128,000 are hospitalized, and 3000 people die.[1] With some 300 million people eating three meals per day, not counting snacks, however, the likelihood of getting sick from eating a single meal is extremely small.

Many government agencies—local, state, and federal—are involved with regulating

food safety. The challenge is enormous: An analysis published in 1992 estimated that some 6100 meat and poultry plants, more than 50,000 food processing establishments, about 537,000 commercial restaurants, 172,000 institutional food programs, 190,000 retail food stores, and 1 million food vending locations are subject to government inspection, and the numbers have certainly grown since this analysis was performed.[2]

The need for government oversight of the food supply, like many other public health measures, arose with the urbanization of the population. City dwellers neither grew their own food nor knew its source and history. Demands for action arose as the public became aware of unhygienic conditions such as those in meatpacking plants—conditions revealed in Upton Sinclair's 1906 novel, The Jungle. Other widespread practices that outraged the public included adulteration of supposedly pure food with cheaper materials and the use of sometimes toxic additives to improve color and conceal spoilage. The Federal Food and Drugs Act and the Meat Inspection Act, both passed in 1906, established a program to supervise and control the circumstances of manufacture, labeling, and sale of food.[3]

Because similar abuses occurred in the sale of medicines, the 1906 Federal Food and Drugs Act also included provisions to control the manufacturing, labeling, and sale of drugs. The U.S. Food and Drug Administration (FDA), created to oversee regulation of food and drugs, was later given authority over cosmetics, medical devices, and feed and drugs for pets and farm animals.

Causes of Foodborne Illness

Foodborne diseases are most often caused by contamination of foods with bacteria, viruses, or parasites due to breakdowns in sanitation and/or proper food handling practices. *Salmonella* bacteria, for example, are common contaminants of poultry, meat, and eggs. Infected hens may transfer the pathogens to the eggs as they are being formed in the chicken's ovary. Although the bacteria are killed when the food is thoroughly cooked, people who prefer their meat rare or their egg yolks runny are at risk of salmonellosis, especially if the food has been kept at room temperature long enough for the bacteria to flourish. Caesar salad dressing made with raw eggs and homemade eggnog are particularly risky. The symptoms of salmonellosis, like the symptoms of most types of food poisoning, include vomiting, diarrhea, and abdominal pain.

Like *Salmonella* in poultry and eggs, *Escherichia coli* 0157:H7 is widespread in beef, probably due to the way livestock are raised and processed. To prevent illness and deaths such as those that occurred in 1993 in Seattle,

hamburgers must be cooked more thoroughly than the previous standard required. In addition to its discovery in ground beef, *E. coli* 0157:H7 has turned up in other foods, including salami, raw milk, lettuce, alfalfa sprouts, and unpasteurized apple juice. These bacteria are common in the intestinal tracts of cows and are excreted with their feces. The contaminated apple juice may have been made from apples that fell onto ground where cows had wandered, and the contaminated lettuce was prepared under unsanitary conditions near a cow pen.[4,5] The alfalfa sprouts could have been contaminated by being grown in fields near cattle feed lots and irrigated with water contaminated by manure.[6]

In fact, fresh produce is responsible for an increasing proportion of foodborne illness. In 2017, the most common single-food categories causing outbreaks were mollusks (41 outbreaks), fish (37), and chicken (23). The categories causing the most individual illnesses were turkey (609 illnesses), fruits (521), and chicken (487).[7] In 2008, the largest foodborne disease outbreak in the previous decade was attributed to *Salmonella*-contaminated jalapeño and serrano peppers imported from Mexico. Investigators traced the infection to two farms, where a pool of water used for irrigation was found to contain the bacteria. This investigation was especially difficult because few of the interviewed victims recalled eating peppers, which were probably a minor ingredient in dishes that were remembered to contain tomatoes. The outbreak sickened 1442 people and contributed to 2 deaths in 43 states, the District of Columbia, and Canada.[8] In 2011, an outbreak caused by *Listeria*-contaminated cantaloupe produced by a Colorado company killed 30 people and sickened 148 more in 28 states.[9]

Fish and shellfish are likely to harbor pathogenic microbes if they are harvested from waters polluted by human sewage. Raw clams and oysters are especially dangerous: Because they grow in shallow coastal waters, which are likely to be polluted, these shellfish may carry cholera and related bacteria, hepatitis A virus, and the common Norwalk virus, all of which are capable of causing disease in humans. Fish used uncooked for Japanese dishes such as sushi and sashimi and South American ceviche may also carry parasites harmful to humans.[3]

Some bacteria cause illness by way of **toxins** they produce rather than by simple infection. Thus these contaminants are hazardous even after the food is cooked. The best known—and deadliest—of these are the bacteria that cause botulism. They flourish in the absence of oxygen and are most commonly associated with home-canned vegetables that were inadequately cooked before canning, although a number of botulism outbreaks have been traced to commercially canned foods. Once the toxin forms, it can be destroyed only by boiling for 15 to 20 minutes—not a common practice with canned foods. Certain fish and shellfish may also contain toxins—for example, ciguatoxin or scombroid poison—produced by bacteria or algae that the fish feed on or that grow on them, thereby poisoning the flesh for human consumption.[3]

Food may also be contaminated by the actions of food handlers, either if they themselves are infected or if they transfer pathogens from one food to another. For example, a salad might be contaminated with *Salmonella* if the raw vegetables are chopped on a cutting board that had previously been used to cut up uncooked chicken. A number of other bacterial or viral infections tend to be transferred by infected food handlers to raw or cooked foods, such as salads, hot dogs, and delicatessen takeout items. The famous case of Typhoid Mary illustrates how an infected food handler can spread pathogenic bacteria even when she herself has no symptoms. Hepatitis A virus is also frequently transmitted by food handlers who are careless about hygiene. This disease is most contagious 10 to 14 days before the onset of symptoms, so it may spread silently before people become visibly ill.

Government Action to Prevent Foodborne Disease

A variety of federal, state, and local agencies are responsible for protecting the safety of the U.S. food supply. Because of patchwork legislation, division of responsibility, and lack of coordination, there are major inconsistencies among different types of foods in terms of the way food safety is regulated. Increasingly, it has become clear that the overall system depends too heavily on detecting and correcting problems after they occur rather than preventing them. As nutritionist Marion Nestle stated in her 2010 book, *Safe Food: The Politics of Food Safety*, "Today, an inventory of federal food safety activities reveals a system breathtaking in its irrationality."[10(p.55)] Some of the shortcomings were remedied by the FDA Food Safety Modernization Act, signed by President Barack Obama in January 2011, though many problems remain.

The FDA and the U.S. Department of Agriculture (USDA) share the primary responsibility for ensuring that foods are safe, wholesome, and properly labeled. The laws governing the actions of these two agencies are highly inconsistent. The USDA is responsible for the safety of meat and poultry, including prepared products that contain more than 2% cooked meat or poultry, as well as for the safety of processed eggs. The law requires inspection of all meat- and poultry-processing plants daily, and an inspector must be on site whenever a slaughtering plant is in operation. The plants that the USDA inspects account for about 20% of federally regulated foods and 26% of foodborne illness outbreaks. The USDA's budget for food safety in 2018 was $1.04 billion.[11]

The FDA is responsible for ensuring the safety of the other 80% of federally regulated foods, including seafood and produce, which account for 66.5% of reported foodborne illness outbreaks. By 2018, the FDA's annual budget for food safety had grown to $1.05 billion.[12] Because of budgetary constraints, the FDA can inspect food-processing facilities under its jurisdiction only once every 10 years, on average. This leads to the paradox that a plant making frozen cheese pizza may be inspected (by the FDA) only once every 10 years, while a plant making frozen pepperoni pizza will be inspected (by the USDA) almost every day. The Food Safety Modernization Law put additional responsibilities on the FDA, including expanded inspections and setting standards for the safe growing, harvesting, sorting, packing, and storage of fresh fruits and vegetables. However, in today's climate of congressional budget cutting, it is not clear whether the FDA's budget will be adequate for carrying out these tasks.

An increasing proportion of Americans' food is imported from other countries, especially developing countries, which poses a challenge to the food safety system. Approximately 50% of fresh fruits, 20% of fresh vegetables, and 80% of seafood sold in the United States are imported.[13] The USDA has the power to bar importing of meat and poultry from countries with inferior food safety systems—a power the FDA lacked for fruits, vegetables, grains, and fish until the passage of the Modernization Act in 2011. The FDA still must rely on port-of-entry inspections, an expensive and ineffective approach, but it now has the authority to deny entry of food from a facility that refuses to permit FDA inspection and it can detain for testing shipments of food that it has reason to believe may be harmful.[13]

Because they are often eaten raw, fruits and vegetables imported from countries with inadequate safety systems are especially risky. In the 1990s, for example, a hepatitis A outbreak was caused by Mexican green onions, a *Salmonella* outbreak by Mexican peppers, and a *Cyclospora* (parasite) outbreak by Guatemalan raspberries. As one CDC official is quoted as saying, "We used to believe you had to travel overseas to get travelers' diarrhea. It's a classic example of emerging infections common in Latin America becoming a problem here."[14]

Fish and shellfish cause more outbreaks than any other food category except produce.[7] Regulation of the fish industry, which falls mainly under jurisdiction of the FDA, is especially difficult because most fish are caught in the wild by independent fishermen in relatively small boats. Fish may have been exposed to viruses or bacterial toxins in polluted waters, or they may have been contaminated with scombroid toxin due to inadequate cooling on the boat. Currently no techniques are available that would allow inspectors on the docks to test for these problems. Shellfish should, in theory, be easier to regulate because their source can be determined. However, much of the enforcement is left to the states, and some of them are lax about enforcing standards.

Fish also have the potential to be contaminated with nonmicrobial toxins. Research published in 2004 revealed that farmed salmon contained potentially dangerous levels of polychlorinated biphenyls (PCBs), as well as dioxin and several organochlorine pesticides. It turned out that farmed fish were fed a concentrated feed that was tainted with the chemicals. Since the news broke, fish farmers have been experimenting with new feeds that will eliminate the PCB problem.[3] Another hazard from fish was revealed in 2008, when *The New York Times* published a report describing high levels of mercury in sushi made from tuna in 20 Manhattan stores and restaurants.[15] It has long been known that pregnant women and children should limit their consumption of some varieties of canned tuna because they contain mercury, but the levels found in the sushi were significantly higher. Mercury gets into the ocean from industrial sources, especially coal-burning power plants; is absorbed by bacteria; and makes its way up the food chain to larger fish such as tuna. The extent of the risk from farmed salmon or tuna continues to inspire debate, because these risks must be balanced against the many health benefits of eating fish.

Because of concerns about seafood, as well as repeated outbreaks caused by meat, including an *E. coli* outbreak from Jack-in-the-Box hamburgers in 1993, the Bill Clinton administration implemented a new preventive approach to meat and seafood safety, which took effect in December 1997.[16] Called the **hazard analysis critical control point** or **HACCP** ("hassip"), the new system was developed in the 1960s by food processors in cooperation with the National Aeronautics and Space Administration to ensure that foods prepared for the astronauts were safe. Rather than relying on inspections, which can never be done frequently or thoroughly enough to ensure complete safety, the HACCP system focuses on procedures, putting the responsibility on food businesses to analyze their procedures and requiring government inspectors to verify compliance. The system involves identifying potential sources of contamination and devising ways to avoid them. HACCP requires an analysis of every step in the process of food production, processing, and preparation (**Box 24-1**). It seeks to identify each possible hazard and, for each, one or more "control points," which are practices and procedures that will eliminate, prevent, or minimize the hazard.[16]

Many companies were already using HACCP, and the FDA and USDA in the late 1990s moved to encourage more reliance on the system. When fully implemented, HACCP is intended to reduce the need for inspections, relying instead on frequent reviews of procedures to make sure the system is being carried out. The USDA now has a mandatory HACCP system for meat and poultry, including a requirement that the foods be tested for common pathogens. The FDA has also implemented HACCP for seafood, making it mandatory in 1999. Raw sprouts, eggs, and fresh juice were added later, but for them, use of the system is voluntary.[3,16]

The FDA, in addition to its oversight of food production on a national scale, issues recommendations that state and local governments can use to regulate establishments that deal with food, including retail stores, restaurants, and institutions such as schools and nursing homes. These rules emphasize the importance of hand washing by food service workers and restricting sick workers from direct contact with food. They also include strict guidelines concerning the temperatures at which food may be stored, cooked, and kept in heating trays. To prevent bacterial growth, foods should be refrigerated at a temperature of 40°F or below, or heated thoroughly so that internal temperatures are above 140°F. Special rules apply to large pieces such as roast meats and stuffed poultry because their internal temperatures may lag behind the external changes in temperature, allowing pathogens to grow during roasting or after refrigeration.[3] Local health departments usually enforce these rules by conducting periodic inspections of stores, restaurants, and institutions, and they are usually authorized by local and state laws to close facilities that are significantly in violation.

One potential solution to the problem of foodborne disease is the use of radiation to kill microbial contaminants in food. The idea of irradiating food frightens many people, and the proposal has aroused great opposition among some consumer groups—yet it leaves no radioactive residue, and more than 40 years of research has shown it to be safe. Irradiation

---

Box 24-1 HACCP Principles

1. Conduct a hazard analysis.
2. Determine the critical control points.
3. Establish critical limits.
4. Establish monitoring procedures.
5. Establish corrective actions.
6. Establish verification procedures.
7. Establish record-keeping and documentation procedures.

Data from U.S. Food and Drug Administration, "HACCP Principles & Application Guidelines," December 19, 2017, www.fda.gov/food /hazard-analysis-critical-control-point-haccp/haccp-principles -application-guidelines#princ, accessed October 8, 2019.

is already used for some foods in the United States and is widely used in some other countries. Radiation treatment kills pests in dried herbs, spices, and tea; controls insects in wheat and flour; and kills the parasites that cause trichinosis when undercooked pork is eaten. It has been shown to greatly reduce the contamination of chicken breasts with *Salmonella*, ground beef with *E. coli* 0157:H7, and shrimp with cholera-causing bacteria. Because microbial contamination of food is such a common hazard, with potentially deadly consequences, many experts believe that widespread use of irradiation could greatly increase the safety of the food supply. The FDA has approved irradiation of a variety of foods including red meat, poultry, shellfish, fruits and vegetables, seeds, herbs and spices, and eggs.[17,18] All foods that have been irradiated are required to be labeled as such. Some experts believe that irradiation should be used routinely for many foods. The CDC has estimated that irradiation of high-risk foods could prevent as many as 1 million cases of bacterial foodborne disease each year in North America.[19]

A very important component of any food safety program is epidemiologic surveillance and prompt follow-up of any foodborne outbreak to prevent further spread of disease. With a nationwide food distribution network, local public health authorities may not recognize that a number of seemingly isolated cases of an illness might be caused by contamination at a single source. The CDC's **PulseNet** program utilizes public health laboratories in all 50 states and Canada to do DNA "fingerprinting" of foodborne bacteria. This network permits timely comparisons of pathogens that may cause outbreaks in various parts of the country, identifying common sources and enabling public health officials to take quick action to halt the distribution of a contaminated food.[20]

The system worked in November 2008, when PulseNet staff noted that an unusual strain of *Salmonella* had been reported from 12 states. As CDC epidemiologists, working with state and local health departments, began to investigate the cluster of cases, more case reports flooded in. Interviews with patients suggested an association with peanut butter. After noting that several of the patients had eaten in institutional settings, including nursing homes and an elementary school, the source of the problem was identified in early January 2009 as peanut butter produced by a Georgia company, which supplied the product to institutions and to producers of other foods, including cookies, crackers, cereal, candy, ice cream, and pet treats. The company voluntarily recalled all products, leading to a cascade of recalls of peanut butter–containing products made by other companies. As of the end of January 2009, 529 people from 43 states had been reported with laboratory-confirmed cases of the same unusual strain; 116 of them had been hospitalized and 8 had died. The outbreak was probably considerably larger than the official numbers, since only about 3% of *Salmonella* infections are laboratory confirmed. The Georgia plant was found to be severely deficient, with investigators discovering rodents, a leaky roof, demoralized workers, and previous evidence of *Salmonella* contamination that had not been addressed. The plant is now closed and the company filed for bankruptcy. The company's former president was convicted on dozens of criminal counts and sentenced to 28 years in prison.[21–23] In 2018, PulseNet was instrumental in the investigation of 25 outbreaks, including those involving *Salmonella* in Achdut brand Tahini and Hy-vee brand Spring Pasta Salad; *E. coli* in romaine lettuce; and *Cyclospora* in McDonald's Fresh Express Salad Mix and Del Monte's Fresh Produce Vegetable Trays.[24]

Another program developed by the CDC is an active surveillance network called **FoodNet**, which is designed to help public health officials better understand the epidemiology of foodborne diseases in the United States.[25] In contrast to the usual epidemiologic surveillance, called passive surveillance, in which the public health agency waits for information to be reported by doctors, hospitals, and laboratories, FoodNet investigators proactively seek out potential cases. They contact laboratories to ask about every case of diarrheal illness they have conducted tests on; send surveys to physicians to determine how often and under what conditions they send stool specimens to laboratories; and even call members of the general population to ask if they have had recent diarrheal illnesses, what they think might have caused it, and whether they sought treatment. The data collected through these methods provide information on less severe foodborne illnesses that are often not reported to public health authorities and help officials at the USDA and FDA identify where their regulatory systems should be improved. The FoodNet network, implemented in 1996, includes, in addition to the CDC, investigators at the USDA, the FDA, and 10 state health departments.

Data collected through these efforts show that *Salmonella* was the leading cause of hospitalization and death in 2015,[25] and its incidence has remained steady since at least 1996.[26] The incidence of *Vibrio* infection, caused by eating contaminated seafood, had increased significantly, while cases involving Shiga toxin-producing *E. coli* have declined.[26]

Despite some signs of improvement, the patchwork system of federal food safety regulation remains, and there have been repeated calls to establish a single, independent agency that would administer a unified, science-based food safety system. The National Academy of Medicine (formerly called the Institute of Medicine), the President's Council on Food Safety, and the U.S. General Accountability Office (GAO) have all conducted studies on the current system and concluded that laws should be revised to give one federal official responsibility and authority to keep the nation's food supply safe. Part of the problem is resistance by the powerful food industry, which has great influence in Congress.[9] In 2015, President Obama proposed consolidating the food safety components of the USDA and the FDA into a single new agency.[27] The need became even more urgent when the threat of bioterrorism became more prominent. In December 2004, when then-Secretary of the U.S. Department of Health and Human Services announced his resignation, he warned of the problem. "For the life of me, I cannot understand why the terrorists have not attacked our food supply because it's so easy to do," Secretary Tommy Thompson said in his final press conference.[28] In 2018, there was another proposal to consolidate federal food safety efforts, this time by the Donald Trump administration, although efforts were still ongoing as of late 2019.[29]

Additives and Contaminants

Food safety standards include limits on contaminants, unwanted substances that accidentally get into food, as well as on additives, which are purposely incorporated into food to improve its taste, color, and resistance to deterioration. Contaminants that can be detected by inspection include dirt, hairs, rodent feces, and insect parts. Pesticide residue may be left on food as a result of crop spraying or when livestock eat pesticide-contaminated fodder. A pesticide law passed by Congress in 1996 requires the Environmental Protection Agency (EPA) to establish tolerance levels—the maximum allowable residues—for all pesticides used on food crops. While earlier health concerns focused on cancer, the new law requires testing of pesticides for damage to the endocrine system and for effects on developing fetuses, infants, and young children. The FDA and the USDA are then required to monitor foods to ensure that pesticide residues are within the allowed tolerance levels.[30]

This monitoring system has been criticized on several fronts: Only a fraction of the food supply is tested, tests are available for only some of the pesticides, and when contaminants are detected, it is often too late to prevent the food from being marketed. This is especially a problem with imported foods, which may contain residues of pesticides that are banned in the United States.

Other possible contaminants include hormones and antibiotics. The use of antibiotics in livestock feed is believed to have led to increased antibiotic resistance in many bacteria. In the past, the sex hormone diethylstilbestrol, a form of estrogen, was fed to chickens to promote their growth. Because of concerns that hormone residues in the meat might increase human breast cancer risk, this practice was banned in 1977. In 1994, the FDA approved the use of bovine growth hormone in dairy cows to increase their milk production. Although hormone residues are generally not found in the milk, many consumers are concerned about the safety of the practice.[3]

Many people choose foods labeled as "organic," believing that these foods are safer than foods grown by common commercial methods. Until 2000, however, no federal standard regulated which foods could carry this label. A 1990 law required the USDA to set standards, but there was so much controversy and objections from the conventional food industry that it took more than a decade for the standards-setting process to be completed and the standards to finally become fully effective in 2002. The standards require that organic meat, poultry, eggs, and dairy products must be grown without antibiotics or growth hormones, and organic produce must be grown without pesticides, synthetic fertilizers, or sewage sludge. Genetically engineered products and radiation are also not allowed for organic foods. Then in early 2004, the George W. Bush administration "clarified" the standards, weakening some of the prohibitions on antibiotics and pesticides.[31,32] Such a clamor of protest arose that the agriculture secretary reversed the new ruling the next day. Studies have shown that organic produce contains only one-third as many pesticide residues as conventionally grown foods and that children fed organic produce and juice have only

one-sixth the level of pesticide by-products in their urine compared with those who eat conventionally farmed foods.[33,34] A law passed in 2014 expanded federal support for organic farming and encouraged consumer access to local produce by means such as farmers markets.[35]

Additives are put into food for a variety of reasons. One purpose is to prevent deficiency diseases that historically caused serious public health problems in the United States. For example, the addition of iodine to table salt has virtually eliminated goiter; vitamin D added to milk has done away with rickets; and niacin, a B vitamin, is added to bread to prevent pellagra. The FDA mandates that folic acid be added to flour and rice products to prevent some birth defects. Other food additives work as preservatives, retarding spoilage or preventing fats from turning rancid. Other additives are used to improve color or to enhance flavor or texture.[3]

Because of public concern about the safety of many food additives, in 1958 Congress passed legislation that required FDA approval for any proposed food additive. Additives already in use were exempted and placed on the GRAS ("generally recognized as safe") list. Since then, several additives on the list have been removed because they turned out not to be safe, including several food colors that were shown to be carcinogenic.

Drugs and Cosmetics

As its name makes clear, the FDA is also responsible for the safety of drugs. This responsibility includes both prescription drugs and over-the-counter drugs—those available without a prescription. Both types of drugs must be proven safe and effective before they can receive marketing approval from the FDA.

The FDA does not test drugs itself. Instead, companies seeking to market new drugs are required by law to conduct the tests and submit the evidence to the agency. FDA staff then review the data and determine whether the evidence supports the new drugs' safety and efficacy.

There is an orderly procedure for collecting the evidence on new prescription drugs. Several stages of exchange of information between the pharmaceutical company and the FDA are required. The company files a new drug application (NDA) for an investigational new drug, providing evidence that the drug has the desired effect in animals and satisfies some basic safety criteria. If the FDA approves the NDA, the company is allowed to test the drug in humans in three phases of **clinical trials**. In phase 1, the new drug is given to a small number of people who are extensively tested to measure the drug's absorption, distribution, metabolism, and excretion, and to look for side effects and toxicities. Phase 2 tests a larger number of patients for signs that the new drug is effective. Phase 3 is a full-scale controlled trial in which patients are assigned randomly to two groups. People in the experimental group receive the new drug, whereas members of the control group receive either a placebo or the standard treatment.[36]

The FDA also has a system of postmarketing surveillance, through which doctors and patients can report adverse reactions to an approved drug. On occasion, after a drug is on the market, evidence emerges that it has risks that were not recognized in preapproval studies. The FDA has revoked its approval of a number of drugs based on such evidence. For years, the agency's drug approval process has involved great political controversy, as described later in this chapter.

Cosmetics are more loosely regulated by the FDA. They do not need preapproval. In fact, there is no requirement for safety testing of cosmetics, other than testing of color additives, but a warning label must be attached to any product that has not been tested. A number of ingredients that were used in cosmetics in the past have been shown to be harmful to health, and their use is prohibited by law. These include several chlorinated compounds as well as some color additives and most compounds containing mercury.

Food and Drug Labeling and Advertising

The scandals that inspired passage of the original Pure Food and Drugs Act of 1906 were cases of economic fraud as much as they were threats to public health. Expensive imports such as tea, coffee, and spices were frequently adulterated with dried leaves of native trees or ground native nuts and berries.[37] Thus, accurate labeling was one of the important provisions of the 1906 act. Labeling requirements have become increasingly elaborate over the years. Recently, as it has become clear that overall dietary behavior has far more impact on health than food contamination does, the FDA has placed more emphasis on empowering consumers to eat a healthy diet. Regulations established in 1994 require labels on prepared foods to contain information on fats, fiber, vitamins, and other nutrients, along with recommended daily intakes for these nutrients. Because the kinds of fats in the diet have an important effect on health, especially heart disease, labels are required to list the amount of artery-clogging saturated fat, the kind found in butter, whole milk, beef, and pork. Also, since January 2006, foods have been required to identify the amount of trans fats in a serving of the product. Trans fats, which have been used since the 1980s as substitutes for saturated fats in margarine, fried foods, and baked goods, have been found to be at least as harmful to our arteries as saturated fats are. In 2015, the FDA announced a ban on adding trans fats to food. The current deadline for compliance is January 1, 2020.[38]

The FDA also requires drugs to carry accurate labels. With these products, the emphasis is on ensuring that claims of safety and efficacy are accurate and communicate information about hazards directly to the consumer. This is especially important for over-the-counter drugs, for which the label may be the sole basis on which consumers choose to buy and consume the product. Oddly, advertising—a form of labeling—of over-the-counter drugs is regulated by the Federal Trade Commission rather than the FDA. However, the labeling of prescription drugs falls under the authority of the FDA. Prescription drugs are increasingly being advertised directly to consumers, and critics have become concerned that these ads are often misleading, overemphasizing the benefits and underemphasizing the risks. If the FDA determines that an ad is misleading, it may send a notice of violation to the drug company; however, the agency's authority is limited, and it has been criticized for not enforcing the law vigorously.[39]

Unfounded claims for health benefits from certain foods, drugs, and vitamins have had popular appeal in the United States since the nation's birth, despite governmental efforts to enforce accuracy in labeling and advertising. In the late 19th and early 20th centuries, patent medicines contained alcohol and sometimes opium, which helped patients feel better but did little to cure the underlying problems. Even today, desperate patients suffering from incurable diseases may turn to quack therapies, at best just wasting their money, but in some cases turning their backs on therapies that might do some good. The FDA can act when labels on a food or drug contain false or misleading claims; any accompanying leaflets are also considered labels. However, nothing can be done to suppress articles, books, and websites containing unsubstantiated health claims about foods and "nutritional supplements" if the writings cannot be classified as labels.

Among the most persistent nutritional misconceptions has been the belief that if a product is "natural," it must be safe. Accordingly, Congress in 1994 succumbed to intense lobbying by the health food industry and passed the **Dietary Supplement Health and Education Act**, which was signed by President Clinton. The act forbids the FDA from requiring safety testing of herbs and food supplements. Consequently, a number of products known to have quite potent physiological effects are readily available in health food stores, although they may turn out to be harmful once they are better understood. For example, St. John's wort, promoted as an aid for depression, is sold as a nutritional supplement even though studies have found only mixed results for its effectiveness. Unfortunately, it also contains chemicals that have been shown clearly to interact in dangerous, sometimes life-threatening ways, with prescription medications. For example, the substance can weaken the effect of prescription antidepressants, birth control pills, some HIV drugs, some cancer medications, and warfarin, a blood thinner used to prevent blood clots and stroke.[40]

In 1996, people were shocked by news stories that a college student on spring break had died after taking an herbal product called "Ultimate Xphoria" (also called "Herbal Ecstasy"), which contained ephedra, a potent natural stimulant that is similar to amphetamines. Ephedra-containing compounds were marketed as energy boosters, as weight-loss aids, as sexual stimulants, and as a way to get high.[41] Soon afterward, the CDC reported that 8 deaths and 500 adverse health effects, including heart attacks, seizures, and psychoses, had occurred nationwide among people who had consumed ephedra-containing products.[42] While some state and local governments banned these products, the FDA could not stop their sale and use. Finally, after the highly publicized death in early 2003 of a 23-year-old Baltimore Orioles pitcher who used ephedra to lose weight at the beginning of spring training, the FDA banned the substance. It was the first time that the FDA had removed a dietary supplement from the market since 1994, and the action succeeded only after the agency had reviewed some 16,000 reports of adverse reactions, commissioned a study by a nonprofit research agency, and received tens of thousands of comments from the public.[43]

Ephedra is not the only natural substance that has proven to be unsafe. A federal law passed in 2007 requires supplement manufacturers to report serious adverse effects to the FDA.[44] The Modernization Act requires manufacturers to notify the FDA of plans to include a new dietary ingredient and to submit evidence that the ingredient would reasonably to expected to be safe.[45] The agency now posts warnings and can issue bans. For example, in 2015 it warned that some supplements labeled as "bee pollen" and sold as weight-loss products contained illegal stimulants that are dangerous to people with cardiovascular disease as well as phenolphthalein, a laxative known to be carcinogenic.[46] In 2013, the FDA ordered a Texas company to recall OxyElite Pro, advertised as an aid to losing weight and building muscle, because it caused dozens of cases of acute liver failure and hepatitis. One victim died and several others needed liver transplants.[45]

Politics of the FDA

The FDA regulates products that account for more than 25% of all consumer dollars spent in the United States.[47] Not surprisingly, it has made itself unpopular with some of the industries financially impacted by its decisions. These industries can place intense political pressures on Congress and the White House to rein in the agency's actions, as illustrated by the success of the dietary supplement industry in getting itself exempted from FDA oversight.

One of the most frequent criticisms of the FDA has been that it is too slow in approving new drugs. This complaint comes from the pharmaceutical industry, which argues that companies must wait too long to recoup their investments in research and development, as well as from patients with intractable diseases, who feel they are being denied promising new

treatments. AIDS activists were especially critical of the FDA's caution early in the epidemic, arguing that they would inevitably die if the process of new drug approval was not accelerated. Citing the thalidomide disaster that was averted in the United States by a cautious FDA official was no longer enough to deter calls for "reform." In 1992, Congress acted to speed up the approval process by requiring drug companies to pay a fee for the processing of NDAs, which allowed the agency to hire more reviewers, but this situation has given rise to other problems.

Consumer advocates claim that the FDA is now too ready to approve new drugs, a claim supported by the necessity in recent years to recall several drugs because of adverse effects that became evident only after they were on the market. For example, the diet drug known as "fenphen," approved in 1996, had to be recalled a year later because it caused serious heart valve problems.[48,49] Other drugs that were withdrawn included the allergy drug Seldane in 1997 because of cardiac arrhythmias, the diabetes drug Rezulin in 2000 because of liver problems, and the cholesterol-lowering drug Baycol in 2001 because of injury to muscle tissue.

Further doubts about the drug-approval and drug-monitoring processes surfaced in 2004, when the Merck pharmaceutical company withdrew Vioxx from the market. This painkiller was one of the most widely advertised drugs in the world and had earned $2.5 billion for the company since it was approved by the FDA in 1999. Merck had found in a new study that taking the drug doubled the study participants' risk of heart attacks and strokes. Questions were raised about why the FDA had not recognized the problems with Vioxx and recalled it earlier. In a hearing held by the Senate Finance Committee, FDA employees disagreed with one another on whether the agency was too likely to surrender to the demands of the industry. As described in a *New York Times* news report on the hearing, "the clash was a rare public airing of tensions that have simmered in the agency for decades."[50] The conflict is clearly one that also reflects the opposing views Congress has held on the agency. After years of congressional pressure on the FDA to protect the interests of the pharmaceutical industry, the FDA was now accused of neglecting the safety of consumers.[50] As the newly appointed commissioner and principal deputy commissioner wrote in a 2009 article, "It has been said that the FDA has just two speeds of approval—too fast and too slow."[51]

Drugs sold in the United States, like foods, are increasingly being manufactured in and imported from other countries, especially China and India. The FDA has a mandate to inspect the producers of drugs and chemicals used to manufacture drugs for the American market, but it has been overwhelmed with the increasing number of foreign producers, estimated to now number between 3200 and 6800. That challenge was illustrated by the 2008 recall of large quantities of heparin, a blood thinner commonly used to prevent clotting during surgery or other medical procedures, because of allergic reactions to an impurity introduced during manufacturing at a plant in China. At least 62 people in the United States died as a result. The Chinese plant had not been inspected by the FDA.[52]

The FDA's difficulties inspired a review by the Institute of Medicine, which recommended a number of reforms.[53] Its report emphasized the need for improved monitoring of the safety of drugs after they have been approved and introduced into the marketplace. The report authors recommended both more funding for that purpose and greater authority for the FDA to require companies to conduct follow-up clinical studies on newly detected adverse effects. They also proposed that newly approved drugs should carry labeling that indicates safety information is incomplete, and that direct-to-consumer advertising should be banned

for the first two years after a drug's approval. Another proposal called for the mandatory registration of clinical trials.[54]

In 2007, Congress passed legislation that addressed some, but not all, of the criticisms. It reauthorized the use of user fees for the drug-approval process, and significantly increased funding for postmarketing studies of drugs already on the market. It also granted the FDA authority to require companies to do studies on approved drugs for adverse side effects. The law requires registration of all clinical trials and public posting of their results. In addition, it includes incentives for testing drugs in children, as well as provisions designed to limit conflicts of interest of advisors.[55]

Nevertheless, concerns persist about the safety of drugs manufactured abroad, especially in India, which provides approximately 40% of the generic and over-the-counter drugs used in the United States. In 2014, the FDA banned the importation of products from three Indian pharmaceutical companies, after several recalls and import bans. Ranbaxy Laboratories recalled more than 64,000 bottles of a generic cholesterol-lowering drug after doses were mixed up in a bottle. Sun Pharmaceuticals recalled 2528 bottles of a diabetes drug after a bottle was found to contain an epilepsy drug. Another Indian company had to recall more than 58,000 bottles of a heartburn drug due to microbial contamination.[56]

Conclusion

Confidence in the safety of the U.S. food supply has been shaken in recent years by widely publicized outbreaks of illnesses caused by foods, ranging from bagged spinach to peanut butter. Common sources of illness include *Salmonella* bacteria in poultry, meat, and eggs, as well as a variety of viruses and parasites in fish and shellfish. Over the past two decades, *E. coli* 0157:H7 has emerged as a serious threat in ground beef and other foods as well as in unpasteurized fruit juice.

Governmental responsibility for food safety is distributed among a variety of federal, state, and local agencies. Unfortunately, the laws related to this issue are inconsistent and, in many cases, paradoxical. The USDA has significant authority over meat and poultry safety. The FDA is responsible for most other foods, including fish and seafood, but its financial resources for inspection and monitoring are limited, and it has limited power to act. The increasing proportion of imported foods in the American market has posed serious challenges to food safety regulation.

As the problem of food contamination became more apparent in the 1990s, the FDA and the USDA began to advocate for a system focused on preventing problems before they occur rather than depending on inspections to detect food that is already contaminated. This system, called HACCP, analyzes every step in the food production, processing, and preparation chain, with the objective of identifying possible hazards and instituting practices that will eliminate or minimize them. Notably, the FDA has approved irradiation of many foods to kill microbial contaminants. Although many consumers are distrustful of irradiated food, this practice has been shown to be safe, and many experts believe routine irradiation would greatly improve the safety of our food supply. Strengthened surveillance for rapid detection of foodborne disease outbreaks is another feature of the food safety system; in the event of an outbreak, surveillance allows sources to be identified so that distribution can be halted rapidly.

In addition to its role in the prevention of microbial contamination of food, the FDA regulates food additives and chemical contaminants, as well as food labeling and advertising. It sets standards for foods to be labeled "organic."

The FDA also has oversight of the safety of drugs and medical devices. This responsibility has led to considerable controversy, as the pharmaceutical industry and patient groups frequently complain about the slow pace of new drug approval. Conservatives in the U.S. Congress have made repeated efforts to weaken the agency's authority and to force it to act more quickly on drug approvals. One result was legislation passed in 1992 that allowed the FDA to assess fees on the pharmaceutical industry to be used for processing new drug approvals. Critics believe that this practice has led to too cozy a relationship between the agency and the drug companies. Another law that has been controversial is the Dietary Supplement Health and Education Act of 1994, which prohibits the FDA from regulating herbs and food supplements, although it can step in once a problem is apparent. Consumer groups are concerned that these laws, together with the climate of pressure to speed up drug approvals, endanger public health by allowing unsafe products on the market.

Several scandals occurred in the late 1990s and the 2000s that confirmed fears that drugs are approved too easily and that the system for detecting safety problems after approval is inadequate. The trend toward increasing importation of drugs from foreign countries has made regulation more difficult. Evidence that pharmaceutical companies selectively publicize clinical trials that show benefits of their drugs while suppressing negative results led to mandatory registration of clinical trials at the outset, so that all the evidence will be available publicly. This requirement was part of legislation passed in 2007 that also included a number of other measures designed to increase the FDA's funding and authority.

References

1. Centers for Disease Control and Prevention, "Estimates of Foodborne Illness in the United States," November 5, 2018, https://www.cdc.gov/foodborneburden/index.html, accessed October 8, 2019.

2. W. M. Laydon, "Food Safety: A Patchwork System," *GAO Journal* (Spring–Summer 1992): 48–59.

3. A. Nadakavukaren, *Our Global Environment: A Health Perspective*, 7th ed. (Prospect Heights, IL: Waveland Press, 2011).

4. C. Drew and P. Belluck, "Deadly Bacteria: A New Threat to Fruit and Produce in U.S.," *The New York Times*, January 4, 1998.

5. P. Belluck and C. Drew, "Tracing Bout of Illness to Small Lettuce Farm," *The New York Times*, January 5, 1998.

6. T. Breuer et al., "A Multistate Outbreak of Escherichia coli 0157:H7 Infections Linked to Alfalfa Sprouts Grown from Contaminated Seeds," *Emerging Infectious Diseases Journal* 7 (2001): 977–982.

7. Centers for Disease Control and Prevention, "Surveillance for Foodborne Disease Outbreaks, United States, 2017: Annual Report," 2019, https://www.cdc.gov/fdoss/pdf/2017_FoodBorneOutbreaks_508.pdf, accessed October 8, 2019.

8. Centers for Disease Control and Prevention, "Outbreak of *Salmonella* Serotype Saintpaul Infections Associated with Multiple Raw Produce Items—United States, 2008," *Morbidity and Mortality Weekly Report* 57 (2008): 929–934.

9. Center for Science in the Public Interest, "Outbreak Alert! 2014: A Review of Foodborne Illness in America from 2002 to 2011," April 2014, https://cspinet.org/sites/default/files/attachment/outbreakalert2014.pdf, accessed October 8, 2019.

10. M. Nestle, *Safe Food: The Politics of Food Safety* (Berkeley, CA: University of California Press, 2010).

11. U.S. Department of Agriculture, "FY 2018 Budget Summary," https://www.usda.gov/sites/default/files/documents/USDA-Budget-Summary-2018.pdf, accessed October 8, 2019.

12. U.S. Food and Drug Administration, "2018 Operating Plan," https://www.fda.gov/about-fda/budgets/2018-fda-budget-summary, accessed October 8, 2019.

13. U.S. Food and Drug Administration, "Background on the FDA Food Safety Modernization Act (FSMA)," https://www.fda.gov/food/food-safety-modernization-act-fsma/background-fda-food-safety-modernization-act-fsma, accessed October 8, 2019.

14. M. Burros, "President to Push for Food Safety," *The New York Times*, July 4, 1998.

15. M. Burros, "High Mercury Levels Are Found in Tuna Sushi Sold in Manhattan," *The New York Times*, January 23, 2008.

16. U.S. Food and Drug Administration, "Guidance for Industry: HACCP Regulation for Fish and Fishery Products," January 1999, https://www.fda.gov/regulatory-information/search-fda-guidance-documents/guidance-industry-questions-and-answers-guidance-facilitate-implementation-haccp-system-seafood, accessed October 8, 2019.

17. M. T. Osterholm and A. P. Norgan, "Role of Irradiation in Food Safety," *New England Journal of Medicine* 350 (2004): 1898–1901.

18. U.S. Food and Drug Administration, "Food Irradiation: What You Need to Know," January 4, 2018, https://www.fda.gov/buy-store-serve-safe-food/food-irradiation-what-you-need-know, accessed October 8, 2019.

19. D. G. Maki, "Coming to Grips with Foodborne Infection: Peanut Butter, Peppers, and Nationwide *Salmonella* Outbreaks," *New England Journal of Medicine* 360 (2009): 949–953.

20. Centers for Disease Control and Prevention, "About PulseNet," February 16, 2016, https://www.cdc.gov/pulsenet/about/index.html, accessed October 8, 2019.

21. Centers for Disease Control and Prevention, "Multistate Outbreak of *Salmonella* Infections Associated with Peanut Butter and Peanut Butter-Containing Products—United States, 2008–2009," *Morbidity and Mortality Weekly Report* 58 (2009): 85–90.

22. M. Moss, "Peanut Case Shows Holes in Food Safety Net," *The New York Times*, February 9, 2009.

23. A. Blinder, "Georgia: 28-Year Sentence in Tainted Peanut Case," *The New York Times*, September 21, 2015.

24. Centers for Disease Control and Prevention, "List of Selected Multistate Foodborne Outbreak Investigations," August 22, 2019, https://www.cdc.gov/foodsafety/outbreaks/multistate-outbreaks/outbreaks-list.html, accessed October 8, 2019.

25. Centers for Disease Control and Prevention, "Foodborne Diseases Active Surveillance Network (FoodNet): Final Data," 2017, https://www.cdc.gov/foodnet/pdfs/FoodNet-Annual-Report-2015-508c.pdf, accessed October 8, 2019.

26. Centers for Disease Control and Prevention, "FoodNet Fast," https://wwwn.cdc.gov/foodnetfast/, accessed October 8, 2019.

27. U.S. General Accountability Office, "Food Safety," https://www.gao.gov/key_issues/food_safety/issues_summary, accessed October 8, 2019.

28. R. Pear, "Departing Health Secretary Warns of Flu Risk and Attacks on Food," *The New York Times*, December 3, 2004.

29. Executive Office of the President of the United States, "Reform Plan and Reorganization Recommendations," 2018, https://www.performance.gov/GovReform/Reform-and-Reorg-Plan-Final.pdf, accessed October 8, 2019.

30. U.S. Environmental Protection Agency, "Accomplishments Under the Food Quality Protection Act (FQPA)," August 3, 2006, https://archive.epa.gov/pesticides/regulating/laws/fqpa/web/html/fqpa_accomplishments.html, accessed October 8, 2019.

31. M. Burros, "Last Word on Organic Standards, Again," *The New York Times*, May 26, 2004.

32. M. Burros, "Agriculture Dept. Rescinds Changes to Organic Food Standards," *The New York Times*, May 27, 2004.

33. B. P. Baker, C. M. Benbrook, E. Groth 3rd, and K. Lutz Benbrook, "Pesticide Residues in Conventional, Integrated Pest Management (IPM)-Grown and Organic Foods: Insights from Three US Data Sets," *Food Additives and Contaminants* 19 (2002): 427–446.

34. C. Curl , R. A. Fenske, and K. Elgethun, "Organophosphorus Pesticide Exposure of Urban and Suburban Preschool Children with Organic and Conventional Diets," *Environmental Health Perspectives* 111 (2003): 377–382.

35. U.S. Department of Agriculture, "Agricultural Act of 2014," https://www.ers.usda.gov/agricultural-act-of-2014-highlights-and-implications.aspx, accessed October 8, 2019.

36. U.S. Food and Drug Administration, "The FDA's Drug Review Process: Ensuring Drugs Are Safe and Effective," November 24, 2017, https://www.fda.gov/Drugs/ResourcesForYou/Consumers/ucm143534.htm, accessed October 8, 2019.

37. R. M. Deutsch, *The New Nuts Among the Berries: How Nutritional Nonsense Captured America* (Palo Alto, CA: Bull Publishing, 1977).

38. U.S. Food and Drug Administration, "Trans Fat," May 18, 2018, https://www.fda.gov/food/food-additives-petitions/trans-fat, accessed October 9, 2019.

39. S. M. Wolfe, "Direct-to-Consumer Advertising: Education or Emotion Promotion?" *New England Journal of Medicine* 346 (2002): 524–526.

40. National Institutes of Health, National Center for Complementary and Integrative Health, "St. John's Wort," December 1, 2016, https://nccih.nih.gov/health/stjohnswort/ataglance.htm, accessed October 8, 2019.

41. M. Burros and S. Jay, "Concern Grows Over Herb That Promises a Legal High," *The New York Times*, April 10, 1996.

42. Centers for Disease Control and Prevention, "Adverse Events Associated with Ephedrine-Containing Products—Texas, December 1993–September 1995," *Morbidity and Mortality Weekly Report* 45 (1996): 689–692.

43. S. G. Stolberg, "U.S. to Prohibit Supplement Tied to Health Risks," *The New York Times*, December 31, 2003.

44. D. Hurley, "Diet Supplements and Safety: Some Disquieting Data," *The New York Times*, January 16, 2007.

45. U.S. Food and Drug Administration, "Public Notification: Oxy ELITE Pro Super Thermogenic contains hidden drug ingredient," February 28, 2015, https://www.fda.gov/drugs/medication-health-fraud/public-notification-oxy-elite-pro-super-thermogenic-contains-hidden-drug-ingredient, accessed October 8, 2019.

46. National Institutes of Health, National Center for Complementary and Integrative Health, "Some Bee Pollen Weight Loss Products Are Dangerous Scams," June 19, 2014, https://nccih.nih.gov/node/6190, accessed October 8, 2019.

47. A. J. J. Wood, "Playing 'Kick the FDA': Risk-Free to Players but Hazardous to Public Health," *New England Journal of Medicine* 358 (2008): 1774–1775.

48. J. Couzin, "Gaps in the Safety Net," *Science* 307 (2005): 196–198.

49. W. A. Ray and C. M. Stein, "Reform of Drug Regulation: Beyond an Independent Drug-Safety Board," *New England Journal of Medicine* 354 (2008): 194–201.

50. G. Harris, "FDA Failing in Drug Safety, Official Asserts," *The New York Times*, November 19, 2004.

51. M. A. Hamburg and J. M. Sharfstein, "The FDA as a Public Health Agency," *New England Journal of Medicine* 360 (2009): 2492–2495.

52. S. O. Schweitzer, "Trying Times at the FDA: The Challenge of Ensuring the Safety of Imported Pharmaceuticals," *New England Journal of Medicine* 358 (2008): 1773–1777.

53. Institute of Medicine, *The Future of Drug Safety: Preserving and Protecting the Health of the Public* (Washington, DC: National Academies Press, 2006).

54. G. D. Curfman, S. Morrissey, and J. M. Drazen, "Blueprint for a Stronger Food and Drug Administration," *New England Journal of Medicine* 355 (2006): 1821.

55. G. Harris, "House Passes Bill Giving More Power to the FDA," *The New York Times*, September 20, 2007.

56. T. Clarke and B. Berkrot, "Unease Grows Among U.S. Doctors over Indian Drug Quality," *Reuters*, March 18, 2014.

CHAPTER 25

The Population Bomb

Population: The Ultimate Environmental Health Issue

KEY TERMS

Carrying capacity
Global warming
Human immunodeficiency
  virus (HIV)

Intergovernmental Panel on
  Climate Change (IPCC)

Urbanization

Population biology is a science in itself. Studies of animal, plant, and microorganism populations have yielded some concepts and insights that can be applied to human populations. However, application of these studies' findings to human populations is an inexact science, and predictions are always highly controversial. Interest in the dynamics of the human population arises from concern about its continuing growth and its increasing impact on the environment.

All organisms tend to produce more offspring than would be needed to maintain a stable population. Pressures from the environment, such as availability of food and prevalence of predators, tend to limit the survival of those offspring. The difference between the birth rate and the death rate is the population's rate of growth.

Studies of organisms newly introduced into a closed environment have shown two general patterns of population growth: the S curve and the J curve (**Figure 25-1**). Both patterns start out with a rapidly expanding population, but they differ in their response to environmental limitations. In the more common S pattern, environmental pressures increase gradually as the population approaches the number known as the **carrying capacity**—the number of organisms that can be supported in a given environment without degrading that environment. In the J pattern, the population expands rapidly past the carrying capacity and then crashes, because once the carrying capacity is exceeded, the environment is degraded, and the carrying capacity is reduced. For example, the J pattern is seen in lemmings and locusts, species famous for

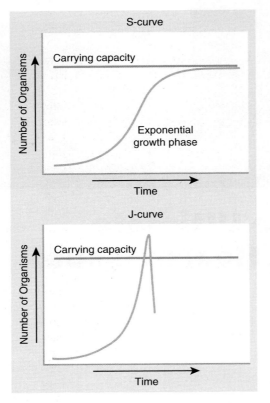

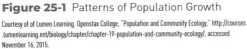

Figure 25-1 Patterns of Population Growth

Courtesy of of Lumen Learning. Openstax College, "Population and Community Ecology," http://courses .lumenlearning.net/biology/chapter/chapter-19-population-and-community-ecology/, accessed November 16, 2015.

huge population explosions followed by massive numbers of deaths when the food supply is exhausted.[1(Ch.2)]

It is not yet clear whether the human population is growing in an S or a J pattern. The world population has grown steadily, with minor irregularities, for the past million years, with a major surge beginning about 200 years ago. About that time, when the population of the earth was approximately 1 billion, the British clergyman and economist Thomas Malthus raised an alarm that population growth was outpacing the food supply; he predicted that the resulting crowding would lead to famine, war, and disease. However, Malthus's dismal predictions were not realized, and his warnings

were discredited. Progress in agricultural technology and migrations from highly populated areas in Europe to the open spaces of the Americas and southern Africa relieved pressures on populations, allowing the expansion to continue.[1(Ch. 21)]

In 1968, when the world's population was 3.5 billion, Paul Ehrlich, an American ecologist, published *The Population Bomb*, a best seller that repeated and expanded upon Malthus's warning.[2] Perhaps in part due to the attention paid to Ehrlich's book, the rate of the world's population growth has slowed since then, from an all-time high of 2.1% per year between 1965 and 1970 to 1.1% per year over the period 2015 to 2020. In 2019, the world's population was 7.7 billion.[3] Population growth has a tremendous momentum, however, and the number of people living on earth continues to increase dramatically. In 1990, when the population had reached 5.3 billion, Ehrlich and his wife, Anne, published another book, *The Population Explosion*, arguing that many of his dire predictions have already begun to be realized.[4] In 2004, with the world's population at 6.4 billion, they published *One with Nineveh*, which further examines the consequences of overpopulation and the linked problems of overconsumption and political and economic inequity—consequences that include the prospect of increasing terrorism.[5] Most recently, in 2010 when the population was approaching 7 billion, Paul Ehrlich, with Robert E. Ornstein, published *Humanity on a Tightrope*, in which the authors argue that, to balance on the tightrope of sustainability suspended over the collapse of civilization, people need to recognize that we are all part of one family.[6]

Most environmentalists and public health experts agree with Ehrlich. However, like Malthus, he also has his detractors. Some pro-growth advocates—mostly economists—argue that human ingenuity will always find ways of overcoming any problems created by crowding. In response, Paul and Anne Ehrlich quote Kenneth Boulding: "Anyone who believes exponential growth can go on forever in a finite world is either a madman or an economist."[4(p.159)] Some of the world's major religions oppose population control measures, making it easier for politicians to listen to growth advocates and to simply ignore the problems created by overpopulation.

It is very difficult to predict what the world population will be in the future. Some evidence indicates, as the Ehrlichs point out, that environmental pressures opposing population growth are increasing, especially in developing regions of the world. Other evidence suggests that international family planning efforts are paying off in slowing growth rates in many parts of the world. In 2019, the United Nations predicted that, if current trends continue, the population will reach 9.7 billion by 2050.[3] The vast majority of this growth will occur in the poorest countries of Africa and southern Asia. Projections after that point in time are uncertain. It is not clear whether the earth's carrying capacity is large enough to support so many people. If not, irreversible forces may be building for a sudden J-type population crash. By the time the Ehrlichs would be proved right, it would be too late to do anything to prevent the disaster.

Public Health and Population Growth

Public health has had a major role in bringing about the dramatic growth in the world's population that has occurred over the past several decades. Public health improvements—including clean water, immunization, pest control measures, and inexpensive oral rehydration treatment of diarrheal diseases—in developing countries have led to major declines in death rates, especially among children. According to the World Health Organization, the number of children who die before reaching their fifth birthday declined by more than 59% between 1990 and 2018, from 93 deaths per 1000 children to 39 deaths per 1000 children.[7] Because birth rates remained roughly constant, populations grew rapidly in developing countries over that span.

In developed countries, which instituted public health measures over a period of many decades in the 19th and 20th centuries, birth rates tended to fall in response to falling death rates, a process known as the "demographic transition." The fall in birth rates is a rational response to parents' knowledge that their children are likely to survive to adulthood. In an industrialized, urban society, children are an economic liability—expensive to feed, clothe, and educate.

In the developing world, however, many public health measures were introduced by international agencies over a short period of time after World War II. International aid for population control efforts has not been as generous. This is, in part, because of cultural resistance to contraception within some societies and, in part, because of the religious and political controversy surrounding family planning, especially in the United States, which has limited the amount of aid this nation provides.

Because of continued high birth rates, the public health in many developing countries is now, ironically, threatened by the crowding that has resulted from public health improvements. In all parts of the world, there has been a trend toward **urbanization**: Put simply, rural areas whose main industries are agricultural in nature no longer need the increasing numbers of workers. This trend has been most marked in developing countries, where migrants from rural areas have flocked to the cities. From 1950 to 2018, the percentage of people living in cities increased from less than one-third to more than one-half; if current trends continue, the world will be two-thirds urban by 2050.[8] According to the United Nations, 43% of Africa's population now lives in cities, and that percentage will continue to increase; Asia's rate of urbanization is 50% and also increasing.[8] Governments struggling to provide adequate drinking water and sewage services to their citizens cannot keep up with the influx. Many of the migrants settle on the outskirts of the cities in shantytowns totally lacking in water and sanitation. Others are completely homeless, simply living on the streets.

These conditions threaten to reverse all the progress in public health made through earlier efforts. Cholera and other diarrheal diseases are rampant in the developing-country slums. Malaria and tuberculosis are also common. Intensive public health efforts have had some benefits. Immunization campaigns have reduced the incidence of measles, diphtheria, and other infectious diseases, including polio. In fact, the World Health Organization announced that there were just 33 reported cases of polio worldwide, in Afghanistan and Pakistan, and none elsewhere, in 2018—down from 350,000 cases in 125 countries in 1988.[9]

The acquired immunodeficiency syndrome (AIDS) epidemic in Africa is also waning, due to intensive efforts to provide antiretroviral treatment as widely as possible. In 2018, 61% of people infected with the **human immunodeficiency virus (HIV)** were receiving therapy, up from 24% in 2010 and 2% in 2000. By 2018, new infections had fallen by 42% from the peak in 1997, and AIDS-related deaths fell by 55% from the peak in 2004.[10] Nevertheless, 4.8% of the adult population of sub-Saharan Africa is infected with HIV. In some countries, prevalence is shockingly high: In 2018, the percentage of adults living with HIV in Eswatini (formerly known as Swaziland) was 27.3%; in Botswana, it was 20.3%.[11] An estimated 15 million African children have been left orphaned by AIDS.[12] In fact, AIDS has dwarfed all other public health problems in Africa. Life expectancy in the hardest-hit countries in southern Africa has fallen by as much as 10 years, and the rate of population growth has decreased, although not enough to relieve the pressures of too many people.[1(Ch.2),13]

The desperate conditions in the urban slums of developing countries lead to the disruption of traditional lifestyles and to the breakdown of normal social constraints, including sexual and parental restraints. Prostitution is common; children are abandoned to fend for themselves. These conditions are believed to have led to the origin of AIDS as an epidemic threat, and they contribute to the continuing disaster of the epidemic. Such conditions may be the breeding ground for other emerging infections in the future. In addition, these conditions encourage crime and violence. Even if, as predicted, population growth rates continue to decline, 95% of the 2 or 3 billion people added to the world in the next 25 to 50 years will be in the poorest countries, and most of that growth will occur in cities.[1(Ch.2)]

Even the United States and other developed countries are affected by some of the pressures just described, although the rate of population growth in the United States is less than 1% annually; in Japan and most European countries, it is close to zero. Russia and some other Eastern European countries have negative population growth.[3] The American population is becoming increasingly urban, with some 82% living in communities with more than 2500 residents in 2018.[8] In 2016, 18% of American children lived in families with incomes below the poverty line; a high percentage of these children live with both housing and food insecurity.[14]

The United States is also affected by the social consequences of population growth in developing countries. Highly publicized problems with illegal immigration from Mexico and Central America are linked with poverty and with social problems caused by population growth in those countries. As conditions in those areas become more crowded and residents become more desperate in the future, the pressures on people to seek less crowded, more prosperous surroundings will increase, making it more difficult for the United States to remain isolated. Infectious diseases have no respect for political boundaries. With international travel and commerce so rapid and widespread, Americans are at risk from diseases imported from anywhere in the world.

Furthermore, as discussed in the following section, human population growth threatens to change the environment of the entire globe, posing health threats that no one can escape, even if the nation's borders are sealed.

Global Impact of Population Growth: Depletion of Resources

The carrying capacity of the earth—the population size that the earth can support without being degraded—is determined by a number of factors, some of which can be altered by technological intervention and human behavior. These factors, which are related, include the availability of fresh water, the availability of fuel, the amount and productivity of arable land, and the amount and disposition of wastes, both biological and technological. Some signs indicate that the carrying capacity has already been exceeded in some parts of the world: As the environment is degraded, the size of the population that can be supported shrinks, leading to further environmental degradation and a vicious circle of hunger, disease, and death.

The supply of fresh water, which is basic to human life, is one of the factors that limits the earth's carrying capacity. Water is essential for drinking, cooking, and washing. It is also used for agriculture, irrigating dry fields to grow the increasing amounts of food required by expanding populations. Water is a renewable resource, due to cycles of evaporation and precipitation, but the rate at which water supplies are renewed is fixed. Only a small percentage of the water on earth is suitable for human use: While scientists have developed methods of removing the salt from seawater, the technology is expensive and uses large amounts of energy. Pollution resulting from the use of fresh water supplies for disposal of wastes also renders potential sources of water unsuitable for human use.

Availability of fresh water is highly variable according to geographic area and precipitation patterns. In drier parts of the world, especially the Middle East, water rights have become volatile international issues because some countries depend on water sources that originate beyond their borders. For example, the Nile River flows into Egypt from Ethiopia and Sudan, and the flow of the Tigris–Euphrates rivers into Syria and Iraq may be altered by dam construction in Turkey.

In the United States, water supplies have been sufficiently plentiful so that Americans are accustomed to lavish consumption, watering lawns, washing cars, and filling private swimming pools, even in relatively dry areas of the Southwest. For example, much of the water used in that part of the country comes from the Ogallala Aquifer, the world's largest underground water reserve, which underlies portions of six southwestern states. This water accumulated during the last ice age and cannot be replenished. Yet it is being used, among other things, for industry and irrigation, attracting people to the area who will be left literally high and dry when the water runs out.[1(Ch.15)]

California, too, is used to an abundant supply of water provided by snow melt from the Sierra Nevada mountains. However, after several years of record hot and dry weather, as well as snow-less winters in the Sierras, wells began going dry in some parts of the state and wildfires burned out of control. Governor Jerry Brown declared a state of drought emergency in January 2014 and called for a 20% voluntary reduction in water use. In April 2015, Governor Brown ordered a mandatory 25% reduction in water use.[15] Communities have begun efforts at desalination of seawater and recycling of wastewater. Lawns have been replaced with rocks and cactus. Gardens and golf courses have needed to find ways to get by with less water. Because 80% of California's water goes to agriculture, farmers needed to develop more efficient irrigation methods. Finally, in March 2019, following a particularly wet winter, the state became drought-free after 376 consecutive weeks under some form of official drought.[16,17] However, in October 2019, California's largest utility company, Pacific Gas and Electric, shut off power to the northern part of the state because of dry, windy conditions. That left an estimated 2.5 million people without electricity and, among other consequences, caused multiple motor vehicle crashes at intersections where traffic lights went dark. The utility's equipment had been blamed for a major fire that killed 86 people the previous year and the company had declared bankruptcy in January 2019.[18]

The amount of fresh water on earth is theoretically sufficient to support a population of 20 billion people if evenly distributed.[19] Many countries have taken steps to conserve their fresh water supplies and to clean up the pollution. In poorer, drier countries, however, the available water is insufficient to support the population growth that is occurring. The lack of water for cooking and washing, and the pollution of drinking water with human and industrial wastes, is already harming public health in these areas. According to the United Nations, 40% of the world's people, mostly in Africa and south Asia, live in regions with water shortages, and that number will grow to two-thirds by 2025.[1(Ch.15)]

Predictions about the earth's carrying capacity have most often centered on food, attempting to estimate the limits of agricultural productivity. Malthus's warnings were built on concerns about limited growth in food supplies, which nevertheless continued to grow rapidly for almost two centuries. It appears that Malthus was to some degree correct. According to the United Nations' Food and Agriculture Organization (UNFAO), in 2015 nearly 11% of the world's population was chronically or acutely malnourished. In sub-Saharan Africa, the prevalence of hunger is about 23%; in southern Asia, it is 16%.[20]

With increasing populations needing greater amounts of food, the amount of land used for agriculture grew quickly during the period between 1850 and 1950. Then, despite continued population growth, the expansion of arable land slowed down and ceased altogether in the late 1980s.[21] Food production continued to keep pace with population growth during the 1960s and 1970s, however, because of the "green revolution"—that is, the development of genetic strains of wheat and rice that yielded harvests two to three times greater than conventional strains. Crop yields also grew because of increasing use of fertilizers, irrigation, and chemical pesticides.

Such increases in yields are unlikely to continue because of water shortages, depletion of soil, and the development of resistance by pests to chemical pesticides. The amount of land under cultivation has declined in some parts of the world, especially Africa. According to one estimate, 40% of the world's agricultural lands are strongly or very strongly degraded.[1(Ch.5)] In part this trend reflects spreading urban centers; in part it is because the soil is depleted of nutrients or has become salty from irrigation. Both erosion of topsoil due to overgrazing and poor agricultural practices contribute to the loss of arable land. The demand for agricultural land for farming has led to widespread clearing of forests, although forested land may be only marginally suitable for cultivation. Deforestation also occurs as a result of people gathering wood for fuel. Growing populations' need for firewood for cooking and, in colder climates and mountainous regions, for heating as well, has resulted in vast treeless areas around towns and villages throughout Africa, Asia, and Latin America. The loss of forests increases soil erosion and contributes to catastrophic flooding in areas subject to monsoons.[1(Ch.5)]

Population growth has also caught up with the seemingly limitless supply of food from the sea. Fish catches increased dramatically between 1950 and 1989, but have declined since then. The UNFAO has concluded that 33% of the world's marine fish stocks are overfished in an unsustainable way, and another 60% are maximally sustainably fished. Pollution of coastal waters has also contributed to the decline of harvests, especially those of shellfish. On the bright side, the practice of aquaculture is growing rapidly, and by the early 21st century almost half of all fish eaten worldwide was raised on fish farms.[1(Ch.4),22] Fish farming has some notable drawbacks, however. Farmed salmon, for example, are fed fish meal and fish oil made from large amounts of smaller fish such as sardines, anchovies, and herring, thus depleting fisheries that might otherwise feed people. The waste from penned fish pollutes coastal waters. In addition, saltwater fish farms incubate microbes and parasites that threaten to infect wild stocks.

Global Impact of Population Growth: Climate Change

Perhaps the most threatening effects of population growth are the changes in the composition of the earth's atmosphere that it brings, with potentially drastic consequences. The depletion of the ozone layer, which protects the earth's surface from ultraviolet radiation, is known to increase risks in humans of skin cancer, melanoma, and cataracts. It may also have a harmful impact on plant and animal life.

Although international agreements have led to policies effective in slowing and possibly even reversing damage to the ozone layer, there is less hope of preventing climate change caused by other human activities. Alterations in the relative concentrations of the four major constituents of air—nitrogen, oxygen, argon, and carbon dioxide—are causing **global warming** due to the "greenhouse effect," in which the energy of sunlight is absorbed by carbon dioxide in the air and turned into heat rather than radiating back into outer space.

The balance of atmospheric gases has been maintained over the millennia by the photosynthetic activities of green plants, which take up carbon dioxide and release oxygen. The reverse process occurs during combustion of wood, coal, oil, and gas: Oxygen is consumed and carbon dioxide is released. Since the beginning of the Industrial Revolution, with humans' ever-increasing use of fossil fuels, the levels of carbon dioxide in the atmosphere have been rising. The trend is made worse by the loss of photosynthetic action that accompanies widespread destruction of forests through logging and, worse, by the burning of vegetation, including tropical rain forests, to clear land for agriculture and human settlement. Green plants are being lost from the ocean as well, through poisoning of phytoplankton by pollution of the seas. The concentration of atmospheric carbon dioxide has increased by 45% since the beginning of the Industrial Revolution and is continuing to grow at an accelerating rate.[23,24] Other gases also contribute to the greenhouse effect, especially methane, which is released by microbial activity in the intestines of cattle and in paddy fields where rice is grown.

Although the evidence was strongly disputed for many years, it is becoming increasingly clear that global climate change has begun: The earth's average combined land and ocean temperature rose by more than 1°F over the past century and is approaching a 1°C increase (**Figure 25-2**). Predictions for temperatures in the year 2100 range from 3°F to 7°F higher than today.[24] The temperature increase is widespread over the globe and is greatest in the northern arctic region. According to the **Intergovernmental Panel on Climate Change (IPCC)**, which won the Nobel Peace Prize in 2007 along with former U.S. Vice President Al Gore, the effects of global warming are already being felt. Sea levels rose during the second half of the 20th century and have continued to rise as glaciers and Arctic ice sheets melt. The IPCC predicts a rise of 1 to 2.7 feet by the end of the 21st century. Shifting precipitation patterns have increased dryness in the southwestern United States,

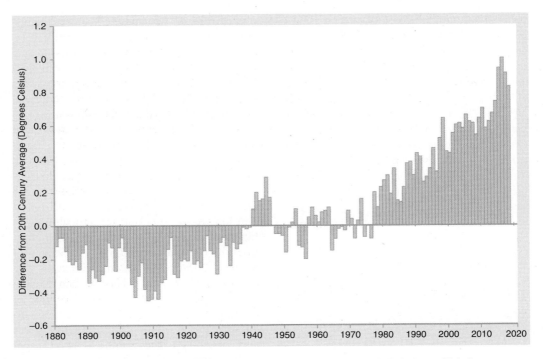

Figure 25-2 Global Land and Ocean Temperature Anomalies, 1880–2018, Relative to 20th Century Average

Data from NOAA National Centers for Environmental Information, "Climate at a Glance: Global Time Series," September 2019, https://www.ncdc.noaa.gov/cag/, accessed October 8, 2019.

northern Mexico, the Mediterranean region, and sub-Saharan Africa, while increasing wetness in northern North America and northern Europe.[24] The California drought that began in 2012 and continued until 2019 is due, at least in part, to global warming.[25]

As the oceans continue to rise, seawater will inundate coastal towns and cities, threatening tens of millions of people living in coastal regions of Africa, Asia, and small island nations.[26] The intensity of storms and hurricanes will increase. In the United States, 53% of the population lives in counties that include coastal areas, many of which—especially in the Southeast, Texas, and California—already suffer from the effects of hurricanes and tropical storms. The impact of higher sea levels will threaten many airports, rail lines, roads, ports, and pipelines.[27]

The implications for human health are complex and far-reaching. Food supplies will be affected, as optimal temperature and

rainfall conditions for agriculture shift northward, and marginally dry lands turn to desert. Insect pests will become more active, adversely affecting crops even further. As temperate zones become hotter, vector-borne diseases that now plague tropical regions will enlarge their territory, spreading even to industrialized countries. Mosquitoes that carry the dengue and yellow fever viruses and malaria parasites threaten to move northward into the United States from Central America. A warmer climate may have been responsible for the emergence of hantavirus infections in the United States, and the 1991 outbreak in South America of epidemic cholera, the first such event seen in the Western hemisphere in more than a century.[1(Ch.6)] The earth may also experience more extreme heat waves, such as the ones that occurred in Europe in July 2019, in which the continent broke its all-time heat record by an astonishing 5.6°F, and in the southwestern United States in May 2019, in which many locations reached 100°F earlier in the season than ever before.[28,29]

Prospects for significantly slowing the process of global warming appear dim, in part because population pressures in developing countries contribute to continuing deforestation but, more importantly, because the United States, Canada, and other industrialized countries contribute disproportionately to the production of greenhouse gases (**Figure 25-3**). The United States, with less than 4.3% of the world's population, contributes 15.5% of the world's greenhouse emissions. By contrast, India has 17.5% of the people in the world but is responsible for only 6.7% of the world's greenhouse emissions. **Figure 25-4** shows per capita carbon dioxide production for the top per capita emitting countries, providing

a different view of the problem. Australia and Canada look considerably more problematic in this light. The high per capita production of carbon dioxide is part of the affluent lifestyle— the lifestyle that poorer countries strive to emulate and may begin to achieve if they can control population growth. China, with 18.2% of the world's population, is rapidly improving the standard of living of its people and now contributes 29.0% of emissions, an amount that is growing.[30] It is probable that environmental damage caused by the continued rise in the earth's temperature will cause increases in human suffering, especially in the poorest countries.

Recognizing the dangers of global climate change, delegates to the United Nations' Earth Summit in 1992 negotiated an agreement that called for voluntary reductions in greenhouse

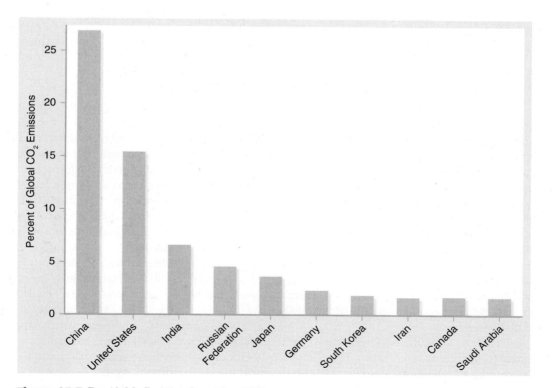

Figure 25-3 Top 10 CO_2 Emitting Countries, 2016

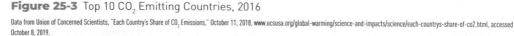
Data from Union of Concerned Scientists, "Each Country's Share of CO_2 Emissions," October 11, 2018, www.ucsusa.org/global-warming/science-and-impacts/science/each-countrys-share-of-co2.html, accessed October 8, 2019.

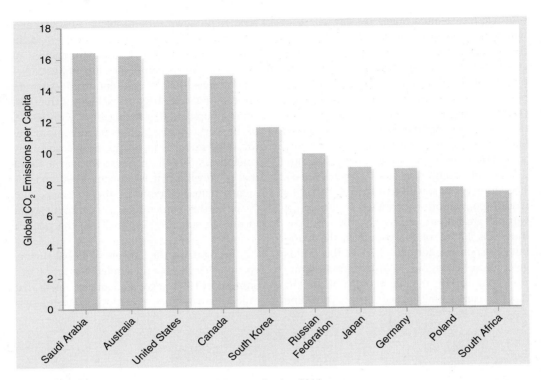

Figure 25-4 Top 10 CO_2 Emitting Countries per Capita, 2016

Data from Union of Concerned Scientists, "Each Country's Share of CO_2 Emissions," October 11, 2018, www.ucsusa.org/global-warming/science-and-impacts/science/each-countrys-share-of-co2.html, accessed October 8, 2019.

gas emissions. It soon became obvious, however, that the nations were failing miserably at achieving any reduction in emissions, and negotiations were resumed in 1997 in Kyoto, Japan. At that conference, representatives from 171 nations agreed on mandatory reductions, with individualized goals for each country. The United States was assigned the goal of reducing its emissions to 7% less than the 1990 levels by 2012. The Kyoto Protocol was to become legally binding after being ratified by 55 countries representing 55% of the 1990 emissions.[1(Ch.11)]

Prospects for ratification by the U.S. Congress looked bleak even when Bill Clinton was president, but upon the election of George W. Bush, it was clear that the United States would not participate. President Bush withdrew the nation from the Kyoto Protocol soon after he was inaugurated. He rejected evidence that global warming is occurring, to the extent that political pressures forced all references to climate change to be removed from a major Environmental Protection Agency (EPA) report on environmental quality.[31] In 2004, Russia became the 127th nation to ratify the Kyoto Protocol, allowing it to take effect in early 2005. However, without the participation of the world's leading emitters of greenhouse gases, the United States and China—which was not assigned limits under the Kyoto Protocol—the treaty was unlikely to make much difference. Even if all the signatories met their targets, the achievement would be only a small step toward reducing the impact of climate change.[1(Ch.11)]

Another United Nations conference on climate change took place in Copenhagen in

December 2009. Diplomats had worked hard over the preceding two years to negotiate a new treaty, which President Barack Obama made a top priority. Nevertheless, major differences between rich nations and poor nations remained, and no hard agreement was reached. Negotiators agreed to keep trying, but prospects for reaching an international agreement to control greenhouse gas emissions in the foreseeable future did not look promising.[32]

In December 2015, another conference took place in Paris. In preparation, countries submitted pledges of specific cuts in greenhouse gases. President Obama promised that the United States would cut its emissions 26% to 28% by 2030.[33] Despite many Republican congressional members' denials that climate change is even occurring, and their labeling of the president's plans as "a war on coal," the United States, along with China, agreed to ratify the Paris Climate Accord in 2016. Four days after the accord came into effect, Donald Trump was elected president of the United States. In June 2017, he announced that the United States was withdrawing from the accord, leaving global climate planning in the lurch.[34,35]

Dire Predictions and Fragile Hope

According to a moderate estimate, the United Nations expects the world's population to reach 9.7 billion in 2050 and be increasing by about 42 million persons annually at that time. The populations of some countries are growing much more rapidly than others: The population of the 48 least-developed countries is growing at 2.4% per year and is expected to double by 2050. The 10 countries with the highest fertility rates in 2017 are all located in Africa, except for Afghanistan. Populations in the more-developed regions are expected to decrease or increase only slightly by 2050, with most of that increase due to immigration. Most of the 10 countries with the lowest fertility rates are found in East Asia and Eastern Europe. China, the most populous country in 2019, has a fertility rate of only 1.60, and its population is expected to decline 2% by 2050. The United States, with a fertility rate of 1.87, expects its population to grow by about 20% over that same period, mostly due to immigration.[3,36]

Many developing countries are already suffering from shortages of natural and economic resources, including limited agricultural land and a lack of nonagricultural employment. Such regions may have already passed a threshold of irreversibility. The speed and magnitude with which populations are outstripping the available resources are unprecedented in history. The result is expected to be an increase in migrations and violent conflicts. Hundreds of millions of people may be compelled to relocate. Already, wars and civil violence are being fought over scarce resources such as water, farmland, forests, and fish. For example, droughts in the Middle East caused by climate change, together with population growth, have contributed to recent unrest in Egypt, Syria, and Libya, which has led to massive migrations of people into Turkey, as well as boatloads of refugees attempting to reach Europe by crossing the Mediterranean.[37,38]

Any hope for saving the earth from the most dire of these predicted fates must include cooperation between rich and poor countries, and some control of population growth. Unfortunately, international agreement of this kind is exceedingly difficult. Three United Nations conferences on population were held at 10-year intervals, beginning in 1974; all were fraught with ethical, religious, and political controversy. Rich countries blamed poor countries for the destruction of natural resources, while poor countries blamed the rich for profligate consumption. Poor countries demanded help from the rich, which attached unwelcome conditions to the aid they provided. Opposition to contraception by Roman Catholic and Muslim authorities, as well as the incendiary politics of abortion in the United States, obstructed rational attempts at limiting population growth.

Although the 1994 International Conference on Population and Development (ICPD) held in Cairo was as contentious as the two previous meetings, a consensus emerged on a new approach to population policy—one that focused on individual rights, especially women's rights, including their right to make reproductive decisions. The conference produced a 20-year "Programme of Action" that included, among other goals, education for women.[39] Educated women prefer fewer children, and they have more bargaining power in the family and in society, studies have shown. Other goals agreed upon at Cairo were universal access to safe and reliable family-planning methods, universal access to and completion of primary education, reduction of infant mortality rates, reduction of maternal mortality rates, and increased life expectancy. The philosophy underlying the "Cairo Consensus" was that if needs for family planning and reproductive health care are met, along with other basic health and education services, then population stabilization will occur naturally, not as a matter of coercion or control.

In 2014, the 20th anniversary of the Cairo conference, the United Nations conducted an in-depth review of the status of the Programme of Action, conducting the "ICPD Beyond 2014 Global Survey." This survey concluded that, although progress had been made in some countries, it was uneven and the agenda remained unfinished. The United Nations agreed to extend the goals indefinitely.[40] It issued a "Framework of Action" as a follow-up to the Programme of Action, reaffirming the importance of sexual and reproductive health and rights of all people as a critical foundation for sustainable development.[41]

The United States is sheltered from some of the realities of the population problem because of the nation's relative isolation from the most crowded regions of the planet. However, Americans cannot afford to be complacent about the dangers posed by world crowding. Global warming, air and ocean pollution, and loss of biodiversity are environmental effects of overpopulation that are certain to affect public health in the United States, even if the nation could close its borders to all international travelers. Without global population control, other public health efforts would ultimately be a losing battle.

Population control cannot be imposed by force, however. As Paul and Anne Ehrlich point out in their book *One with Nineveh*, stabilization of the world's population is closely tied to modernization and economic viability of the poorest countries.[5] This agrees with the conclusions of the 1994 Cairo conference, and it is the goal that the United States and other developed nations have agreed to strive toward. The Ehrlichs quote Lester Pearson, former prime minister of Canada and president of the United Nations General Assembly: "A planet cannot, any more than a country, survive half slave, half free, half engulfed in misery, half careening along toward the supposed joys of almost unlimited consumption. Neither our ecology nor our morality could survive such contrasts."[5(p.234)]

Conclusion

The earth's human population has been growing rapidly and continuously for centuries. While the rate of growth appears to be slowing, the science of population biology suggests that a disastrous population crash is possible, as a result of environmental pressures.

Paradoxically, public health measures such as clean water, immunization, and pest control have contributed to population growth by saving lives. While improved life expectancy has led to a fall in birth rates in industrialized countries, in the developing world population control efforts have not kept up with other public health efforts. The resulting crowding threatens to reverse the advances that have been made in public health. In developing countries, migrants from rural areas, in search of jobs, often settle in urban shantytowns that lack adequate drinking water and sewage services. These conditions lead to frequent epidemics of infectious diseases, and the accompanying social breakdown contributed to the rise of the AIDS epidemic. The AIDS epidemic is so severe in parts of Africa that it has slowed population growth in those countries.

Many analysts believe that the carrying capacity of the earth—the population size that the earth can support without being degraded—is being reached. Factors that limit carrying capacity include the availability of fresh water, the availability of fuel, the amount and productivity of arable land, and the amount and disposition of wastes. Fresh water is already in short supply in some parts of the world, and many sources of fresh water are being degraded by pollution with human and industrial wastes. Arable land is being depleted through overcultivation and erosion. Deforestation is occurring on all continents, and even the sea is being depleted of fish.

In addition to the impact of resource shortages on human populations, overpopulation is bringing about global climate change. Increased atmospheric concentrations of greenhouse gases brought about by human activities are causing warming of the earth's surface. This, in turn, causes melting of the polar ice caps and a rise in ocean levels. Weather patterns are already changing. Warming of temperate zones may account for the recent emergence in the United States of a number of infectious diseases

formerly confined to more tropical regions. At an international conference in Kyoto, Japan, in 1997, an agreement was reached for countries to reduce their greenhouse gas emissions. However, President Bush tried to cast doubt on the evidence for global warming and withdrew U.S. support for the Kyoto Protocol. At another climate conference that took place in Copenhagen in December 2009, President Obama expressed his support for climate control measures, but there was little agreement on details. At another conference in December 2015, all major countries of the world, including the United States and China, for the first time pledged specific emissions cuts, but the Trump administration pulled the United States out of the accord, leaving global climate planning in the lurch.

The United Nations has held three conferences on population, all fraught with ethical, religious, and political controversy. At the third conference, held in Cairo in 1994, a new approach to population control was agreed upon with a 20-year plan of action. This consensus builds on evidence that education and empowerment of women lead them to choose smaller families and brings a fragile hope that stabilization of the population may be achieved by helping the poorest nations to modernize and become economically stronger. On the 20-year anniversary of the Cairo conference, the United Nations assessed progress toward reaching the goals, concluding that progress was uneven and the agenda remained incomplete, and reaffirmed the importance of continuing to try.

References

1. A. Nadakavukaren, *Our Global Environment: A Health Perspective*, 7th ed. (Long Grove, IL: Waveland Press, 2011).
2. P. R. Ehrlich, *The Population Bomb* (New York, NY: Ballantine Books, 1975).
3. United Nations, Department of Economic and Social Affairs, Population Division, "World Population Prospects 2019: Highlights," 2019, https://population.un.org/wpp/Publications/Files/WPP2019_Highlights.pdf, accessed October 8, 2019.
4. P. R. Ehrlich and A. H. Ehrlich, *The Population Explosion* (New York, NY: Simon and Schuster, 1990).
5. P. R. Ehrlich and A. H. Ehrlich, *One with Nineveh: Politics, Consumption, and the Human Future* (Washington, DC: Island Press, 2004).

6. P. R. Ehrlich and R. E. Ornstein, *Humanity on a Tightrope: Thoughts on Empathy, Family, and Big Changes for a Viable Future* (Lanham, MD: Rowman & Littlefield, 2010).

7. World Health Organization, "Children: Reducing Mortality," September 19, 2019, https://www.who .int/news-room/fact-sheets/detail/children-reducing -mortality, accessed October 8, 2019.

8. United Nations, Department of Economics and Social Affairs, "2018 Revision of World Urbanization Prospects," https://www.un.org/development/desa /publications/2018-revision-of-world-urbanization -prospects.html, accessed October 8, 2019.

9. World Health Organization, "Polio," 2019, https://www .afro.who.int/health-topics/polio, accessed October 8, 2019.

10. Joint United Nations Programme on HIV and AIDS (UNAIDS), "How AIDS Changed Everything: Fact Sheet," https://www.unaids.org/sites/default/files/media _asset/UNAIDS_FactSheet_en.pdf, accessed October 8, 2019.

11. UNAIDS, "Countries," 2019, https://www.unaids.org /en/regionscountries/countries, accessed October 8, 2019.

12. AVERT: Averting HIV and AIDS, "Children Orphaned by HIV and AIDS," https://www.avert.org/professionals /hiv-social-issues/key-affected-populations/children, accessed August 16, 2015.

13. The World Bank, "Data by Country," https://data .worldbank.org/country/, accessed October 8, 2019.

14. Federal Interagency Forum on Child and Family Statistics, "America's Children: Key National Indicators of Well-Being, 2018," https://www.childstats.gov/pdf /ac2018/ac_18.pdf, accessed October 8, 2019.

15. A. Nagourney, "California Imposes First Mandatory Water Restrictions to Deal with Drought," *The New York Times*, April 1, 2015.

16. C. Fishman, "How California Is Winning the Drought," *The New York Times*, August 14, 2015.

17. Phil Helsel, "California Drought Officially over After More Than Seven Years," *NBC News*, March 14, 2019, https://www.nbcnews.com/storyline/california -drought/california-drought-officially-over-after-more -seven-years-n983461, accessed October 8, 2019.

18. T. Fuller, "Facing Fire Risk, Expanses of California Go Dark," *The New York Times*, October 10, 2019.

19. J. W. Maurits la Rivière, "Threats to the World's Water," *Scientific American* 261 (1989): 80–97.

20. Food and Agriculture Organization of the United Nations, "The State of Food Insecurity in the World—2015," http://www.fao.org/3/a-i4646e.pdf, accessed October 8, 2019.

21. J. Bongaarts, "Can the Growing Human Population Feed Itself?" *Scientific American* (March 1994): 36–42.

22. Food and Agricultural Organization of the United Nations, "The State of the World Fisheries and Aquaculture," 2018, http://www.fao.org/3/I9540EN /i9540en.pdf, accessed October 8, 2019.

23. National Oceanic and Atmospheric Administration, Earth System Research Laboratory, Global Monitoring Division, "Trends in Atmospheric Carbon Dioxide," https://www.esrl.noaa.gov/gmd/ccgg/trends/global .html, accessed October 6, 2019.

24. Intergovernmental Panel on Climate Change, "Climate Change 2014: Synthesis Report—Summary for Policymakers," https://www.ipcc.ch/report/ar5 /syr/, accessed October 8, 2019.

25. J. Gillis, "California Drought Is Made Worse by Global Warming, Scientists Say," *The New York Times*, August 20, 2015.

26. R. A. Kerr, "Global Warming Is Changing the World," *Science* 316 (2007): 188–190.

27. National Research Council Transportation Research Board, *Potential Impacts of Climate Change on U.S. Transportation* (Washington, DC: National Academies Press, 2008).

28. I. Magra, "Europe Suffers Heat Wave of Dangerous, Record-High Temperatures," *The New York Times*, July 24, 2019.

29. K. Pydynowski, "Heat Wave Tightens Grip on Southeast US as Dozens of High Temperature Records Fall," *AccuWeather*, September 4, 2019, https://www .accuweather.com/en/weather-news/unrelenting-heat -wave-to-keep-breaking-records-in-southeast-into -beyond-memorial-day/70008360, accessed October 8, 2019.

30. Union of Concerned Scientists, "Each Country's Share of CO_2 Emissions," October 11, 2018, https://www .ucsusa.org/global-warming/science-and-impacts /science/each-countrys-share-of-co2.html, accessed October 8, 2019.

31. E. Stokstad, "EPA Report Takes Heat for Climate Change Edits," *Science* 300 (2003): 201.

32. J. M. Broder, "Many Goals Remain Unmet in 5 Nations' Climate Deal," *The New York Times*, December 18, 2009.

33. J. Gillis, "Pledges to Cut Emissions Lag as Climate Talks Get Underway," *The New York Times*, November 29, 2015.

34. C. E. Lee and W. Mauldin, "U.S., China Agree on Implementing Paris Climate-Change Pact," *The Wall Street Journal*, September 3, 2016.

35. Michael D. Shear, "Trump Will Withdraw U.S. from Paris Climate Agreement," *The New York Times*, June 1, 2017.

36. Central Intelligence Agency, "The World Factbook, Total Fertility Rate, 2017," www.cia .gov/library/publications/the-world-factbook /rankorder/2127rank.html, accessed October 8, 2019.

37. Center for American Progress, "The Arab Spring and Climate Change: A Climate and Security Correlations Series," February 28, 2013, https://www.americanprogress.org/issues/security/report/2013/02/28/54579/the-arab-spring-and-climate-change/, accessed October 8, 2019.

38. P. Boehler and S. Peçanha, "The Global Struggle to Respond to the Worst Refugee Crisis in Generations," *The New York Times*, July 1, 2015.

39. J. DeJong, "Role and Limitations of the Cairo International Conference on Population and Development," *Social Science and Medicine* 51 (2000): 941–953.

40. United Nations, International Conference on Population and Development, "Programme of Action: Twentieth Anniversary Edition," 2014, https://www.unfpa.org/publications/international-conference-population-and-development-programme-action, accessed October 8, 2019.

41. United Nations Commission on Population and Development, "Framework of Action for the Follow-Up to the Programme of Action of the International Conference on Population and Development (ICPD) Beyond 2014," January 2014, https://www.unfpa.org/publications/framework-actions-follow-programme-action-international-conference-population-and, accessed October 8, 2019.

Medical Care and Public Health

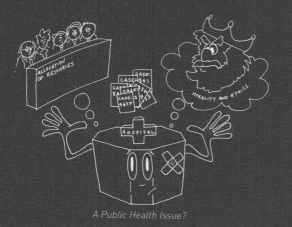

CHAPTER 26

A Public Health Issue?

Is the Medical Care System a Public Health Issue?

KEY TERMS

Advance directive
Affordable Care Act
Children's Health Insurance
   Program (CHIP)
Communicable diseases

Community health centers
Copayment
Department of Veterans
   Affairs (VA)
Fee-for-service

Health insurance
Medicaid
Medicare
United Network of Organ
   Sharing (UNOS)

Even in an ideal world where public health functioned perfectly, there would be a need for medicine. The medical system provides preventive care: immunizations against infectious diseases, monitoring of pregnancies and provision of "well-baby care" to ensure that children develop normally, testing of adults for risk factors (such as high cholesterol and blood pressure) that lead to cardiovascular disease, and secondary prevention measures—screening for early detection of diabetes and cancer, for example, and early interventions to correct problems. Even people with the healthiest lifestyles may get sick or injured. Medical care saves lives and prevents suffering and disability and, therefore, must be considered necessary for public health.

Medical care is even more necessary when public health is not functioning perfectly. There are many gaps in the public health system because of a lack of resources, lack of political will, and the emergence of new health threats. Also, competing values in society lead people to behave in unhealthy ways. The medical system is called upon to deal with the consequences of failures in public health. Doctors are asked to repair the damage when an unvaccinated child contracts an infectious disease, when a community is sickened by water or food contaminated because of deficiencies in sanitary practices, when someone is injured in a motor vehicle accident caused by a drunk driver, or when a smoker develops cancer after years of exposure to tobacco smoke.

The fact that medical care can and does make a difference in people's health raises a number of fundamental social questions. Who is responsible for providing medical care when it is needed? Medical care is expensive, and the costs have been rising dramatically over the past several decades. Who should pay for that care? Vastly greater sums of public money are spent each year on medical care than on public health measures aimed at preventing disease and disability. Is that a rational allocation of resources? Should U.S. citizens have the same right to medical care as they have to education in childhood? And, if there are limits on the community's responsibility for providing medical care, how should those limits be determined?

The medical profession has fought governmental involvement in addressing these questions, regarding itself as the ultimate authority over all matters of health.[1] However, public health concerns have repeatedly forced government action on a piecemeal basis to challenge medicine's sovereignty. Public health has always seen a role for itself as the provider of last resort, offering needed medical care to people who cannot afford to pay for it. This is part of the assurance function that the Institute of Medicine identified as one of public health's core functions. Government regulation has also been necessary to set standards for the practice of various healthcare services, to discipline medical professionals when they are thought to be acting unethically or incompetently, and to establish policy when ethical dilemmas have arisen that transcend the individual sickroom.

When Medical Care Is a Public Health Responsibility

Some forms of medical care are more important to the health of the community than are others. Medical treatment of **communicable diseases** is particularly important because of the possibility that one sick individual could infect many others. Consequently, public health has taken a major interest in all aspects of infectious disease control, from the early days when quarantines were the only effective way of controlling epidemics, to immunization programs, to the provision of free medical treatment for those who do not have health insurance and cannot afford to pay for care. City and county health departments have traditionally operated clinics for diagnosis and treatment of infectious diseases. In the early 1990s, the threat of reemerging tuberculosis was taken seriously enough that, for example, the New York City Department of Health provided a program of directly observed therapy in which public health nurses were sent to track down patients and make sure they took their medicine. The fact that acquired immunodeficiency syndrome (AIDS) is a communicable disease accounts, at least in part, for the major investment that the federal and some state governments have made not only in research, but also in providing treatment for patients.

A second area in which communities have an undisputed interest in the universal availability of medical care is the provision of emergency services. Emergencies are, by definition, unpredictable and can strike individuals at any time and in any place. In an increasingly mobile society, heart attacks and motor vehicle crashes may occur when people are far from home, with no family or friends present to provide first aid or call the doctor. It is in the interest of everyone to save lives first and ask questions later. Beginning with the Highway Safety Act of 1966, the federal government began to pressure states and localities to develop procedures for providing quick access to emergency care. Since then, in accordance with federal standards, communities have developed 911 phone-response networks, trained emergency medical technicians, dispatched ambulances using a centralized system, regulated the availability of hospital emergency rooms, identified trauma centers, and provided evacuation helicopters in rural areas. Even so, the quality and the effectiveness of emergency response systems vary considerably in different parts of the country.[2]

A number of federal and state laws require that emergency rooms provide treatment to any patient who arrives with a life-threatening condition until he or she is stabilized, regardless of ability to pay. When the emergency situation has passed, however, many hospitals transfer poor and uninsured patients to public or charity hospitals. Some states have laws that prohibit hospitals from denying admission based solely on inability to pay, but in many parts of the country hospitals can and do turn away patients for financial reasons. Once medical treatment is under way, however, a patient's rights are greatly enhanced. Laws against "abandonment" ensure that hospitals cannot simply discharge patients because they are poor and uninsured.

Although most U.S. citizens do not have a general right to medical care, there are several exceptions, including veterans and prisoners. The hospitals and clinics of the U.S. **Department of Veterans Affairs (VA)** were designed to treat war-related injuries, but they also serve as a safety net for low-income veterans who do not have other sources of medical care. While funding for the VA system has historically been inadequate, a recent study found that VA hospitals perform at least as well as private hospitals.[3] Many veterans suffer from psychiatric disabilities or have substance abuse problems—conditions that the VA has special expertise to treat. In 2019, the Donald Trump administration loosened rules so that VA enrollees can obtain medical care outside the VA system: Veterans who have to wait at least 14 days for care in the VA system can now seek private care instead, with the VA covering the costs. Previously, the rules allowed for private care only after a 30-day wait.[4] Prisoners are entitled to medical care because, as wards of the state, they are unable to seek care on their own. The courts have ruled that to deny them care would be the

cruel and unusual punishment forbidden by the Constitution.[5] The medical care provided in prisons, however, is often substandard.

The Conflict Between Public Health and the Medical Profession

Most Americans get **health insurance** as part of an employee benefit package. Such insurance covers the worker and his or her family. This approach to paying medical bills became dominant after World War II, when unions bargained actively to obtain health benefits for workers. The resulting arrangement satisfied most groups over the next three or four decades. Workers and their families could receive necessary medical care without worrying about the cost; doctors and hospitals were happy because they could provide care as they saw fit and not worry about getting paid; unions took credit for forcing employers to provide the benefits; employers did not object because the cost at first was modest and the benefits inspired loyalty in their workers.

Traditional health insurance—the kind of insurance provided by most employers until quite recently—is like car insurance. Regular premiums are paid to the insurance company to cover the worker and his or her family. When covered individuals get sick, they go to the doctor or other medical provider of their choice, and that provider then sends them bills for services rendered. The patients pay the bills and are reimbursed by the insurance company. Sometimes the policy, like many car insurance policies, calls for a deductible that the patient must pay first before the insurance kicks in. Sometimes the patients must also pay a flat fee or a fixed percentage of the remainder of the bill, called a **copayment**. This way of paying for medical care is called "**fee-for-service**." The fee-for-service approach permits doctors to make decisions about a patient's care with no consideration of cost. Unfortunately, this freedom has led to escalating medical costs and increasing numbers of uninsured citizens whose access to care is limited.

The medical profession has strongly resisted efforts to be included in the domain of public services. Since the end of the 19th century, with the discovery of bacterial causes of diseases, public health has claimed the prevention and treatment of infectious disease as its responsibility, and doctors have resisted that claim. While tolerant of public health's efforts to clean up the environment, private practitioners regarded diagnosing and curing sick people as their domain. Early in the 20th century, they fought reporting requirements for cases of tuberculosis and venereal disease, and they opposed the creation of public health clinics and centers, which they perceived as an attack on their economic interests. This struggle continued throughout the century, and although public health had some victories, the medical establishment was able to prevent the United States from providing for its citizens the public assurance of needed medical care.[1]

Nevertheless, the United States has a long history of providing charity care for the nation's poor. Often, treatment was provided by part-time volunteer physicians who combined their services with research and the teaching of medical students. This practice began in the late 18th century, with the establishment of free dispensaries in eastern cities, many of them connected with medical schools. At the time, these services were quite controversial. On the one hand, private practitioners were suspicious that free care was being provided to those who could afford to pay for it, and there was great concern about "dispensary abuse." On the other hand, the poor were distrustful of the dispensaries, where they were forced to wait hours for hasty and superficial attention.[1]

In the early 20th century, city health departments began setting up clinics for the control of infectious diseases and the prevention of infant mortality. Baby clinics emphasized the teaching of hygienic practices and promotion of improvements in child care,

diet, and living patterns. Clinics for tuberculosis and venereal disease provided diagnosis and advice about hygiene and diet but left treatment to private physicians, who objected strongly when they felt that the clinics were trespassing on their territory. The New York City Department of Health ran into trouble when its diagnostic bacteriologic laboratory began producing diphtheria antitoxin, selling it to drugstores, and making it available to poor patients for free, prompting complaints of socialism and unfair competition that forced it to cease all sales of the antitoxin. Despite the early opposition of the medical profession, however, an uneasy truce has evolved that allows city and county health departments to provide treatment for the poor, often under the uncomfortable conditions that prevailed in the old dispensaries.[1]

Community health centers serve as another source of basic medical care for the poor. These centers are supported by federal grants as well as by payments by public and private health insurance for services provided. There are about 1400 community health centers in the United States. They are located in inner cities and isolated rural areas where there are shortages of medical and social services. Community health centers provide primary and preventive care to people who might otherwise not be able to afford it. Services may be paid for by government programs (see the next section), or patients may pay a fee based on a sliding scale according to income. Community health centers serve as an important safety net for low-income families; the numbers of patients seen at these facilities have been increasing, and they now serve approximately 20% of low-income uninsured persons, or about 8% of the U.S. population.[6]

The health of schoolchildren has been a public health concern since the late 19th century. To control the spread of communicable diseases, cities began to employ medical inspectors to examine children who showed signs of illness and exclude them from school if they had a communicable disease. School doctors and nurses also began testing children for eye problems and other physical impairments that might interfere with learning. Because of the opposition of the medical establishment, they were not allowed to provide medical treatments. With the development of effective vaccines, the law began requiring that children be immunized—by their private physicians or in public clinics—before they started school, and the threat of epidemics in the schools has receded. In some cities, school health programs treat minor problems; sometimes they merely send notes recommending treatment home to parents. It is a source of frustration to public health practitioners that school health programs are not integrated with medical services, leaving many children with health problems that are repeatedly diagnosed but go untreated.[1]

Throughout the 20th century, there were repeated attempts in the United States to provide some kind of national health insurance plan to ensure that everyone would have access to needed medical care. During this period, most industrialized countries were setting up such programs—some of them run by the national government, others more loosely organized. Germany established the first national system of compulsory sickness insurance in 1883. Over the next 30 years, Austria, Hungary, Norway, Serbia, Britain, Russia, and the Netherlands followed Germany's example. Canada implemented a national health insurance plan in the 1970s.[1]

In the United States, efforts to establish a national health program were made before World War I but were derailed by the war. Another attempt was made during the 1930s as part of President Franklin D. Roosevelt's New Deal, but health insurance was not included in the Social Security Act. After World War II, President Harry S. Truman proposed a single health insurance system that would apply to everyone; again the attempt failed. Each time, the medical profession opposed governmental involvement in medical care as "socialized medicine," and various other political interests joined to defeat the proposals.[1]

In 1965, a significant victory over the medical establishment's opposition was achieved under President Lyndon Johnson: Laws establishing Medicare, which provides insurance for the elderly, and Medicaid, a welfare-type program for the poor, were passed. These programs were designed to remedy what people considered the main problems with employer-based insurance: It stopped when a worker retired, and it left the poor and unemployed out of the system.[1]

Medicare, created in 1965 as a mandatory insurance program for people older than age 65, is part of the Social Security system. (Younger people who are entitled to Social Security benefits because of disability are also eligible for Medicare.) Workers pay into the system through deductions from their paychecks; employers pay a tax on their payroll, and workers are entitled to benefits when they reach retirement age. The Medicare program has two main parts: Part A, which covers hospital insurance, and Part B, which pays doctor bills and other outpatient costs. Virtually all people are automatically enrolled in Medicare Part A when they reach age 65. Part B is voluntary and requires participants to pay a monthly premium. Medicare is much like traditional health insurance, in that most doctors and other providers are paid on a fee-for-service basis. Like private insurance, the patient is required to pay deductibles and copayments. Medicare Part C (also called Medicare Advantage) was added in 1997, and gives beneficiaries more flexibility in which health plans they use. In 2003, legislation was passed that created a new Medicare prescription drug plan, Part D. This benefit, which became effective in 2006, is optional and requires an additional monthly premium.

Medicaid was created, also in 1965, as a welfare program for the poor, with costs shared by the federal government and the states. Eligibility is determined by income and varies from one state to another. Medical bills are paid directly by the state or local government to the provider, usually at a low, fixed rate for each service. Alternatively, states may fund managed care companies to cover Medicaid patients.

In the early 1970s, President Richard Nixon tried to expand these programs, proposing a national plan to cover everyone, but his efforts were derailed by the Watergate scandal. No further efforts were made until President Bill Clinton was elected in 1992, promising to provide health insurance for all; his proposal was also defeated. However, because of increasing concern about the problem of children without access to medical care, President Clinton and Congress negotiated a program called the **Children's Health Insurance Program (CHIP)**. This joint federal–state program, similar to Medicaid, expanded coverage to children in families that earn too much to qualify for Medicaid, usually up to 200% of the federal poverty level.[7] In 2010, President Barack Obama succeeded in persuading Congress to pass the **Affordable Care Act**, an attempt to ensure that all Americans are covered by medical insurance. This program is discussed elsewhere in this text.

Before the Affordable Care Act, the United States was the only industrialized nation, except South Africa, that did not have a national plan for providing medical care to all its citizens. In 2008, more than 20% of the American population ages 18 to 64 had no health insurance.[8] For many of these people, there was no guaranteed access to health care except for emergency care. While most public health advocates believe that the government should ensure access to basic medical care for anyone who needs it, the American political system traditionally has not supported that view. Clinical medicine, always more prestigious and better financed than public health, was generally able to fend off public health's attempts to integrate medical treatment into a rational system that would maximize the health of all Americans. However, in response to increasing evidence that the U.S. healthcare system was dysfunctional, even the American Medical Association endorsed President Obama's efforts to change the system.[9]

Licensing and Regulation

While the medical profession, until recently, has resisted government efforts to ensure and fund medical care for all Americans, it has been willing to submit to some forms of government regulation. Licensure of qualified medical practitioners, including physicians, nurses, and other health professionals, protects the prerogatives of the professionals from encroachment by unlicensed practitioners and also ensures quality of care for patients. Physicians, nurses, and dentists must be licensed to practice in every state. Licensing requirements for other healthcare professionals vary from state to state. States may establish requirements, such as continuing medical education, for physicians and nurses to maintain or update their skills to retain their licenses. States also have the power to discipline medical professionals for incompetence or misconduct, with the ultimate threat being revocation of their licenses.

States also license and regulate medical facilities such as hospitals and nursing homes. To confirm that they provide high-quality care, healthcare institutions also may seek accreditation by a private organization, generally The Joint Commission.[10] Given that Medicare, Medicaid, and many private health insurers usually require institutions to be accredited before they will pay them for patient services, maintaining accreditation is important to these facilities. Schools of medicine, nursing, and public health as well as training programs for advanced medical specialties also seek accreditation as a measure of their quality. As medical care is increasingly being provided by managed care organizations and as methods are developed to evaluate the quality of care provided by these organizations, accreditation of managed care organizations is becoming more widespread.

Governments have attempted to use regulatory approaches to restrain the growth of medical costs by requiring certificates of need before new facilities can be built or expensive new equipment purchased. These efforts have generally proved ineffective and most have been abandoned.

Ethical and Legal Issues in Medical Care

Although the United States throughout the 20th century chose not to establish a broad right to medical care, it has been forced repeatedly to deal with individual cases that attract public attention and demand community response. Consequently, there are many legal requirements and restrictions on medical care that have arisen from specific cases. Usually, such cases have come to the attention of the courts when medical professionals disagreed with each other or with patients' families. Decisions in these cases have set legal precedents for how medicine can be practiced in certain situations. Many of these situations involve the beginning and end of life, and many of the precedents have profound implications for public health.

Abortion is one of the most controversial medicolegal issues, pitting the "right to life" of the fetus against the right of the pregnant woman to control her own body. Abortion was illegal in most states until 1973, when the U.S. Supreme Court decided in *Roe v. Wade* that women have a constitutional right to an abortion, at least in the first trimester of pregnancy. The controversy continues, however, with right-to-life activists trying, with some success in some state legislatures, to place limits on the circumstances under which women can exercise their rights.

Similar controversy raged in the late 1990s over whether mentally competent, terminally ill patients have the right to physician-assisted suicide. Dr. Jack Kevorkian was making a career of helping to end the lives of people who were suffering or were afraid that they would suffer painful or degrading deaths. While laws were passed outlawing Kevorkian's

activities, juries sympathized with the patients and refused to convict him. However, in 1999, he was convicted of second-degree murder because he went beyond assisting suicide and actually administered a lethal drug to a patient who wished to die. The death of a 52-year-old man with Lou Gehrig's disease was aired on the CBS program *60 Minutes*. Kevorkian served eight years in prison and was released in 2007 after assuring authorities that he would never conduct another assisted suicide. He died of natural causes in 2011 at the age of 83. Meanwhile, seven states—California, Colorado, Hawaii, New Jersey, Oregon, Washington, Vermont—and the District of Columbia have passed laws that allow physicians to assist patients to commit suicide by prescribing lethal doses of drugs. The patients must be mentally competent adults, terminally ill with less than six months to live, and capable of taking the medications by themselves. In Montana, the courts have decided that doctors may prescribe such drugs.[12,13]

Ironically, while there is no legal requirement to provide medical care to people who want and could benefit from it, many of the most contentious legal cases have concerned the system's insistence on providing expensive, intrusive, and unwanted treatment to patients whose conditions are judged medically hopeless. In the 1976 case of Karen Ann Quinlan, a young woman left permanently unconscious from an overdose of drugs and alcohol, the New Jersey Supreme Court eventually ruled that she could be removed from a ventilator at the request of her parents over the objections of hospital personnel. However, in the 14 months of the court battle, the young woman had been weaned from the ventilator and was able to breathe on her own, although she remained unconscious. She was transferred to a nursing home, where she survived for 10 years in a persistent vegetative state.[14]

In the similar case of Nancy Cruzan, a young Missouri woman in a persistent vegetative state resulting from an automobile crash, the U.S. Supreme Court decided in 1990 that states could set the standards for when life support could be removed. Cruzan's father had to move her to another state to remove the feeding tube and let her die.[15] Now, after a number of other cases have been tried in the courts, the precedent is well established that competent patients can refuse medical treatment and that life-support measures are not required for an incompetent patient who has specified in advance the conditions under which he or she would not want them. The most reliable way for an individual to ensure that his or her wishes will be followed is to sign a durable power of attorney over to a trusted friend or family member who can make medical decisions if he or she becomes incompetent.

The lack of such an **advance directive** led to the politically charged battle in early 2005 over removing a feeding tube from Terri Schiavo, a young Florida woman who had been in a persistent vegetative state for 15 years. Florida law provided that Ms. Schiavo's husband was entitled to decide that the feeding tube should be removed; he contended that she would not have wanted to be kept alive in this condition. However, Ms. Schiavo's parents objected, maintaining that she recognized them and that she might improve with treatment. Inspired by "right-to-life" political pressures, the Florida governor—Jeb Bush—and legislature, the U.S. Congress, and President George W. Bush attempted to block removal of the feeding tube; however, the Florida courts, the federal appeals court, and the Supreme Court upheld the husband's right to decide. Ms. Schiavo died 13 days after the tube was removed. Such family disputes over withdrawing life support, while common, would be easily resolved if the individual had prepared a "living will" that specified her or his wishes.[16]

But what happens if a patient indicates that he or she wants all possible measures taken to preserve his or her life, even if there is no hope of regaining consciousness? This is what happened in 1991 in the case of Helga Wanglie, an 87-year-old woman in a persistent

vegetative state who was being kept on a ventilator and feeding tube in a Minneapolis hospital. Her husband and children refused to allow life support to be removed, stating that they were praying for a miracle. The hospital went to court, claiming that the treatment was futile and merely prolonged death. The court refused to intervene, and the patient remained on life support until she died three days later.[17,18] In some states, including California and Texas, the law allows healthcare institutions to withdraw life support when further treatment is judged futile, even against the wishes of the patient as expressed in an advance directive.[16] Not often mentioned in the legal arguments is the cost of the care. Most often, the costs of caring for brain-damaged patients are borne by the taxpayer, since few families have the resources to pay for such long-term care.

Similar quandaries occur at the beginning of life, when decisions must be made about treating infants whose prospects are limited. Several notable cases occurred in the 1970s and 1980s involving babies born with Down syndrome, a condition characterized by mental retardation and often accompanied by physical defects that are lethal but correctable by surgery. The difficult question with which parents are confronted, while still reeling from the news that their infant is not normal, is whether to authorize the surgery, allowing the infant a chance to live although his or her quality of life will be uncertain. In 1982, the Infant Doe case drew public attention to this particular problem. Infant Doe was a Down syndrome baby born in Bloomington, Indiana, with tracheoesophageal fistula, a hole between the respiratory and digestive tracts. The parents chose not to operate, but hospital administrators and pediatricians went to court to force the surgery. The judge ruled that the parents had the right to make the decision; each level of appeal supported the parents, and the baby died before the case reached the Supreme Court.[14]

However, the publicity over Infant Doe attracted the attention of the Ronald Reagan administration, which firmly supported the right-to-life viewpoint. On the grounds that nontreatment of newborns constituted discrimination against people with disabilities, the Justice Department implemented the so-called Baby Doe rules, which mandated treatment of all newborns with birth defects. Large posters were to be displayed outside all neonatal intensive care units stating that "Discriminatory failure to feed and care for handicapped infants in this facility is prohibited by federal law." A toll-free 800 number, the "Baby Doe hotline," was posted to report abuses, and "Baby Doe squads," composed of lawyers, government administrators, and physicians, investigated complaints. Later court action struck down the Baby Doe rules. Nevertheless, in 1984, Congress passed a law declaring that nontreatment in Baby Doe cases is child abuse except when the child is chronically and irreversibly comatose, the child is inevitably dying, or treatment would be "futile and inhumane."[12]

It is not only infants with Down syndrome that must be given aggressive medical treatment. Many of the 543,000 infants born preterm every year also must be provided with advanced, high-technology care. Although most of these infants survive to lead normal lives, many others—especially those with very low birth weight (less than 3.4 pounds)—die or are left with permanent impairments. Infants with very low birth weight who survive are at increased risk of such long-term disabilities as cerebral palsy, autism, mental retardation, vision and hearing impairments, and other developmental problems.[19] In most cases, decisions about care for very-low-birth-weight infants are made by parents in consultation with their doctor. However in 2002, Congress passed and President George W. Bush signed the Born Alive Infant Protection Act, which mandated that infants born with any signs of life be treated as suffering from an emergency medical condition, no matter how futile that treatment might be. This law and the 1984 Baby Doe rules have rarely been enforced despite a statement by President Bush's Secretary of Health and Human Services that his department would investigate all circumstances where the law appeared to be violated.[20,21]

The costs of medical treatment for these infants, like the costs of providing life support for nearly dead adults, are not generally considered when decisions are made about whether aggressive treatment should be given. If these babies survive with major handicaps, medical and caretaking costs will continue throughout their lives. According to the most recent estimates, calculated by the Institute of Medicine, preterm births cost the nation $26 billion annually, mostly for medical care, but also for early intervention, special education, and lost productivity.[19] Much of the costs, like those for brain-damaged adults, is borne by taxpayers.

From a public health perspective, the American healthcare system is unfair and unethical. Vast resources are spent on relatively few, desperately ill patients, many of whom have no prospect of a reasonable quality of life, while millions of Americans have no access to the most basic medical services that could relieve pain and prevent long-term disability. Richard Lamm, a former governor of Colorado who was an outspoken critic of the inequities of the system, lamented that medical ethicists debate agonizingly over the treatment of a few individuals yet pay little attention to social ethics, a neglected and much-needed examination of the allocation of resources for the entire system. Lamm argued that "it is axiomatic that public funds should buy the most health for the most people,"[22(p.14)] a view consistent with that of public health.

Ethical Issues in Medical Resource Allocation

While public health advocates believe that the inequities in access to care are the most important ethical dilemmas concerning the medical system, numerous other situations call for public participation in medical decisions.

Sometimes the issue is access to scarce resources other than money. For example, when hemodialysis (blood-cleansing) was first developed in 1970 to help patients with failing kidneys, there was a shortage of dialysis machines. To choose which patients should receive dialysis, "God Committees" were formed. The committees consisted of laypeople who would select the most worthy candidates for the life-saving treatment. The committees tended to favor those who had jobs, family responsibilities, youth, good general health, and strong motivation. The judgment process made many people uncomfortable.[13] After dramatic publicity about the plight of patients with kidney failure who were denied the dialysis treatment, Congress passed the 1972 End-Stage Renal Disease (ESRD) Act, which funded dialysis treatment for all Americans who needed it without selection criteria. Subsequently, the program's funding was extended to include kidney transplants, which can obviate patients' need for dialysis.

The ESRD Act created a new group of citizens with a right to medical care based on their diagnoses. Advocates for patients with other conditions, such as hemophilia and heart and lung disease, tried to persuade Congress to fund their diseases as well; however, the cost of kidney dialysis and transplants skyrocketed due in part to the open-ended funding, and Congress declined to extend the benefit to people other than kidney patients.[13]

As organ transplantation has become increasingly successful due to improved antirejection drugs, the problem of how to distribute scarce resources has resurfaced, since the number of donor organs is never adequate to fill the need. Livers are in especially short supply, and there is no substitute treatment, like kidney dialysis, for failing livers. Approximately 6000 patients receive liver transplants each year, but in 2015, there were more than 5000 people on regional waiting lists.[23]

The policy on distributing organs has been controversial. The task of matching available organs with waiting patients is handled by a nonprofit organization under contract with the U.S. Department of Health and Human Services. This organization, called the **United Network of Organ Sharing (UNOS)**, maintains a computerized network of 58 organ recovery centers in 11 geographic regions of the nation. Patients are prioritized according to how urgently they need the organ. When an organ becomes available, a suitable recipient—one who is compatible according to blood type and other characteristics—is sought among the most urgent candidates within the same region. If a suitable match is not made within the region, the computer looks at waiting lists in other regions.[23]

In 2009, the issue of priority for transplants arose when Steve Jobs, the chief executive of Apple, unexpectedly received a liver transplant some time after he had been diagnosed with pancreatic cancer, possibly because the cancer had spread to his liver. Questions were raised about whether he had jumped to the head of the waiting list because of his wealth and celebrity, as had apparently happened when baseball star Mickey Mantle had a liver transplant in 1995 after only one day on the list. In a *New York Times* article, transplant specialists were quoted as saying that, although jumping ahead of others would not have been allowed for Jobs, there were ways of working the system that he could have used. Because waiting times vary at different transplant centers around the country, Jobs could have registered at more than one center and, having access to a private jet, could have arrived at a center promptly when an organ became available.[24] The allocation process is a life-or-death matter because, on average, 18 people die every day while waiting for an organ.[25]

The acrimony over rationing of organs, which is unavoidable because of obvious shortages, demonstrates how difficult it is politically to make rational decisions in the allocation of medical care. An argument can be made that rationing currently exists throughout the medical system and should be addressed openly, although very few politicians or medical professionals are willing to face this fact.

Conclusion

While public health's focus on prevention of disease aims to minimize the need for medical care, access to medical care is an important part of the assurance function of public health. Medicine has always resisted attempts to include it as part of the public health system, with considerable success. Most Americans have private health insurance provided through their employers. However, public health concerns have overcome the opposition of the medical profession on some issues.

The urgent need to control the spread of communicable diseases has led to significant government involvement at the local level in providing medical care. Governments also coordinate, and often provide, emergency services to ensure prompt response when lives are at stake. Public health clinics that provide care for the poor have been grudgingly accepted by organized medicine, but there is no general right to medical care for Americans, as there is in most other industrialized countries.

There have been repeated attempts throughout the 20th century to enact a universal health insurance system in the United States. All were defeated. However, in the 1960s, the U.S. Congress created the Medicare program, which guarantees medical care for the elderly, and the Medicaid program, which provides health care for the poor. In the 1990s, a joint federal–state program called Children's Health Insurance Program was created to provide medical care for poor children. In 2010, President Obama succeeded in persuading Congress to pass a law intended to ensure that all Americans will be covered by insurance.

Public health has a role in monitoring and ensuring the quality of medical care through licensing of physicians, nurses, and other health professionals. Healthcare institutions such as hospitals and nursing homes also must be licensed by states. By requiring institutions to be accredited to receive Medicare and Medicaid payment for services, the government can help ensure that the services provided meet a standard of quality. Government involvement in medical issues also occurs in connection with ethical and legal debates about life and death—issues that impact both medicine and public health. Such questions are especially painful when they concern removal of life support from permanently unconscious patients or nontreatment of severely handicapped newborns—situations that involve the provision of costly and probably futile care, usually at the public's expense.

Public participation in medical decisions is also necessary when scarce resources other than money are distributed. When hemodialysis for kidney failure was developed, there was a shortage of dialysis machines, and committees were formed to decide which patients could have the life-saving treatments. This was such a difficult political issue that Congress decided on the expensive solution of funding treatment for all Americans with kidney failure. Currently, patients with failing livers are in similar life-and-death situations, with liver transplants being their only hope of survival. However, there is a shortage of livers available for transplant, and there is always controversy over how organs should be distributed.

References

1. P. Starr, *The Social Transformation of American Medicine* (New York, NY: Basic Books, 1982).

2. M. Peisert, *The Hospital's Role in Emergency Medical Services Systems* (Chicago, IL: American Hospital Publishing, 1984).

3. W. B. Weeks and A. N. West, "Veterans Health Administration Hospitals Outperform Non–Veterans Health Administration Hospitals in Most Health Care Markets," *Annals of Internal Medicine* 170, (2019): 426–428.

4. J. Steinhauer, "V.A. Prepares for Major Shift in Veterans' Health Care," *The New York Times*, June 5, 2019.

5. L. I. Palmer, Law, Medicine, and Social Justice (Louisville, KY: Westminster/John Knox Press, 1989).

6. National Association of Community Health Centers, "Annual Report, 2016-2017," http://www.nachc.org/wp-content/uploads/2018/03/NACHC_20162017AnnualReport_FNL.pdf, accessed October 9, 2019.

7. Centers for Medicare & Medicaid Services, "CHIP: Financing,"https://www.medicaid.gov/chip/financing/index.html, accessed December 30, 2019.

8. E. Eckholm, "Last Year's Poverty Rate Was Highest in 12 Years," *The New York Times*, September 10, 2009.

9. D. D. Kirkpatrick, "A.M.A. Endorses a Health Care Overhaul," *The New York Times*, September 9, 2009.

10. The Joint Commission, https://www.jointcommission.org, accessed August 30, 2015.

11. K. Schneider, "Dr. Jack Kevorkian Dies at 83; A Doctor Who Helped End Lives," *The New York Times*, June 3, 2011.

12. E. Barone, "Brittany Maynard Was One of Hundreds of People in Five States Who've Taken Advantage of Death with Dignity Laws," *Time*, November 3, 2014, https://time.com/3551560/brittany-maynard-right-to-die-laws/, accessed December 30, 2019.

13. I. Lovett and R. Perez-Pena, "California Governor Signs Assisted Suicide Bill into Law," *The New York Times*, October 5, 2015.

14. G. E. Pence, *Classic Cases in Medical Ethics: Accounts of the Cases That Have Shaped Medical Ethics*, 5th ed. (Boston, MA: McGraw-Hill, 2008).

15. G. J. Annas, "Nancy Cruzan and the Right to Die," *New England Journal of Medicine* 323 (1990): 670–672.

16. L. O. Gostin, "Ethics, the Constitution, and the Dying Process: The Case of Theresa Marie Schiavo," *Journal of the American Medical Association* 293 (2005): 2402–2407.

17. M. Angell, "The Case of Helga Wanglie: A New Kind of 'Right to Die' Case," *New England Journal of Medicine* 225 (1991): 511–512.

18. S. H. Miles, "Sounding Board: Informed Demand for 'Non-Beneficial' Medical Treatment," *New England Journal of Medicine* 225 (1991): 512–515.

19. Institute of Medicine, *Preterm Birth: Causes, Consequences, and Prevention* (Washington, DC: National Academies Press, 2007).

20. L. M. Kopelman, "Are the 21-Year-Old Baby Doe Rules Misunderstood or Mistaken?", *Pediatrics* 115 (2005): 797–802.

21. J. C. Partridge, M. D. Sendowski, E. A. Drey, and A. M. Martinez, "Resuscitation of Likely Nonviable Newborns: Would Neonatology Practices in California Change if the Born Alive Infant Protection Act Were Enforced?", *Pediatrics* 123 (2009): 1083–1094.

22. R. D. Lamm, "Ethics of Excess," *Hastings Center Report* 24 (1994): 14.

23. UNOS: United Network of Organ Sharing, https://unos.org/, accessed December 30, 2019.

24. D. Grady and B. Meir, "A Transplant That Is Raising Many Questions," *The New York Times*, June 22, 2009.

25. LiveOnNY, "All About Donation: Frequently Asked Questions," https://www.liveonny.org/be-an-organ-donor/, accessed December 30, 2019.

CHAPTER 27

Inequalities in Access

Why the U.S. Medical System Needs Reform

KEY TERMS

Access to medical care
Consumer-directed health plans
Deductibles
Gross domestic product (GDP)
Health maintenance
 organization (HMO)

Healthcare reform
Health savings accounts
Insurance exchanges
Malpractice
Managed care

Preferred provider organizations
 (PPOs)
Quality of medical care
Rationing

It was obvious almost as soon as the Medicare and Medicaid programs were established that the U.S. healthcare system still had problems. Medical costs in the United States, which had been rising more rapidly than general inflation, rose even more rapidly, putting a strain on all forms of health insurance. **Access to medical care** was difficult for many Americans to obtain because they lacked insurance. And despite the high costs, some evidence suggested that the **quality of medical care** might not be as high as Americans liked to believe. A variety of attempts have been made to reform the system, aimed at controlling costs and improving access. None had significant success until the most recent attempt, described later in this chapter—President Barack Obama's 2010 Affordable Care Act (ACA), which took full effect in 2014.

Figure 27-1 shows the growth in medical care expenditures in the United States since 1960. In that year, approximately $27 billion was spent on medical care. In 1970, the figure had grown to $74 billion. By 2016, national health expenditures had reached $3.34 trillion dollars per year.[1] Historically, the rate of increase has exceeded the overall growth rate of the economy, so that medical costs have constituted an increasingly larger percentage of the nation's **gross domestic product (GDP)**. In 1960, medical expenditures amounted to approximately 5% of the GDP; in 2018, they were 16.9%.[1]

Although expenditures on health have risen all over the world, the United States spends far more on medical care per person than any other country in the world. In 2018, an average of $10,586 was spent on health costs for each

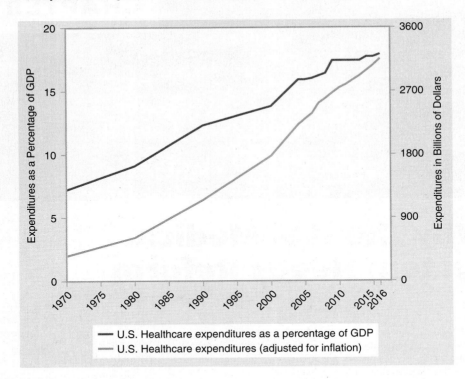

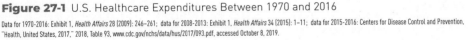

Figure 27-1 U.S. Healthcare Expenditures Between 1970 and 2016

Data for 1970-2016: Exhibit 1, *Health Affairs* 28 (2009): 246–261; data for 2008-2013: Exhibit 1, *Health Affairs* 34 (2015): 1–11; data for 2015-2016: Centers for Disease Control and Prevention, "Health, United States, 2017," 2018, Table 93, www.cdc.gov/nchs/data/hus/2017/093.pdf, accessed October 8, 2019.

American, more than twice the average of a group of 29 industrialized countries that are members of the Organization for Economic Cooperation and Development (OECD) (**Figure 27-2**). Healthcare spending as a percentage of GDP is also higher in the United States, amounting to 16.9% in 2018; Switzerland followed at 12.2%, with France and Germany next at 11.2%. The average for the 29 OECD countries for which data was available was 8.8%.[2]

There is no evidence that Americans are healthier as a result of the greater expenditures. In fact, as measured by the common indicators of health status used for international comparisons, the United States does poorly. Of OECD countries compared in 2017, the United States ranked 32nd out of 36 in terms of infant mortality; its life expectancy at birth was 27th out of 36 countries.[2]

Problems with Access

Despite the large expenditures, many Americans have difficulty getting access to medical care when they need it. Approximately 27.5 million people, or 8.5% of the population, lacked health insurance for the entire year in 2018.[3] Many more may be uninsured for part of the year. The numbers were increasing and were predicted to continue to rise before the ACA was implemented. In 2010, the year the ACA legislation was passed, 15.5% of the population lacked health insurance. Most of the uninsured are poor, and the percentage of uninsured citizens decreases as their income increases. The percentage of children who were uninsured declined to 5.5% in 2018 because of the Children's Health Insurance Program (CHIP), which was established in the 1990s,

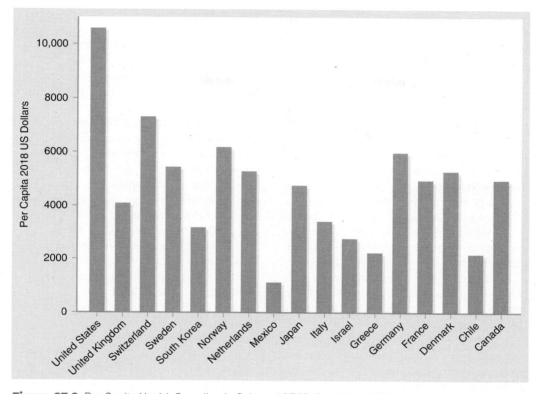

Figure 27-2 Per Capita Health Spending in Selected OECD Countries, 2018

Data from OECD.Stat, Health Expenditure and Financing table, stats.oecd.org/index.aspx?DataSetCode=HEALTH_STAT#, accessed October 10, 2019.

and because of provisions of the ACA. In contrast, young adults are the group most likely to be uninsured: Approximately 13.7% of those ages 19 to 24 are uninsured, as are 14.0% of those ages 25 to 34. Members of racial and ethnic minority groups are more likely to be uninsured than are white Americans: Approximately 9.7% of blacks and 17.8% of Hispanics were uninsured in 2018, compared with 5.4% of non-Hispanic whites.[3] Before the ACA, many of the uninsured were patients with chronic diseases who were closed out of the market because of policies that denied coverage for preexisting conditions. That practice is prohibited by the ACA.

The decade-long effort to repeal or weaken the ACA made by Republicans in the U.S. Congress and, more recently, by the Trump administration has halted the decline in the number of insured. After dramatic reductions in the number of uninsured between 2013 and 2016, the size of the uninsured population increased in both 2017 and 2018.[3,4]

The problem of access to medical care is closely related to the problem of its cost. As monthly premiums have risen in proportion to wages, it has become increasingly expensive for employers, especially small businesses, to provide health insurance for employees and their families. Employers have cut back on their coverage, shifting more of the costs to the employees by requiring them to pay a larger share of the premiums, higher deductibles, and higher copayments. Some low-wage workers may choose to remain uninsured because their share of the premiums is too high—yet these workers earn too much to qualify for Medicaid in most states. In 2014, 77% of the uninsured lived in families that had full-time workers, but were middle-class or lower income.[4]

No other industrialized country has such large numbers of uninsured citizens as the United States. The western European countries, Japan, and Canada have national health plans that virtually guarantee coverage to all citizens. They spend less per capita and devote a smaller percentage of their economies to medical costs.

Lack of insurance clearly leads to poorer outcomes when people are sick. People who are uninsured tend to postpone seeking medical care when they need it, and they may be denied care. If they are sufficiently sick, they may go to an emergency room, which is required by law to treat them, and the cost of their care may be borne by shifting it to other payers, increasing the charges for insured patients. This is certainly not the most effective form of medical care. The uninsured are more likely to be hospitalized for preventable illnesses than are insured patients, and they are less likely to survive a serious illness.[5] A study published in 2009 found that people without health insurance had a 40% higher risk of death than those with private insurance, leading to an extra 45,000 deaths each year.[6]

Although Medicare has ensured that most older adults have access to medical care when they need it, escalating costs have had an impact among this group, too. Each year, the Medicare program pays out more than it collects in premiums, and Congress has repeatedly tried to make adjustments to save the system from bankruptcy. In 2018, 15% of the federal budget went to Medicare, and spending on this program is growing, although more slowly since the passage of the ACA.[7] Attempts to cut costs are politically delicate because older adults are fiercely protective of their entitlements. Because of the overall growth of medical expenses generally, together with requirements for beneficiaries to pay deductibles

and copayments, older adults spent, on average, 14% of their income on out-of-pocket medical expenses in 2012. Most have some form of supplemental insurance plan.[8]

Medicaid, a joint federal–state program, has never worked as well as expected, but since the passage of the ACA, it covers many more poor Americans. The ACA as originally written expanded Medicaid to cover all low-income adults, but a U.S. Supreme Court decision allowed states to opt out of the expansion. Thirty-seven states implemented the expansion: In these states, even childless adults with incomes below a median of 138% of the federal poverty level are eligible for Medicaid.[9] In states that decided not to participate, childless adults are not covered. All but two states cover children in families with incomes at or above 200% of the poverty level with either Medicaid or CHIP. In 33 states, pregnant women with incomes at or above 200% of the poverty level are eligible for Medicaid.[10]

In some states, the fixed fees that Medicaid pays to providers are so low that doctors are unwilling to participate in the program, making it difficult for families that have coverage to find someone to treat them other than poor-quality "Medicaid mills." Even so, the growing costs of Medicaid are placing a strain on many state budgets, using funds that might otherwise be devoted to education or other services. Although almost 85% of Medicaid beneficiaries are children, their parents, and pregnant women, 25% of the spending goes to long-term care for the elderly and disabled.[11,12]

Overall, although the American medical system is the most expensive in the world, it is highly inefficient. The United States spends a higher proportion of its resources on health care than do other countries; at the same time, a significant proportion of the population is denied services, a situation almost unheard of in other countries. Moreover, the health status of the American population fares poorly in international comparisons—evidence that all the spending on medical care cannot compensate for failures in the public health system.

Why Do Costs Keep Rising?

A number of factors are responsible for the high and rising cost of medical care in the United States—some of them common to all industrialized countries, some unique to the American system. The aging of the population, for example, is a problem common to most countries. Because older people generally have a greater need for medical care, aging populations are driving up medical expenditures everywhere. In fact, several other countries have older populations than the United States.

Another factor that increases costs everywhere is the continual development of new medical technology and high-tech procedures. Current instruments such as computed tomography (CT) scanners and magnetic resonance imaging (MRI) devices and newer procedures such as arthroscopic and laparoscopic surgery and cardiac catheterization are expensive. They can be very effective in diagnosing and treating illness, so they are used widely—perhaps too widely. However, these technologies are available in all advanced countries, and it is not clear that they are more widely used in the United States.[13]

When inflationary factors that are unique to the American system are considered, administrative costs are one of the favorite targets of blame. Indeed, a study published in 2019 in the *Journal of the American Medical Association* found administrative complexity, primarily the mounds of billing and reporting paperwork involved, was the largest source of healthcare spending waste. This study found that 25% of American healthcare spending overall—between $760 billion and $935 billion per year—is waste. The authors categorized this waste into six domains: $102–166 billion is due to failure of care delivery, such as patients acquiring infections in the hospital; $27–78 billion is due to failure of care coordination, which includes items such as unnecessary hospital admissions; $76–101 billion is from overtreatment or low-value care; $231–241 billion is pricing failure, primarily overpricing; $59–84 billion is Medicare fraud; and $266 billion is due to the administrative complexity mentioned earlier.[14] In regard to the last domain, because many different insurers pay for medical care, each with its own forms and documentation requirements, the process of billing and paying for care in the United States is much more time consuming and expensive than in countries where the government pays for everything. Moreover, some insurance companies, in trying to control costs, institute additional administrative procedures—for example, requiring doctors to justify the need for certain treatments. This has the paradoxical effect of increasing paperwork and the percentage of effort and expense that goes toward administration. As one eminent health economist lamented: "I look at the U.S. healthcare system and see an administrative monstrosity, a truly bizarre mélange of thousands of payers with payment systems that differ for no socially beneficial reason."[15]

Another peculiarly American characteristic that adds to medical costs is our tendency to sue for **malpractice** when something goes wrong. Doctors complain about the exorbitant price of malpractice insurance, and occasional news stories tell of a multimillion-dollar jury award to an unfortunate patient who was harmed by some medical procedure. Although these costs do not in themselves have a significant overall impact, the fear of malpractice suits may affect a physician's decisions. In particular, some doctors may practice "defensive medicine," ordering more diagnostic tests and medical procedures than necessary, to document in court that they did "everything possible" for the patient.

In fact, studies have shown that the whole system of malpractice compensation is inefficient and unjust. Most patients who are harmed by poor medical treatment are not compensated, and many patients who have suffered a bad outcome sue and win, even when the medical provider was not negligent.[16]

However, because many Americans still lack health insurance, winning a malpractice suit may be the only way an injured patient will be able to pay for treatment of his injury.

One analysis of why medical spending in this country is higher than in other OECD countries found that the United States has higher rates of chronic diseases associated with obesity, including diabetes and heart disease. More than two-thirds of Americans are overweight or obese, far exceeding the prevalence in other countries.[13]

Among the most significant factors driving up medical costs are financial incentives for medical providers. In the "fee-for-service" system of payment, doctors and hospitals are motivated to provide more services so as to increase their income. Moreover, performing surgical procedures and using high-tech diagnostic equipment are more profitable than the more time-consuming practices of talking, listening, observing, and touching.

Along with the growth of new medical technologies has come the growth of specialization among physicians. Fewer than 50% of doctors in the United States work in primary care, which includes family practice, general internal medicine, pediatrics, and obstetrics/gynecology. The majority of American physicians practice more lucrative technological specialties such as radiology, anesthesiology, ophthalmology, cardiology, gastroenterology, and urology. Because of the relatively low pay for primary care providers, many patients looking for an internist or pediatrician may not be able to find one.[17] There is concern that the new healthcare law will exacerbate this problem.

Conspiring with providers in forcing up costs are the expectations of the medical care "consumer"—the patient. Patients with traditional insurance do not have to consider the costs of their care in making decisions on how they should be treated, because the bills are paid by their insurance company. Thus they demand "the best" in technology, treatment by specialists, and prompt service. Economists point out that the medical marketplace is different from classical markets, which are sensitive to the price of goods and services. In the medical marketplace, the seller (the doctor) rather than the buyer (the patient) determines what the buyer needs. Sellers also set the price, and because the bill is paid by a third party (the insurance company), there is no incentive for the buyer to select less expensive options.

Approaches to Controlling Medical Costs

Of the total amount spent on medical care in the United States in 2016, 36% was paid by private health insurance (typically sponsored by employers), 22% was paid by Medicare, and 18% was paid by Medicaid.[1] Thus, both governments and employers have reason to control costs, and they have tried a variety of approaches to achieve that goal. The first cost control effort by the federal government was the imposition of price controls by President Nixon from 1971 to 1974. Although this policy moderated cost increases temporarily, providers adapted to the lower fees paid for each service by increasing the quantity of services. In turn, total spending continued to rise.

Another regulatory approach to cost control focused on limiting spending on new facilities and technology. This is a major strategy used by other OECD countries to control their costs. In the 1970s, the federal and some state governments tried to constrain the supply of hospital beds and high-tech equipment by establishing regional planning agencies that would assess the need for capital expenditures and issue certificates-of-need for new investments. Without limits on budgets, however, state or local governments had few incentives to control these expenditures. Considerable political pressure was also exerted to force approval of new projects. In the 1980s, certificate-of-need programs were gradually abandoned as ineffective.

In the 1980s, the Medicare program tried a different approach to cost control. Because its greatest expenditures were payments to hospitals, the program devised a payment system designed to provide incentives for hospitals to limit the length of hospital stays. Medicare paid a flat fee for each hospital stay—an amount based on the illness category of the patient, or diagnosis-related group (DRG), and the average cost of treating similar patients throughout the country. If a hospital could cure the patient in a shorter time than average, it could keep the extra cash. If a longer stay was necessary, the hospital had to swallow the additional cost. Hospitals, in response, began charging private insurance companies more to make up for their losses from the government. Several states eventually adopted DRG-type rate-setting systems for all payers, forcing hospitals to accept the same rates for everyone. One result of policies limiting payments to hospitals was to move more treatment out of the hospital. Hospital stays are, on average, much shorter now than they were three decades ago, and outpatient surgery and diagnostic testing have become the rule. The DRG system was effective in reducing expenditures for hospital care, but overall costs continued to rise because there was no DRG system for outpatient care.

Managed Care and Beyond

Employer-based private insurance plans have tried a number of approaches to limit costs by bargaining with providers—doctors and hospitals—for discounts on services. The result is a variety of plans that fall under the category of **managed care**. For example, in **preferred provider organizations (PPOs)**, patients are required to seek care from participating providers who have agreed to provide services at lower rates. In some of these plans, patients are not allowed to see a specialist without a referral from a primary care physician, a strategy for limiting access to expensive, high-tech care as well as for ensuring coordination of the care received by the patient from various providers. A variation on the PPO arrangement allows patients to go to nonparticipating providers but requires them to pay a higher percentage of those costs out of their own pockets.

The most stringent form of managed care is the **health maintenance organization (HMO)**, so called because—in theory at least—the organization has a financial incentive to maintain the health of its members. An HMO acts as both insurer and provider. In return for a fixed monthly or annual payment, the HMO agrees to provide all the medical care the individual needs. Conventional HMOs hire a staff of physicians, nurses, and other healthcare workers who earn a salary and thus have no incentive to provide expensive treatments when they are not necessary. Moreover, HMOs have incentives to provide preventive care and health promotion programs, adopting some of the goals and objectives of public health.

Managed care flourished in the 1990s. With the continued rise of medical costs and the failure to enact President Clinton's plan for healthcare reform, employers moved to restrict the choices of their employees to plans that incorporated cost-control measures. In 1995, almost three-quarters of all workers covered by employer-sponsored insurance were in managed care plans.[18] States began to move Medicaid recipients into managed care plans in hopes of providing them with a higher quality of care and more continuity of care, as well as controlling Medicaid costs. The Medicare program also tried to encourage more of its elderly beneficiaries to enroll in managed care plans. The result was a dramatic slowing of medical inflation in the 1990s.[19] However, the slowdown did not last.

With the success of managed care came some major criticism and what was called "the HMO backlash."[20] Patients understood that the financial incentives encouraged denial of treatment, and they were outraged, even when some of the treatments denied were of unproven efficacy. Some for-profit HMOs had especially objectionable practices of giving bonuses to those physicians who were most successful in denying care. Patients also objected to limits on their choice of doctors to consult. News stories told of HMO "gag rules" that forbade physicians from recommending treatments for which the HMO would not approve payment. Many state legislatures passed laws prohibiting gag rules. Similarly, states passed laws regarding "drive-through deliveries" and "drive-through mastectomies" in response to managed care plans that limited hospital stays for women giving birth or having cancer surgery. In 1996 alone, 56 laws were passed in 35 states aimed at regulating or weakening HMOs.[19] The result of such laws, together with some important decisions in federal courts that favored consumers' right to sue HMOs for denial of care, meant that managed care organizations lost much of their ability to manage medical care in a cost-conscious way.[21]

Despite the complaints about managed care, including well-publicized instances of patients being denied expensive procedures that might have saved their lives, there is no evidence that patients are harmed by the cost-control measures overall. In many ways, managed care has an advantage over fee-for-service plans in providing high-quality care. Its emphasis on prevention and health education may indeed help keep members healthy. Coordination of care and use of interdisciplinary teams for disease management can help prevent patients with chronic diseases from developing severe and costly complications. The use of primary care physicians as gatekeepers for controlling patient access to specialists may help prevent unnecessary procedures that could put patients at risk. Managed care organizations, because of their centralized recordkeeping, have the ability to monitor patients' health and to evaluate the quality of care they receive.

The result of the weakening of cost-control methods used by managed care organizations was that medical spending began to grow again in the late 1990s and early 2000s, although at a slower rate. Plans became less restrictive, and PPOs became more popular because they allow more choices. Health insurance, however, became less affordable. More of the costs were shifted to the patients, and the problems of the uninsured grew worse. When fee-for-service reimbursement was the norm, hospitals could charge higher rates to insured patients to cover the costs of treating the uninsured, as they are often required to do by law. However, managed care organizations, even the weaker ones, negotiated reduced payments for treatment of their members, and hospitals were less able to cost-shift, causing financial pain for the hospitals. While some states provided disproportionate-share payments to hospitals to cover bad debt and charity care, antitax sentiment discouraged such public funding for the poor. Private hospitals selected the most profitable patients, and stories of patient "dumping" became common. Public hospitals in inner cities tend to bear the brunt of caring for the sickest uninsured patients, and many cut back on services or threatened to close because of lack of funding.

The passage of the ACA promised to improve the solvency of public hospitals due to the prospect that virtually all patients would be able to pay their bills. Accordingly, states that had provided disproportionate-share payments to safety-net hospitals reduced or stopped these payments. However, because a significant number of people remain uninsured, and because Medicaid payments fall short of the actual costs of patient care, the financial stability of these hospitals remains under threat.[22]

The approach to controlling medical costs called **consumer-directed health plans** is popular among political conservatives and was encouraged during the George W. Bush administration. These plans try to make consumers more cost-conscious when they seek medical care by providing them with information on cost and quality and requiring them to share more of the cost. The plans tend to have high **deductibles**, so that insurance payments do not kick in until after patients have paid for a significant amount of services, and they tend to be combined with **health savings accounts**, in which individuals set aside funds tax-free to be used for paying medical expenses. A number of drawbacks have been noted with these plans, including that they are most likely to be used as a tax haven for healthy and wealthy individuals. Another difficulty is that they motivate people to avoid, skip, or delay health care because of costs, sometimes leading to more serious disease and increased risk of needing hospitalization.[23]

The Patient Protection and Affordable Care Act

In 2010, President Obama persuaded Congress to pass a **healthcare reform** law, colloquially known as "Obamacare," aimed at addressing many of the problems with the American medical care system. A key component of the law was the individual mandate, a requirement that all Americans have health insurance or pay a fine. Many employees of large businesses already receive insurance through their employers. The law did not require employers to provide insurance, but any business with 50 or more workers that did not provide coverage was required to pay an assessment of $2000 per employee. Small businesses received tax credits to provide insurance to their workers.[24]

The ACA required states to have affordable **insurance exchanges**, whereby individuals can shop for a plan that meets their needs. As of 2018, 11 states and the District of Columbia had established their own exchanges. The other states rely to varying extents on the federal government to run their exchanges.[25] The law also included a requirement to expand Medicaid, which had different eligibility rules in different states, to cover low-income adults.

Some other provisions of the ACA have proved popular, including an expansion of coverage for young adults on their parents' plan up to age 26. Medicare now provides older adults with preventive benefits including a yearly wellness visit and a range of no-cost screenings for cancer, diabetes, and other chronic diseases. Among the preventive services required by the law is contraception, a provision that has proved controversial. Seniors benefit from savings in the Medicare prescription drug plan. A number of insurance company abuses, such as cancellation of policies of patients when their medical costs rise, are outlawed by the new law.[23] The ACA also established a Center for Medicare and Medicaid Innovation to begin testing new ways of delivering care aimed at improving quality of care and reducing the rate of growth in costs for Medicare, Medicaid, and the Children's Health Insurance Program.

The ACA was scheduled to be fully implemented by the beginning of 2015, but the constitutionality of the law was challenged in court by 26 states, with the individual mandate being the most hotly contested issue. The Supreme Court largely upheld the law in 2012. Chief Justice John Roberts, generally a conservative, cast the decisive vote in favor of the ACA, ruling that the fine for not having insurance amounted to a tax, which the government has the power to impose. However, the Court's decision restricted the expansion of Medicaid, allowing some states to not expand eligibility.[26] Another Republican challenge in 2015 questioned subsidies for people buying insurance through exchanges that were run by the federal government, based on a phrase in the law that provided for subsidies when people buy insurance on "an exchange established by the states." The Supreme Court again upheld the ACA.[27] These decisions, together with the reelection of President Obama in 2012, ensured that the reform of the medical care system would survive. However, the fact that 17 states have chosen not to expand Medicaid eligibility has left a still significant proportion of Americans without health insurance. As of the beginning of 2018, the uninsured rate was 8.5%.[3]

The Trump administration and congressional Republicans have done whatever they could to further damage the ACA. In 2017, they eliminated subsidies for low-income individuals and families who bought policies on the exchanges. Also in 2017, Congress passed a major tax reform law that abolished the individual mandate. Without a mandate, younger, healthier people are less likely to buy insurance, driving up premiums for everyone else.[28]

Rationing

In the late 1980s, the state of Oregon tried an experiment. Realizing that its Medicaid budget was not large enough to provide comprehensive coverage for all of its poor citizens, the state legislature undertook a plan to spread its resources over a larger number of people by limiting the services for which it would pay. Its first move was highly controversial: It decided not to pay for organ transplants, with the justification that the funds required for 34 transplants could provide for prenatal care and delivery for 1500 pregnant women.[29] When a young boy with acute leukemia was denied a bone-marrow transplant and died as a result, a national uproar ensued.

The legislature, led by John Kitzhaber, a physician who was then president of the state senate and later became governor, decided to develop a more acceptable policy for broadening Medicaid eligibility. The new approach focused on life-saving treatments for serious conditions and tried to eliminate less effective therapies for less serious conditions. The state decided to develop a prioritized list of health services and draw a line below which treatments would not be covered. The goal was to cover all citizens whose incomes were below the poverty level, and to use managed care plans to provide medical care.

A commission was formed to develop the list by consulting as much as possible with the citizens of the state. Public hearings and town meetings were held to determine the relative value placed on various medical services by the public. The commission established 17 categories of health problems according to 13 criteria, including life expectancy, quality of life, the cost-effectiveness of a treatment, and the probable number of people who would benefit. The highest priority was placed on acute problems that could be fatal and for which treatment would provide full recovery. Maternity care and preventive care for children are examples of high-priority services. At the bottom of the list were treatments known to be ineffective, or those that did not improve quality of life or extend life, including some treatments for cancer and acquired immunodeficiency syndrome (AIDS).[30]

The Oregon plan provoked opposition on legal, social, and ethical grounds. In 1991, the Department of Health and Human Services denied permission for Oregon to implement the plan on the basis that it violated the Americans with Disabilities Act, because the list undervalued the quality of life of people with disabilities. After some revisions, the plan was finally approved by the Clinton administration in 1993. More than 100,000 Oregonians were added to the Medicaid program as a result.[30]

Many critics have pointed out that Oregon's policy would be more equitable and that the decisions would be much less difficult if everyone—not just the poor—were included in the **rationing** proposal. The U.S. medical system as a whole is rich enough to provide necessary care for everyone; the need to ration care for the poor is a consequence of failures of the system to provide adequate and affordable care for everyone. Health policy experts have praised the Oregon plan's focus on medical necessity so that all appropriate care and no inappropriate care is covered. In addition, the plan called attention to the need for more research on outcomes of various treatments to permit better-informed decisions on medical necessity.

However, the Oregon plan struggled and eventually collapsed. In part, its difficulties stemmed from an attempt in 2002 to expand it further to include additional uninsured residents, which happened at a time when the state was experiencing an economic downturn. Oregonians, as residents of other states have done, resisted increasing taxes to finance the program. In part, the program faltered because Governor Kitzhaber was term limited, and his successor was not such an enthusiastic defender of the plan. Also, in Oregon, as in the rest of the country, medical care costs began growing faster than the general economy, making the provision of health care for all economically and politically increasingly more difficult to achieve.[31]

The Oregon experiment made many people uncomfortable. People do not like to confront the idea that rationing medical care might be necessary or desirable. In reality, rationing medical care has been going on all along: Care has been rationed on the basis of ability to pay, but the rationing has not been explicitly admitted. When a story hits the news about an uninsured child denied treatment for leukemia, for example, the public and politicians purport to be shocked that such a thing could happen in our society. Yet it is politically impossible to raise taxes so that such children could be provided with medical insurance or that public hospitals could afford to provide effective care.

Our society has never been willing to discuss trade-offs between costs and quality of medical care.[31] Because third parties—usually the government or insurance companies—pay for care, people have come to believe that cost should not be considered when making decisions about medical treatments. When asked about a particular patient or situation, people will say that no effort should be spared in trying to achieve the best possible outcome. It is an easy thing to say when they are not paying the bills. At the same time, people naturally seek out insurance plans with the lowest premiums. It is a Catch-22 situation: Society demands that the healthcare system maximize quality while minimizing costs, but it has placed a taboo on the consideration of cost.[32]

Rationing is a dirty word when it applies to medical care—but rationing is inevitable. In economics, "rationing is simply the process of allocating goods in the face of scarcity."[33] Since most people are unwilling to pay an unlimited amount of money to receive a small benefit, decisions are continually being made about the allocation of medical services. What is needed is an open discussion of how those decisions should be made. Should kidney dialysis be denied to the elderly or to people with diabetes so advanced that they have lost their vision? Should we tolerate long waiting lists for hip replacements? Should the rich receive care and the poor be denied it? Should we allow for-profit healthcare systems to make large profits for their stockholders while refusing to care for patients with expensive chronic diseases?[34] These are difficult questions for medicine and for public health, but we need to openly discuss them and decide the appropriate answers on a societal basis.

Conclusion

The U.S. medical care system is the most expensive in the world. At the same time, it has many faults, including lack of access for the uninsured, who made up approximately 16% of the American population before the ACA's implementation. Medical care costs have risen continuously, and the rising costs contribute to the inability of many to afford health insurance.

Many factors are driving the high and rising costs. An aging population needs more medical care; expensive new medical technologies are regularly developed and widely used; administrative costs are high in the United States; malpractice suits lead to defensive medicine; insured patients are shielded from consideration of costs; and financial incentives often favor overtreatment.

A number of attempts to impose cost-containment measures on medical care have been relatively unsuccessful in controlling costs. Managed care slowed the growth in healthcare costs in the 1990s and consequently became the dominant form of employer-sponsored health insurance. Managed care organizations negotiate reduced payments to healthcare providers and employ various strategies to limit patients' access to treatments considered non-essential or too expensive given the expected benefit. Despite its successes, managed care has been unpopular with the public, and it has not improved access for the uninsured. Because of its unpopularity, managed care has suffered legislative and legal setbacks that have weakened its ability to control costs. Medical care expenditures have resumed their escalation, and it is not clear how the nation can pay for medical care in the future.

Many health policy makers believe that some form of rationing will ultimately be necessary to ensure access to high-quality medical care for the whole population. They point out that care is already rationed by cost. In Oregon, the Medicaid program, using an explicit method of ranking various treatments and cutting off access to lower-priority procedures, significantly expanded the number of people covered by the plan; ultimately, however, the plan faltered due to rising costs and state economic setbacks. Discussion of rationing remains largely taboo in the current political climate, but if the problems of the U.S. healthcare system continue to grow, Americans may be forced to consider cost and fairness when making decisions about medical care.

President Obama prioritized efforts to reform the American healthcare system, and in 2010 he succeeded in persuading Congress to pass a plan that would provide health insurance to more of the population and, it is hoped, help control costs. The law was challenged by a number of states, but was substantially upheld by the Supreme Court. The ACA took full effect at the beginning of 2015 and has significantly reduced the number of uninsured Americans.

References

1. Centers for Disease Control and Prevention, "Health, United States, 2017," 2018, Table 93, https://www.cdc.gov/nchs/data/hus/2017/093.pdf, accessed October 8, 2019.

2. Organization for Economic Cooperation and Development, "Health Expenditure and Financing," https://stats.oecd.org/index.aspx?DataSetCode=HEALTH_STAT, accessed October 10, 2019.

3. E. R. Berchick, J. C. Barnett, and R. D. Upton, "Health Insurance Coverage in the United States: 2018," *Current Population Reports*, U.S. Census Bureau, September 2019, https://www.census.gov/content/dam/Census/library/publications/2019/demo/p60-267.pdf, accessed October 9, 2019.

4. Kaiser Family Foundation, "Key Facts About the Uninsured Population," December 7, 2018, https://www.kff.org/uninsured/fact-sheet/key-facts-about-the-uninsured-population/, accessed October 9, 2019.

5. Institute of Medicine, *America's Uninsured Crisis: Consequences for Health and Health Care* (Washington, DC: National Academies Press, 2009).

6. A. P. Wilper, S. Woolhandler, K. E. Lasser, D. McCormick, D. H. Bor, and D. U. Himmelstein, "Health Insurance and Mortality in U.S. Adults," *American Journal of Public Health* 99 (2009): 2289–2295.

7. Kaiser Family Foundation, "The Facts on Medicare Spending and Financing," August 20, 2019, https://www.kff.org/medicare/issue-brief/the-facts-on-medicare-spending-and-financing/, accessed October 10, 2019.

8. Kaiser Family Foundation, "Health Care on a Budget: The Financial Burden of Health Spending by Medicare Households," January 9, 2014, https://www.kff.org/medicare/issue-brief/health-care-on-a-budget-the-financial-burden-of-health-spending-by-medicare-households/, accessed October 10, 2019.

9. Kaiser Family Foundation, "10 Things to Know About Medicaid: Setting the Facts Straight," March 6, 2019, https://www.kff.org/medicaid/issue-brief/10-things-to-know-about-medicaid-setting-the-facts-straight/, accessed October 10, 2019.

10. Kaiser Family Foundation, "Modern Era Medicaid: Findings from a 50-State Survey of Eligibility, Enrollment, Renewal, and Cost-Sharing Policies in Medicaid and CHIP as of January 2015," https://www.kff.org/health-reform/report/modern-era-medicaid-findings-from-a-50-state-survey-of-eligibility-enrollment-renewal-and-cost-sharing-policies-in-medicaid-and-chip-as-of-january-2015, accessed October 11, 2019.

11. Medicaid.gov, "What are Annual Expenditures for Medicaid & CHIP?", https://www.medicaid.gov/state-overviews/scorecard/national-context/annual-expenditures/index.html, accessed October 11, 2019.

12. Kaiser Family Foundation, "Distribution of Medicaid Spending by Service," 2014, https://www.kff.org/state-category/medicaid-chip/medicaid-spending/, accessed October 10, 2019.

13. G. F. Anderson, B. K. Frogner, and U. E. Reinhardt, "Health Spending in OECD Countries: An Update," *Health Affairs* 26 (2007): 1481–1489.

14. W. H. Shrank, T. L. Rogstad, and N. Parekh, "Waste in the US Health Care System: Estimated Costs and Potential for Savings," *Journal of the American Medical Association* 322 (2019): 1501–1509.

15. H. J. Aaron, "Costs of Health Care Administration in the United States and Canada: Questionable Answers to a Questionable Question," *New England Journal of Medicine* 349 (2003): 801–803.

16. T. A. Brennan, C. M. Sox, and H. R. Burstin, "Relation Between Negligent Adverse Events and the Outcomes of Medical-Malpractice Litigation," *New England Journal of Medicine* 335 (1996): 1963–1967.

17. L. G. Sandy, T. Bodenheimer, L. G. Pawlson, and B. Starfield, "The Political Economy of U.S. Primary Care," *Health Affairs* 28 (2009): 1136–1144.

18. G. A. Jensen, M. A. Morrissey, S. Gaffney, and D. K. Liston, "The New Dominance of Managed Care: Insurance Trends in the 1990s," *Health Affairs* 16 (1997): 125–136.

19. A. B. Martin, D. Lassman, B. Washington, A. Catlin; National Health Expenditure Accounts Team, "Growth in U.S. Health Spending Remained Slow in 2010: Health Share of Gross Domestic Product Was Unchanged from 2009," *Health Affairs* 31 (2012): 208–219.

20. T. Bodenheimer, "The HMO Backlash: Righteous or Reactionary?" *New England Journal of Medicine* 335 (1996): 1601–1604.

21. M. G. Bloche and K. M. Studdert, "A Quiet Revolution: Law as an Agent of Health System Change," *Health Affairs* (March/April 2004): 29–42.

22. K. Neuhausen, A. C. Davis, J. Needleman, R. H. Brook, D. Zingmond, and D. H. Roby, "Disproportionate-Share Hospital Payment Reductions May Threaten the Financial Stability of Safety-Net Hospitals," *Health Affairs* 33 (2014): 988–996.

23. A. Dixon, J. Greene, and J. Hibbard, "Do Consumer-Directed Health Plans Drive Change in Enrollees' Health Care Behavior?", *Health Affairs* 27 (2008): 1120–1131.

24. U.S. Department of Health & Human Services, "About the Law," https://www.hhs.gov/healthcare/rights/index.html, accessed October 10, 2019.

25. Kaiser Family Foundation, "State Health Insurance Marketplace Types, 2018," https://www.kff.org/health-reform/slide/state-decisions-for-creating-health-insurance-exchanges/, accessed October 10, 2019.

26. A. Liptak, "Supreme Court Upholds Health Care Law, 5–4, in Victory for Obama," *The New York Times*, June 28, 2012.

27. A. Liptak, "Supreme Court Allows Nationwide Health Care Subsidies," *The New York Times*, June 25, 2015.

28. B. Casselman, M. Sanger-Katz, and J. Smialek, "Share of Americans with Health Insurance Declined in 2018," *The New York Times*, September 10, 2019.

29. R. M. Kaplan, *The Hippocratic Predicament: Affordability, Access, and Accountability in American Medicine* (San Diego, CA: Academic Press, 1993).

30. T. Bodenheimer, "The Oregon Health Plan: Lessons for the Nation," *New England Journal of Medicine* 337 (1997): 651–655.

31. J. Oberlander, "Health Reform Interrupted: The Unraveling of the Oregon Health Plan," *Health Affairs* 26 (2007): w96–w105.

32. D. M. Eddy, "Balancing Cost and Quality in Fee-for-Service Versus Managed Care," *Health Affairs* 16 (1997): 162–173.

33. D. A. Asch and P. A. Ubel, "Rationing by Any Other Name," *New England Journal of Medicine* 336 (1997): 1668–1671.

34. J. P. Kassirer, "Our Endangered Integrity: It Can Only Get Worse," *New England Journal of Medicine* 336 (1997): 1666–1667.

CHAPTER 28

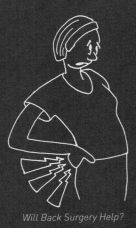
Health Services Research: Finding What Works

KEY TERMS

Agency for Healthcare Research
and Quality (AHRQ)
Health services research

National Committee for Quality
Assurance (NCQA)
Outcomes research

Small-area analysis
Variations in medical practice

In the late 1960s and early 1970s, the medical establishment was shaken by a number of reports that documented wide variations in the way physicians treated their patients for common health problems. One study found that in Morrisville, Vermont, nearly 70% of the children had their tonsils removed by the time they were 15 years old, whereas in nearby Middlebury, only 8% of children underwent the operation. Another study in Iowa reported that more than 60% of the male population of one community had their prostate glands removed by age 85, whereas the rate was only 15% in another area. Similarly, the rates at which women underwent hysterectomy varied from 20% in one part of Maine to 70% in a city less than 20 miles away.[1]

The reasons for these differences were unclear. The populations of the comparison communities were not substantially different from one another, and there was no reason to believe that the residents of one community were sicker than those of another or that their insurance coverage was more comprehensive. It seemed obvious that these procedures were being overused in some geographic areas or underused in others. However, the studies could not determine which is the case or decide what the appropriate use rates should be.

This method of examining how medical practice varies across geographic areas, known as **small-area analysis**, has been applied over the past several decades to a broad range of medical practices and procedures. Repeatedly, wide variations have been found, with no apparent reason for the differences in practice. Beginning in 1996, Dr. John Wennberg, a professor at Dartmouth Medical School and a pioneer in the field, who had conducted the studies in Vermont, Maine, and Iowa along with his colleagues, began publishing the *Dartmouth Atlas of Health Care* series, which examines Medicare and Medicaid data.[2] (Since the Medicare and Medicaid programs maintain files on everything they pay for, including services to virtually all Americans 65 and older, they provide valuable data for this kind of research.) All over the country, variations occur in treatments for prostate cancer, breast cancer, heart disease, and many other common conditions.

For example, a 2015 *Dartmouth Atlas* report found that for the years 2007 to 2011, the rates of bariatric surgery to treat obesity were 9 per 100,000 Medicare beneficiaries in Winston-Salem, North Carolina, but 75 per 100,000 in Great Falls, Montana, even though Great Falls had significantly lower obesity and diabetes rates.[3] A 2019 *Dartmouth Atlas* report found enormous variation in neonatal intensive care unit (NICU) use across the country. NICUs offer life-saving treatment for many seriously ill newborns; while once relatively rare, they are now common in hospitals. The study found that nearly half of newborns admitted to NICUs now have a normal weight and often may not need such intensive and expensive care. In fact, this care can do more harm than good because the newborns are separated from their natural post-birth connection with their mothers and are exposed to prolonged bright light and noise. Yet 15% of very-low-birth-weight babies (those less than 3.3 pounds), who would typically rely on such care, do not receive high-level NICU treatment. As examples of the regional variations, normal-birth-weight babies were admitted into the NICU at a rate of 1.6% in Richmond, Virginia, and 1.7% in Laredo, Texas, but 8.9% in El Paso, Texas, and 9.2% in Newark, Delaware. The study's principal author concluded that "newborn and NICU care varied markedly across regions and hospitals. Little of the variation was explained by differences in newborn health needs."[4,5]

Small-area analysis called attention to the lack of scientific evidence on which doctors and patients base decisions about how various medical conditions should be treated. The surprising results of the early studies were part of a new field of research—**health services research**. This research attempts to understand the reasons for the observed variations in medical practice and to determine, from observations of the everyday practice of medicine, what treatments lead to the most desirable outcomes. Health services research studies the effectiveness, efficiency, and equity of the healthcare system. It is a way of trying to assess the quality of medical care, but may also lead to insights on how to control costs and improve access.

Reasons for Practice Variations

A number of explanations have been suggested for **variations in medical practice**, most of which can be tested, and most of which can be shown to play a role in the observed differences. It is clear that the variability in the use of specific treatments reflects the degree of uncertainty facing physicians regarding their relative efficacy. Variations in practice are far greater for some medical conditions than for others. For example, most physicians agree that surgery is the appropriate treatment for a broken hip. Correspondingly, the geographic variability in the treatment of this condition is much smaller than the variability in the surgery rates for tonsillitis and disorders of the uterus, for which there is much less evidence about when surgery is needed.

In many cases, doctors are unaware that their way of treating a condition is unusual, and they will change their patterns of practice when presented with evidence that they are deviating from the norm. In the early 1970s, Wennberg confronted the physicians of Morrisville, Vermont, with data showing that they were doing tonsillectomies far more frequently than other doctors in the state. The Morrisville physicians reconsidered the indications for the procedure, instituted a policy of obtaining second opinions before deciding on surgery, and ended by reducing the tonsillectomy rate to less than 10% of what it had been.[1] Similarly in 2009, Atul Gawande published an exposé on the very high rate of healthcare spending in McAllen, Texas. Medicare patients there were receiving 40% more surgeries, almost twice the number of heart tests, and more than twice as many pacemakers, cardiac bypass operations, and other treatments compared with similar patients in nearby El Paso, Texas. In the years that followed, after some local introspection and a bit of outside pressure, the medical community in McAllen was able to reduce the amount of government-funded healthcare spending by as much as half a billion dollars by 2015.[6]

It is easy to suspect that inappropriate use of tests and procedures is responsible for the observed variations in the frequency with which they are done. While this suspicion is supported by the Vermont experience in reducing tonsillectomy rates and for some of the excessive spending in McAllen, Texas, other studies have found that inappropriate use explains only a small part of the wide variability observed for many procedures.

In one small-area study of three procedures commonly done on Medicare patients, panels of expert physicians examined the files of a random sample of patients who had undergone each procedure. The experts compared the indications for the procedure in a high-use area with those in a low-use area. They were asked to determine, for each patient, whether the decision to do the procedure was appropriate, equivocal, or inappropriate. Coronary angiography—used to identify blockages in the blood vessels of the heart—was performed more than twice as frequently in the high-use area as in the low-use area. Yet even in the high-use area, the experts considered it inappropriate in only one-sixth of the cases. Carotid endarterectomy (CEA), which had an

almost fourfold variation in frequency, was the procedure most often judged inappropriate. A risky procedure intended to remove blockages in the arteries that carry blood to the brain, CEA was deemed inappropriate in approximately one-third of the cases done in the high-use area. However, the procedure was considered by the experts to be inappropriate almost as frequently in the low-use area.[7]

This evidence suggests that, for many medical conditions, more than one response may be appropriate. When faced with a patient suffering from a specific illness, one physician may prefer conservative treatment using drugs and "watchful waiting," whereas another physician may believe that immediate surgery is indicated. These opinions tend to be shared by the physicians within a community. Wennberg has called these differences the "practice style" factor. For most of the conditions in question, there was not enough scientific evidence to determine which treatment yields a better outcome for the patient. In many cases, the choice of treatment involves weighing benefits against risks, a trade-off that different patients might evaluate differently if they are given the opportunity to choose.

The high variability and frequent inappropriate use of CEA, together with the high risks associated with this procedure, inspired several large randomized controlled trials, involving more than 10,000 patients, to clarify the indications for and efficacy of CEA. The trials demonstrated that, among carefully selected patients and surgeons, the procedure reduced the risk of stroke and death compared with medical therapy alone. In a later analysis to determine whether the evidence provided by the trials changed medical practice, researchers in New York State conducted a cohort study of all Medicare patients who had a CEA over an 18-month period in 1998 and 1999. The results showed a great improvement over the earlier study: Overall 87.1% of the procedures had been done for appropriate reasons; 4.3% had been done for uncertain reasons; and 8.6% had been done for inappropriate reasons.[8]

As for coronary angiography, another procedure studied earlier, no such randomized trials have been performed to determine its appropriateness. It remains a high-variability procedure: A recent study comparing rates in different states found a 53% higher rate of coronary angiography in Florida than in Colorado. The rate depended in part on the density of specialists in the area.[9]

The Field of Dreams Effect

One factor that has consistently been shown to influence practice styles is the availability of services in a community, as shown in the rates of coronary angiography discussed earlier. For example, the presence of a greater number of surgeons is accompanied by the performance of a larger number of surgeries. This effect was dramatically illustrated in Maine during the early 1980s, when two neurosurgeons moved to a community and devoted themselves to performing laminectomies—disc surgery for low back pain. The number of laminectomies for the whole state nearly doubled as a result of the work of these two surgeons, although only 20% of the population of Maine lived in that community and the adjacent referral area.[10] This high rate of surgery, like the tonsillectomies in Vermont, was reduced after the surgeons were confronted with data on practice patterns in other communities.

Research has consistently demonstrated an influence of supply on usage when hospital beds are concerned. A study done in the 1980s comparing Boston, Massachusetts, with New Haven, Connecticut, found that Boston had 4.5 hospital beds per thousand people, whereas New Haven had only 2.9 beds per thousand, even though mortality rates and other measures of quality of care were almost the same in the two cities. Approximately the same percentage of beds was filled in the two cities, meaning that the population of Boston was hospitalized at a higher rate than that

of New Haven. When Wennberg and his colleagues interviewed physicians in the two cities, they found that New Haven doctors were not purposely trying to ration care and that neither group of doctors knew that they hospitalized patients more or less frequently than average.[10]

The Dartmouth researchers' analysis of Medicare data found that the number of hospital beds in a community significantly influences the kind of care received by dying elderly people.[11] Medicare patients in New York City; Newark, New Jersey; and Memphis, Tennessee, are much more likely to spend their final days in a hospital, often in an intensive care unit, than are elderly patients in Portland, Oregon, or Salt Lake City, Utah, who are more likely to die at home. Based on 1994 and 1995 data, the rates at which Medicare patients die in the hospital correlate closely with the number of hospital beds per thousand residents in their community. Researchers call this correlation the "Field of Dreams Effect," after the line in the 1989 movie about a baseball field: "If you build it, they will come."

While there is little evidence to show that patients are helped or harmed by the more intensive care they receive in Boston, Memphis, and other high-use areas of the country, such differences in use have a major impact on medical care costs. For example, the average hospital bill for each Medicare enrollee's final six months of life was $16,571 in the New York City borough of Manhattan, as opposed to an average of only $6793 in Portland, Oregon.[11] In the Boston–New Haven comparative study, Boston's per capita hospital expenditures were about double those of New Haven.[12]

Wennberg does not specifically argue that conflict of interest or pecuniary motives enter into decisions that determine use rates of medical services. However, many studies suggest that financial considerations may influence some physicians' medical decision making. For example, evidence indicates that when physicians stand to profit from the performance of diagnostic tests, they are much more likely to order such tests. Until the practice was outlawed by Congress, physicians who owned an interest in clinical laboratories were more likely to refer patients for laboratory tests compared to similar physicians who referred patients to labs in which they had no financial interest.[13] Similarly, physicians who own diagnostic imaging equipment are more likely to use it than are comparable physicians who must refer patients elsewhere for such examinations. Physicians in Japan, who are legally permitted to sell prescription drugs directly to patients (unlike in the United States), appear to favor higher-profit drugs.[14,15] A recent surge in complex spinal-fusion operations has been linked to the high rates that Medicare pays to surgeons and hospitals for these surgeries, although there is no evidence that the procedure is more effective at curing back pain than laminectomy or even less invasive approaches.[16]

Outcomes Research

As we have seen, variations in medical care are greatest for medical conditions for which the least is known about the effectiveness and appropriateness of various diagnostic and treatment approaches. To resolve the uncertainties raised by small-area analysis, the best approach is to study outcomes of these various diagnostic and treatment approaches to determine what works. Many policy makers believe that such research will allow the development of guidelines for medical practice, leading not only to more effective medical care but also to cost savings through the elimination of unnecessary care.

The epidemiologic study of medical care is called **outcomes research**. Whereas epidemiology usually examines the disease-causing effects of exposure to agents such as viruses and toxic chemicals, outcomes research examines the health effects of exposure to medical interventions. Controlled clinical trials are one form of outcomes research, but practical, financial, and ethical barriers prevent researchers from conducting controlled trials aimed at answering many important questions about medical care. Outcomes research collects and analyzes data generated by the everyday practice of medicine in an effort to reach conclusions on benefits and risks of various interventions for various types of patients.

One of the early questions examined by John Wennberg's group dealt with prostatectomy, the surgical removal of men's prostate glands. It was a high-variation procedure: In some parts of Maine, 60% of the men had their prostates removed by age 80; in other parts, fewer than 20% underwent this surgery.[17] The procedure is used as a treatment for cancer of the prostate and for benign prostatic hyperplasia (BPH), a common condition in older men that causes difficulties with urination. Other treatments are available for both conditions, including watchful waiting, as many cases of prostate cancer never progress to become life threatening. In patients with BPH, proponents of the surgical procedure argued, it could reduce symptoms and improve the quality of men's lives. Skeptics pointed out that surgery often has unwelcome side effects.

Wennberg and his colleagues conducted a major analysis of Medicare records to determine outcomes of surgery for BPH. They found that published reports significantly overstated the benefits of prostatectomy and understated the complications. Although only approximately 1% of men undergoing this procedure died in the hospital, 2% to 5% of the patients died in the weeks following the surgery. Moreover, within four years of the surgery, almost half of the patients required further treatment for urinary tract problems. After eight years, about one in five needed a second prostatectomy.[10] Having the surgery did not increase life expectancy, and the effect on quality of life was mixed: It improved urinary tract symptoms, but had a negative impact on sexual function.[17]

The results of these studies indicate a need for better informing patients about their choices and about the probable outcomes of each choice.[18] Feelings about symptoms, willingness to accept risks of the surgery, and personal assessment of the possible outcomes vary substantially among individuals. Outcomes research should enable these patients to make informed decisions based on their own values. Effective drug therapies have been developed for BPH, and the number of surgeries performed for this condition declined in the 1990s, perhaps due in part to evidence contributed by outcomes research.[19]

The number of prostatectomies for cancer has increased, however, due in part to the development of a new screening method that became widely used in the 1990s. This test measures prostate-specific antigen (PSA) in the blood, levels of which have been correlated with the presence of cancer. However, low-grade prostate cancer is very common in older men, and many cases never progress to cause a problem. The follow-up testing and treatment of men whose PSA levels are elevated is invasive and may have undesirable side effects. The problem with the use of PSA screening is that no evidence shows that it reduces mortality from prostate cancer.

In a study conducted by the Dartmouth researchers, Medicare data were used to compare two cohorts of men who lived in areas with different practice patterns for screening and treatment. In the Seattle–Puget Sound area, men were tested at a rate 5.4 times the rate in Connecticut. The researchers found that more than twice as many men in the Seattle area, compared with Connecticut men, were subjected to biopsies of the prostate to confirm the presence of cancer. The Seattle area men were more than five times more likely to have a prostatectomy than were the Connecticut men. However, after 11 years of follow-up, there was no significant difference in the mortality rates from prostate cancer between the two groups of men.[20] This finding was confirmed in 2009 with the publication of results from two clinical trials that followed a total of 259,000 men in the United States and Europe for 7 to 10 years. In both trials, men were randomly assigned to groups with and

without PSA screening, and there was little difference in mortality between the two groups.[21]

In 2011, the U.S. Preventive Services Task Force, an independent panel of experts appointed and funded by the Agency for Healthcare Research and Quality, reviewed the findings from these trials as well as other studies and recommended against routine PSA screening. Similarly, a 2014 *Dartmouth Atlas of Health Care Series* review of the evidence concluded that PSA screening results in, at best, only a small reduction in mortality from the disease and is associated with unnecessary harms.[22,23] The problem with finding prostate cancers through screening is that there is no good way to determine which ones are likely to progress rapidly and cause harm and which are indolent and can be left alone.

Inspired in part by Wennberg's work, Congress in 1989 established the federal Agency for Healthcare Policy and Research (AHCPR), hoping that studies such as those on BPH would encourage a reduction in use of high-technology medicine and save money on medical costs, especially for Medicare and Medicaid. The agency was mandated to examine the reasons for the wide variations in healthcare practices around the country, develop guidelines for treatment, and find effective ways to disseminate its research findings and guidelines.[24] However, the agency—and Congress—discovered to their surprise that the research results were not always welcome.

One health condition that the AHCPR tackled early was low back pain. It is a widespread problem, ranking second only to the common cold as a reason that people go to the doctor. Treatment of back and neck problems cost more than $80 billion in the United States in 2011.[3] Surgery for low back pain is a high-variability procedure, ranging from a low in the Northeast to a rate in the Northwest that is more than three times higher. The guidelines developed by AHCPR's panel of experts and released in December 1994 recommended treating most acute, painful low back problems with nonprescription painkillers and mild exercise, followed in about two weeks by conditioning exercises. Surgery benefits only about 1 in 200 people with acute low back problems, according to the chairman of the panel, a professor of orthopedic surgery at the University of Washington School of Medicine.[25]

Back surgeons responded with both rage and political action. With the Republican Congress intent on budget cutting in 1995, legislators were sympathetic to claims by the back surgeons' lobbying group that AHCPR was a waste of money, that the government should not be telling doctors how to practice medicine, and that the agency should be eliminated.[26] Defenders of the AHCPR pointed out that the guidelines could save billions of dollars and accused back surgeons of merely trying to protect their incomes. When the federal budget was finally approved that year, AHCPR had survived, although its budget was cut substantially. Its leaders decided that developing clinical guidelines was too dangerous politically, but the agency continued collecting evidence that allowed other organizations to do so, and it maintains a national clearinghouse of evidence-based clinical guidelines developed by other organizations. A new emphasis was placed on quality of care and patient safety, and the agency's name was changed to the **Agency for Healthcare Research and Quality (AHRQ)**. Four years after its "near-death experience," AHRQ had regained all the funding it lost, and the agency's budget held roughly steady at more than twice this original level through 2019 (after accounting for inflation).[27,28] Wennberg has argued for an expanded role for AHRQ, noting that outcomes research has the potential to restrain wasteful spending and could help control costs.[12]

In fact, the federal government is increasingly interested in supporting comparative effectiveness research to evaluate the efficacy of competing drugs and to compare the effectiveness of different treatment options. For example, the American Recovery and Reinvestment Act of 2009 allocated $1.1 billion to the AHRQ, the National Institutes of Health, and the U.S. Department of Health and Human Services to conduct such research, and also provided funds to the Institute of Medicine to recommend priorities for spending the money.[29] The Patient Protection and Affordable Care Act of 2010 included the establishment of a Patient-Centered Outcomes Research Institute aimed at helping patients make better-informed healthcare decisions.

As for treatment of low back pain, surgery rates in the Medicare population increased by 220% between 1988 and 2001, though the rates varied dramatically across geographic areas.[30] To determine what an appropriate rate might be, a prospective study was conducted in Maine, where surgery rates were four times higher in some areas than in others. The researchers followed all patients who had surgery to see whether their symptoms improved after the operation. They found that the best outcomes occurred in the areas where the rates were lowest; conversely, the worst outcomes occurred in the areas with the highest rates. The evidence suggested that surgeons in the low-use area used more stringent criteria for recommending surgery. In these areas, patients with more severe disease were more likely to benefit, and those with less severe disease avoided the risks of surgery, which are significant. The authors concluded: "Outcomes research has the potential to provide information that will enable each patient to better understand the outcomes, risks and benefits of an operation and other treatment."[31(p.761)] Unfortunately, these findings do not seem to have reduced the number of back surgeries. Two Dartmouth researchers found in 2017 that the rate of back surgeries had increased by 28% since 2006, and that the large regional variation persists.[32]

Quality

The AHCPR drama came at a time when there had been a series of highly publicized medical errors. A 39-year-old health reporter for the

Boston Globe died after receiving an overdose of a chemotherapy drug while being treated for breast cancer at one of the most prestigious hospitals in the country. A 51-year-old diabetic man had the wrong leg amputated in a Florida hospital. In another Florida hospital, an 8-year-old boy died due to a drug mix-up during minor surgery.

A number of studies were published in the 1990s documenting that preventable medical errors occurred in 1.5% to 2% of hospitalizations, and that many of these errors caused the patient's death. The Institute of Medicine (IOM) was asked to investigate the issue and recommend a strategy that would lead to improvements in quality of care. Its study led to the publication in 1999 of a landmark report, *To Err Is Human: Building a Safer Health System.*[33] The report estimated that 44,000 to 98,000 deaths per year in the United States were caused by medical errors—more than the deaths from motor vehicle accidents, breast cancer, or acquired immunodeficiency syndrome (AIDS), placing medical errors among the top 10 causes of death. Within a few years, even this enormous estimated number was recognized as being too low. In 2004, an AHQR study of Medicare patients found that 195,000 deaths per year were due to medical errors. In 2008, a U.S. Department of Health and Human Services study of hospital records found that 180,000 deaths per year were due to medical errors—among Medicare-covered patients alone. Another study, extrapolating from North Carolina data, found that 135,000 deaths per year nationwide were due to hospital medical errors. Notably, none of these studies accounted for medical-error deaths in nursing homes or outpatient care centers such as ambulatory surgery centers. A recent review of this literature concluded that the actual annual number of medical-error deaths in the United States was at least 251,000 and likely much higher because so many of them go unrecorded. This figure would make medical errors the third leading cause of death in the United States, behind heart disease and cancer.[34]

Before the IOM report was published, medical errors were blamed on failures by individual doctors and nurses; practitioners who made mistakes were sued for malpractice, and some were even prosecuted as criminals. The report shifted the blame to the medical care system—or nonsystem, according to some critics—characterizing it as decentralized and fragmented, rife with confusion, miscommunication, and lack of incentives for improvements in safety. The IOM committee compared the medical care industry unfavorably with other high-risk industries that had been much more successful at improving safety and preventing injury, especially the commercial airline industry. The report made a number of recommendations, beginning with the creation of a Center for Patient Safety within the AHRQ, which would set national goals, track progress, develop a research agenda, evaluate methods for identifying and preventing errors, and disseminate information. Another recommendation was that, as in the airline industry, accidents and near-misses should be reported so that errors could be investigated, leading to an understanding of the underlying factors that contribute to them. A mandatory, nonpunitive system should be developed that encourages providers to learn from their mistakes.[33]

Recognizing that many adverse events involve medication errors, the report recommended that the U.S. Food and Drug Administration (FDA) should require that drug naming, packaging, and labeling be designed to minimize confusion. Because of doctors' notoriously poor handwriting, procedures should be developed to ensure accurate communication of prescriptions and other orders.

In 2009, Consumers Union (CU), the non-profit agency that publishes *Consumer Reports,* published an evaluation of progress in implementing the IOM report's recommendations 10 years later. The report gave the country a failing grade in implementing procedures that CU believed necessary to create a healthcare system free of preventable medical harm. In particular,

CU reported that few hospitals had adopted measures to prevent medication errors and that the FDA rarely intervened. Computerized prescribing and dispensing systems have not been widely adopted, despite evidence that they make patients safer. There is no national system of reporting medical errors. Where such reporting does occur, it is generally confidential, meaning that patients do not have access to information on how to compare the performance of doctors and hospitals, so these providers face little pressure to improve. Another IOM recommendation was to raise standards for competency of doctors, nurses, and other healthcare professionals by requiring them to periodically pass examinations demonstrating skills, knowledge, and use of best-practice care to maintain their certification. Most specialty boards now have this requirement but, according to the CU report, there is no mechanism in place to ensure the competency of the 15% of physicians not certified by one of these boards, as well as those "grandfathered" prior to the adoption of the standards.[35]

In 2015, the National Patient Safety Foundation published a follow-up to the IOM report. It found that some progress had occurred over the past 15 years. Notably, there was increased recognition of the problem, and a survey of experts in the field of medical care safety revealed a belief that progress was being made. At the same time, the follow-up report highlighted that major problems remain: In the United States, about 10% of hospital inpatients incur an adverse event such as a fall, a hospital-acquired infection, or a preventable negative drug effect; roughly half of surgeries involve a medication error or a dangerous drug event; and more than 5% of outpatient diagnoses, affecting 12 million American adults, are in error each year.[36]

One example of a system that works was established as part of a safety initiative in Michigan called the Keystone ICU project. The project was funded by AHRQ and was instituted in 2004 in 103 Michigan intensive care units. One of the goals was to prevent some

of the estimated 80,000 catheter-associated bloodstream infections and 28,000 deaths associated with these infections that occur in the United States each year. The intervention consisted of a short checklist of best practices related to catheter use; nurses were empowered to ensure that doctors were following these practices. Researchers tracked catheter-associated infections and found that the incidence dropped to less than 20% of what it had been before the procedures were implemented.[37]

The CU report argues that among the most important of the IOM recommendations is "increased accountability through mandatory, validated and public reporting of preventable medical harm, including healthcare-acquired infections." According to the report, "It is a fundamental principle of quality control that if a process cannot be measured, it cannot be improved."[35(p.6)]

Medical Care Report Cards

The rise of managed care contributed to an increasing interest in the measurement of the quality and efficiency, or cost-effectiveness, of medical care. Managed care's focus on cutting costs, however, conflicted with the common assumption that, when it comes to medical care, more is better—an assumption that is challenged by outcomes research, which suggests that sometimes less may be better as well as less expensive.[38] However, many people are suspicious that managed care companies, which have a financial incentive to do less for their patients, may have an inherent conflict of interest. The suspicion is especially strong in the case of for-profit managed care plans, which have an obligation to maximize profits for their investors, perhaps at the expense of the patients.

In the medical care marketplace, where economic factors are becoming increasingly significant, outcomes research has an important role to play in evaluating the quality and efficiency of different medical plans. In theory, when given enough information, customers—both the employers who choose which plans to offer and the employees who must choose among the plans that are offered—can make informed decisions, weighing quality and cost.[39] Moreover, patients are increasingly becoming more active participants in their own care. In part because of growing distrust of the medical system, patients want information on risks and benefits of available treatments and, if possible, on the competence of their physicians and other medical providers. Outcomes research provides some of this information.

Although managed care is often regarded with skepticism, it is more easily evaluated than the traditional fee-for-service form of medical practice. The organization of services that allows care to be "managed" makes it possible for those services to be assessed in a formal way, something that is not realistic when each medical provider acts independently. Through an accreditation process conducted by the nonprofit **National Committee for Quality Assurance (NCQA)**, it is possible to rate managed care plans on their performance with respect to a number of standards. Information on the accreditation status of a plan can influence a business's decision about whether to offer the plan to its employees, and the information can be used by employees to choose among plans offered. In its 2018 State of Health Care Quality report, more than 1000 health plans provided data to NCQA on a multitude of different measures of healthcare quality. NCQA reported that most of the health plans had improved on many of the measures. For example, the rate of body mass index (BMI) assessments, an important monitor of patient health, rose steadily from 2011 to 2017; rates of colorectal cancer and diabetes screening also improved, as did osteoporosis management in women who have experienced fractures. However, little recent progress has been made in reducing overuse and inappropriate

medical procedures—for example, imaging (x-ray, magnetic resonance imaging [MRI], computed tomography [CT] scans) for lower back pain, which has not been shown to improve outcomes and exposes patients to unnecessary radiation.[40] Consumers can access "report cards" of plans on the NCQA website and compare their performance.

Many of the most easily measured standards used by NCQA focus on preventive care, such as whether children receive a full set of immunizations and whether women get mammograms and Pap tests. Other standards evaluate how a plan manages care for patients with common diseases. The findings of outcomes research can be used, for example, to measure performance of a health maintenance organization in treating elderly patients who experience heart attacks. Research supported by AHCPR found that patients 65 years of age and older were 43% less likely to die after a heart attack if they were treated with beta blockers than if they did not receive these drugs.[41] Using that information, NCQA established, as one of its standards for evaluating a plan, the use of beta blockers for treatment of heart attacks. Since the agency began reporting on this measure, the percentage of patients with heart attack who received the drugs went from 60% to about 90%.[42]

Outcomes research can also be used in some circumstances to evaluate the performance of individual medical providers. The findings offer a basis not only for patients to choose where to go for treatment, but also how providers perform relative to their peers. Since 1989, New York State has measured the outcomes of coronary artery bypass surgery for treatment of blocked arteries in the heart, monitoring each of the hospitals where the operations are performed. Mortality rates in 1989, adjusted for patient-related risk factors such as age, diabetes, and hypertension, varied widely, from 0.88% to 10.02%.[43] Data have also been collected on outcomes achieved by individual surgeons.

One of the study's findings was that hospitals that perform large volumes of coronary surgery have better outcomes than those that perform few of the operations, a relationship that has also been found to hold for other types of surgery. The New York study also revealed that surgeons who perform more than 150 bypass operations per year have only half the patient mortality rate of surgeons who perform fewer than 50 such procedures. The publicity that followed the release of the 1989 data on individual hospitals led to a dramatic decline (41%) statewide in mortality rates associated with the surgery over the next three years.[44] Thus, the information provided by outcomes research led to improved quality of surgical care statewide. An analysis of how the improvements were accomplished show that hospitals identified as performing poorly reacted strongly, for example, by restricting the surgical privileges of some low-volume surgeons whose patients were more likely to die from the operation.[45] Several other states, including Pennsylvania, California, and Massachusetts, now maintain similar data sets for coronary surgery in their hospitals.[46]

Despite the successes, health services research has a long way to go before it can be widely used to help people make decisions about health care based on quality. Most of the indicators of managed care quality measured by accrediting agencies focus on preventive care for the healthy. Although this approach is important from a public health perspective, what matters most to individual patients is the quality of care they receive when they are ill.[33] Detailed analyses of providers' performance are available for only a limited number of procedures in New York and the few other states that carry out such ambitious programs. The New York State Health Department publishes annual reports on its cardiac surgery data (available at https://www.health.state.ny.us/statistics/diseases/cardiovascular), and the data are increasingly being used: Managed care organizations are more likely to contract with surgeons who have lower risk-adjusted mortality rates, and

surgeons who are rated poorly are more likely to discontinue performing the procedures.[46]

Inequities in Medical Care

Health services research has shed light on an unpleasant reality that pervades the American medical care system: Not only is care rationed by ability to pay, but there are racial inequities in how care is delivered even when individuals are able to pay for it. As documented in a 2002 IOM report, *Unequal Treatment: What Healthcare Providers Need to Know About Racial and Ethnic Disparities in Healthcare*,[47] blacks and Hispanics are less likely than whites to receive the most effective treatments for heart disease, human immunodeficiency virus (HIV) infection, asthma, breast cancer, and many other conditions, even when their income and insurance status are equal to whites.

Examining all patients with fee-for-service Medicare coverage in 1999, for example, researchers found that whites underwent coronary artery bypass surgeries at 2.1 times the rate of blacks. By 2014, this multiple had fallen to 1.7 times, shrinking the gap, which nevertheless remains large. The gap in 30-day mortality after the surgery, however, has not decreased over the period, consistently remaining about 1.2 times higher for blacks than whites over the study period.[48]

Childhood asthma is a chronic disease that can usually be kept under control by providing patients and their families with prescriptions for inhaled medications and education on how to use them. A study that examined records of children found that blacks had twice the rate of emergency room visits as whites for asthma attacks, but were 64% less likely to receive timely follow-up care after this visit. Black children with asthma also visited physicians for routine care at a significantly lower rate than did white children. Thus, black children seem to be receiving poorer-quality care than white children do, an observation that is especially disturbing because the prevalence of asthma in black children is higher than in whites—81% higher, according to the National Health Interview Survey.[49–51]

According to the American Cancer Society, blacks have the highest death rate and the shortest survival of any racial and ethnic group in the United States for most cancers. Although the overall racial disparity in cancer death rates is decreasing, the death rate for all cancers combined is 20% higher in black men and 13% higher in black women than in white men and women, respectively. Blacks are less likely to survive five years after diagnosis, most likely due to their tendency to be diagnosed at a later stage, when the disease has spread. Blacks are also less likely to receive timely and high-quality treatment.[52]

There are signs of promise in some areas and little progress in other areas. AHRQ's *National Healthcare Quality and Disparities Report*, which has been provided to Congress annually since 2001, tracks disparities in healthcare access and quality across racial, ethnic, and economic groups. On the question of access to care, the report shows that the percentage of white adults ages 18 to 64 without health insurance continues to be much lower than the percentages for blacks and Hispanics, although this gap is shrinking. In 2010, 16.4% of whites were uninsured compared to 27.2% of blacks and 43.2% of Hispanics. By 2018, 9.0% of whites were uninsured, while 15.2% of blacks and 26.7% of Hispanics were uninsured.[53]

As for quality of care, the report shows that the gap between whites and minorities has generally persisted. For example, in 2001, black smokers who had a medical checkup were less likely than white smokers to be given advice by a doctor on quitting smoking. By 2018, this gap between black and white smokers in what advice is provided had increased. By contrast, when effective treatments are widely adopted in the healthcare system, patients of all races and socioeconomic characteristics often benefit significantly. In some cases, the gap has disappeared almost entirely. One example is the rate at which patients experiencing heart attack receive fibrinolytic medication to prevent or break down blood clots. In 2005, white patients were over 11% more likely to receive this medication compared to black patients; by 2013, however, this difference had been cut by more than half. The AHRQ report shows that the gap in healthcare quality is larger when measured along economic lines. Households below the poverty line receive worse care compared to high-income households on the majority of quality measures that are tracked in the *National Healthcare Quality and Disparities Report*, and better care on almost none of these measures. Even worse, the overall gap increased between 2001 and 2017.[53]

These studies provide evidence that inequities in medical care extend significantly beyond disparities in health insurance status. The IOM report concluded that "although myriad sources contribute to these disparities, some evidence suggests that bias, prejudice, and stereotyping on the part of healthcare providers may contribute to differences in care."[46] Other recent analyses indicate that the situation may be more complex. Health services research by the Dartmouth group, discussed earlier in this chapter, has found evidence that some of the differences are due more to geographic variations than to racial disparities within the same area. Some of the disparities in treatment may be due to blacks living disproportionately in regions with low rates for all patients. Others may be due to higher-than-average surgery rates among whites rather than lower-than-average rates among blacks.[54]

Finally, it is useful to keep in mind that the causes of disparities in health are not limited to disparities in health care. For example, there is a threefold difference in diabetes mortality rates between college graduates and those with only a high school education. No diabetes drug makes such a large difference.[55]

The Relative Importance of Medical Care for Public Health

Health services research, in addition to studying medical care epidemiology, has tried to answer questions about the proper place of medical care within the public health system. To what extent does medical care contribute to improving the health of the population as a whole? Some skeptics have argued that medicine's effectiveness is limited and that its impact on health is marginal at best. The improvement in life expectancy over the past century resulted more from public health measures and improvements in the population's economic status than from improvements in medical interventions.

In focusing on the population perspective, analysts weigh the contribution of medical care with other factors that contribute to people's health (**Figure 28-1**). No consensus has been reached on the relative importance of the various factors, which include genetics; behavioral patterns such as diet, exercise, and substance abuse; social circumstances such as education and housing; and environmental pollution, in addition to medical care. But researchers have tried to estimate the importance of these factors, and have identified that a shortfall in medical care is far from the most important cause of premature death. Behavioral patterns are particularly important, and any consideration of these factors calls attention to the fact that, in the United States, resources devoted to medical care are far out of proportion to their contribution to health. In fact, the enormous American investment in medical care uses up resources that would otherwise be available to address other factors that affect health, such as

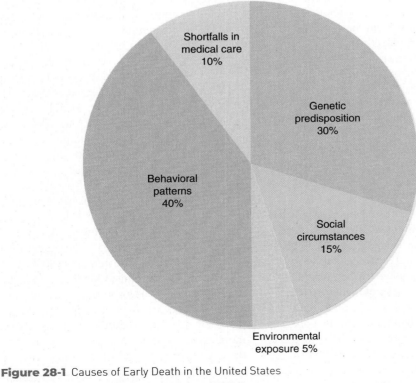

Figure 28-1 Causes of Early Death in the United States

Data from "The Case for More Active Attention to Health Promotion," *Health Affairs*, 21 (2002): 78–93.

education, housing, and the environment. In that sense, it may be that the greater the expansion of the medical care system, the more negative the impact on the population's health.[56]

Evidence from small-area comparisons in the United States, as well as comparative studies of industrialized nations, has clearly indicated that health is not correlated with resources devoted to medical care. This was true, for example, in Wennberg's comparison of healthcare costs and the population's health status in Boston and New Haven. Similarly, international studies of mortality rates in developed nations have found no consistent relationship with levels of medical care resources.[57] The United States has higher rates of chronic disease prevalence and mortality compared to other developed countries, despite its high spending on medical care. The fact that more medical care does not lead to better health is supported by a 2003 study by Wennberg's group that looked at U.S. patients with heart attacks, hip fractures, or colorectal cancer who lived in geographic areas with high Medicare spending compared with similar patients in areas with lower spending. The researchers found that patients in the high-spending areas had more physicians' visits, underwent more tests and procedures, and spent more time in the hospital than those in the low-spending areas, but the outcomes were not better and, in fact, included a small increase in the risk of death. Apparently, the higher-intensity practice patterns caused harm to patients.[58]

The United States does not get its money's worth for the resources allocated to medical care. Health services research that focuses on the efficiency of the healthcare system can offer evidence on how the nation could keep costs under control while achieving better health. A number of studies have investigated the effects of different methods of paying for care on the use of care and on health outcomes. One influential study was the RAND Health Insurance Experiment,[59] which compared use of services, expenditures, and health outcomes among several groups of consumers who were assigned randomly to receive free care or to pay copayments of varying amounts. The evidence showed, not surprisingly, that higher copayments discouraged patients from seeking care. The more consumers had to pay, the less medical care they consumed, and the free-care group used services costing 50% more than those who had to pay the most. For most of the participants, the extra services were not found to have any impact on their health status. Thus, many healthcare services provided to Americans with generous insurance policies may be wasted in that they do not contribute to better health.

However, for those individuals who were both poor and chronically ill, free care did provide significant benefits in health status. These are the people most likely to lack access to medical care because of financial barriers despite their great need for care. This has been the tragedy of the American health system, which, despite the highest rate of healthcare spending in the world—much of it probably of limited benefit—has left a significant fraction of the population uninsured and without high-quality access.

It remains to be seen just how much the full implementation of the Affordable Care Act will change this characterization of the U.S. healthcare system, but early results suggest it has prompted some improvements. A 2019 study that compared mortality of older Americans in states that expanded Medicaid eligibility under the Affordable Care Act compared to states that did not expand Medicaid eligibility found almost a 10% reduction in mortality in the expansion states.[60] Nevertheless, since the significant reforms in the American medical care system were put in place, a great deal more remains to be learned from health services research. The research thus far has demonstrated that a significant proportion of the resources spent on medical care in the United States does not contribute to better health in the population. But if the reformed system can be made more efficient and equitable than it is today, then the health of the American population can be significantly improved.

Conclusion

One hope for reducing costs of medical care and improving its quality is health services research, which studies the effectiveness, efficiency, and equity of the healthcare system. Small-area analysis, a form of health services research, has found that physicians in different geographic areas vary widely in how they treat common health problems. This observation suggests that for some conditions, decisions on treatment are somewhat arbitrary, and that different treatments may be equally valid—or invalid. Large variations are most likely to occur in the absence of clear evidence showing which treatments are most effective.

The observed differences may be due in part to the varying availability of services in a community. Larger numbers of surgeries are done in communities with higher numbers of surgeons. More people are hospitalized in communities with higher per capita numbers of hospital beds. Other variations seem to be merely variations in practice style, which tends to be shared by all physicians in a community. Comparisons of high-usage areas with low-usage areas have not found significant differences in health status, indicating that the variations are not caused by greater severity of illness in some areas, and there is no evidence that high usage helps or harms people's health. However, medical costs are proportionately high in the high-usage areas, suggesting that adopting the practices of low-usage areas could save substantial sums.

Outcomes research—the epidemiologic study of the everyday practice of medicine—holds hope for reaching conclusions about the benefits and risks of treatment approaches, especially those with a high variation. For example, prostatectomy for benign prostatic disease is a common surgery performed on older men. However, it is not always effective in relieving symptoms, and it can have undesirable complications such as impotence and incontinence. Results of outcomes research have made it clear that people should be informed of the risks of surgery and the possible outcomes before they make choices about their treatment. Surgery for BPH is now used less often than in the past. PSA screening for prostate cancer is also of questionable value since it leads to many biopsies and prostatectomies but does not appear to meaningfully lower mortality rates.

The federal agency formerly called AHCPR got into political trouble in the 1990s when it published evidence recommending less use of back surgery for low back pain. Now known as AHRQ, the agency has regained its funding and more, and healthcare reformers are hoping that its comparative effectiveness research will help save money for the American healthcare system as a whole.

Outcomes research can be used to evaluate the quality of managed care plans, assessing whether those plans provide services that have been demonstrated to be effective. Such research can also be used to compare the performance of hospitals and surgeons. Health services research has documented extensive evidence that the delivery of medical care is inequitable and that ethnic and racial minorities may receive poorer-quality care than do white Americans. This is true even after differences in health insurance status have been taken into consideration.

Although health services research is certainly capable of improving the quality of medical care, it also shows that medical care is a less important influence on people's health than some other factors, including diet and exercise, education, and the environment. In fact, health services research suggests that if the United States spent less on medical care, and instead invested the savings in these other risk factors, the population's health might be improved.

References

1. J. E. Wennberg, "Dealing with Medical Practice Variations: A Proposal for Action," *Health Affairs* 3 (1984): 6–32.

2. J. E. Wennberg and M. M. Cooper, eds., *Dartmouth Atlas of Health Care 1996* (Chicago, IL: American Hospital Publishing, 1996).

3. P. R. Goodney et al., "Variations in the Care of Surgical Conditions," *A Dartmouth Atlas of Health Care Series* (Hanover, NH: Trustees of Dartmouth College, 2015), https://www.dartmouthatlas.org/downloads/atlases/Surgical_Atlas_2014.pdf, accessed October 15, 2019.

4. D. C. Goodman, G. A. Little, W. N. Harrison, A. Moen, M. E. Mowitz, C. Ganduglia Cazaban, et al., eds., *The Dartmouth Atlas of Neonatal Intensive Care* (Lebanon, NH: Dartmouth Institute of Health Policy & Clinical Practice, Geisel School of Medicine at Dartmouth, 2019).

5. Dartmouth Institute for Health Policy & Clinical Practice, "Once Scarce, Neonatal Care Proliferates," September 4, 2019, https://www.dartmouthatlas.org/downloads/press/NICU_report_press_release_090419.pdf, accessed October 10, 2019.

6. A. Gawande, "Overkill," *The New Yorker*, May 11, 2015, https://www.newyorker.com/magazine/2015/05/11/overkill-atul-gawande, accessed October 10, 2019.

7. M. R. Chassin, J. Kosecoff, R. E. Park, C. M. Winslow, K. L. Kahn, N. J. Merrick, et al., "Does Inappropriate Use Explain Geographic Variations in the Use of Health Care Services? A Study of Three Procedures," *Journal of the American Medical Association* 258 (1987): 2533–2537.

8. E. A. Halm, S. Tuhrim, J. J. Wang, M. Rojas, E. L. Hannan, and M. R. Chassin, "Has Evidence Changed Practice? Appropriateness of Carotid Endarterectomy After the Clinical Trials," *Neurology* 68 (2007): 187–194.

9. E. L. Hannan, C. Wu, and M. R. Chassin, "Differences in Per Capita Rates of Revascularization and in Choice of Revascularization Procedure for Eleven States," *BMS Health Services Research* 6 (2008): 35.

10. J. E. Wennberg, "Small Area Analysis and the Medical Care Outcome Problem," in L. Sechrest, E. Perrin, and J. Bunker, *Conference Proceedings: Research Methodology: Strengthening Causal Interpretations of Nonexperimental Data* (AHCPR, May 1990), 177–201.

11. J. E. Wennberg and M. M. Cooper, eds., *Dartmouth Atlas of Health Care 1998* (Chicago, IL: American Hospital Publishing, 1998).

12. J. E. Wennberg, "Outcomes Research, Cost Containment, and the Fear of Health Care Rationing," *New England Journal of Medicine* 323 (1990): 1202–1204.

13. M. Waldholtz and W. Bogdanich, "Warm Bodies: Doctor-Owned Labs Earn Lavish Profits in a Captive Market," *Wall Street Journal*, March 1, 1989.

14. B. J. Hillman, C. A. Joseph, M. R. Mabry, J. H. Sunshine, S. D. Kennedy, and M. Noether, "Frequency and Costs of Diagnostic Imaging in Office Practice: A Comparison of Self-Referring and Radiologist-Referring Physicians," *New England Journal of Medicine* 323 (1990): 1604–1608.

15. T. Iizuka, "Experts' Agency Problems: Evidence from the Prescription Drug Market in Japan," *Rand Journal of Economics* 38 (2007): 844–862.

16. R. Abelson and M. Petersen, "An Operation to Ease Back Pain Bolsters the Bottom Line, Too," *The New York Times*, December 31, 2003.

17. F. Mullan, "Wrestling with Variation: An Interview with Jack Wennberg," *Health Affairs* (2004): VAR-71-80, Web Exclusive.

18. F. J. Fowler, J. E. Wennberg, R. P. Timothy, M. J. Barry, A. G. Mulley Jr, D. Hanley, "Symptom Status and Quality of Life Following Prostatectomy," *Journal of the American Medical Association* 259 (1988): 3018–3022.

19. J. H. Wasson, T. A. Bubolz, G. L. Lu-Yao, E. Walker-Corkery, C. S. Hammond, M. J. Barry, "Transurethral Resection of the Prostate Among Medicare Beneficiaries: 1984–1997. For the Patient Outcomes Research Team for Prostatic Diseases," *Journal of Urology* 164 (2000): 1212–1215.

20. G. Lu-Yao, P. C. Albertsen, J. L. Stanford, T. A. Stukel, E. S. Walker-Corkery, and M. J. Barry, "Natural Experiment Examining Impact of Aggressive Screening and Treatment on Prostate Cancer Mortality in Two Fixed Cohorts from Seattle Area and Connecticut," *British Medical Journal* 325 (2002): 740–746.

21. M. J. Barry, "Screening for Prostate Cancer: The Controversy That Refuses to Die," *New England Journal of Medicine* 360 (2009): 1351–1354.

22. R. Chou, J. M. Croswell, T. Dana, C. Bougatsos, I. Blazina, and R. Fu, "Screening for Prostate Cancer: A Review of the Evidence for the U.S. Preventive Services Task Force," *Annals of Internal Medicine* 155 (2011): 762–771.

23. E. S. Hymans, P. R. Goodney, N. Dzebisashvili, D. C. Goodman, and K. K. Bronner, "Variation in the Care of Surgical Conditions: Prostate Cancer," *Dartmouth Atlas of Health Care Series*, 2014, https://www.dartmouthatlas.org/downloads/reports/Prostate_cancer_report_12_03_14.pdf, accessed October 15, 2019.

24. J. Kosterlitz, "Cookbook Medicine," *National Journal* (March 9, 1991): 574–577.

25. Agency for Health Care Policy and Research, "AHCPR Releases Low Back Pain Guideline," *Research Activities* (January 1995): 15–16.

26. N. A. Lewis, "Agency Facing Revolt After Report: Enraged Back Surgeons Recruiting Republicans for a Battle," *The New York Times*, September 14, 1995.

27. B. H. Gray, M. K. Gusmano, and S. R. Collins, "AHCPR and the Changing Politics of Health Services Research," *Health Affairs* 22 no. Suppl 1 (2003), Web exclusive.

28. U.S. Department of Health & Human Services, Agency for Healthcare Research and Quality, "Operating Plan for Fiscal Year 2019," https://www.ahrq.gov/cpi /about/mission/operating-plan/index.html, accessed October 10, 2019.

29. M. Mitka, "Studies Comparing Treatments Ramp Up," *Journal of the American Medical Association* 301 (2009): 1975.

30. R. A. Deyo, S. K. Mirza, J. A. Turner, and B. I. Martin, "Overtreating Chronic Back Pain: Time to Back Off?" *Journal of the American Board of Family Medicine* 22 (2009): 62–68.

31. R. B. Keller, S. J. Atlas, D. N. Soule, D. E. Singer, and R. A. Deyo, "Relationship Between Rates and Outcomes of Operative Treatment for Lumbar Disc Herniation and Spinal Stenosis," *Journal of Bone and Joint Surgery* 81-A (1999): 752–762.

32. A. Frakt and J. Skinner, "The Puzzling Popularity of Back Surgery in Certain Regions," *The New York Times*, February 13, 2017.

33. Institute of Medicine, *To Err Is Human: Building a Safer Health System* (Washington, DC: National Academy Press, 1999).

34. M. A. Makaray and M. Daniel, "Medical Error: The Third Leading Cause of Death in the US," *British Medical Journal* 353 (May 3, 2016).

35. Consumers Union, "*To Err Is Human—To Delay Is Deadly,*" accessed July 29, 2015.

36. National Patient Safety Foundation, "Free From Harm: Accelerating Patient Safety Improvements Fifteen Years after *To Err Is Human*," 2015, http:// www.aig.com/content/dam/aig/america-canada/us /documents/brochure/free-from-harm-final-report .pdf, accessed October 15, 2019.

37. P. Pronovost, D. Needham, S. Berenholtz, D. Sinopoli, H. Chu, S. Cosgrove, et al., "An Intervention to Decrease Catheter-Related Bloodstream Infections in the ICU," *New England Journal of Medicine* 355 (2006): 2725–2732.

38. C. R. Gaus and L. Simpson, "Reinventing Health Services Research," *Inquiry* 32 (1995): 130–133.

39. M. Angell and J. P. Kassirer, "Quality and the Medical Marketplace: Following Elephants," *New England Journal of Medicine* 335 (1996): 883–885.

40. National Committee for Quality Assurance, "The State of Health Care Quality 2018," https://www.ncqa.org/wp -content/uploads/2018/12/20181214_State_of_Health _Care_Quality_2018.pdf, accessed December 12, 2019.

41. S. B. Soumerai, T. J. McLaughlin, D. Spiegelman, E. Hertzmark, G. Thibault, and L. Goldman, "Adverse Outcomes of Underuse of Beta-Blockers in Elderly Survivors of Acute Myocardial Infarction," *Journal of the American Medical Association* 277 (1997): 115–121.

42. National Committee for Quality Assurance, "Persistence of Beta-Blocker Treatment After a Heart Attack," https://www.ncqa.org/hedis/measures/persistence -of-beta-blocker-treatment-after-a-heart-attack/, accessed October 16, 2019.

43. E. L. Hannan, H. Kilburn Jr, M. Racz, E. Shields, and M. R. Chassin, "Improving the Outcomes of Coronary Bypass Surgery in New York State," *Journal of the American Medical Association* 271 (1994): 761–766.

44. E. L. Hannan, A. L. Siu, D. Kumar, H. Kilburn Jr, and M. R. Chassin, "Decline in Coronary Artery Bypass Graft Surgery Mortality in New York State: The Role of Surgeon Volume," *Journal of the American Medical Association* 273 (1995): 209–213.

45. M. R. Chassin, "Achieving and Sustaining Improved Quality: Lessons from New York State and Cardiac Surgery," *Health Affairs* (July/August 2002): 40–51.

46. E. L. Hannan, K. Cozzens, S. B. King 3rd, G. Walford, and N. R. Shah, "The New York State Cardiac Registries: History, Contributions, Limitations, and Lessons for Future Efforts to Assess and Publicly Report Healthcare Outcomes," *Journal of the American College of Cardiology* 59 (2012): 2309–2316.

47. Institute of Medicine, *Unequal Treatment: What Healthcare Providers Need to Know About Racial and Ethnic Disparities in Healthcare* (Washington, DC: National Academy Press, 2002).

48. S. Angraal, R. Khera, Y. Wang, Y. Lu, R. Jean, R. P. Dreyer, et al. "Sex and Race Differences in the Utilization and Outcomes of Coronary Artery Bypass Grafting Among Medicare Beneficiaries, 1999–2014," *Journal of the American Heart Association* 7, no. 14 (2018).

49. A. E. Shields, C. Comstock, and K. B. Weiss, "Variations in Asthma Care by Race/Ethnicity Among Children Enrolled in a State Medicaid Program," *Pediatrics* 113, no. 3 (2004).

50. H. S. Zahran, C. M. Bailey, S. A. Damon, P. L. Garbe, and P. N. Breysse, "Vital Signs: Asthma in Children— United States, 2001–2016," *Morbidity and Mortality Weekly Report* 67, no. 5 (2018).

51. Centers for Disease Control and Prevention, "2015 National Health Interview Survey Data, Asthma Prevalence Data," February 10, 2017, https://www.cdc .gov/asthma/nhis/2015/data.htm, accessed October 15, 2019.

52. American Cancer Society, "Cancer Facts and Figures for African Americans 2019–2021," 2019, http:// www.cancer.org/content/dam/cancer-org/research /cancer-facts-and-statistics/cancer-facts-and-figures -for-african-americans/cancer-facts-and-figures-for

-african-americans-2019-2021.pdf, accessed October 15, 2019.

53. U.S. Department of Health & Human Services, Agency for Healthcare Research and Quality, "2018 National Health Care Quality and Disparities Report," 2018, https://www.ahrq.gov/research/findings/nhqrdr/nhqdr18/index.html, accessed October 15, 2019.

54. K. Baicker, A. Chandra, J. S. Skinner, and J. E. Wennberg, "Who You Are and Where You Live: How Race and Geography Affect the Treatment of Medicare Beneficiaries," *Health Affairs* (October 7, 2004): Web exclusive.

55. S. H. Woolf, "Social Policy as Health Policy," *Journal of the American Medical Association* 301 (2009): 1166–1169.

56. R. G. Evans and G. L. Stoddart, "Producing Health, Consuming Health Care," *Social Science and Medicine* 31 (1990): 1347–1363.

57. G. F. Anderson, B. K. Frogner, and U. E. Reinhardt, "Health Spending in OECD Countries in 2004: An Update," *Health Affairs* 26 (2007): 1481–1489.

58. E. S. Fisher, D. E. Wennberg, T. A. Stukel, D. J. Gottlieb, F. L. Lucas, and E. L. Pinder, "The Implications of Regional Variations in Medicare Spending. Part 2: Health Outcomes and Satisfaction with Care," *Annals of Internal Medicine* 138 (2003): 288–298.

59. L. A. Aday, *Evaluating the Medical Care System: Effectiveness, Efficiency, and Equity* (Ann Arbor, MI: Health Administration Press, 1993).

60. S. Miller, S. Altekruse, N. Johnson, and L. R. Wherry, "Medicaid and mortality: New evidence from linked survey and administrative data," *National Bureau of Economic Research Working Paper Series*, No. w26081, 2019.

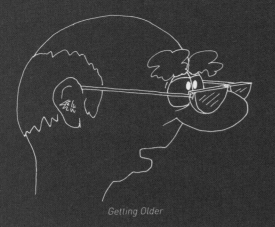

CHAPTER 29

Getting Older

Public Health and the Aging Population

KEY TERMS

Alzheimer's disease
Arthritis
Chronic obstructive pulmonary
  disease (COPD)

Dementia
Hospice
Morbidity

Osteoporosis
Social Security

The U.S. population is getting older. The "baby-boom" generation, many of whom are now older than 65, is in the process of retiring. This situation is causing great alarm among health planners because of the increasing pressure it places on medical costs. Medicare spending has grown dramatically since the program began, both because of growing medical care costs and because of the aging population. Politicians know that they must do something to remedy the situation, but there is no agreement about how or what should be done.

Older people tend to have poorer health than do younger ones. They tend to have more chronic illnesses, and are more likely to suffer limitations of their ability to participate fully in the activities of their community. These truths have two unhappy consequences: The quality of life of the elderly is, on average, poorer

than that for younger people, and their medical costs are higher. Both issues are of great concern for public health.

Quality of life in later years depends significantly on lifestyle in youth and middle age. Therefore, to the extent that public health succeeds in promoting healthy behavior throughout the lifespan, there is a payoff in improved health and quality of life for older people. Public health must also address the inevitability that there will be limits to society's willingness to pay the medical costs of the aged. Although the Medicare program was created in hopes of enabling all older people to receive adequate care, the financial barriers it faces are increasing and, as in the healthcare system as a whole, medical care for the elderly is being rationed. The challenge for public health is twofold: (1) to improve the health of older people by prevention of disease and disability and (2) to confront the issue of how costs can be controlled in an equitable and humane way. Although these public health goals for older people are no different from those for other age groups, the case of the elderly creates special urgency because society has made a unique commitment to this group through the Social Security and Medicare programs—a commitment that is now under stress.

The Aging of the Population: Trends

The population is getting older, as defined by a number of measures. The median age of the American population—the age at which half the population is younger and half older—increased from 22.9 years in 1900 to 38.2 years in 2018 and is predicted to continue increasing through 2030. In 2018, 16.0% of the population was 65 years or older. As the baby-boom cohort grows older, the proportion of people older than age 65 is expected to reach 20.3% of the population by 2030. The increased number of older people has generally been accompanied by an increase in life expectancy at birth, from 47.3 years in 1900–1902 to 78.6 years in 2017.[1-3] The number of centenarians in the U.S. population increased from 37,000 in 1990 to more than 86,000 in 2017.[4,5]

As people are living longer, most people aged 65 —the traditional retirement age—are still relatively vigorous. To reflect this reality, the elderly are categorized into three component groups, which have quite different characteristics and needs: the "young old," ages 65 to 74; the "aged," who are 75 to 84; and the "oldest old," those 85 and older. In 2017, there were 6.5 million oldest-old people in the United States, and this is the fastest-growing age group in the population other than the baby boomers.[1,5] The U.S. Census Bureau predicts that there will be about 9 million people age 85 and older by the year 2030.[1] Obviously, these projections have important implications for the Social Security and Medicare systems, because the numbers of working-age people—who will be expected to pay to support the elderly—are growing at much slower rates.

Figure 29-1 shows the age distribution of the U.S. population in 2017. The baby-boom generation—those born between 1946 and 1964—is making its way through the age groups like the proverbial pig through a python and accounts for an explosive increase in the number of elderly persons that began in 2011. Predictions of future population size depend both on the birth rate—which is currently fairly stable—and immigration rates, which are somewhat unpredictable and depend on federal policies.

Females increasingly outnumber males in older age groups. Among the oldest old, there are almost twice as many women as men, and there are almost four times as many female centenarians as male centenarians. This is a consequence of the fact that women have a longer life expectancy than men, although the difference is decreasing. After the age of 80, most women are widowed and live alone, while most men are married and live with their wives.

Racial and ethnic diversity among the elderly is expected to increase: Non-Hispanic whites constituted 77% of the older population in 2017, but that proportion is projected to shrink to 55% in 2060. The proportion of Hispanics will grow to 22%; blacks will account for 12%; and Asians will represent 9% of the elderly population. As in younger age groups, older whites are in better health than older people of racial and ethnic minorities. Life expectancy at age 65 is 1.1 years longer for whites than for blacks. However, racial differences in health grow smaller in the oldest populations, and blacks who survive to join the oldest-old category have a

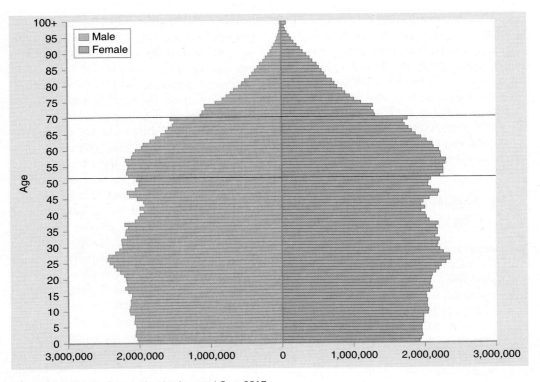

Figure 29-1 U.S. Population by Age and Sex, 2017

Data from U.S. Census Bureau, "American FactFinder, Annual Estimates of the Resident Population by Sex, Single Year of Age, Race, and Hispanic Origin for the United States: 2017 Population Estimates," July 1, 2017, https://factfinder.census.gov/faces/tableservices/jsf/pages/productview.xhtml?src=bkmk#, accessed October 16, 2019.

slightly longer life expectancy than whites of the same age.[6]

Social Security and Medicare have helped most of the older population stay out of poverty. The percentage of people 65 and older living in poverty declined from 15% in 1974 to about 10% in 2014. Older women (12%) were more likely to be poor compared to older men (7%). Poverty rates were higher for older blacks (19%) and Hispanics (18%) than for whites (8%). The percentage that have a high school diploma increased from 24% in 1965 to 84% in 2015; college graduates increased from 5% to 27%.[6] This increased level of education is generally expected to correlate with better health.

Health Status of the Older Population

The greatest public health concern for Americans older than age 65 is long-term chronic illness, disability, and dependency. The majority of the older population, especially those in the younger groups, are in good health. In national surveys of noninstitutionalized persons, 80% of the young old who are white consider their health to be good to excellent, as do 78% of those in the 75 to 84 age group and 68% of those ages 85 and older. Blacks and Hispanics report poorer health than do whites. With more advanced age, many older people have chronic conditions that cause them to require assistance with the activities of daily living. Overall, approximately 1.5% of people ages 65 to 75 live in nursing homes or have home health care, but that proportion increases to about 11% of the oldest old.[6]

The causes of death of older people are essentially the same as the causes of death in the overall population, with cardiovascular disease and cancer leading the list (**Figure 29-2**). Motor vehicle crashes and suicide are also significant causes of death, among older men far

more than older women. Men are likely to die at a younger age, whereas older women are more likely to suffer from chronic, disabling diseases. Heart disease, cancer, and stroke, in addition to killing people, can contribute to chronic health problems and dependency. Many of the elderly, especially women, suffer from **arthritis**, diabetes, osteoporosis, and Alzheimer's disease—conditions that limit their independence and may force them into nursing homes.

A still-unanswered question with very important implications for public health is

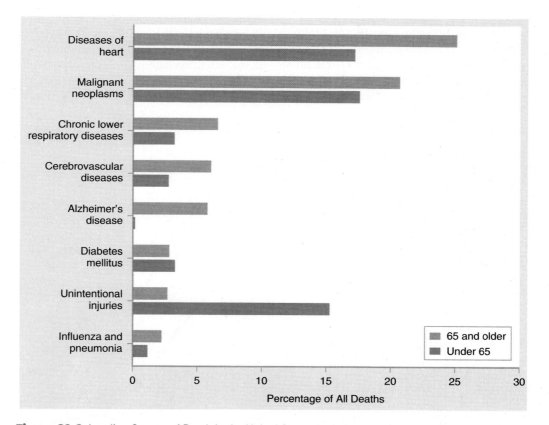

Figure 29-2 Leading Causes of Death in the United States for Individuals Younger Than 65 Years and Individuals 65 Years and Older, 2017

Data from Centers for Disease Control and Prevention. "Deaths: Final Data for 2017." Table 6. *National Vital Statistics Report* 68(9). June 24, 2019. https://www.cdc.gov/nchs/data/nvsr/nvsr68 /nvsr68_09-508.pdf, accessed October 16, 2019.

whether longer life expectancy means more healthy years for most people or, alternatively, if it leads to longer periods of chronic illness and disability. The financial solvency of the Medicare system will be highly dependent on the answer. Experts on aging agree that the trend in the 20th century was a "compression of mortality" (**Figure 29-3**), meaning that deaths increasingly became concentrated in a relatively short age range at about the biological limit of lifespan. What is less certain is whether the compression of mortality will be accompanied by a compression of **morbidity**—the rates of chronic disease and disability. Ideally, most people would prefer to live a long, healthy life and then suddenly drop dead, like Oliver Wendell Holmes's "wonderful one-hoss shay," a scenario that would also save massive amounts of Medicare money.

Evidence is beginning to emerge that a compression of morbidity is, indeed, taking place.[7] An ongoing national survey of Medicare recipients indicates that disability rates among those older than age 65 declined steadily, from 26.5% in 1982 to 19.0% in 2004.[8] Other national surveys have produced similar findings. Surveys by the Centers for Disease Control and Prevention (CDC) have shown that the percentage of older people living in nursing homes declined significantly between 1977 and 2004, especially for whites.[9] The Framingham Heart Study, which tracks the health of a cohort of original participants and their offspring, found that the younger generation had less disability than their parents at the same ages.[10] Conversely, the prevalence of many diseases has increased in the older population. For example, chronic cardiovascular disease has become more prevalent as deaths from cardiovascular disease

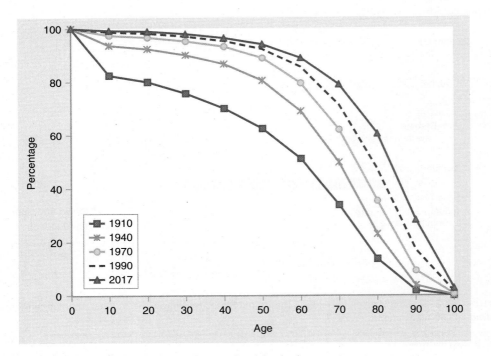

Figure 29-3 Compression of Mortality: Percent Surviving by Age

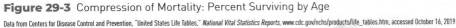
Data from Centers for Disease Control and Prevention, "United States Life Tables," *National Vital Statistics Reports*, www.cdc.gov/nchs/products/life_tables.htm, accessed October 16, 2019.

have declined. Having a disease appears to be less disabling than in the past.[11] At the same time, concern has arisen that increased obesity in the American population may lead to increased disability rates.

General Approaches to Maximizing Health in Old Age

There is still a great deal to learn about how public health can continue to achieve a compression of morbidity, thereby improving quality of life for those who benefit from the compression of mortality that has already occurred. Although a variety of factors might influence the risk of disability in old age, health-related behavior is one important variable that would be expected to make a difference. A study that tracked 1741 older alumni of the University of Pennsylvania found that, indeed, a healthy lifestyle reduced not only their risk of dying but also their disability in later years. The study subjects, who had attended the university in 1939 and 1940, were surveyed on their smoking habits, body mass index (BMI), and exercise patterns and, beginning in 1986, chronic conditions, use of medical services, and extent of disability. The alumni were classified into three risk groups, with the highest risk being associated with obese, inactive smokers. Those in the highest risk group had twice the cumulative disability of those with low risk, and the onset of disability was postponed by almost eight years in the low-risk group.[7,12]

This evidence indicates that, as in younger age groups, the behaviors that most significantly affect health in older people are smoking, obesity, and physical inactivity.[7] However, the recently observed compression of morbidity cannot entirely be explained by improvements in these factors. Undoubtedly, the reduced prevalence of smoking over the past several decades is partly responsible for the fact that the elderly are healthier than they used to be. But the increased prevalence of overweight, obesity, and physical inactivity would be expected to have the opposite effect, leading to increased disability in older people.

Smoking is always a major risk factor for cardiovascular disease and cancer, which remain the leading causes of death in persons older than age 65. **Chronic obstructive pulmonary disease (COPD)** is caused almost entirely by smoking. Osteoporosis and disorders of the mouth are also made worse by smoking. It is significant that prevalence of smoking drops off with increasing age, in part because many older people have succeeded in quitting and in part because many smokers die before they reach old age. In 2016, only 10.1% of American men age 65 and older smoked. The rate among older women was 7.7%.[13,Table 47]

Nutrition and physical activity are the other most important determinants of health in old age. Diet and exercise affect the risk of both cardiovascular disease and cancer. Overweight and obesity—the result of overnutrition and lack of exercise—increase the risk not only of these leading killers, but also of diabetes and arthritis of the weight-bearing joints. Interestingly, the percentage of the population that is overweight and obese decreases after age 75 (**Figure 29-4**). The reason for this finding is not known, but one theory suggests that, like cigarette smokers, obese people die at an earlier age. This may explain in part the apparent paradox between the obesity epidemic and the trend toward better health in the older population. Because obese people are more likely to report poor health than people of normal weight, it is likely that the compression of morbidity seen in recent years will be reversed unless the obesity epidemic can be halted.[14] However, some studies suggest that the health effects of obesity in older people may be less harmful.[8]

Obesity is not the only outcome of poor diet and lack of exercise. Elderly individuals need physical activity to maintain muscle

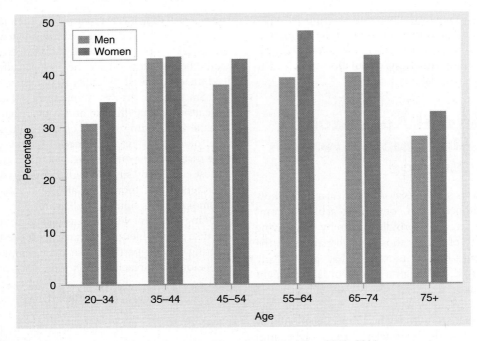

Figure 29-4 Percentage of U.S. Population Obese by Age and Sex, 2013–2016

Data from Centers for Disease Control and Prevention, "Health, United States, 2017," Table 58, www.cdc.gov/nchs/data/hus/2017/058.pdf, accessed October 16, 2019.

strength, balance, and cardiovascular fitness, which protect them against osteoporosis and falls. The special nutritional needs of the elderly are not well understood, but adequate calcium and vitamin D are clearly important to maintain strong bones and teeth. Little evidence exists regarding the special effects of other nutrients in protecting against the diseases of the elderly; thus, the best advice is, as for younger people, to eat a varied diet low in fat and rich in fruits and vegetables.

Through the 1990s, an increasing body of evidence appeared that suggested hormone replacement therapy (HRT) might have broad health advantages for older women in addition to its well-known efficacy in fending off the symptoms of menopause. On the one hand, a number of epidemiologic studies, including research involving the cohort of 60,000 women in the Nurses' Health Study, showed that estrogen therapy was associated with lower rates of heart disease and osteoporosis and perhaps

Alzheimer's disease as well. On the other hand, the hormone increases the risk of breast and uterine cancer. In a 1997 publication, the investigators concluded that HRT reduced women's overall risk of dying as long as they took the hormones.[15] The hopes for estrogen's antiaging effects were crushed, however, with the publication of the clinical trial conducted as part of the Women's Health Initiative. This trial found that although HRT helped prevent osteoporosis and the symptoms of menopause, it actually increased the risk of heart disease, stroke, and even Alzheimer's disease. It seems that the apparent benefits of estrogen were caused by the confounding factor that women who chose HRT were healthier and more likely to have a healthy lifestyle than those who chose not to use the hormone.[16]

Other aspects of medical care have probably contributed to reductions in disability among the elderly. For example, secondary prevention approaches such as the use of drugs to treat diabetes, high blood pressure, and high cholesterol have undoubtedly reduced morbidity and mortality in many older people. The number of total knee replacements for arthritis and cataract surgeries doubled over the period of 1991 to 2010, greatly reducing disabilities and improving quality of life.[17,18]

Preventing Disease and Disability in Old Age

Much of the disease and disability common in later life is linked to unhealthy behavior in earlier years. However, the elderly and their caregivers can certainly take some preventive measures to improve their quality of life and prospects for independence even after health has begun to fail. Some of these measures are well known and readily available, such as vaccination against pneumonia and influenza. Some are beneficial and appropriate for people of any age, such as smoking cessation and blood pressure control. Others are not widely recognized or well understood.

Research is needed on how to prevent many of the debilitating conditions and how to minimize their impact on quality of life for the elderly. In a 1990 report, the Institute of Medicine (IOM) identified a number of the most common problems of the elderly and made recommendations for combating them.[19] These problems commonly and uniquely afflict the elderly and have a severe impact on their quality of life, but are not among the leading causes of death. Despite the passage of 30 years since the IOM report, these problems continue to cause trouble for many older people.

Medications

Although the chronic conditions that afflict many of the elderly can often be treated with prescription drugs, some of these treatments have unwanted side effects that may seriously impair health and quality of life. Little is known about how the body's ability to metabolize drugs changes with age. Kidney and liver function are often impaired in older people, leading to increased sensitivity to drugs. In older bodies, a higher percentage of body weight is contributed by fat, which metabolizes drugs less actively, causing an increased risk of overdoses. Moreover, older people often take a number of medications for various chronic conditions. This could lead to unexpected interactions between drugs, including over-the-counter drugs, because patients tend not to inform their doctors about their use of these medications.

Reducing the risks from adverse drug reactions requires education and vigilance by everyone involved. Elderly patients' needs for medications should be reassessed regularly. In some cases, the potential benefit provided by a drug—for example, improved heart function—may not be worth the damage it could cause to other aging organs—for example, the brain. According to the IOM, there is an urgent need for more research on the risks versus benefits of various types of drugs in the elderly. Better coordination and monitoring of medical care are also necessary—a need that might be better filled by managed care than by fee-for-service care, which currently dominates in serving the Medicare population.

Osteoporosis

Bone loss is common with age, especially in women. This loss sometimes leads to **osteoporosis**—a condition characterized by "porous bones," which tend to break easily. Bone loss among women is greatest in the years following menopause. Smoking and alcohol consumption increase the risk of osteoporosis, whereas obesity reduces the risk (one of the few health benefits of being overweight). White women have the greatest risk for the condition; black men have the lowest risk, and Asians have an intermediate risk. A number of medications commonly used by older people cause bone loss, as do some diseases.

The degree of osteoporosis depends on bone density earlier in life, which is determined by a number of factors including genetics, diet, and physical activity. Thus, drinking milk and exercising during youth can protect women against osteoporosis in old age. Unfortunately, girls tend to not take the threat seriously when these habits could do them the most good. Surveys have found that the average amount of calcium women obtain in their diet is significantly less than the recommended amount.[20]

Osteoporosis itself has no symptoms, and most older people are unaware that they have the problem until they suffer a broken bone. Hip fractures are the most serious consequence of osteoporosis: There is a significant risk that a hip fracture might lead to substantial disability and death. Of those individuals age 60 or older who suffer a hip fracture, approximately 20% die within a year.[20,21] Wrist fractures are also a frequent result of osteoporosis, but there are few data on their frequency. Fractures of the vertebrae, which are even more common, might go unrecognized but often lead to progressive loss of height and the curvature of the upper spine called "dowager's hump." Some osteoporotic fractures are untreatable and cause chronic, debilitating pain. A Surgeon General's report on bone health, published in 2004, estimated that approximately 1.5 million people per year suffer a bone fracture related to osteoporosis, and the cost of caring for these patients amounts to an estimated $18 billion per year.[20]

Considerable research has been done on osteoporosis prevention. The Framingham Study, among others, found that taking estrogen after menopause can protect women from bone loss and reduce the risk of hip fracture.[22] However, HRT is no longer recommended for older women. The Surgeon General's report makes a number of recommendations for preventing osteoporosis. These include getting adequate amounts of calcium (1000 mg per day for adults younger than 50 years and 1200 mg for those older than 50) and vitamin D (200 mg per day for everyone up to 50 years, 400 mg for those ages 51 to 70, and 600 mg for those older than 70). Good sources of calcium include milk, leafy green vegetables, soybeans, yogurt, and cheese. Vitamin D is produced in the skin following exposure to the sun and is found in fortified milk and other foods. Other recommendations include being physically active at least 30 minutes per day for adults and 60 minutes per day for children, including engaging in weight-bearing activities, which have been shown to increase bone strength.[20]

Bone scan tests can screen for risk of osteoporosis, and the Surgeon General's report recommends that the test be used to screen all women older than 65 and younger men and women who have risk factors, including previous fractures. When the test shows bone thinning, drugs are available that can help prevent further loss of bone mass. The drugs have been found to reduce the fracture rate by approximately 50%.

Falls

Most osteoporotic fractures occur when elderly people fall. Thus, in addition to osteoporosis prevention, public health efforts focus on preventing falls. More than one-third of people age 65 and older fall each year; many of them fall repeatedly. About 1 fall in 10 results in a serious injury, such as a fracture or head injury. Many older people have a high risk of falls because of medical conditions that affect their mobility, such as arthritis, stroke, and Parkinson's disease. Other risk factors include vision impairment, muscular weakness, problems with balance, and the side effects of medications. The use of four or more prescription drugs is considered a risk factor for falls. Psychoactive drugs such as antidepressants, tranquilizers, and sleeping pills are especially dangerous.[22]

The Mayo Clinic recommends six measures that older people can take to prevent falls. They should consult with their physician in forming a plan. People should have their medications reviewed, as discussed earlier, to reduce drug interactions and side effects. They should also exercise regularly. Muscle strengthening exercises can significantly increase their mobility, strength, and balance. Older adults should improve the lighting in their homes, and should reduce fall hazards in the home. A home environment can be fall-proofed by such means as covering floors with tacked-down carpets, keeping walkways clear of obstacles, equipping bathrooms with grab bars around toilets and tubs, keeping stairways well lit, and using night lights. Elderly people should also wear comfortable sturdy shoes, avoiding high heels, flip flops, and shoes with slick soles. Finally, they should make use of assistive devices like hand rails on stairs and grab bars in the shower or bathtub.[23]

Clinical trials have shown that vitamin D supplements can reduce the risk of falls independently of their value in osteoporosis prevention. The vitamin appears to directly improve muscle strength.[24]

Impairment of Vision and Hearing

Loss of vision and hearing are among the most prevalent conditions among elderly Americans. Either condition may be disabling, limiting the individual's ability to interact with the environment and communicate with others. Loss of vision increases the risk of falls and other injuries. It may restrict the individual's ability to drive, which represents a significant handicap in many parts of the country. Impairment of either vision or hearing is likely to lead to social isolation, a risk factor for poor health at any age and an even greater risk factor in the elderly. Sensory loss also is associated with depression and cognitive impairment in the elderly.

The leading causes of visual impairment among the elderly are cataracts, glaucoma, macular degeneration, and diabetic retinopathy. Cataracts—clouding of the lens—are the most prevalent cause of eye disease; by age 80,

more than half of Americans either have a cataract or have had cataract surgery. Exposure to sunlight contributes to the lens damage, so wearing sunglasses and hats with brims can help protect the eyes. Smoking increases the risk of cataracts, as does diabetes. Most cataracts can be effectively corrected by surgery in which the clouded lens is removed and replaced with a synthetic lens.[25]

Glaucoma is a gradual increase in pressure within the eye that causes damage to the optic nerve. It is not known why this condition occurs or how it can be prevented. Glaucoma is a common cause of blindness, especially in blacks and Hispanics. People with a family history of the disease have an increased risk. Secondary prevention is the best approach to controlling glaucoma: Regular eye checkups can catch the increase in pressure before it causes harm, and the pressure can be reduced with medication in the form of eye drops.[25]

Age-related macular degeneration involves the breakdown of the light-sensing cells in the macula, the central part of the retina. The risk of macular degeneration increases with age. People with a family history have a greater risk. Whites are at greater risk than blacks, and women have a higher risk than men. Smoking may increase the risk. The cause of macular degeneration is not well understood, and there is no known way to prevent the disease. Progression of some forms of the disease can be slowed by drugs that are injected into the eye. Researchers are studying whether certain vitamins and minerals might help slow the progress of the disease.[25] Some evidence suggests that high levels of vitamin D in the blood may protect against macular degeneration.[26]

Diabetic retinopathy is a common complication of diabetes that poses a major risk to vision. In this condition, high blood sugar damages the tiny blood vessels in the retina. Strict blood sugar control helps reduce the extent of this damage, and the condition can be treated with laser surgery.[25]

The most common form of hearing loss among the elderly is characterized by reduced sensitivity to higher frequency tones and, therefore, difficulty in comprehending speech. This pattern is similar to that associated with exposure to excessive noise. In fact, populations living in relatively noise-free environments are less likely to suffer age-related hearing loss. The proportion of Americans affected by hearing impairment ranges from about one-third of individuals ages 65 to 74 to nearly half of those ages 75 and older, and that proportion is expected to increase with the aging of generations that thrive on rock concerts and listening to music through headphones at high volume. Many products can help people to hear better, including hearing aids, telephone amplifying devices, and assistive listening devices in public places such as movie theaters, churches, mosques, and synagogues, and auditoriums.[27]

One barrier that limits the access of many older individuals to services and devices that correct the effects of sensory loss, such as glasses and hearing aids, is that Medicare does not cover them.[28]

Oral Health

As people age, they suffer increasingly from diseases and impairments of the mouth, including tooth loss, dental caries, periodontal disease, salivary dysfunction, cancer and precancerous conditions, and chronic pain. Such problems can have a severe impact on quality of life. They may impair the individual's ability to chew, taste, and swallow, thereby posing a threat to physical health and nutrition far beyond the anatomical parts that are primarily affected. Like sensory impairments, disorders of the mouth may diminish social functioning by affecting speech, facial esthetics, and self-esteem.

Oral health in old age, like overall health, depends on healthy behaviors throughout life, but older people can improve their health status by instituting healthier habits at any time.

For example, they can quit smoking, use better oral hygiene self-care practices, and use professional dental services. Unfortunately, many of the elderly do not have access to dental services for financial reasons, and Medicare does not cover them.[28]

Alzheimer's and Other Dementias

Alzheimer's disease is one of the most dreaded afflictions of old age. It robs the individual of memory and individuality, and eventually reduces him or her to the helplessness of an infant. Caring for someone with Alzheimer's disease imposes a crushing emotional, physical, and financial burden on a family. **Dementia** among the elderly is a major public health problem, currently affecting at least 5 million people in the United States at a cost of nearly $300 billion per year; much of that expense goes for long-term care in nursing homes. Even so, a great deal of the care of patients with dementia is unpaid care provided by family members, often people who are themselves elderly. The estimated value of this informal care is nearly equal to the medical and long-term care costs of dementia patients.[29,30]

Alzheimer's disease is the most common cause of dementia in the elderly. Other causes include vascular dementia, which may stem from a stroke or a series of mini-strokes that impair blood circulation in the brain. Dementia can also be caused by traumatic brain injury, certain infections, and certain toxic exposures. Diagnosing Alzheimer's disease and differentiating it from other forms of dementia is done by taking a clinical history and administering question-and-answer tests of memory and skills at language and arithmetic. Brain imaging studies such as computed tomography (CT), positron emission tomography (PET), and magnetic resonance imaging (MRI) scans are also useful.[31]

The risk of dementia increases with age, becoming especially high in the oldest age group. The Alzheimer's Association estimates that 3% of people ages 65 to 74 have the disease, 17% of people ages 74 to 85, and 32% of people older than age 85. Blacks are twice as likely to develop Alzheimer's disease as whites, and the prevalence among Hispanics is 1.5 that of whites. With the rapid increase in the oldest-old population, it is estimated that by the middle of the 21st century, as many as 14 million Americans could be suffering from Alzheimer's disease unless a way can be found to prevent or effectively treat the disease.[30]

While a few types of dementia are treatable, there is no cure for Alzheimer's disease. Until recently, almost nothing was known about its cause or means to prevent it. However, the magnitude of the problem has stimulated a great deal of research. Biomedical scientists have learned much about the changes in the brain that typically occur with Alzheimer's disease, including the characteristic tangles of fibers within brain cells and deposits of the protein beta-amyloid, called plaques, in extracellular spaces. These changes lead to the loss of connections between nerve cells, which eventually die, so that the brain atrophies. Several genes have been identified that influence the risk that an individual will develop Alzheimer's disease. Much of what is known about this disease has come from studies of a rare early-onset form of the disease, which is largely determined by genetics.[31] In some families, this form is inherited as an autosomal dominant mutated gene, causing symptoms to appear between ages 30 and 60. An animal model of Alzheimer's disease has been developed by genetically engineering a mouse with a mutant human gene so that it produces amyloid plaques and develops memory loss as it ages. These animals can be used to study methods of preventing plaque formation. An experimental vaccine was developed by injecting beta-amyloid into the mice, which stimulated antibodies to the protein and reduced the number of plaques. This success led to a clinical trial in humans, but the trial had to be stopped when the vaccine caused harmful side effects.[31]

Risk for the more common late-onset form of Alzheimer's disease is also affected by genes, a few of which have been identified. However, nongenetic factors play a significant role in the development of the late-onset form, as well as other forms of dementia. This offers hope that it will be possible to prevent, or at least postpone, the onset of the disease. Some experts predict that merely delaying the onset of Alzheimer's disease by an average of five years could reduce the number of cases by half, as many potential victims would then be nearing the end of their lives for other reasons. Factors that increase the risk of dementia include the risk factors for cardiovascular disease. This suggests that preventive measures against heart disease, such as weight control, physical activity, avoidance of smoking, treatment of high blood pressure and cholesterol, and aspirin, might help ward off dementia as well. Diabetes increases the risk of Alzheimer's disease, just as it does other dementias and cardiovascular disease.[31]

A number of studies have followed cohorts of people to try to determine which factors might influence their risk of developing Alzheimer's disease. Several of these studies have found that formal education seems to protect the brain, providing people with "cognitive reserve." According to this theory, when aging begins to cause pathology in the brain, people with a larger reserve may be better able to function normally. The theory is supported by evidence from the Swedish Twin Registry of 109 pairs of identical twins, in which one twin had been diagnosed with dementia and the other had not. The twin with the dementia had significantly less education than the healthy one.[32]

However, a different theory comes from the Nun Study of 678 Sisters of Notre Dame, who had similar lifestyles and medical care throughout their lives. The nuns, all born before 1917, had been required to write an autobiographical essay when they entered the convent. It turned out that the nuns who had demonstrated the lowest linguistic skills in their essays, written in their early 20s, were most likely to develop Alzheimer's disease as they aged. This evidence suggests that the nuns with higher linguistic ability were more resistant to developing brain pathology in the first place.[32]

Other studies have suggested that all forms of mental activity—reading, puzzles, cards, board games, crafts, playing a musical instrument—are protective. Conversely, watching television is correlated with an increased risk. It is not clear, however, whether less participation in intellectually demanding activities is merely an early symptom rather than a cause of the disease.

Physical exercise has been found in a number of studies to protect against Alzheimer's disease. The Nurses' Health Study, for example, found that women who got the most exercise showed less cognitive decline over the years compared to less active women. This finding is consistent with evidence, discussed earlier, that the brain is protected by the same factors that protect the heart. Participating in social activities also appears to help protect people's brains.[32]

A number of medical approaches are being tested to treat or prevent Alzheimer's disease. Vaccines against beta-amyloid were tested in clinical trials that had to be halted, as discussed earlier. Drugs that act on the neurotransmitters—chemicals that carry signals between nerve cells—have been shown to delay progression of some symptoms, and several of these drugs have been approved by the U.S. Food and Drug Administration.[31] There was great hope that HRT would protect against Alzheimer's disease, but the Women's Health Initiative found evidence to the contrary.

The National Institute on Aging is conducting other studies aimed at helping people maintain mental functioning and managing symptoms common in Alzheimer's disease, such as sleeplessness, aggression, and agitation. As more is learned about the risk factors, some studies are seeking to determine whether interventions against cardiovascular disease and diabetes will be effective against dementia as well.[31]

Medical Costs of the Elderly

Medicare, the federal program that pays medical bills for elderly Americans, as well as for the disabled, is already feeling the strain of the aging population. The number of people enrolled for Medicare coverage has more than tripled since 1966, from 19 million then to 58.5 million in 2017, and the numbers will continue to swell as more baby boomers reach age 65.[33] The number of workers whose earnings contribute to the system is growing at a much slower pace. The same problem applies to **Social Security**, the retirement system for the elderly. In 2018, there were 2.8 workers supporting every retiree; by the year 2036, only 2.2 workers are expected to support each retiree.[34] From a financial standpoint, the Social Security system went into the red in 2010, but the government projects that the Social Security trust fund will keep the program solvent until 2035.[34] Medicare's problems are worse than Social Security's, however, because its costs are less predictable. Not only is the number of people enrolled growing, but the cost per enrollee is also rising, although at a slower rate than overall health-care cost inflation. The average annual expenditure for each Medicare enrollee rose from about $1200 in 1980 to $10,986 in 2014.[35] If present trends continue, Medicare spending is projected to nearly double from $605 billion in 2018 to $1.278 trillion in 2029.[36]

Despite the large expenditures that threaten Medicare's solvency, the program has major benefit gaps and cost-sharing requirements.[37] In 2018, 34% of Medicare beneficiaries were enrolled in Medicare Advantage Plans, which are private plans that require higher premiums than traditional Medicare but generally offer extra benefits.[38] Other beneficiaries have purchased "Medigap" insurance policies that help pay for expenses not covered by Medicare. Employer-sponsored retiree health plans provide supplemental coverage for approximately 30% of beneficiaries.

Medicaid, with funding provided jointly by federal and state governments, acts as a Medigap policy for poor elderly persons. The Medicaid program, which was intended to serve the poor, and poor children in particular, has increasingly been called on to pay for services for the elderly that Medicare does not cover, especially nursing home care and home health care. Because of the high costs of nursing home care, most patients in these facilities have rapidly depleted their savings and become poor enough to qualify for Medicaid, which does cover such care. Almost half of all nursing home costs are paid by Medicaid, which like Medicare, has seen its budget mushroom, from $26 billion in 1980 to $582 billion in 2017. While the elderly constituted only 15% of the persons enrolled in Medicaid in 2014, they consumed 34% of the Medicaid budget.[39] This aspect of the crisis in healthcare costs for the elderly has received less attention than the problems of Medicare.

Past efforts to rein in the growth of government expenditures for the elderly's medical bills have meant that these patients bear a higher percentage of the costs through higher premiums and copayments. Half of all Medicare beneficiaries have annual incomes less than $26,200.[37] This trend threatens the Medicare population with rationing by ability to pay, a matter of great concern to them.

Another approach to controlling growth of costs has been to reduce reimbursement to medical providers—a strategy that, it is feared, could induce some providers to refuse treatment to Medicare patients. In 1997, Congress tried to control Medicare costs by providing incentives for the elderly to enroll in managed care plans, an approach that had been successful in younger groups. However, over the next few years, many problems arose with these plans, in part because of Congress's efforts to control costs. The plans raised premiums and reduced benefits; providers withdrew from the plans; and a large number of plans withdrew from the Medicare program. The 2003 legislation that established prescription drug benefits also contained provisions meant to encourage the use of Medicare Advantage plans, which may offer supplemental benefits, such as vision or hearing or prescription drugs. Such plans have been criticized because they cost the government more money than regular fee-for-service Medicare.[38] One provision of the Affordable Care Act is that government payments to Medicare Advantage plans will be reduced.

The Medicare prescription drug plan, or Medicare Part D, which became effective in 2006, was inspired by news stories of older adults having to choose between drugs and food. The plan has indeed helped many older people to pay for their medicines, but it has many drawbacks and sources of confusion. In contrast to traditional Medicare, Part D is optional and is offered exclusively through private plans. These vary widely, offering different choices of drugs, with widely varying premiums, a situation that can be very confusing to the elderly. Most bizarre, the benefit structure features a coverage gap, dubbed the "doughnut hole," which was instituted to prevent the new benefit from costing more than Congress wanted to spend. The exact dollar amounts vary from one year to another, but for 2019, the maximum deductible amount was $415, which beneficiaries must pay out of pocket. Then there is a coverage gap between $3820 and $5100 in spending. Above that, catastrophic coverage kicks in and beneficiaries pay only a small percentage of the costs of the drugs. In 2018, 72% of Medicare beneficiaries were enrolled in Part D. The program has added to the growth in Medicare costs, amounting to 13% of Medicare spending in 2018.[40,41]

On the Medicaid side, costs for the program have increased faster than those of Medicare, putting immense strain on state budgets. Approximately one-third of Medicaid spending is for long-term care—not only for the elderly, but also for the disabled.[42] Many states set low reimbursement rates for long-term care providers in an attempt to save money.

Some states try to control costs through regulations limiting the number of available nursing home beds. In response, nursing homes tend to preferentially admit patients who can pay their own bills, usually at higher rates than allowed by Medicaid. Consequently, there is a large and growing unmet need among the less affluent elderly for nursing home care.

Unless the baby-boom generation turns out to be significantly healthier and more independent than the aged and oldest old of today, their need for nursing homes and other forms of long-term care is likely to reach critical proportions. In the past, and even today, most elderly Americans who need help with the activities of daily living have been cared for by their families, with the primary responsibility typically borne by a daughter or daughter-in-law. A number of trends make these arrangements less feasible in the future. Baby boomers have fewer children to share the burden of caring for them in old age than did previous generations. The increased divorce rate has led to more complicated family arrangements, which may make it more difficult for the younger generation to take their parents into their homes. A more mobile society also means that many children live far away from their parents. Moreover, most women work outside the home. Thus, just as the government is reducing social services for the elderly, older adults may be less able to depend on their families for the help they need.

Proposals for Rationing

As it has become obvious that the growth in healthcare costs for the elderly is unsustainable, various proposals have been made for controlling those costs through a systematic process that would be fair and equitable, such as rationing. Richard Lamm, a former governor of Colorado, was one of the first to draw attention to the idea by suggesting in 1984 that older persons have a duty to die and get out of the way.[43] His concern was that, as the elderly consume increasing amounts of medical care, society is cutting back on care for children and working people, jeopardizing their future and the productivity of society as a whole. Moreover, as medical costs—largely for the elderly—consume an increasing proportion of the national budget, the government is cutting back other social programs, such as education and food programs targeted for the young, that are important for the future health and prosperity of the country.

Most of the proposals for rationing involve denying expensive life-prolonging technology to people older than a set age, which seems unfair because it appears to punish people who have taken care of their health, or denying it to people who are not expected to achieve a substantial improvement in quality of life from the treatment, an approach that has many defenders. In some cases, expensive treatments are denied to people who are seen as causing their own medical problems through unhealthy behavior. For example, liver transplants are often denied to alcoholics who cannot or will not stop drinking, with the denial justified by the reality that the new scarce organ is likely to be similarly destroyed.

Considering how the nation should care for its increasing numbers of elderly citizens requires examination of our ethics and values as a society. The questions raised are difficult to answer and most people would prefer not to think about them. However, refusal to take responsibility for solving the problems that will inevitably face us will lead to desperation among the elderly and those who must care for them, especially people who do not have the resources to pay for needed care.

The current interest in assisted suicide is one consequence of ill and elderly patients' fear that they will not receive humane care as they lose control and independence. Euthanasia is only a step further, and its widespread use would certainly cut the costs of caring for the dying, an incentive feared by its opponents. Desperate families might increasingly resort to "granny dumping"—abandoning in a public place an unidentified elderly person, most often someone with Alzheimer's disease—when they feel they can no longer cope with caring for a difficult dependent.

Although Governor Lamm's statement outraged some, evidence says his suggestion makes sense. He explained his reasoning by saying that he was referring to the terminally ill—that they should not attempt to prolong their lives by artificial means, generating high medical costs and often adding to their suffering. According to John Wennberg and his Dartmouth research group, geographic variations in end-of-life care demonstrate that a significant amount of the spending on these patients is wasted. The work also shows that more aggressive care is not necessarily better quality care.

The Dartmouth group compared the care of patients dying of chronic diseases, such as cancer and heart failure, in different geographic areas. The studies confirmed that there are wide variations in Medicare spending, determined largely by the aggressiveness of care. Patients in high-spending areas spent more time in the hospital and more time in intensive care, and had more visits to physician specialists. These patients do not have better survival. In fact, evidence shows that a higher-intensity pattern of care may have worse outcomes.[44] Examples of expensive care that could be considered futile include kidney dialysis for frail nursing home residents with end-stage renal disease, which offers little benefit for most of them, and burdensome interventions in patients with Alzheimer's disease in the last three months of life, when **hospice** or "comfort" care would have been more appropriate.[45,46] As Wennberg is quoted as saying, "Some chronically ill and dying Americans are receiving too much care—more than they and their families actually want or benefit from."[47] The Dartmouth researchers note that Medicare costs could be greatly reduced, and end-of-life care might be more humane, if all parts of the country used the same patterns of care as the low-cost areas.

Applying lessons from the study of regional variations is not what is usually considered rationing; it is merely common sense. It requires patients and their families to consider what they want at the end of their lives and discuss it with their doctors. The issue is still highly controversial, however. During the 2009 debate over healthcare reform, a proposal calling for Medicare reimbursement for doctors who counseled patients about end-of-life care provoked accusations that President Barack Obama was advocating "death panels."

Perhaps the greatest hope for reducing costs in an aging population is the possibility of improved health for the elderly—that is, the compression of morbidity that most people would wish for as they look forward to longer lives. This is a realistic hope in that the baby-boom generation is relatively well educated as compared to preceding generations, and more education correlates with better health in the elderly as in other age groups. A consortium of opinion leaders has proposed that this goal could be more readily achieved through a conscious policy of integrating public health and medical services with the aim of reducing the need and demand for medical care.[48] The advocates include James F. Fries, author of the University of Pennsylvania alumni study described earlier in this chapter, who has long argued that compression of morbidity is already occurring, and former Surgeon General C. Everett Koop. Fries and Koop propose that the goal of an integrated healthcare system should be to postpone the onset of chronic infirmity—which accounts for the bulk of illness in the population—by reducing risk factors such as smoking, dietary fat intake, lack of exercise, and failure to wear seat belts; all of these measures would reduce the need for medical care. In addition, they suggest that demand for medical care could be reduced by educating individuals to assume more responsibility for their own health, including self-management of chronic disease. The Fries–Koop consortium's proposal is, in effect, an integration of the missions of public health and medicine, a "doubly positive policy goal," they write; "it promises better health for the individual and lowering of the medical costs that now consume a dangerously high share of our nation's productivity."[48(p.82)]

Conclusion

The American population is aging. Because older people tend to use medical services more than younger people, there are fears that the reliance of an increasing percentage of the population on Medicare to pay for their medical costs will overwhelm the system.

Factors that increase the risk of chronic disability in the elderly—and thus drive up medical costs—are similar to those that cause premature mortality in younger people. These factors include smoking, poor diet, physical inactivity, and unsafe driving practices. Public health aims to prevent the major killers, such as cardiovascular disease, cancer, diabetes, and injuries, but it also has a role in secondary and tertiary prevention of a number of problems common in elderly patients that can adversely affect their independence and quality of life. These include over-medication, osteoporosis, falls, impairment of vision and hearing, impairments of the mouth, and Alzheimer's disease and other dementias.

A key question in planning for the future is whether the compression of mortality—the increasing probability that people will survive until the biological limit of lifespan—will be accompanied by a compression of morbidity, permitting people to remain healthy until shortly before they die. As medical costs of the elderly have grown, and as the baby-boom generation has begun to retire, it has become clear that current trends will cause the system to be overwhelmed. To address this situation, various proposals for rationing medical care have been put forward. Evidence on geographic variations in end-of-life care intensity and cost suggests that care could be delivered much more efficiently without sacrificing quality. The best hope for avoiding the need for rationing, while simultaneously improving quality of life for the elderly, would be to devise a way of integrating public health measures with the medical system to prevent chronic disease in the elderly, thereby reducing the need and demand for medical care.

References

1. U.S. Census Bureau, "65 Plus in the United States: 2010," June 2014, https://www.census.gov/content /dam/Census/library/publications/2014/demo/p23 -212.pdf, accessed October 16, 2019.

2. U.S. Census Bureau, "Population Estimates Show Aging Across Race Groups Differs," June 20, 2019, https:// www.census.gov/newsroom/press-releases/2019 /estimates-characteristics.html, accessed October 16, 2019.

3. Centers for Disease Control and Prevention, "United States Life Tables, 2017," *National Statistics Vital Reports*, June 24, 2019, https://www.cdc.gov/nchs/data/nvsr /nvsr68/nvsr68_07-508.pdf, accessed September 14, 2019.

4. U.S. Census Bureau, "Centenarians in the United States, 1990," July 1999, https://www.census.gov/prod /99pubs/p23-199.pdf, accessed October 16, 2019.

5. U.S. Census Bureau, "American FactFinder, Annual Estimates of the Resident Population by Sex, Single Year of Age, Race, and Hispanic Origin for the United States: 2017 Population Estimates," July 1, 2017, https://factfinder .census.gov/faces/tableservices/jsf/pages/productview .xhtml?src=bkmk, accessed October 16, 2019.

6. Federal Interagency Forum on Aging-Related Statistics, "2016 Older Americans: Key Indicators of Well-Being," https://agingstats.gov/docs/LatestReport /Older-Americans-2016-Key-Indicators-of -WellBeing.pdf, accessed October 16, 2019.

7. J. F. Fries, "Measuring and Monitoring Success in Compressing Morbidity," *Annals of Internal Medicine* 139 (2003): 456–459.

8. K. G. Manton, "Recent Declines in Chronic Disability in the Elderly U.S. Population: Risk Factors and Future Dynamics," *Annual Review of Public Health* 29 (2008): 91–113.

9. Centers for Disease Control and Prevention, "Nursing Home Residents per 1,000 Population by Age, Sex, and Ethnicity, U.S., 1977–2004," slide 24, https://www.cdc.gov/nchs/ppt/aging/aging_english.ppt, accessed October 16, 2019.

10. S. H. Allaire, M. P. LaValley, S. R. Evans, G. T. O'Connor, M. Kelly-Hayes, R. F. Meenan, et al., "Evidence for Decline in Disability and Improved Health Among Persons Aged 55 to 70 Years: The Framingham Heart Study," *American Journal of Public Health* 89 (1997): 1678–1683.

11. E. M. Crimmins, "Trends in the Health of the Elderly," *Annual Review of Public Health* 25 (2004): 79–98.

12. A. J. Vita, R. B. Terry, H. B. Hubert, and J. F. Fries, "Aging, Health Risks, and Cumulative Disability," *New England Journal of Medicine* 338 (1998): 1035–1066.

13. Centers for Disease Control and Prevention, "*Health, United States, 2017*," 2017, https://www.cdc.gov/nchs/data/hus/hus17.pdf, accessed October 16, 2019.

14. R. Sturm, J. S. Ringel, and T. Andreyeva, "Increasing Obesity Rates and Disability Trends," *Health Affairs* 23 (2004): 199–205.

15. F. Grodstein, M. J. Stampfer, G. A. Colditz, W. C. Willett, J. E. Manson, M. Joffe, et al., "Postmenopausal Hormone Therapy and Mortality," *New England Journal of Medicine* 336 (1997): 1769–1775.

16. F. Goodstein et al., "Understanding the Divergent Data on Postmenopausal Hormone Therapy," *New England Journal of Medicine* 348 (2003): 645–650.

17. P. Cram, X. Lu, S. L. Kates, J. A. Singh, Y. Li, and B. R. Wolf, "Total Knee Arthroplasty Volume, Utilization, and Outcomes Among Medicare Beneficiaries, 1991–2010," *Journal of the American Medical Association* 308 (2012): 1227–1235.

18. Mayo Clinic, "Incidence of Cataract Surgery Continues to Increase Steadily," April 2013, https://www.mayoclinic.org/medical-professionals/clinical-updates/ophthalmology/incidence-cataract-surgery-continues-increase-steadily, accessed October 12, 2019.

19. Institute of Medicine, *The Second 50 Years: Promoting Health and Preventing Disability* (Washington, DC: National Academies Press, 1990).

20. U.S. Department of Health and Human Services, *Bone Health and Osteoporosis: A Report of the Surgeon General* (Washington, DC: U.S. Government Printing Office, 2004).

21. S. Schnell, S. M. Friedman, D. A. Mendelson, K. W. Bingham, and S. L. Kates, "The 1-Year Mortality of Patients Treated in a Hip Fracture Program for Elders," *Geriatric Orthopaedic Surgery & Rehabilitation* 1 (2010): 6–14.

22. M. E. Tinetti, "Preventing Falls in Elderly Persons," *New England Journal of Medicine* 348 (2003): 42–49.

23. Mayo Clinic, "Healthy Aging, Fall Prevention: Simple Tips to Prevent Falls," October 4, 2019, https://www.mayoclinic.org/healthy-lifestyle/healthy-aging/in-depth/fall-prevention/art-20047358/, accessed October 16, 2019.

24. H. A. Bischoff-Ferrari, B. Dawson-Hughes, W. C. Willett, H. B. Staehelin, M. G. Bazemore, R. Y. Zee, and J. B. Wong, "Effect of Vitamin D on Falls: A Meta-Analysis," *Journal of the American Medical Association* 291 (2004): 1999–2006.

25. National Eye Institute, "Eye Health Topics," https://www.nei.nih.gov/health/, accessed October 12, 2019.

26. N. Parekh, R. J. Chappell, A. E. Millen, D. M. Albert, and J. A. Mares, "Association Between Vitamin D and Age-Related Macular Degeneration in the Third National Health and Nutrition Examination Survey, 1988 Through 1994," *Archives of Ophthalmology* 125 (2007): 661–669.

27. National Institute on Deafness and Other Communication Disorders, "Age-Related Hearing Loss," July 17, 2018, https://www.nidcd.nih.gov/health/hearing/Pages/Age-Related-Hearing-Loss.aspx, accessed October 12, 2019.

28. Medicare.gov, "Your Medicare Coverage: Is My Test, Item or Service Covered?", https://www.medicare.gov/coverage/, accessed October 15, 2019.

29. Alzheimer's Association, "2019 Alzheimer's Disease Facts and Figures," https://www.alz.org/media/documents/alzheimers-facts-and-figures-2019-r.pdf, accessed October 15, 2019.

30. Centers for Disease Control and Prevention, "Alzheimer's Disease and Healthy Aging," https://www.cdc.gov/aging/aginginfo/alzheimers.htm, October 15, 2019.

31. National Institute on Aging, "Alzheimer's Disease: Unraveling the Mystery," January 22, 2015, https://adrccares.org/wp-content/uploads/2016/01/alzheimers_disease_unraveling_the_mystery_0.pdf, accessed October 15, 2019.

32. J. Marx, "Preventing Alzheimer's: A Lifelong Commitment?", *Science* 309 (2005): 864–866.

33. U.S Centers for Medicare and Medicaid Services, "CMS Program Statistics: 2017 Medicare Enrollment Section," April 26, 2019, https://www.cms.gov/Research-Statistics-Data-and-Systems/Statistics-Trends-and-Reports/CMSProgramStatistics/2017/2017_Enrollment.html, accessed October 15, 2019.

34. U.S. Social Security Administration, "Fast Facts & Figures About Social Security, 2019," https://www.ssa.gov/policy/docs/chartbooks/fast_facts/2019/fast_facts19.html#contributions, accessed October 15, 2019.

35. Kaiser Family Foundation, "Medicare Spending Per Enrollee, by State," https://www.kff.org/medicare/state-indicator/per-enrollee-spending-by-residence/, accessed October 15, 2019.

36. Kaiser Family Foundation, "The Facts on Medicare Spending and Financing," August 20, 2019, https://www.kff.org/medicare/issue-brief/the-facts-on-medicare-spending-and-financing/, accessed October 15, 2019.

37. Kaiser Family Foundation, "An Overview of Medicare," February 13, 2019, https://www.kff.org/medicare/issue-brief/an-overview-of-medicare/, accessed October 15, 2019.

38. Kaiser Family Foundation, "Medicare Advantage," June 6, 2019, https://www.kff.org/medicare/fact-sheet/medicare-advantage, accessed October 16, 2019.

39. Centers for Medicare and Medicaid Services, "NHE Fact Sheet," April 26, 2019, https://www.cms.gov/research-statistics-data-and-systems/statistics-trends-and-reports/nationalhealthexpenddata/nhe-fact-sheet.html, accessed October 15, 2019.

40. Kaiser Family Foundation, "An Overview of the Medicare Part D Prescription Drug Benefit," October 12, 2018, https://www.kff.org/medicare/fact-sheet/the-medicare-prescription-drug-benefit-fact-sheet/, accessed October 16, 2019.

41. Kaiser Family Foundation, "Medicare Part D in 2018: The Latest on Enrollment, Premiums, and Cost Sharing," May 17, 2018, https://www.kff.org/medicare/issue-brief/medicare-part-d-in-2018-the-latest-on-enrollment-premiums-and-cost-sharing/, accessed October 15, 2019.

42. Medicaid.gov, "Medicaid Expenditures for Long-Term Services and Supports in FY 2016," May 2018, https://www.medicaid.gov/medicaid/ltss/downloads/reports-and-evaluations/ltssexpenditures2016.pdf, accessed October 16, 2019.

43. Associated Press, "Gov. Lamm Asserts Elderly, If Very Ill, Have 'Duty to Die,'" *The New York Times*, March 29, 1994.

44. D. C. Goodman et al., "Trends and Variations in End-of-Life Care for Medicare Beneficiaries with Severe Chronic Illness," April 12, 2011, https://www.dartmouthatlas.org/downloads/reports/EOL_Trend_Report_0411.pdf, accessed October 16, 2019.

45. R. M. Arnold and M. L. Zeidel, "Dialysis in Frail Elders: A Role for Palliative Care," *New England Journal of Medicine* 361 (2009): 1597–1598.

46. G. A. Sachs, "Dying from Dementia," *New England Journal of Medicine* 361 (2009): 1595–1596.

47. R. Pear, "Researchers Find Huge Variations in End-of-Life Treatment," *The New York Times*, April 7, 2008.

48. J. F. Fries, C. E. Koop, J. Sokolov, C. E. Beadle, and D. Wright, "Beyond Health Promotion: Reducing Need and Demand for Medical Care," *Health Affairs* 17 (1998): 70–84.

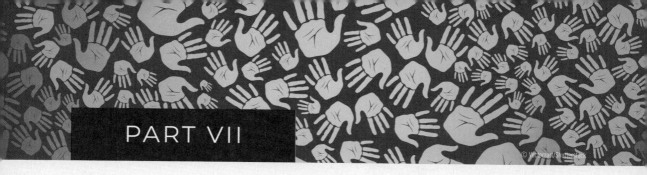

The Future of Public Health

CHAPTER 30

Emergency Response

Emergency Preparedness, Post-9/11

KEY TERMS

Bioterrorism
Department of Homeland
    Security
Federal Emergency
    Management Agency (FEMA)

Incident Command System (ICS)
Model State Emergency Health
    Powers Act
National Incident Management
    System (NIMS)

Office of Emergency
    Management (OEM)
Pandemic
Strategic National Stockpile

The events of September 2001 confronted the United States with a new awareness of its vulnerability. The attacks on the World Trade Center and the Pentagon made it clear that the nation was threatened by enemies who wished to terrorize it using nonconventional weapons and that military and intelligence agencies were unequipped to defend against them. A series of anthrax-containing letters sent through the mail, while causing only minimal loss of life, exposed a threat from another nonconventional weapon, suggesting the equally terrifying possibility of epidemics for which health agencies were unprepared. The successes and, mostly, the failures of the nation's response to these events forced national soul-searching and mobilization of resources to ensure that the United States would not again be caught by surprise. However, the nation again proved to be unprepared in August 2005, when

New Orleans and the surrounding areas were hit with a natural disaster in the form of Hurricane Katrina. Despite extensive planning for emergencies by federal, state, and local governments, especially after 9/11, it became apparent during and after the hurricane that important segments of the New Orleans population had not been considered in the plans, with tragic consequences.

The terrorism-driven plane crashes and the intentional spread of pathogenic bacteria required law-enforcement responses aimed at identifying responsibility, punishing the perpetrators, and preventing further harmful actions. These events also prompted public health responses to deal with the consequences of the incidents and to prevent further injury and illness. In responding to natural disasters, such as hurricanes, public health has always had an important role. However, important lessons have been learned from the failures related to Hurricane Katrina, and it is hoped that further planning will better prepare the nation to deal with future emergencies of all kinds.

Types of Disasters and Public Health Responses

Disasters cause death, injury, disease, and property damage on a scale beyond the routine emergencies to which the health system is accustomed. However, many natural disasters are predictable—for example, hurricanes, blizzards, and forest fires—and vulnerable areas generally have plans to deal with them—although the adequacy of these plans may not become obvious until they are put to the test. These plans usually include prior evacuation of the population in affected areas to minimize negative health effects and loss of life. Other natural disasters may be unpredictable, like earthquakes, but even these unpredictable disasters tend to occur in specific geographic areas—California, for example—and therefore allow communities to be prepared through strict building codes, requirements that appliances be secured, easy turn-off of gas and electricity, and so on.

Human-made and technological disasters are generally unpredictable, although the potential for these events can sometimes be identified and the possibility minimized through government regulation and community planning. Typical technological disasters include industrial explosions, hazardous material releases, building and bridge collapses, and transportation crashes that may also cause a chemical or radioactive release. The presence of an industrial facility or a nuclear power plant should prompt a community to conduct emergency planning appropriate to the facility and the possible exposures. Detailed planning is more complicated for plane crashes and crashes of trains or trucks carrying hazardous materials, which may occur at unforeseen sites. Most terrorist events fall into the category of technological disasters. An act of bioterrorism could cause a disaster, but it would be expected to mimic a natural disease outbreak and demand the same public health response that a natural epidemic would require.

Most disasters, natural or human-made, cause immediate injury to many residents of the affected area. Sometimes specially trained and equipped rescue personnel are needed to locate and extricate people buried in the rubble of collapsed buildings or to move people out of harm's way in fires or floods. Police and firefighters are often on the front line in combating a disaster. The injured require emergency medical care and transportation to hospitals. If hazardous materials are involved, measures must be taken to protect the rescuers and medical personnel. The situation can get even more complex when volunteers join the rescue efforts. In some cases, family members might be wandering around anxiously searching for loved ones. These individuals may also need protection from hazards in the affected environment. When an incident involves many deaths, procedures must be established to identify victims and to communicate with their families. In all disaster situations, there is a critical need for coordination of activities.

Disasters also create conditions that cause health risks for the survivors. These tend to be amplifications of the general environmental hazards that public health deals with routinely: contamination of air, water, and food; exposure to toxic chemicals or radioactivity; and injury hazards such as fallen power lines and unstable buildings. The survivors need food and potable water; some people with chronic diseases may urgently need medications such as insulin or cardiac drugs. People may be left homeless by the disaster, or they may be displaced and need temporary shelter.

What is the role of public health in all these activities? One of its most important functions is planning in advance of the emergency, working with other agencies to ensure coordination of all the activities of the responders. Local public health authorities should be knowledgeable about the community and its resources because they have the responsibility to protect the health of the survivors. One of the outcomes of the 9/11 attacks was the recognition of weaknesses in coordination and communication of the emergency responders. This led to a concerted effort, organized by the federal government, to ensure that all communities have disaster-response plans in place so that any future attack may be met by an effective response. This planning process is intended to have the added benefit of preparing the nation to deal with other natural or human-made disasters. In fact, many private and public organizations actively promote the need for "all-hazards planning." Unfortunately, the response by all levels of government to Hurricane Katrina demonstrated the weaknesses in the previous planning.

New York's Response to the World Trade Center Attacks

When two jet planes hit the World Trade Center towers on September 11, 2001, at 8:46 and 9:02 a.m., New York City police, firefighters, and emergency medical workers rushed to the site. The firefighters and police launched rescue and evacuation efforts, and emergency medical workers set up temporary medical posts to treat injured survivors. The city's **Office of Emergency Management (OEM)** began directing activities from its headquarters nearby at 7 World Trade Center. Ambulances came from all over the city, and hospitals in all five boroughs prepared to receive large numbers of casualties.

Between 13,000 and 15,000 people were successfully evacuated from the towers before the south tower collapsed at 9:59 a.m. and the north tower at 10:28 a.m.[1] Tragically, 2801

people died, including 149 passengers on the planes.[2] The fact that so many people survived the disaster showed that, in many ways, the emergency response efforts were successful. Subsequent to the 1993 bombing at the World Trade Center, improvements in fire safety measures had been established, including better lighting in the stairways and evacuation drills. However, many things also went wrong on September 11. The building housing the OEM headquarters was severely damaged by the collapse of the north tower soon after the attack and had to be evacuated, significantly undermining OEM's ability to coordinate the rescue efforts. Moreover, OEM's communication depended on an antenna located on the roof of the north tower.[3] The police department and the fire department each had its own radio communications system, but they used different frequencies and could not communicate with each other. Poor communication led to confusion for some evacuees when some stairways were blocked, and they were not informed of alternative routes down. Doors to the roof were locked, trapping people who worked above the impact sites and tried to escape by climbing upward. Tragically, the fire department radios worked only sporadically in the high-rise buildings, so, despite attempts to warn them, at least 121 of the 343 firefighters who died were in the north tower when it collapsed. They had not realized that the south tower had fallen.[4]

After the buildings collapsed, the air was filled with dust, soot, and smoke, posing a threat to the thousands of rescue workers, cleanup workers, and later, residents and people who worked in downtown Manhattan, who were allowed to return to their homes and offices. An estimated 5000 tons of asbestos had been released into the air due to the destruction of the buildings.[5] Lead, other metals, dioxin, and polychlorinated biphenyls (PCBs) were also detected in the soot, as fires continued to burn for months after the disaster. Although workers at the site should have been wearing respirators to protect their lungs, few of them did in the early days, and many of them developed the notorious "World Trade Center cough." It was not clear which agencies were responsible for determining when the area was safe. A priority at the highest levels of government was to get the downtown area back in business, especially Wall Street, which was reopened only six days after the collapse. Politicians rushed to reassure New Yorkers that the environment was safe, but there was no scientific basis for these reassurances, and their statements were received with appropriate skepticism.[6] The U.S. Environmental Protection Agency was accused of covering up the risk.

The Departments of Health of New York City and New York State had the responsibility to carry out routine public health functions, under not-so-routine conditions, during the period after the disaster. They issued death certificates and burial permits. They monitored food and drinking water served to emergency workers to ensure that it was safe. They cleaned up food in abandoned restaurants at the site to prevent outbreaks of rodents. Because of concerns that the attack might have included biological agents, the Centers for Disease Control and Prevention (CDC) sent officers to monitor hospital emergency rooms for patients with unusual symptoms. Later ongoing surveillance activities included sampling of dust and debris near the site to assess risk and monitoring of symptoms of cleanup workers and area residents. In addition to respiratory symptoms, insomnia, headaches, and dizziness, millions of survivors and workers suffered from psychological distress suggestive of post-traumatic stress disorder. Mental health agencies arranged for counseling. Victim location services were established for families with missing relatives, and shelters for displaced residents were set up. At least 19 city, state, and federal government agencies, as well as several academic, medical, and other organizations, were involved in the public health and medical response to the disaster.[2]

Response to Hurricane Katrina

In 2005, Hurricane Katrina became the costliest natural disaster to ever hit the United States, inflicting $169 billion in damage after adjusting for inflation. (In comparison, the next three most expensive natural disasters—Hurricane Harvey in Texas in 2017, Hurricane Maria in Puerto Rico in 2017, and Hurricane Sandy in New York in 2012—caused $130 billion, $94 billion, and $74 billion in damage, respectively.[7]) Hurricane Katrina was not a surprise. Hurricanes regularly make landfall along the Gulf Coast, frequently threatening Louisiana. Parts of New Orleans were flooded by Hurricane Betsy in 1965, and the city was threatened by Hurricane Camille in 1969, Hurricane Andrew in 1992, and Hurricane Ivan in 2004.[8] Some 80% of New Orleans is below sea level and the city is essentially surrounded by water, bordered by the Mississippi River on the south and Lake Pontchartrain on the north, which is connected with the Gulf of Mexico on the East.[9] The city is kept dry by levees, built by the U.S. Army Corps of Engineers, that have long been known to be inadequate to withstand a major storm; funds for planned upgrades have been repeatedly cut from the federal budget.

Tropical Storm Katrina was identified and named on Wednesday, August 24, 2005, while it was in the vicinity of the Bahamas. On Thursday, August 25, the storm was upgraded to a category one hurricane as it passed through Florida into the Gulf. At that point, the **Federal Emergency Management Agency (FEMA)** National Coordination Center was activated. On Friday, the National Hurricane Center forecasted that the hurricane would strike east of New Orleans, and Louisiana governor Kathleen Blanco declared a state of emergency. On Saturday, Katrina was upgraded to category three and several parishes and coastal areas were ordered to evacuate. Contraflow traffic was instituted on all highways in southeastern Louisiana, allowing outgoing travel only. Governor Blanco called into duty 4000 National Guard troops. Early Sunday morning, Katrina was upgraded to a category four storm; a few hours later it was upgraded to category five, with winds of 160 miles per hour. At 10:00 a.m., the governor and Mayor Ray Nagin ordered mandatory evacuation of the city of New Orleans.[8,10]

On Sunday morning, the Superdome opened as a shelter of last resort. Cars were leaving Greater New Orleans at the rate of 18,000 per hour, and the highways were clogged. By the end of the day, an estimated 80% of the city's population of 458,000 had left, but more than 100,000 people did not have a car and were unable or unwilling to evacuate. Approximately 10,000 people were in the Superdome, and an unknown number were waiting out the storm in houses and other buildings in the region. Rain began to fall in the city around 9:00 p.m.

By early Monday morning, New Orleans was being pounded by wind and rain; power and telephone service had failed, and some of the levees had been breached. Generators provided dim light to the Superdome, but no air conditioning, and the air was stifling and stinking. Two holes opened up in the roof of the Superdome, which was a cesspool of human waste and garbage. Refugees taking shelter there faced a lack of food, water, and medicines. In various parts of the city the water was 4 to 15 feet deep. People were trapped in attics and clinging to rooftops. The Coast Guard and the Louisiana Department of Wildlife and Fisheries began going around in boats, rescuing people and taking them to the Convention Center, which did not have food, water, or other provisions for sheltering people. As the day progressed, the hurricane began to move away from the city.[8,10]

As of Tuesday morning, there were 20,000 people in the Convention Center. Patients and staff members were stranded in New Orleans hospitals, all but one of which were without power, and conditions were deteriorating.

There were dead bodies in the street, floating in polluted water. Some people drowned in their beds because they were old or disabled and could not get up and go to higher ground; others drowned in their attics because there was nowhere higher to go. In one nursing home that did not evacuate, 35 elderly or handicapped people died in the flood; five more died within a week, probably from the stress of the ordeal. Although some hospitals evacuated before the storm and others were on high enough ground to escape flooding, three of the poorest hospitals suffered through the storm in primitive conditions, in stifling heat, without electricity to run ventilators or other medical equipment; some ran out of food and medicines.[8,10]

As of Wednesday morning, 26,000 people were in the Superdome. U.S. Secretary of Health and Human Services Michael Leavitt declared that a public health emergency existed in the states affected by Katrina. At 2:00 p.m., buses began evacuating seriously ill and disabled people from the Superdome. On Thursday through Sunday, patients and medical personnel were evacuated from hospitals by helicopter or boat to a makeshift field hospital at the airport. Many patients did not survive that long.[8,10]

An accurate death toll from Katrina will probably never be known. According to a report by the National Hurricane Center, the number of fatalities exceeded 1200.[11] Most of these victims were poor and black. In fact, 68% of the pre-Katrina population of New Orleans was black, 23% had incomes below the poverty level, and 21% lacked a vehicle—all factors that contributed to the high death toll.[12] The majority of the fatalities were people who did not or could not evacuate ahead of the storm. This raises a question: Why did so many people apparently ignore orders to evacuate?

Later surveys of survivors from New Orleans who were evacuated after the storm to shelters elsewhere found several common themes in people's decisions. One study analyzed the findings according to the Health Belief Model (HBM).[13] In regard to the first factor in the HBM, the extent to which people felt susceptible to the threat, many long-time residents felt they could survive because they had survived many previous hurricanes without serious problems. Another source of optimism was religious faith: Many people believed God would take care of them.

In terms of the second factor in the HBM, the perceived severity of the threat, many interviewees reported that they were confused about the messages from the governor and the mayor. The early evacuation orders were not mandatory, and residents interpreted this recommendation as meaning that the threat was not severe. By the time the officials made the order mandatory, they said, it was too late to leave.

In regard to the third factor in the HBM, barriers to action, poor blacks perceived many barriers—financial, logistical, and community. Orders to evacuate were not clear on how or where to go. Even families that had a car may have lacked money for gas or worried about paying for necessities while traveling, or their family might have been too large to fit comfortably in the car. Family members who were old or had health problems made it difficult for the whole family to evacuate. Some people were reluctant to leave their homes without their pets, making it difficult even to go to a shelter. Some people were afraid they would lose their jobs if they left the city. Others felt they needed to stay behind to protect their property from looters.[13–15]

Many of those individuals who stayed in New Orleans during the storm felt they were victims of racism. This feeling was reinforced by incidents in which residents of black neighborhoods were prevented by police from entering richer, white neighborhoods when they tried to get to safer ground. One rumor suggested that levees in poorer areas had been purposely dynamited to protect whiter, richer areas of the city.[9] One later survey found that 68% of survivors thought that government would have responded more quickly if more New Orleans residents had been wealthy and white.[14]

The scale of the disaster was well beyond the coping ability of a single city or even a single state. Not only was 80% of New Orleans flooded, but widespread destruction occurred throughout southern Louisiana, Mississippi, Alabama, and Florida. Katrina turned out to be the deadliest hurricane since 1928 and the costliest natural disaster on record in the United States.[7,16] Then, 26 days later, Hurricane Rita made landfall near the Texas–Louisiana border, interfering with hurricane-response activities in New Orleans and forcing evacuation of coastal regions of Louisiana and Texas, including some areas where New Orleans evacuees had taken shelter.

In New Orleans itself, there was a desperate need for help from outside the city—a need that should have been filled by FEMA and the National Guard. Help from these fronts was tragically inadequate, for a number of reasons. Governor Blanco called up the Louisiana National Guard on Friday before the storm struck, but the ranks were depleted because 35% to 40% of the members had been called to active duty in Iraq and Afghanistan, along with much of their equipment. The troops patrolled the streets of the city, provided security at the Superdome and the Convention Center, and delivered what food and water were available. Eventually, National Guard troops from other states were sent to New Orleans to help with evacuation and cleanup.[8,10]

FEMA was a weaker agency than it had been during the Bill Clinton administration, when it was a cabinet-level agency with a professional disaster-relief professional as a director. Under President George W. Bush, FEMA had been incorporated into the U.S. Department of Homeland Security, where the focus was on terrorism; its budget had been cut repeatedly, and it had lost many of its experienced staff.[10,17] Moreover, its director, Michael Brown, was a political crony of the president, clearly incompetent for the job. Despite the notoriously untrue Bush remark on his visit to New Orleans Friday, September 2—"Brownie, you're doing a heck of a job"—Brown was severely criticized in the press, by Congress, and within the administration, and he resigned in mid-September.[10]

President Bush himself was mostly absent from the early days of the crisis. He had been on an extended vacation at his ranch in Crawford, Texas, throughout August, and he had not seemed to pay much attention to the hurricane as it developed. On Tuesday, August 30, he delivered a speech on Iraq in San Diego, making only brief, reassuring comments on Hurricane Katrina. He returned to Washington, D.C., on Wednesday, declaring that he was cutting his vacation two days short. Vice President Richard Cheney was on vacation in Wyoming.[10]

Hurricanes Katrina and Rita left many public health problems in New Orleans and the surrounding area, some of which are still unaddressed. Because most of the city's population, estimated at 485,000 in 2000, was evacuated either before or after the hurricanes, it stood at fewer than several thousand by the end of the first week in September 2005. A RAND Corporation study found that, as of December 2005, approximately 91,000 people had returned to their homes, and it was estimated that this number would rise to about 198,000.[18] The population has continued to grow, and the U.S. Census Bureau estimated the population to be 391,006 in 2018, with somewhat smaller proportions of whites and blacks, more Hispanics and Asians, and fewer children than before the storm.[19] Many New Orleans evacuees are still living in communities throughout the country.

Many homes in New Orleans were destroyed by the floods and many damaged houses remain, especially in the poorer areas of the city that were badly inundated. Housing problems account for some health problems among hurricane survivors. FEMA had supplied trailers for people whose homes had been destroyed, and it later became apparent that the air in these trailers was contaminated with unhealthy levels of formaldehyde. Mold, common in many homes that had been under water during the floods, caused respiratory problems in people with allergies. Wells were contaminated. Mosquito-borne diseases posed a threat, as did home invasions by rodents and snakes. An estimated 50% of survivors are expected to suffer from persistent psychological trauma and post-traumatic stress disorder.[20] The full extent of the health consequences of the disaster may never be known.

Principles of Emergency Planning and Preparedness

The weaknesses evident in the response to the 9/11 attacks called attention to the need for advance planning for possible future disasters. After 9/11, the federal government funded planning efforts throughout the nation, but obviously the results were not adequate to be ready for Hurricane Katrina. Two essential ingredients of an emergency plan missing in both New York and New Orleans were coordination and communication. The lack of these functions in New York resulted in part from the fact that the emergency management headquarters and communication antenna were disabled in the event. Likewise, in New Orleans, communication was disabled by the loss of electricity and telephones throughout the region. This situation highlights the importance of emergency system redundancy. A backup plan for managing the crisis in the absence of these resources should have been in place in both places. Redundancy in the communication system would have ensured, for example, that critical information about evacuation routes could be shared with everyone in the World Trade Center towers. In New Orleans, an unambiguous message to evacuate did not come until too close to the time the hurricane struck for the most vulnerable members of the population to act on it. The situations were aggravated in New York by a history of competition between the police and fire departments and the OEM, and in New Orleans by the lack of a competent federal official with whom the governor and mayor could coordinate.

Because any disaster will require a coordinated response from a number of different agencies, the basic principle used in the immediate response to an emergency is the **Incident Command System (ICS)**.[21] This approach puts a single person, who has responsibility for managing and coordinating the response, in charge at the scene. Disaster response is generally managed by authorities from local government agencies, because the response must be immediate and local authorities are closest to the scene and know the territory. The lead agency is often the fire department or the police department, while the state and federal governments provide technical assistance and backup resources.

Agencies involved in the ICS might include an emergency operations center, the fire department, the police department, the emergency medical system, the public health agency, the American Red Cross, the electric company and gas company, and, sometimes, the highway department or, as in the case of the World Trade Center, the Port Authority and the manager of the buildings. Most of these agencies would know their responsibilities in an emergency and would have practiced them as part of their planning and preparedness process. Different agencies might have different communication networks, but it is critically important that all communications be integrated. The public health agency, in coordination with emergency medical services and hospitals, is responsible for directing patients to the appropriate level of care and for dispatching ambulances according to the availability of appropriate resources such as operating rooms and intensive care units. On September 11, one nearby hospital was swamped with "walking wounded" and critical patients, while a trauma center located only three miles away sat idle.[3] In New Orleans, hospitals and nursing homes lacked plans for evacuating their patients, and governments were not prepared to assist in these efforts. FEMA has now developed a system called the **National Incident Management System (NIMS)**, which standardizes the organizational structures, processes, and procedures that communities should employ in planning for an emergency. It also provides guidelines and protocols for integration of all levels of government and the voluntary and private sectors in coping with a disaster.[22]

In a guide to public health management of disasters published by the American Public Health Association, the author lists 12 tasks or problems likely to occur in most disasters.[21] All of these tasks depend on effective interorganizational coordination and should be sorted out and practiced ahead of time.

- Sharing information: Two-way radios are often the most reliable way to communicate, but it is important to choose a common frequency.
- Resource management: Personnel should identify themselves at a check-in area and should be given an assignment and a radio; arrival of equipment and supplies should be logged in, and these resources should be distributed where they are most needed.
- Warnings should be issued and evacuations ordered by the appropriate agencies. The warnings should be delivered, usually by the mass media, in a manner that will prompt appropriate action by the population.
- Warnings must be unambiguous and consistent, and must include specific information about who is at risk and what actions should be taken.
- Search and rescue operations should be coordinated so that casualties are entered into the emergency medical services system and the healthcare system.
- The mass media should be used to warn the public about health risks after the disaster as an effective public health measure.

- Triage, a method for sorting survivors based on the severity of their injury and the need for treatment, should be established at the scene by trained medical personnel.
- Casualty distribution: Protocols should be established to ensure that patients are distributed among available hospitals or other facilities.
- Tracking of patients and other survivors is difficult but, to the extent it is possible, should be done to avert later difficulties.
- Establishing methods to care for patients with all levels of need should be part of the advance planning. Many survivors seek care for minor injuries or may need prescription medications for chronic medical conditions. Backup arrangements should be made for care of patients when hospitals and other healthcare centers are damaged, including backup supplies of power and water and plans to evacuate to alternative sites.
- Management of volunteers and donations should be planned for; resources should be collected, organized, and distributed at a site outside the disaster area to avoid disrupting ongoing emergency operations.
- Expect the unexpected. Be ready to respond to unanticipated problems.

The plan should be practiced at least once, and preferably once per year. The exercises can be desktop simulations, field exercises, or drills. The time for partners to meet each other is before—not after—the disaster strikes.

Since September 11, the federal government has provided substantial resources to states and major metropolitan areas to assure public health preparedness, including preparedness for natural disasters, bioterrorism, and chemical and radiological disasters. Since 2002, the CDC has invested more than $9 billion in state, local, tribal, and territorial public health departments to upgrade their ability to respond to a range of public health threats.[23] These funds are used for planning, training,

improving communication and coordination, strengthening hospitals and laboratories, and improving epidemiology and disease surveillance in state and local areas. A **Strategic National Stockpile** includes medical supplies, antibiotics, vaccines, and antidotes for chemical agents. In the event of an emergency, federal personnel can deliver these supplies to the people who need them anywhere in the United States within 12 hours.

An evaluation of the progress made by 12 metropolitan areas between September 11, 2001, and May 2003 found that emergency preparedness had improved, but gaps still remained. The researchers highlighted three communities of different sizes that they found to be especially strong in their level of preparedness: Syracuse, New York; Indianapolis, Indiana; and Orange County, California.[24] The success of these three communities is credited in part to previous experience with public health threats. Syracuse, for example, has a nuclear power plant nearby, which had stimulated the local population's concern about a nuclear accident or a terrorist attack. Indianapolis has done extensive planning over the years for the annual Indianapolis 500 auto races and other large sporting events. Orange County has experience in disaster planning because of the ongoing threat of earthquakes and fires; a nuclear power plant is also located nearby. Other factors that contribute to readiness, the researchers concluded, are strong leadership, successful collaboration, and adequate funding.[24]

Congressional hearings on the response to Hurricane Katrina, however, noted in early 2006 that whatever improvements had been made to our capacity to respond to natural or human-made disaster more than four years after 9/11, U.S. disaster preparedness remained dangerously inadequate. A report by a bipartisan committee of the U.S. House of Representatives identified failures at all levels of government. "All the little pigs built houses of straw," the report said. "Katrina was a national failure, an abdication of the most solemn obligation to provide for the common welfare."[25] Whether the nation would be better prepared today will not be known until the next emergency.

Bioterrorism Preparedness

The anthrax letters attack of fall 2001 constituted a terrorist attack just as surely as the 9/11 hijackings and plane crashes, and similarly spread terror in the American population, although it caused far fewer deaths. The anthrax letters were recognized to be a terrorist attack in part because of the heightened alertness created by the events of 9/11, and in part because anthrax is such a rare pathogen in humans. Anthrax had been identified as a possible agent of biowarfare in the planning that the federal government had been carrying out during the late 1990s. If a less conspicuous pathogen had been used, the attack might not have been recognized as quickly. For example, a 1984 *Salmonella* outbreak in Oregon was not recognized as a deliberate attack until much later, when the cult members who carried it

out quarreled publicly about the attack, and a criminal investigation was launched.[26]

Bioterrorism requires a very different kind of preparedness strategy than the response needed for dramatic disasters such as a hurricane or the attack on and collapse of the World Trade Center towers. The greatest challenge in bioterrorism preparedness might be the ability to recognize that an attack is under way. Accordingly, the CDC has coordinated extensive efforts throughout the nation to improve the public health infrastructure, understanding that the response to a biological attack must be the same as that for a natural disease outbreak. As Dr. Julie Gerberding, then director of the CDC said, "We are building . . . capacity [to handle biological terrorism] on the foundation of public health, but we are also using the new investments in [combating] terrorism to strengthen the public health foundation" because "these two programs are inextricably linked."[27]

The CDC has listed the pathogens most likely to be used in a terrorist attack. Category A agents include smallpox, anthrax, Ebola, and other hemorrhagic fever viruses (**Table 30-1**). These agents can be easily disseminated

Table 30-1 **Category A Bioterrorism Agents and Diseases**

Category A

The U.S. public health system and primary healthcare providers must be prepared to address varied biological agents, including pathogens that are rarely seen in the United States. High-priority agents include organisms that pose a risk to national security for the following reasons:

- They can be easily disseminated or transmitted person-to-person.
- They cause high mortality, with potential for major public health impact.
- They might cause public panic and social disruption.
- They require special action for public health preparedness.

Category A Agents/Diseases

- Anthrax (*Bacillus anthracis*)
- Botulism (*Clostridium botulinum* toxin)
- Plague (*Yersinia pestis*)
- Smallpox (*Variola major*)
- Tularemia (*Francisella tularensis*)
- Viral hemorrhagic fevers (filoviruses [e.g., Ebola, Marburg] and arenaviruses [e.g., Lassa, Junin])

Modified from Centers for Disease Control and Prevention, "Emergency Preparedness and Response, Bioterrorism Agents/Diseases," https://emergency.cdc.gov/agent/agentlist-category.asp, accessed October 16, 2019.

Table 30-2 **Steps in Preparing for Biological Attacks**

- Enhance epidemiologic capacity to detect and respond to biological attacks.
- Supply diagnostic reagents to state and local public health agencies.
- Establish communication programs to ensure delivery of accurate information.
- Enhance bioterrorism-related education and training for healthcare professionals.
- Prepare educational materials that will inform and reassure the public during and after a biological attack.
- Stockpile appropriate vaccines and drugs.
- Establish molecular surveillance for microbial strains, including unusual or drug-resistant strains.
- Support the development of diagnostic tests.
- Encourage research on antiviral drugs and vaccines.

Reproduced from Centers for Disease Control and Prevention, "Biological and Chemical Terrorism: Strategic Plan for Preparedness and Response, Recommendations of the CDC Strategic Planning Workshop," *Morbidity and Mortality Weekly Report* 49 (2000): RR-4: 5, www.cdc.gov/mmwr/preview/mmwrhtml/rr4904a1.htm, accessed October 17, 2019.

---

or transmitted person-to-person and cause high mortality, with potential for major public health impact. Recommendations for preparing for biological attacks are shown in **Table 30-2**.

The public health capacities that are being strengthened to improve recognition of a disease outbreak include the following:

- Educating physicians and other medical workers to recognize unusual diseases (unfortunately, the system failed in the case of Thomas Eric Duncan, whose Ebola infection was not suspected by medical workers when he showed up at the emergency room in Texas in 2014, although fortunately this was not a bioterrorist event)[28]
- Monitoring emergency rooms for certain patterns of symptoms
- Opening new laboratories with the capability of identifying unusual viruses and bacteria
- Improving communication between public health agencies at the local, state, and federal levels and the professionals and facilities most likely to first encounter affected patients

Surveillance activities include emergency room visits, calls to 911 and poison control centers, and pharmacy records to detect increased use of antibiotics and/or over-the-counter drugs. (One early indication of the 1993 cryptosporidiosis outbreak in Milwaukee was that pharmacies were selling out of medications for diarrhea.) Similar measures are important for recognizing chemical attacks as well, and the CDC coordinates an integrated network of state, local, federal, military, and international public health laboratories that can respond to both bioterrorism and chemical terrorism.[29] The U.S. Department of Agriculture is similarly conducting surveillance for animal diseases and other agricultural threats. Animal health is an important component of homeland security, both because of the need to protect the food supply and because many animal diseases also pose a threat to humans. An estimated 75% of emerging infections that have recently been identified in humans originate in animals—for example, bird flu, SARS, hantavirus, mad cow disease, and *Escherichia coli* O157:H7.[30] Computer networks serve to alert public health officials about significant or unusual findings from surveillance data. In addition to public health efforts to improve the ability to recognize a bioterrorist attack and identify the agent, the CDC has taken steps to improve response to the event, including establishing the Strategic National Stockpile, as previously described.

The spread of West Nile encephalitis across the country provided an opportunity and a challenge for the public health and medical care systems to develop and practice their response to a new infectious disease. When West Nile virus first appeared in 1999 in New York City, bioterrorism was considered as one possible explanation for its origin. That hypothesis was soon discarded, but the disease was closely monitored as it spreads to areas where it was unfamiliar. The mechanisms used to deal with the spread of West Nile virus are the same as those that would be used in a bioterrorist event.

The prospect of bioterrorism has raised other issues that affect the nation's ability to respond effectively. Among the most important of these is that public health officials need to have the legal power to take action to protect the public and contain an outbreak of an infectious disease. For example, these officials have to be able to isolate and quarantine people. Public health activities are, for the most part, controlled by state law, and the public health laws in many states predate modern scientific understanding of disease. Such laws may be outdated, inadequate, and inconsistent. For example, some states have laws that prevent sharing of surveillance information with other states; private property laws might prevent destruction of contaminated property or the imposed distribution of drugs and medical supplies to where they are needed; privacy laws might interfere with public health agencies' ability to obtain information from hospitals or pharmacies; and quarantine laws might be challenged by affected individuals and thus prevent prompt action.[31]

After the anthrax attacks of 2001, the CDC requested a group of legal and public health scholars to develop a **Model State Emergency Health Powers Act** that state legislatures could follow to update their laws. The suggested provisions include measures to encourage planning for emergencies; surveillance; managing property to ensure availability of vaccines, pharmaceuticals, and hospitals; powers to compel vaccination, testing, treatment, isolation, and quarantine when

necessary; and provision of information to the public. These measures would be activated when a public health emergency is declared and would include legal safeguards to protect personal rights while promoting the common good.[31] The model act was released in December 2001, and most states have passed at least some of the measures. The CDC has a public health law program that seeks to improve the understanding and use of law as a public health tool, to develop CDC's capacity to apply law to achieve public health goals, and to develop the legal preparedness of the public health system to address public health priorities.[32]

Another issue that has been raised but not so readily addressed is the problem of the nearly 30 million Americans who lack health insurance. If the first individuals to be exposed to an infectious agent are uninsured, they may choose not to seek medical care or may delay visiting an emergency room, thus spreading the pathogen and delaying the recognition that an outbreak is under way. "Their lack of insurance is a known risk to their own health, but it must now also be recognized as a risk to the nation's health," noted two public health experts.[33] The problem is compounded by a federal law, passed in 1996, that prohibits federally funded medical clinics from treating illegal immigrants. Unless it is made clear to the whole population that everyone with symptoms of a contagious illness should seek treatment and that they will not suffer legal or financial consequences from presenting themselves for a medical evaluation, the United States will be vulnerable to bioterrorism in a way different from any other developed country. The Affordable Care Act has helped to address this problem by reducing the number of uninsured Americans, but the problem of treating illegal immigrants remains because they are not covered by the act.

While the CDC is taking a major role in planning for bioterrorism, the **Department of Homeland Security** has been developing technological methods of detecting biological and chemical attacks, in hopes of recognizing an attack faster, even before people begin developing symptoms, and of identifying the biological or chemical agent. Monitoring devices with sensors that can detect bacteria, viruses, and toxins have been installed in more than 30 major American cities. These devices suck air through filters, which are periodically changed, and the filter paper taken to a laboratory for testing. It is not clear how effective these detectors would be in an attack, and many scientists are skeptical about the value of the monitoring systems. The Department of Homeland Security is supporting research to develop more sophisticated systems for environmental monitoring.[34]

Smallpox is the most dreaded of the possible bioterrorism agents. Thus, after the initial shock of the anthrax events in 2001, significant government planning efforts were devoted to the possibility of a bioterrorist attack using smallpox. Concerns have arisen that, although smallpox was officially eradicated in the 1970s, rogue nations might have obtained stocks of the virus from the former Soviet Union. A smallpox attack would be devastating. This disease is highly contagious, and there is no effective treatment. Approximately 30% of those infected with smallpox die. Virtually everyone in the world is susceptible to some extent, because immunizations have not been given in more than 40 years. A tabletop exercise, assuming that anonymous terrorists covertly sprayed smallpox virus in three shopping malls, had predicted 3 million hypothetical cases of the disease, of whom 1 million died.[35] Lessons learned from the exercise, which was conducted in June 2001 by policy scholars and former senior government officials, concluded that such an attack could cause breakdowns in essential institutions, disruption of democratic processes, civil disorder, loss of confidence in government, and reduced U.S. strategic flexibility. One of the participants testified to Congress that the exercise taught us that public health is a major national security issue.[36]

Pandemic Flu

Since the emergence of the avian flu in Asia in the 1990s, concerns have focused on the possibility of its turning into a **pandemic**. The virus had a frighteningly high mortality rate among people who were infected, but so far has not demonstrated easy transmissibility from one human to another. The prospect of a mutated avian flu virus that readily spreads within the population, however, has prompted governments to make plans for how to respond if this should occur. Measures that would be needed include rapid development and manufacture of a vaccine targeted to the specific pandemic strain, surveillance of the virus's spread, and stockpiling of antiviral drugs and antibiotics to combat the secondary bacterial infections that killed many of the victims of the 1918 flu. In part due to bioterrorism planning, the CDC has intensified its surveillance activities, and the Strategic National Stockpile would be as useful in a flu pandemic as it would in the event of a bioterrorism attack. Most flu vaccines are produced by growing viruses in eggs, a months-long process that requires large numbers of eggs.[37] Newer methods have been developed that require less time. A vaccine using cells grown in culture was approved by the Food and Drug Administration in 2012. Most efficient in the event of a pandemic is a vaccine using recombinant DNA technology that was approved in 2013.[38]

Other concerns in planning for a severe pandemic include hospital capacity and the need for mechanical respirators. Symptoms of the 1918 flu were similar to those of the severe acute respiratory syndrome (SARS) epidemic, which required intensive care for those affected. It is assumed that more lives of flu patients could be saved by modern medical treatments than was possible in 1918. However, because flu spreads much more readily than SARS does, the medical system would be quickly overwhelmed by a flu epidemic of the severity that occurred in 1918. Planning for pandemic flu has included discussions of how to allocate scarce medical resources when not everyone can be helped.

Unexpectedly, the pandemic that appeared in 2009—the first flu pandemic since the Hong Kong flu of 1968—was not the avian flu but a swine flu, H1N1 instead of H5N1, that turned out to be much less severe than avian flu. The United States was relatively prepared to put its plans into effect. The H1N1 pandemic emerged in the spring, at the end of the normal influenza season, and a public health emergency was declared. The virus was quickly isolated and provided to manufacturers, which were encouraged to begin producing vaccines. Immunizations began in October, but production of the vaccine proceeded more slowly than expected. The regular seasonal flu vaccine was expected not to provide protection against H1N1 flu, so both immunizations were necessary for complete protection.[39,40]

Conclusion

Public health has an important role in preparing for and responding to all kinds of emergencies and disasters, natural and human-made. The immediate response to a disaster must include emergency medical care for the injured and evacuation of survivors. In cases where the disaster can be predicted, such as a hurricane, the safest response is to evacuate people in advance. Later needs focus on ensuring that air, water, and food are not contaminated and eliminating injury hazards such as fallen power lines and unstable buildings. Generally the disaster response is carried out by a number of agencies, so coordination among them is very important. After 9/11, the federal government provided funding for all communities to develop disaster plans, in which all the relevant agencies should participate.

The response in New York to the World Trade Center attacks demonstrated a number of weaknesses, offering lessons that should be incorporated in planning for any future emergencies. The most serious problem was poor communication among response agencies. The city's emergency management center was damaged by the attack, as well as the antenna it used for communication, and the fire department and police department could not communicate with each other. Although more than 13,000 people escaped from the towers, some of the 2801 deaths could have been prevented by better communication and coordination. The air in lower Manhattan was contaminated for months after the attacks, and many of the cleanup workers at the site did not use respiratory protection devices. Critics complained that government agencies were more intent on reassuring the population than on telling them the truth about health risks.

The response to Hurricane Katrina, the costliest natural disaster in U.S. history, was inadequate at all levels of government. The New Orleans mayor and the Louisiana governor hesitated before ordering a mandatory evacuation, and they did not provide information or the means for the most vulnerable members of the population to evacuate. The federal government agency that should have been providing assistance and resources, FEMA, had been weakened by its incorporation into the new Department of Homeland Security; its budget had been severely cut; and its director had no knowledge or experience of emergency planning or response.

There are well-established principles for management of disasters that should be understood by all medical and safety responders. All agencies involved should participate in planning; all responders should be familiar with the plans; and the response should be practiced at least once a year. Since 9/11, the federal government has invested more than $3.7 billion in strengthening the public health infrastructure. These preparations were intended to improve the nation's ability to respond not only to disasters, but also to naturally occurring disease outbreaks and other public health emergencies. However, the

Hurricane Katrina disaster demonstrated that more planning is needed.

Preparedness for bioterrorism requires that the public health system carry out its normal surveillance functions. A biological attack might be recognized only after patients start showing up in hospitals and doctors' offices, but even then their symptoms may not be unusual—most of the pathogens that might be used as bioweapons first cause flu-like symptoms. The CDC has provided funding for states and major cities to develop surveillance of hospital emergency rooms, 911 calls, calls to poison control centers, and pharmacies. The CDC has also opened new laboratories capable of testing for biological and chemical agents, and it maintains a Strategic National Stockpile of medical and emergency supplies. The Department of Agriculture conducts surveillance for animal diseases.

Pandemic flu has caused concern since the late 1990s, when a lethal strain of avian flu appeared in Asia. Although avian flu is not easily transmitted on a person-to-person basis, public health authorities fear that it could mutate and turn into a deadly pandemic. However, the first pandemic since 1968, which struck in 2009, turned out to be a milder swine flu strain, H1N1. Thanks in part to its preparation for bioterrorism, the United States seemed to cope successfully with the new pandemic.

References

1. Centers for Disease Control and Prevention, "Preliminary Results from the World Trade Center Evacuation Study—New York City, 2003," *Morbidity and Mortality Weekly Report* 53 (2004): 815–817.

2. S. Klitzman and F. Freudenberg, "Implications of the World Trade Center Attack for the Public Health and Health Care Infrastructures," *American Journal of Public Health* 93 (2003): 400–406.

3. R. Simon and S. Teperman, "World Trade Center Attack: Lessons for Disaster Management," *Critical Care* 5 (2001): 317–319.

4. J. Dwyer, K. Flynn, and F. Fessenden, "9/11 Exposed Deadly Flaws in Rescue Plan," *The New York Times*, July 7, 2002.

5. J. Shufro, "Perspective on the Tragedy at the World Trade Center," *American Journal of Medicine* 42 (2002): 557–559.

6. G. D. Thurston and L. C. Chen, "Risk Communication in the Aftermath of the World Trade Center Disaster," *American Journal of Industrial Medicine* 42 (2002): 543–544.

7. National Oceanic and Atmospheric Administration, National Centers for Environmental Information, "U.S. Billion-Dollar Weather and Climate Disasters," 2019, www.ncdc.noaa.gov/billions/, accessed October 16, 2019.

8. D. Brinkley, *The Great Deluge: Hurricane Katrina, New Orleans, and the Mississippi Gulf Coast* (New York, NY: William Morrow, 2006).

9. J. Travis, "Scientists' Fears Come True as Hurricane Floods New Orleans," *Science* 309 (2005): 1545–1548.

10. M. E. Dyson, *Come Hell or High Water: Hurricane Katrina and the Color of Disaster* (New York, NY: Basic Books, 2006).

11. National Weather Service, National Hurricane Center, "Hurricanes in History," May 30, 2012, https://www.nhc.noaa.gov/outreach/history/#katrina, accessed October 17, 2019.

12. Kaiser Family Foundation, "Key Facts: States Most Affected by Hurricane Katrina," August 2006, https://www.kff.org/wp-content/uploads/2013/01/7395-02.pdf, accessed October 17, 2019.

13. K. Elder, S. Xirasagar, N. Miller, S. A. Bowen, S. Glover, and C. Piper, "African Americans' Decisions Not to Evacuate New Orleans Before Hurricane Katrina: A Qualitative Study," *American Journal of Public Health* 97 (2007): S124–S129.

14. M. Brodie, E. Weltzien, D. Altman, R. J. Blendon, and J. M. Benson, "Experiences of Hurricane Katrina Evacuees in Houston Shelters: Implications for Future Planning," *American Journal of Public Health* 96 (2006): 1402–1408.

15. D. P. Eisenman, K. M. Cordasco, S. Asch, J. F. Golden, and D. Glik, "Disaster Planning and Risk Communication with Vulnerable Communities: Lessons from Hurricane Katrina," *American Journal of Public Health* 97 (2007): S109–S115.

16. Centers for Disease Control and Prevention, "Public Health Response to Hurricanes Katrina and Rita—

United States, 2005," *Morbidity and Mortality Weekly Report* 55 (2006): 229–231.

17. D. Rosner and G. Markowitz, *Are We Ready? Public Health Since 9/11* (Berkeley, CA: University of California Press, 2006).

18. K. F. McCarthy, D. J. Peterson, N. Sastry, and M. Pollard, "Repopulation of New Orleans After Hurricane Katrina," 2006, https://www .rand.org/pubs/technical_reports/TR369, accessed October 17, 2019.

19. U.S. Census Bureau, "Community Facts," July 1, 2018, https://factfinder.census.gov/faces/nav/jsf /pages/community_facts.xhtml?src=bkmk, accessed October 17, 2019.

20. M. A. Mills, D. Edmondson, and C. L. Park, "Trauma and Stress Response Among Hurricane Katrina Evacuees," *American Journal of Public Health* 97 (2007): S116–S123.

21. L. Y. Landesman, *Public Health Management of Disaster: The Practice Guide*, 2nd ed. (Washington, DC: American Public Health Association, 2005).

22. Federal Emergency Management Agency, "National Incident Management System (NIMS)," October 3, 2015, https://www.fema.gov/national-incident-management-system, accessed October 17, 2019.

23. Centers for Disease Control and Prevention, "Public Health Emergency Preparedness (PHEP) Cooperative Agreement," September 20, 2019, https://www.cdc .gov/phpr/coopagreement.htm, accessed October 17, 2019.

24. M. McHugh, A. B. Staiti, and L. E. Felland, "How Prepared Are Americans for Public Health Emergencies? Twelve Communities Weigh In," *Health Affairs* (May/June 2004): 201–209.

25. S. S. Hsu, "Katrina Report Spreads Blame," *The Washington Post*, February 12, 2006.

26. T. J. Torok, R. V. Tauxe, R. P. Wise, J. R. Livengood, R. Sokolow, and S. Mauvais, et al., "A Large Community Outbreak of Salmonellosis Caused by Intentional Contamination of Restaurant Salad Bars," *Journal of the American Medical Association* 278 (1997): 389–395.

27. L. K. Altman, "Disease Control Center Bolsters Terror Response," *The New York Times*, August 28, 2002.

28. A. Fernandez and K. Sack, "Ebola Patient Sent Home Despite Fever, Records Show," *The New York Times*, October 10, 2014.

29. Centers for Disease Control and Prevention, "Laboratory Response Network Partners in Preparedness," April 10, 2019, https://emergency .cdc.gov/lrn, accessed October 18, 2019.

30. N. Marano and M. Pappiaoanou, "Historical, New, and Reemerging Links Between Human and Animal Health," *Emerging Infectious Diseases* 10 (2004): 2065–2066.

31. L. O. Gostin , J. W. Sapsin, S. P. Teret, S. Burris, J. S. Mair, J. G. Hodge Jr, and J. S. Vernick, "Model State Emergency Health Powers Act: Planning for and Response to Bioterrorism and Naturally Occurring Infectious Diseases," *Journal of the American Medical Association* 288 (2002): 622–628.

32. Centers for Disease Control and Prevention, "Public Health Law Program: About Us," October 4, 2018, https://www.cdc.gov/phlp/about/index.html, accessed October 18, 2019.

33. M. K. Wynis and L. Gostin, "Bioterrorist Threat and Access to Health Care," *Science* 296 (2002): 1613.

34. U.S. Department of Homeland Security, "Biowatch," https://www.dhs.gov/keywords/biowatch, accessed October 18, 2019.

35. T. O'Toole, M. Mair, and T. V. Inglesby, "Shining Light on 'Dark Winter,'" *Clinical Infectious Diseases* 34 (2002): 972–983.

36. "Avoiding a Dark Winter," *The Economist*, October 25, 2001.

37. M. T. Osterholm, "Preparing for the Next Pandemic," *New England Journal of Medicine* 358 (2005): 1839–1842.

38. Centers for Disease Control and Prevention, "Influenza Vaccine Advances," September 16, 2019, https://www.cdc.gov/flu/prevent/advances.htm, accessed October 18, 2019.

39. Centers for Disease Control and Prevention, "2009 H1N1 Flu," August 11, 2010, https://www.cdc.gov /h1n1flu/, accessed October 18, 2019.

40. Centers for Disease Control and Prevention, "Selecting the Viruses for the Seasonal Influenza Vaccine," September 4, 2018, https://www.cdc.gov/flu /prevent/vaccine-selection.htm, accessed October 18, 2019.

CHAPTER 31

Public Health in the Twenty-First Century: Achievements and Challenges

KEY TERMS

Biotechnology
Health Insurance Portability and
   Accountability Act (HIPAA)

Healthy People 2020
Managed care organizations
   (MCOs)

Public Health Information
   Network (PHIN)

In the 20th century, the United States saw great progress in public health. As a field of practice, public health has advanced in both knowledge and methodology. Biomedical scientists have identified many of the organisms that cause infectious diseases and have developed methods to control them. Epidemiologists have recognized risk factors that lead to many chronic diseases, information that can be used to reduce people's risk of illness. Efforts to clean up the environment have resulted in air and water that are much safer than they were a half-century ago. Intensive health education efforts have even persuaded Americans to improve some health-related behaviors, leading to reductions in tobacco use and drunk driving. The ability to assess the state of the public's health and to evaluate the impact of medical and public health interventions has also advanced dramatically because of vast stores of health-related data and computer software capable of analyzing them. These achievements have greatly improved the health of Americans. The average lifespan has increased by more than 30 years since 1900 (when it was 47 years), and 25 of those years are attributed to improvements in public health.[1]

As the last century ended, the Centers for Disease Control and Prevention (CDC) published a "top 10" list of great public health achievements of the 20th century.[1] These accomplishments were chosen for the positive impact they have had and will continue to have in reducing deaths, illnesses, and disabilities in the United States. Following is the CDC's list (not in order of importance).

- Routine use of vaccinations has resulted in dramatic reductions in infectious diseases, including the eradication of smallpox; the elimination of polio in the Americas; and control of measles, rubella, tetanus, diphtheria, and a number of other infectious diseases in the United States and other parts of the world.
- Improvements in motor vehicle safety have contributed to large reductions in motor vehicle–related deaths. This has been achieved through engineering efforts to make vehicles and highways safer and through success in persuading people to adopt healthier behaviors, such as using seat belts, child safety seats, and motorcycle helmets, and to not drink and drive.
- Safer workplaces have resulted in a dramatic reduction in fatal occupational injuries—down 90% since 1933—and illness. This achievement reflects improvements in safety in mines and in the manufacturing, construction, and transportation industries.
- Control of infectious diseases has been achieved by (in addition to vaccination) improved sanitation, cleaner water, safer food, the discovery of antibiotic drugs, and methods of epidemiologic surveillance and follow-up.
- A decline in deaths from heart disease and stroke has resulted from the identification of risk factors and people's significant success in changing their behaviors to reduce cholesterol levels and to stop smoking. Secondary prevention methods, such as early detection and treatment of high blood pressure, have also contributed to the lower number of deaths from these causes.
- Safer and healthier foods have almost eliminated major nutritional deficiency diseases, such as rickets, goiter, and pellagra,

in the United States. Microbial contamination of food has been reduced, and nutritional supplementation and labeling have made possible a healthier diet.
- Healthier mothers and babies are the result of better hygiene and nutrition; availability of antibiotics; greater access to health care, including prenatal care; and technological advances in medicine. Since 1900, the United States has experienced a 90% reduction in its infant mortality rate and a 99% reduction in its maternal mortality rate.
- Access to family planning and contraceptive services has contributed to healthier mothers and babies through smaller family size and longer intervals between the birth of children; increased opportunities for preconception counseling and screening; and improved control of sexually transmitted diseases.
- Fluoridation of drinking water has reduced tooth decay in children by 40% to 70%, and tooth loss in adults has been reduced by 40% to 50%.
- Recognition of tobacco use as a health hazard and subsequent public health anti-smoking campaigns have helped prevent people from beginning to smoke, have promoted quitting, and have reduced exposure to environmental (second-hand) tobacco smoke. The resulting decrease in the prevalence of smoking among adults has prevented millions of smoking-related deaths.

Challenges for the 21st Century

In the first part of the 21st century, public health faces many challenges, both old and new. There are renewed threats from infectious diseases, such as dangerous strains of influenza, antibiotic resistance, and foodborne pathogens. The global economy has increased Americans' vulnerability to many of the health threats faced by residents of less developed nations, brought about by international travel and by imported agricultural products. Paradoxically, past successes have led to new threats, such as climate change caused by overpopulation and economic development, and rising costs of medical care for the aging population. The challenge of understanding and altering human behavior—the factor that now contributes most substantially to premature mortality—remains to be confronted by the public health practitioners of the 21st century. The decline in cigarette smoking has slowed, and while the rate of alcohol use among adolescents has decreased over the past decades, illicit drug use, vaping, and prescription drug abuse among adolescents and other groups of Americans has increased. Moreover, physical inactivity and unhealthy diets contribute to the increasing prevalence of obesity among Americans, and injury, especially drug overdoses, is a resurgent cause of death.[2]

Ironically, the successes of public health in the 20th century led to cutbacks in resources and support for preventive activities. During the second half of the century, the medical approach—curing health problems rather than preventing them—gained acceptance. Public health's many achievements, including those just described, were taken for granted, while rapidly increasing resources were devoted to medical care. This problem was recognized in the Institute of Medicine's (IOM's) 1988 report, *The Future of Public Health*.[3] This report prompted public health agencies, policy makers, and academic institutions to initiate a national discussion on the role of public health and the steps necessary to strengthen its capacity to fulfill its role. Attempts were made to coordinate public health efforts at various levels of government, to develop public–private partnerships in communities, and to undertake strategic planning aimed at achieving defined goals and objectives. The IOM undertook a new analysis in 2003 to follow up on the 1988 report and made recommendations for enhancing

understanding of public health and developing a framework for assuring the public's health in the new century.[4]

The events of late 2001, particularly the bioterrorist attacks using anthrax, brought new attention to the American public health system and revealed the weaknesses in the public health infrastructure—in its workforce, information systems, laboratories, and other organizational capacity—which was suffering from neglect. It became clear to policy makers and the public that the public health system is the front line of defense in protecting the population from bioterrorism and other threats. Concerns about preparedness led to a flow of federal funds into public health agencies and activities. These funds have helped state and local agencies begin strengthening their capacity to respond to public health challenges; however, public health officials are concerned as to whether these efforts will be sustained. Budget deficits at the federal and state levels threaten to derail the upgrades just when their importance is being recognized.

The IOM's 2003 report, *The Future of the Public's Health in the 21st Century*, includes lessons learned from the 2001 attacks.[4] According to this report, "the public health system that was in disarray in 1988 remains in disarray today."[4(p.100)] The IOM noted that the United States was not meeting its potential in the area of population health, in part because of the nation's emphasis on (1) medical care rather than preventive services and (2) biomedical research rather than prevention research. It also pointed out the serious and persistent disparities in health status among various population groups, according to race and ethnicity, gender, and socioeconomic status. The 2003 report recommended that the public health workforce receive better education and training, that public health laws be changed to bring them up-to-date and to ensure better coordination among states and territories, and that advances in information technology be used more effectively to provide adequate surveillance and communication. Although the resources to rectify some of the deficiencies were provided in the wake of 9/11, the IOM report stressed the need for these efforts to be sustained for the long term.

In 2009, the IOM again considered the state of public health in the United States in a report called *For the Public's Health: Investing in a Healthier Future*. In this report, it concluded that the health system's failure to develop and deliver effective prevention strategies continues to take a toll on the economy and society. Public health departments should be the backbone of the health system, the report said, but they need adequate funding to do so. The report recommended that all public health agencies develop a minimum package of public health services that all health departments should deliver, and that Congress authorize a dedicated, stable, and long-term financing structure to generate the revenue required to deliver this minimum package of services. As a source of this revenue, the report suggested a tax on all health-care transactions.[5]

Strategic Planning for Public Health

With so many different agencies at so many different political and organizational levels involved in implementing public health's mission, it became apparent some time ago that there was a need for planning and coordination. Beginning in 1979, the U.S. Public Health Service adopted "management by objectives," a process that was becoming increasingly widespread in the private sector. This technique requires managers to jointly define a set of measurable goals, use these goals as a guide to their actions, and regularly measure progress toward achieving them. The management-by-objectives approach is especially useful in decentralized organizations, where many different actors must coordinate their efforts, and thus is well suited to the needs of the public health system.[6]

To develop goals for the year 1990, the Public Health Service enlisted a broad range of participants from both within and outside of government to specify a set of health status objectives. The national goals, published as *Healthy People: The Surgeon General's Report on Health Promotion and Disease Prevention*,[7] set targets for reducing mortality rates in different age groups, with specific objectives designed to meet each target. For example, to achieve the goal of a 25% death rate reduction for people ages 25 through 64, progress had to be made in reducing the prevalence of cigarette smoking, high blood cholesterol, and high blood pressure among adults. Any state, community, or research group that applied for federal funds for a public health program had to justify its request by showing how its project would contribute to achieving one or more of the *Healthy People* goals. When the results of the first planning cycle were tallied in 1990, the numerical mortality goals were met for three of the four age groups: infants, children, and adults ages 25 through 64. Only targets for adolescents and young adults were not met, because of continued high rates of fatal motor vehicle injuries, homicides, and suicides.[6]

The *Healthy People* planning process encourages states and local communities to use the national objectives as a basis for developing objectives of their own. One problem that became obvious during the first decade of the program was a lack of data systems that could track progress, especially at the local level.

In 1987, the Public Health Service began the process of setting objectives for the following decade. *Healthy People 2000*, a 692-page book, sets three overall goals, with more than 300 measurable objectives divided into 22 priority areas.[8] As in the previous *Healthy People* publication, these objectives set targets for individual behavioral change, environmental and regulatory protections, and access to preventive health services. *Healthy People 2000* also addressed the problem of inadequate data, which had hindered evaluation of progress toward the 1990 objectives. Implementing, tracking, and reporting on the goals and objectives involved many agencies of the federal government, as well as hundreds of state agencies, national organizations, academic institutions, and business groups. Most states developed their own year 2000 objectives. The individual states' objectives either paralleled or modified the national objectives to suit the states' own needs and priorities.

In 2001, a final review was published that evaluated the nation's progress in meeting the *Healthy People 2000* objectives.[9] Progress was achieved on more than 60% of the objectives. Specifically, targets were met in reducing deaths from coronary heart disease and cancer, reducing AIDS incidence, and reducing homicide, suicide, and firearm-related deaths. Likewise, tobacco-related mortality targets were met. Goals for infant mortality and the number of children with elevated blood lead levels were nearly met, and progress was made toward reducing health disparities. However, for 15% of the *Healthy People 2000* objectives, the nation moved away from the report's targets. Notably, these included the prevalence of overweight and obesity, especially among adolescents—an ominous sign for the future health of Americans.

Healthy People 2010, launched in January 2000, set public health goals and objectives even higher.[10] *Healthy People 2010* had two overall goals:

- Increase quality and years of healthy life.
- Eliminate health disparities.

These were similar to the goals of *Healthy People 2000*, except that the first goal placed a new focus on quality of life, and the second goal no longer set different targets for racial and ethnic minorities, aiming to ensure that all groups in the United States will be equally healthy.

Healthy People 2010 was organized into 28 focus areas, many of which were the same as the priority areas in *Healthy People 2000*.

In addition, a set of 10 leading health indicators were chosen as areas of special focus. These indicators, which included such behavioral factors as physical activity and responsible sexual behavior, as well as environmental quality and access to health care, were based on their ability to motivate action, the availability of data to measure their progress, and their relevance as broad public health issues.

A final review of *Healthy People 2010* was published in 2011, assessing progress in achieving the objectives in each of the 28 focus areas, as well as summarizing progress made toward the leading health indicators and the two goals. Also, for each objective, the review summarized disparities by race and ethnicity, sex, education level, income, geographic location, and disability status whenever data were available.[10]

For eight of the focus areas, progress was made on more than 75% of the objectives—in these areas, the nation moved toward, met, or exceeded the 2010 targets. These areas included health communication, heart disease and stroke, immunization and infectious diseases, occupational safety and health, and tobacco use. For five of the focus areas, more than 30% of the objectives could not be assessed because of lack of data. In two focus areas—arthritis, osteoporosis, and chronic back conditions; and nutrition and overweight—the population moved toward or achieved less than 25% of the targets.

In regard to the first goal of *Healthy People 2010*—quality and years of healthy life—years of life continue to improve, especially in the older population, but measures of quality yielded mixed results. There were slight improvements in "years in good or better health" and "expected years free of activity limitations." However, "expected years free of selected chronic conditions" declined. The second goal, eliminating health disparities, did not show evidence of systematic improvement. Status on the objectives improved for most populations, but the differences among groups generally did not decline.[11]

As 2010 approached, the public health community mobilized to launch the process for **Healthy People 2020**. This initiative has four overarching goals:

- Attain high-quality, longer lives free of preventable disease, disability, injury, and premature death.
- Achieve health equity, eliminate disparities, and improve the health of all groups.
- Create social and physical environments that promote good health for all.
- Promote quality of life, health development, and health behaviors across all life stages.

Final 2020 goals and objectives were released in December 2010.[12] *Healthy People 2020* has replaced the traditional print publication with an interactive website, www.healthypeople .gov. There are 42 topic areas, with more than 1200 objectives. A set of 26 leading health indicators was chosen as high-priority health issues. The website allows ongoing tracking of progress toward meeting the targets. In 2016, a midcourse review, evaluating progress toward achieving the *Healthy People 2020* objectives, was published. The data show that, midway through the decade, the targets were met or exceeded for 8 of the 26 indicators, and progress was being made on another 8 indicators. There was little or no change on 7 indicators, and the status was getting worse on 3 indicators. **Table 31-1** shows the results of the midcourse review.

Planning is now under way for *Healthy People 2030*. An advisory committee of nongovernmental, independent experts has been named, which will advise the Secretary of Health and Human Services on establishing a framework for *Healthy People 2030*, objectives development and selection, leading health indicators, and implementation. Committee meetings are open to the public, and reports on past committee meetings will be posted on the *Healthy People* website.

Table 31-1 *Healthy People 2020* **Midcourse Review: Progress on Leading Health Indicators**

Baseline values are from years between 2005 and 2010, and midcourse values are from years between 2009 and 2014.

	Status	Baseline Value	Midcourse Value	Target for 2020
Air Quality Index >100 (number of days, weighted by population and Air Quality Index value)	Target met	2.20 billion	0.98 billion	1.98 billion
Homicides (age-adjusted, per 100,000 population)	Target met	6.1	5.2	5.5
All infant deaths (per 1,000 live births, <1 year)	Target met	6.7	6.0	6.0
Total preterm live births (percent, <37 weeks gestation)	Target met	12.7%	11.4%	11.4%
Adults meeting aerobic physical activity and muscle-strengthening objectives (age-adjusted, percent, 18+ years)	Target met	18.2%	21.3%	20.1%
Adolescents using alcohol or illicit drugs in past 30 days (percent, 12–17 years)	Target met	18.4%	15.9%	16.6%

	Status	Baseline Value	Midcourse Value	Target for 2020
Adolescent cigarette smoking in past 30 days (percent, grades 9–12)	Target met	19.5%	15.7%	16.0%
Children exposed to second-hand smoke (percent; nonsmokers, 3–11 years)	Target met	52.2%	41.3%	47.0%
Students graduating from high school 4 years after starting 9th grade (percent)	Improving	79.0%	81.0%	87.0%
Persons with medical insurance (percent, <65 years) (percent)	Improving	83.2%	86.7%	100.0%
Adults receiving colorectal cancer screening based on most recent guidelines (age-adjusted, percent, 50–75 years)	Improving	52.1%	58.2%	70.5%
Adults with hypertension whose blood pressure is under control (age-adjusted, percent, 18+ years)	Improving	43.7%	48.9%	61.2%
Knowledge of serostatus among HIV-positive persons (percent, 13+ years)	Improving	80.9%	87.2%	90.0%
Children receiving the DTaP, polio, MMR, Hib, HepB, varicella and PCV vaccines by age 19–35 months (percent)	Improving	68.4%	71.6%	80.0%
Injury deaths (age-adjusted, per 100,000 population)	Improving	59.7	58.8	53.7
Adult cigarette smoking (age-adjusted, percent, 18+ years)	Improving	20.6%	17.0%	12.0%
Persons with a usual primary care provider (percent)	Little change	76.3%	76.5%	83.9%
Persons with diagnosed diabetes whose A1c value is greater than 9 percent (age-adjusted, percent, 18+ years)	Little change	18.0%	21.0%	16.2%
Sexually active females receiving reproductive health services (percent, 15–44 years)	Little change	78.6%	77.3%	86.5%
Obesity among adults (age-adjusted, percent, 20+ years)	Little change	33.9%	35.3%	30.5%
Obesity among children and adolescents (percent, 2–19 years)	Little change	16.1%	16.9%	14.5%
Mean daily intake of total vegetables (age-adjusted, cup equivalents per 1,000 calories, 2+ years)	Little change	0.80	0.80	1.16

(continues)

Table 31-1 *Healthy People 2020* **Midcourse Review: Progress on Leading Health Indicators** *(Continued)*

	Status	Baseline Value	Midcourse Value	Target for 2020
Binge drinking in past month—Adults (percent, 18+ years)	Little change	27.1%	26.9%	24.4%
Suicide (age-adjusted, per 100,000 population)	Getting worse	11.3	12.6	10.2
Adolescents with a major depressive episode in the past 12 months (percent, 12–17 years)	Getting worse	8.3%	10.7%	7.5%
Children, adolescents, and adults who visited the dentist in the past year (age-adjusted, percent, 2+ years)	Getting worse	44.5%	42.1%	49.0%

Modified from U.S. Department of Health and Human Services, *Healthy People 2020*, "Midcourse Review, Progress Made toward Targets for Leading Health Indicators," 2016, www.healthypeople.gov/2020/data-search/midcourse-review/lhi, accessed October 20, 2019.

Dashed Hopes for the Integration of Public Health and Medical Practice

Because of the high and continuously rising costs of medical care, managed care became more prevalent in the 1990s. Managed care moves the incentives of medicine closer to the mission of public health—keeping people healthy. While traditional fee-for-service medicine focuses on people who seek care, offering financial rewards to doctors for providing services to patients, **managed care organizations (MCOs)** are responsible for all their members, and they receive financial rewards when the need for expensive medical services is averted. This shift in medicine's perspective had a number of implications for public health.

The incentives for MCOs to keep their patients healthy encourage medical plans to use public health strategies to prevent disease and to promote healthy behaviors among members. The financial incentives also make medicine economically dependent on public health's effectiveness in preventing unnecessary disease in the community. Public health failures can be expensive. Indeed, the 1993 cryptosporidiosis outbreak in Milwaukee, for example, caused $15.5 million in medical costs.[13] Thus, these changes in how medical care is financed and delivered would encourage the medical sector to support adequate funding for the public health sector.

With managed care, medicine is driven by the same kind of measurable goals and objectives that public health has been developing. MCOs are required to collect data on the effectiveness of their services and the health status of their members. They are evaluated on their success in achieving the same kinds of goals and objectives detailed in the *Healthy People* process. These common goals provide medicine and public health with strong incentives to work together.

Unfortunately from the standpoint of public health, the popularity of managed care has declined since the late 1990s. MCOs faced a backlash against many of their cost-control measures, and the benefits that come from incentives to keep MCO members healthy were not obvious to the public. State Medicaid programs continue to rely heavily on managed care, however.

President Barack Obama's reform of the healthcare system, the Affordable Care Act (ACA), compensates somewhat for the failures of the managed care movement by including a number of prevention and wellness measures. Insurers are required to cover preventive benefits such as screening and counseling for obesity, tobacco use, sexually transmitted diseases, cancer, high cholesterol, and human immunodeficiency virus (HIV) infection, as well as recommended immunizations. Medicare is required to provide many of these preventive services at no cost to its beneficiaries. Preventive services for women, including well-woman visits and contraception, are required free of charge; the latter care is particularly controversial with Republicans. Preventive services for children include recommended immunizations, lead screening for those at risk, and regular monitoring of development throughout childhood.[14]

In addition, the ACA provides for a Prevention and Public Health Fund, which sets aside a specific amount every year "to improve health and help restrain the rate of growth in private and public health care costs." This fund is being used to support a variety of community prevention and clinical prevention programs, to bolster the public health infrastructure and workforce, and to expand public health research and tracking efforts.[15] President Donald Trump and the Republican Congress managed to weaken many provisions of the ACA and have reduced funding for some aspects of the law, despite the overall popularity of the ACA, and its future remains uncertain.

Information Technology

Advances in information technology offer extraordinary opportunities for collaboration between public health and medical care.

For example, epidemiologic surveillance using the Internet would allow a system linking state and local health departments, public health laboratories, hospitals, and doctors' offices to collect data in real time and rapidly analyze those data to detect unusual disease patterns. Such a system could simultaneously disseminate the information among all participants. However, at this time, there is no single system, but rather multiple systems that do not necessarily communicate with each other.[16]

One important step toward integration is the CDC's **Public Health Information Network (PHIN)**, a national initiative to increase the capacity of public health agencies to electronically exchange data and information across organizations and jurisdictions. The PHIN promotes the use of standards and defines functional and technical requirements for management and public health information exchange. Using such information exchange systems, the CDC facilitates a number of programs, including, for example, biosurveillance, outbreak management, and national notifiable disease surveillance.[17]

As the 2003 IOM report noted, the anthrax attacks of fall 2001 demonstrated the weaknesses of public health communication and information systems being used at the time. Only half of the nation's state, local, and territorial health departments had Internet capability. Another 20% of these health agencies lacked e-mail.[4] Federal funding for bioterrorism preparedness has helped bring many of the local health departments up to modern standards of information technology, and by 2006, 93% had continuous, high-speed Internet access.[18]

In addition to being used in epidemiologic surveillance, information technology is transforming the assessment and evaluation activities that are so important to the practice of public health and that promise to improve outcomes in the practice of medicine. States and some counties maintain electronic databases on vital statistics, notifiable diseases, chronic diseases, hospital discharges, and immunizations; many of these are tied into the

PHIN. Billing records on patients covered by the Medicare program have proved useful in assessing outcomes of medical care.

Information networks are also being developed by MCOs and other nongovernmental providers of health services. Giant healthcare companies have streamlined their procedures for storing and exchanging data on medical tests, procedures, costs, and outcomes. However, as noted by Paul Starr, historian of the relationship between medicine and public health, "National policy has yet to resolve two of the most fundamental questions about computerized health information: how to keep private what ought to be private, and how to make public what ought to be public."[19(p.103)]

President Obama's reform of the healthcare system included incentives for physicians, hospitals, and other medical providers to use health information technology to improve the efficiency and quality of medical care for all American citizens. A uniform system of electronic medical records for all patients would help overcome the fragmentation of medical care, which, for example, leads to duplication of services when doctors do not have information about procedures and testing a patient has received during previous visits to other doctors. A uniform system of billing could also reduce some of the administrative costs that contribute to the high medical expenditures in the United States.

An investment of $19.5 billion for health information technology was passed by Congress in early 2009, and President Obama appointed a national coordinator to lead the implementation of a nationwide interoperable, privacy-protected health information technology infrastructure. The U.S. Department of Health and Human Services has developed software that is available to hospitals, physicians' offices, pharmacies, labs, insurance companies, and other components of the healthcare system, to enable them to connect to each other and to share data. It has also published guidelines on securing health information by making it unreadable by unauthorized individuals.[20–22]

A federal law passed by Congress in 1996, which became effective in 2003, was designed to protect the privacy of medical records. The **Health Insurance Portability and Accountability Act (HIPAA)** forbids "wrongful disclosure of individually identifiable health information." While this provision helps eliminate some abuses, it has raised concerns that the privacy measures obstruct the use of medical data for many useful purposes. For example, researchers have complained that they cannot conduct outcomes studies, such as comparisons of different treatments for cancer.[23] The privacy rules also have discouraged the creation of public databases that consumers could use to make optimal decisions concerning their health and health care.[19]

The rise of the Internet has presented major new opportunities and challenges for individuals who wish to understand and make choices concerning their personal health. People have access to vast quantities of health information—and misinformation—on the Internet. Many state and federal public health agencies provide the latest and most accurate information about health issues on their websites. Many nongovernmental sites also offer good advice and information, which can raise people's awareness of health risks, provide them with motivation and skills to reduce these risks, offer a helpful sense of connection to others who are in similar situations, and furnish information about difficult choices. However, caution is necessary in using the information presented on websites that lack authoritative sponsors. This information may be biased because of the website creators' commercial interests, distrust of science, or ignorance.

The Internet poses challenges to government agencies charged with regulating medical care because of the lack of accountability on the part of those who create websites.

For example, doctors may set up websites to diagnose and prescribe medications for patients' ills without examining the patients. Prescription drugs are sometimes sold over the Internet to people without valid prescriptions. Drugs that are not approved in the United States can be ordered from foreign markets. Even prescription drugs that are available in the United States may cost more here than in other countries, including Canada, and many people choose to buy them over the Internet to save money. The traditional role of the U.S. Food and Drug Administration (FDA) and other governmental agencies—to protect consumers from fraudulent and irresponsible medical practice—is made much more difficult by the free-wheeling culture of Internet commerce. At the same time, the FDA's opposition to importing cheaper drugs from Canada has begun to seem like a ploy to protect the American drug industry's profits, generating skepticism about the integrity of the agency's mission.

The widespread use of smartphones provides opportunities for people to receive health information and monitor their behaviors. For example, a program called "Sweet Talk" was successful in supporting young people with type 1 diabetes. Participants were sent text messages tailored to their self-management goals and could use the system to submit data and ask questions.[24] A study of young smokers who wanted to quit found that, after 6 weeks, participants who received regular, personalized text messages providing smoking cessation advice, support, and distraction were twice as likely to not be smoking as members of a control group.[25]

The CDC has a mobile application that allows people to sign up to get emergency alerts, new research and reports, and health tips. People with diabetes, for example, can receive tips and reminders on how to manage their diet and exercise. In the event of an emergency, people in the affected zip codes can be alerted and instructed on how to respond.[26]

The FDA regulates mobile medical apps that it considers medical devices because they would pose a risk to a patient's safety if the app did not function as intended. For example, the agency has approved apps that allow a doctor or nurse to view medical images such as electrocardiograms on a mobile platform, or to monitor vital signs measurements of patients at home.[27]

The Challenge of Biotechnology

Biotechnology promises to solve many medical problems with new drugs and procedures—but those drugs and procedures will also contribute to the skyrocketing costs of medical care. Information from the Human Genome Project, for example, allows the detection of individual differences in people's response to various drugs, with the promise that doctors can choose among medications to prescribe for a patient based on genetic tests. Discoveries in cancer genomics offer to provide information on individual tumors that will allow treatments specifically targeted toward a single patient. These promises of "personalized medicine" come with a caveat, however: At a time when medical costs are spiraling out of control, and when a significant proportion of the American population does not have access to even the most basic health care, who will have access to these expensive treatments? Public health should have a voice in deciding how many of these "miracles" our society can afford, and how priorities should be set when resources are limited.

Biotechnology offers even more unprecedented possibilities, such as the ability to choose the characteristics of future children through genetic engineering and cloning or the ability to slow the aging process. These developments will raise many legal and ethical issues, which will have to be faced through public debate and difficult policy choices.

The Ultimate Challenge to Public Health in the 21st Century

"If public health's mission is to fulfill society's interest in assuring conditions in which people can be healthy (*The Future of Public Health* definition), public health has yet to succeed in fostering a national debate on the relative return on investment to improve population health."[28(p.xxiii)] As Jonathan E. Fielding noted, in a review of public health in the 20th century, the enormous expansion of the medical care system—a system that is largely inaccessible to much of the population that needs it most—occurred without consideration of whether this investment could have yielded more benefits to health if invested elsewhere. Public health agencies are chronically starved for funding to carry out essential public health services that are clearly cost-effective in improving the health status of communities.[28]

Health is determined by the social, physical, and economic environments; health behaviors; and genetics. It is affected only marginally by medical interventions. The challenge for public health continues to be educating the public and policy makers about the role of these nonmedical factors in determining people's health and convincing people of the importance of the core public health functions in protecting and promoting the health of the entire population. As it becomes increasingly apparent that advances in high-technology medical care have become economically unsustainable, the nation must focus on assuring conditions in which people can be healthy—the mission of public health—in the 21st century.

Conclusion

The United States made great progress in public health during the 20th century. The threat of infectious diseases was greatly reduced, risk factors for some chronic diseases became well understood, the environment was substantially cleaned up, and a great deal was learned about how health is affected by behavior. In recent decades, the ability to assess the state of the public's health and to evaluate the impact of medical and public health interventions has advanced dramatically because of the existence of vast stores of health-related data and computer software capable of analyzing it.

During the 20th century, the life expectancy of Americans was extended by 30 years. Much of this improvement came from 10 great public health achievements identified by the CDC: vaccination, motor vehicle safety, safer workplaces, control of infectious diseases, decline in deaths from coronary heart disease and stroke, safer and healthier foods, healthier mothers and babies, family planning, fluoridation of drinking water, and recognition of tobacco use as a health hazard.

Despite these gains, public health faces many challenges in the 21st century. Some of these challenges come from new forms of familiar public health problems such as infectious diseases and environmental pollution. Others are posed by efforts to change people's unhealthy behavior, the factor that now contributes the most to premature mortality.

A trend toward decentralizing governmental responsibilities and authority has prompted public health to adopt a planning process called "management by objectives." This process involves setting measurable goals and objectives and periodically assessing progress. The federal government has led this planning process over the past several decades, but involvement in such planning has also expanded to include state, county, and local communities. The result has been substantial progress toward achieving public health goals, but the goals must be constantly reset.

The trend toward managed care as a strategy for controlling medical care costs moved the incentives of medical practice closer to the mission of public health. However, the unpopularity of managed care and the failure to communicate the health benefits it offers led to a backlash. Consequently, medical costs have resumed their upward spiral, and the number of uninsured Americans has again increased because of the actions of President Trump and Congress.

Advances in information technology have led to great improvements in public health surveillance capabilities. The bioterrorism attacks in fall 2001 stimulated a flow of federal funds to state and county health departments for preparedness, allowing improvements in information systems at all levels of government. Information technology also makes possible much of the assessment and evaluation activity that is becoming important to the practice of public health and medicine. President Obama identified integrated health information systems as a priority in his efforts to reform the healthcare system. The rise of the Internet as a source of information and commerce also poses challenges to individual consumers, who must figure out how to evaluate the information, and to government regulators, who must decide how to protect consumers from fraudulent and irresponsible medical practice.

Perhaps the most important challenge faced by public health in the 21st century will be to encourage a society-wide debate on how public resources should be allocated to most effectively improve the health of the population as a whole.

References

1. Centers for Disease Control and Prevention, "Ten Great Public Health Achievements—United States, 1900–1999," *Morbidity and Mortality Weekly Report* 48 (1999): 241–243.
2. U.S. Department of Health and Human Services, "*Healthy People 2020,*" https://www.healthypeople.gov, accessed October 19, 2019.
3. Institute of Medicine, *The Future of Public Health* (Washington, DC: National Academies Press, 1988).
4. Institute of Medicine, *The Future of the Public's Health in the 21st Century* (Washington, DC: National Academies Press, 2003).
5. Institute of Medicine, "*For the Public's Health: Investing in a Healthier Future,*" April 10, 2012, http://www.nationalacademies.org/hmd/~/media/Files/Report%20Files/2012/For-the-Publics-Health/phfunding_rb.pdf, accessed October 19, 2019.
6. J. M. McGinnis and D. R. Maiese, "*Defining Missions, Goals, and Objectives,*" in F. D. Scutchfield and C. W. Keck, eds., *Principles of Public Health Practice* (Albany, NY: Delmar, 1997), pp. 131–146.
7. U.S. Department of Health, Education, and Welfare, *Healthy People: Surgeon General's Report on Health Promotion and Disease Prevention*, PHS publication 79–55071 (Washington, DC: Public Health Service, 1979.
8. U.S. Department of Health and Human Services, *Healthy People 2000: National Health Promotion and Disease Prevention Objectives*, PHS publication 91–50212 (Washington, DC: Public Health Service, 1990).
9. National Center for Health Statistics, *Healthy People 2000 Final Review* (Hyattsville, MD: U.S. Public Health Service, 2001).
10. U.S. Department of Health and Human Services, *Healthy People 2010: Understanding and Improving Health*, 2nd ed. (Washington DC: U.S. Government Printing Office, November 2000).
11. Centers for Disease Control and Prevention, "*Healthy People 2010 Final Review,*" April 11, 2013, https://www.cdc.gov/nchs/healthy_people/hp2010/hp2010_final_review.htm, accessed October 19, 2019.
12. Centers for Disease Control and Prevention, "Healthy People 2020," October 19, 2019, https://www.cdc.gov/nchs/healthy_people/hp2020.htm, accessed October 19, 2019.
13. R. Lasker, *Medicine and Public Health: The Power of Collaboration* (New York, NY: New York Academy of Medicine, 1997), p. 37.
14. U.S. Department of Health and Human Services, "About the Law: Preventive Care," July 27, 2015, https://www.hhs.gov/healthcare/about-the-law/preventive-care/index.html, accessed October 19, 2019.
15. American Public Health Association, "Prevention and Public Health Fund: Dedicated to Improving Our Nation's Public Health," https://www.apha

.org/~/media/files/pdf/topics/aca/2015_pphf_fact _sheet.ashx, accessed October 19, 2019.

16. G. S. Birkhead, M. Klompas, and N. R. Shah, "Use of Electronic Health Records for Public Health Surveillance to Advance Public Health," *Annual Review of Public Health* 36 (2015): 345–359.

17. Centers for Disease Control and Prevention, "Public Health Information Network (PHIN) Tools and Resources," December 19, 2018, https://www.cdc .gov/phin/index.html, accessed October 19, 2019.

18. C. J. Leep, G. Gorenflo, and P. M. Libbey, *"The Local Health Department,"* in F. D. Scutchfield and C. W. Keck, eds., *Principles of Public Health Practice*, 3rd ed. (Clifton Park, NY: Delmar, 2009), pp. 207–231.

19. P. Starr, "Smart Technology, Stunted Policy: Developing Health Information Networks," *Health Affairs* 16 (1997): 91–105.

20. U.S. Department of Health and Human Services, "Press Release: "HHS Names David Blumenthal as National Coordinator for Health Information Technology," March 20, 2009, https://www.businesswire.com/news /home/20090320005413/en/HHS-Names-David -Blumenthal-National-Coordinator-Health, accessed December 12, 2019.

21. U.S. Department of Health and Human Services, "Press Release: Federal Health Architecture Delivers Free, Scalable Solution Helping Organizations Tie Health IT Systems into the NHIN," April 6, 2009, https://www.tmcnet.com/usubmit/2009/04/07 /4114296.htm, accessed October 19, 2019.

22. U.S. Department of Health and Human Services, "Press Release: HHS Releases Guidance for Securing Health Information and Preventing Harm from Breaches," April 17, 2009, http://wayback.archive -it.org/3926/20131018161701/http://www.hhs.gov /news/press/2009pres/04/20090417a.html, accessed October 19, 2019.

23. J. Kaiser, "Privacy Rule Creates Bottleneck for U.S. Biomedical Researchers," *Science* 305 (2004): 168–169.

24. V. L. Franklin, A. Greene, A. Waller, S. A. Greene, and C. Pagliari, "Patients' Engagement with 'Sweet Talk': A Text Messaging Support System for Young People with Diabetes," *Journal of Medical Internet Research* 10 (2008): e20.

25. A. Rodgers, T. Corbett, D. Bramley, T. Riddell, M. Wills, R. B. Lin, and M. Jones, "Do u smoke after txt? Results of a Randomised Trial of Smoking Cessation Using Mobile Phone Text Messaging," *Tobacco Control* 14 (2005): 255–261.

26. Centers for Disease Control and Prevention, "CDC Mobile App," January 8, 2018, https://www.cdc .gov/mobile/applications/cdcgeneral/promos /cdcmobileapp.html, accessed October 19, 2019.

27. U.S. Food and Drug Administration, "Mobile Medical Applications," September 26, 2019, https://www.fda.gov/medicaldevices/digitalhealth /mobilemedicalapplications/default.htm, accessed October 19, 2019.

28. J. E. Fielding, "Public Health in the Twentieth Century: Advances and Challenges," *Annual Review of Public Health* 20 (1999): xiii–xxx.

Glossary

A

Access to medical/health care The potential for timely use of medical services to achieve the best possible health outcomes. Often limited by lack of health insurance.

Acquired immunodeficiency syndrome (AIDS) The most severe phase of infection with the human immunodeficiency virus (HIV). People infected with HIV are said to have AIDS when they get certain opportunistic infections or when their T4 cell count drops below 200.

Adjusted rate A way of comparing two groups that differ in some important variable (e.g., age) by mathematically eliminating the effect of that variable.

Advance directive A written statement of a person's wishes regarding medical treatment, often including a living will, made to ensure those wishes are carried out should the person be unable to communicate them to a doctor.

Aerosol A suspension of liquid particles in the air; many infectious diseases of the respiratory system are transmitted by pathogen-containing aerosols released when an infected person coughs or sneezes.

Affordable Care Act Often called "Obamacare" and also known as the Patient Protection and Affordable Care Act. A law passed in 2010 and fully implemented by 2015 that was designed to provide health insurance to all Americans.

Age-adjusted rate A rate calculated to reflect a standard age distribution.

Agency for Healthcare Research and Quality (AHRQ) A U.S. government agency that functions as a part of the Department of Health & Human Services (HHS) to support research to help improve the quality of health care.

Alzheimer's disease A degenerative disease of the brain characterized by mental deterioration. It is the most common cause of dementia in the elderly, and its prevalence increases with age.

Antibiotic resistance The ability of bacteria and other microorganisms to resist the effects of an antibiotic to which they were once sensitive.

Antibody A protein produced by cells of the immune system that reacts specifically with invading antigens.

Antigens Proteins on the surface of a pathogen that stimulate the development of antibodies to destroy the pathogen.

Antiretroviral therapy (ART) A medical treatment for people infected with human immunodeficiency virus (HIV) using anti-HIV drugs. The standard treatment consists of a combination of at least three drugs (often called "**highly active antiretroviral therapy**" or **HAART**) that suppress HIV replication.

Anxiety *See* Anxiety disorder.

Anxiety disorder A mental illness characterized by intense fear or dread lacking an unambiguous cause or a specific threat.

Arthritis Inflammation of the joints that often causes limitations of activity due to pain and stiffness. Its prevalence increases with age.

Assessment One of the three core functions of public health as specified by *The Future of*

Public Health. The process by which a public health agency regularly and systematically collects, assembles, analyzes, and makes available information on the health of a community, including statistics on health status, community health needs, and epidemiologic and other studies of health problems.

Association The relationship between two or more events or variables. Events are said to be associated when they occur more frequently together than one would expect by chance. Association does not necessarily imply a causal relationship.

Assurance One of the three core functions of public health as specified by *The Future of Public Health*. The process by which a public health agency ensures its constituents that services necessary to achieve agreed-upon goals are provided, either by encouraging actions by other entities (private or public sectors), by requiring such action through regulation, or by providing services directly.

Asthma A lung disease with recurrent exacerbation of airway constriction, mucus secretion, and chronic inflammation of the airways, resulting in reduced airflow that causes symptoms of wheezing, cough, chest tightness, and difficulty breathing.

Atherosclerosis Hardening of the arteries.

Attention-deficit/hyperactivity disorder (ADHD) A common childhood disorder with symptoms including difficulty staying focused and paying attention, difficulty controlling behavior, and overactivity.

Autism A group of developmental brain disorders, characterized by a wide range of symptoms, skills, and levels of impairment, generally including social impairment, communication difficulties, and repetitive and stereotyped behaviors.

Autosomal dominant disorder One of several ways that a trait or disorder can be passed down through families. If a disease is autosomal dominant, it means you only need to get the abnormal gene from one parent in order for you to inherit the disease.

Autosomal recessive disorder A disorder in which two copies of an abnormal gene must be present in order for the disease or trait to develop.

B

Bacteria A large domain of single-celled microorganisms that lack a nucleus or other membrane-bound organelles. Only a few cause disease.

Behavioral Risk Factor Surveillance Survey (BRFSS) A system of health-related telephone surveys that collect state data about U.S. residents regarding their health-related risk behaviors, chronic health conditions, and use of preventive services.

Benign Not cancerous; does not invade nearby tissue or spread to other parts of the body.

Bias The influence of irrelevant or even spurious factors or associations—commonly called confounding variables—on a result or conclusion.

Biomedical science The study of the biological basis of human health and disease, including genetics, immunology, infectious diseases, chronic diseases, and molecular approaches to treatment.

Biopsy The removal of a sample of tissue that is then examined under a microscope to check for cancer cells.

Biostatistics Statistics applied to the analysis of biological and medical data.

Biotechnology The exploitation of biological processes for industrial and other purposes, especially the genetic manipulation of microorganisms for the production of antibiotics, hormones, etc.

Bioterrorism Terrorism involving the release of toxic biological agents.

Bipolar disorder (manic-depressive illness) A brain disorder that causes unusual shifts in mood, energy, activity levels, and the ability to carry out day-to-day tasks.

Birth defect An abnormality in structure, function, or body metabolism that is present at birth, such as cleft lip or palate, phenylketonuria, or sickle cell disease.

Birth rate Number of births in a year per 100,000 people.

Bisphenol A (BPA) An industrial chemical that has been used to make certain plastics and resins since the 1960s.

Blinding A method of keeping subjects and, if possible, researchers unaware of which subjects are in an experimental group (those getting a new drug, for example) and which are in a control group (those getting an older drug or a placebo).

Body Mass Index (BMI) The ratio of a person's weight in kilograms by the square of his or her height in meters. For most people, a BMI over 25 is considered overweight and BMI over 30 is obese.

C

Calorie labeling An FDA law that went into effect in 2018 that requires calorie and nutrition information for standard menu items.

Cancer Diseases in which abnormal cells divide without control. Cancer cells can invade nearby tissue and can spread through the bloodstream and lymphatic system to other parts of the body.

Carbon dioxide A colorless, odorless gas produced by burning carbon and organic compounds and by respiration.

Carcinogen A substance or agent that is known to cause cancer.

Cardiovascular disease Disease of the heart and blood vessels, most commonly caused by atherosclerosis, deposits of fatty substances in the inner layer of the arteries. *Coronary heart disease* affects the arteries of the heart and may lead to a heart attack. *Cerebrovascular disease* affects the arteries of the brain and may lead to a stroke.

Carrier state A state in which a disease has infected a person and can be transmitted to other people from that person but the person him or herself does not have symptoms.

Carrying capacity The limit of population size that the environment can support without being degraded.

Case-control study An epidemiologic study that compares individuals affected by a disease ("cases") with a comparable group of persons who do not have the disease ("controls") to seek possible causes or associations.

Cases In a case-control study, cases, are people who have the disease being studied.

Census *See* United States Census.

Centers for Disease Control and Prevention (CDC) The main assessment and epidemiologic agency for the nation, directly serving the population as well as providing technical assistance to states and localities.

Chain of infection The pattern by which an infectious disease is transmitted from person to person.

Children's Health Insurance Program (CHIP) Joint federal–state program similar to Medicaid, which covers children in families that earn too much to qualify for Medicaid.

Chlorofluorocarbons (CFCs) A gas that was once commonly used in various products (such as aerosols) but that is believed to cause damage to the ozone layer in the Earth's atmosphere.

Cholesterol A compound of the sterol type found in most body tissues, including the blood and the nerves. Cholesterol and its derivatives are important constituents of cell membranes and precursors of other steroid compounds, but high concentrations in the blood (mainly derived from animal fats in the diet) are thought to promote atherosclerosis.

Chromosome A threadlike structure of nucleic acids and protein found in the nucleus of most living cells, carrying genetic information in the form of genes.

Chronic disease A disease that is marked by long duration or frequent recurrence, usually incurable but not immediately fatal. Common diseases that are considered chronic include cardiovascular disease, cancer, diabetes, Alzheimer's disease, and acquired immunodeficiency syndrome (AIDS).

Chronic obstructive pulmonary disease (COPD) A disease characterized by the presence of airflow obstruction due to chronic bronchitis and emphysema, two diseases that often coexist.

Clean Air Act The primary federal law in the United States governing air pollution.

Clean Water Act The primary federal law in the United States governing water pollution.

Clinical trial At its best, a study of the effect of some treatment on two (or more) comparable, randomly selected groups (e.g., an experimental group that is treated and another group that is untreated and considered a control group).

Cohort study A study of a group of people, or cohort, followed over time to see how some disease or diseases develop.

Common-source outbreak A disease outbreak that was acquired by infected individuals from a common or single source.

Communicable disease Infectious disease that spreads directly from one person to another.

Community A specific group of people, often living in a defined geographical area, who share a common culture, values, and norms and are arranged in a social structure according to relationships the community has developed over a period of time.

Community factor Risk factors common to many disorders related to communities such as living in an area with a high rate of disorganization and inadequate schools.

Community health centers Private, nonprofit organizations that directly or indirectly (through contracts and cooperative agreements) provide primary health services and related services to residents of a defined geographic area that is medically underserved.

Comprehensive Environmental Response, Compensation, and Liability Act (CERCLA), also known as the **Superfund program** A United States federal law designed to cleanup sites contaminated with hazardous substances and pollutants.

Concentrated Animal Feeding Operation (CAFO) Also called factory farms, CAFOs crowd thousands of hogs, cattle, and poultry into confined spaces, where they produce large quantities of waste. A major source of air and water pollution.

Confidence interval A range of values so defined that there is a specified probability that the value of a parameter lies within it.

Conflict of interest A situation in which the concerns or aims of two different parties are incompatible.

Confounding variable A factor or explanation other than the one being studied that may affect a result or conclusion.

Congenital Present at birth.

Congenital anomalies An often-inherited medical condition that occurs at or before birth.

Consumer-directed health plans An approach to controlling medical costs that is popular among political conservatives and was encouraged during the George W. Bush administration. The intent of these plans is to make consumers more cost-conscious when they seek medical care by providing them with information on cost and quality and requiring them to share more of the cost.

Consumer Product Safety Commission (CPSC) An independent agency of the United States government. It was created in 1972 through the Consumer Product Safety Act.

Consumer Product Safety Improvement Act (CPSIA) A United States law signed on August 14, 2008 by President George W. Bush. The legislative bill imposes new requirements on manufacturers of apparel, shoes, personal care products, accessories and jewelry, home furnishings, bedding, toys, electronics and video games, books, school supplies, educational materials and science kits.

Contact tracing Locating individuals who have had contact with an infected person as part of an effort to limit the spread of an infectious disease. Contacts that have been identified through contact tracing can then be monitored, tested, isolated, or handled in other ways.

Contraception (birth control) The means of pregnancy prevention. Methods include permanent methods (i.e., male and female sterilization) and temporary methods (i.e., barrier, hormonal, and behavioral).

Control group (controls) A group of individuals used by an experimenter as a standard for comparison—to see the effect of changing one or more variables in an experimental (or treatment) group.

Controls In a case-control study, controls, are healthy individuals who do not have the disease being studied.

Copayment A modest fixed fee for each medical visit, charged to patients who have health insurance. The remainder of the bill is paid by the health insurance company or the managed care organization.

Core functions of public health Three basic tasks performed by public health agencies to ensure conditions in which people can be healthy. As defined by *The Future of Public Health*, these tasks are assessment, policy development, and assurance.

Correlation The extent to which two or more variables are related—for example, the extent to which one variable changes in response to a change in another.

Cost-benefit analysis An economic analysis in which all costs and benefits are converted into monetary values and results are expressed as dollars of benefit per dollar expended.

Cost-effectiveness analysis An economic analysis assessed as health outcome per cost expended.

Criteria Air Pollutants Six common air pollutants known to be harmful to health and the environment: particulates, sulfur dioxide, carbon monoxide, nitrogen oxides, ozone, and lead.

Crude rate The actual rate of events (births, deaths, cases of a disease or injury, etc.) in a population, without adjustment.

D

Deductible A specified amount of money that an insured person must pay before the insurance company will pay a claim.

Dementia A group of thinking and social symptoms that interferes with daily functioning. Alzheimer's disease is the most common cause of dementia.

Department of Homeland Security A cabinet department of the United States federal government, created in response to the September 11 attacks, and with the primary responsibilities of protecting the territory of the United States and protectorates from and responding to terrorist attacks, man-made accidents, and natural disasters.

Department of Veterans Affairs (VA) The second-largest cabinet department, the VA coordinates the distribution of benefits for veterans of the American armed forces and their dependents. The benefits include compensation for disabilities, the management of veterans' hospitals, and various insurance programs.

Determinants Any of a group of variables, such as specific disease agents and environmental factors, that directly or indirectly influence the frequency or distribution of a disease.

Developmental disabilities A broad spectrum of impairments characterized by developmental delay and/or limitation in personal activity, such as mental retardation, cerebral palsy, epilepsy, hearing and other communication disorders, and vision impairment.

Diabetes A chronic disease due to insulin deficiency and/or resistance to insulin action that is associated with high levels of sugar in the blood. Over time, unless properly treated, organ complications related to diabetes develop, including heart, nerve, foot, eye, and kidney damage and problems with pregnancy.

Dietary Guidelines for Americans Guidelines that offer nutritional advice for Americans. The Guidelines are published every 5 years by the U.S. Department of Agriculture, together with the U.S. Department of Health and Human Services.

Dietary Supplement Health and Education Act A 1994 statute of U.S. Federal legislation which defines and regulates dietary supplements.

Directly observed therapy (DOT) A program in which a trained healthcare worker or other designated individual provides the prescribed medications and watches the patient swallow every dose.

Disability Reduction of a person's capacity to function in society.

Disability-adjusted life years A measure of the overall burden of a disease that captures the number of years of life afflicted by poor health or disability, or lost to premature death.

Disturbances of mood Characteristically manifest themselves as a sustained feeling of sadness or hopelessness (major depression) or extreme fluctuations of mood (bipolar disorder). Mood disturbances are also associated with symptoms such as disturbances in appetite, sleep patterns, energy level, concentration, and memory.

Dose–response relationship The relationship between the dose of some agent, or the extent of some exposure, and a physiological response. A dose–response effect means that the effect increases with the dose.

Double-blind Both the patient and the doctor are blind as to whether the patient is receiving a drug or a placebo in a clinical trial.

E

Eating disorders Any range of psychological disorders characterized by abnormal or disturbed eating habits (such as anorexia nervosa).

Ebola A deadly disease with occasional outbreaks that occur primarily on the African continent.

E-cigarettes Handheld battery-powered vaporizer that simulates smoking and provides some of the behavioral aspects of smoking, including the hand-to-mouth action of smoking, but without burning tobacco.

Ecological model of health behavior A way of considering individual behavior in the context of the social environment, including influences at the interpersonal, organizational, community, and public policy levels. The ecological model is useful in designing interventions to promote healthy behavior; the most effective programs intervene at several levels of influence.

Economic impact Total costs and benefits that a particular event or situation can have on the overall.

Effectiveness The improvement in health outcome that a strategy can produce in typical community-based settings. Also, the degree to which objectives are achieved.

Emergency Planning and Community Right-to-Know Act (EPCRA) A U.S. federal law passed by Congress in response to concerns regarding the environmental and safety hazards posed by the storage and handling of toxic chemicals.

Emerging infectious diseases Infectious diseases in which the incidence in humans has increased within the past few decades or threatens to increase in the near future. Emerging diseases may be caused by microorganisms previously unknown to be human pathogens, foodborne pathogens not expected to occur in particular foods, or pathogens that are dramatically increasing in prevalence.

Emissions standards The legal requirements governing air pollutants released into the atmosphere. Emission standards set quantitative limits on the permissible amount of specific air pollutants that may be released from specific sources over specific timeframes.

Endemic rate The usual prevalence of a disease within a given geographic area.

Environmental health Those aspects of human health, diseases, and injury that are determined or influenced by factors in the environment. This includes the study of the direct pathological effects of various chemical, physical, and biological agents as well as the effects on health of the broad physical and social environment, which includes housing, urban development, land use and transportation, industry, and agriculture.

Environmental Protection Agency (EPA) The federal agency responsible for prevention and cleanup of water pollution and air pollution, control of toxic substances, and other issues of environmental contamination.

Epidemic The occurrence in a community or geographic area of a disease at a rate that clearly exceeds the normally expected rate.

Epidemic curve A plot of time trends in the occurrence of a disease or other health- related event for a defined population and time period.

Epidemic investigation A set of procedures used to identify the cause, i.e. the infectious agent, responsible for a disease.

Epidemiologic surveillance The ongoing and systematic collection, analysis, and interpretation of health data essential to the planning, implementation, and evaluation of public health practice, closely integrated with the timely dissemination of these data to those who need to know. The final link in the surveillance chain is the application of these data to prevention and control.

Epidemiology The study of populations to seek the causes of health and disease; the study of the distribution and determinants of disease frequency in human populations.

Experimental group The treated group in a study, in contrast to an untreated or more conventionally treated control group.

Extensively drug-resistant tuberculosis (XDR-TB) A form of tuberculosis caused by bacteria that are resistant to some of the most effective anti-TB drugs.

F

Factory farms *See* Concentrated Animal Feeding Operation (CAFO).

False negative A mistaken identification of persons as healthy or unaffected when, in fact, they have the disease or condition being tested for.

False positive A mistaken identification of persons as affected by some disease or condition when, in fact, they are unaffected by the disease or condition being tested for.

Family factor Risk factors common to many disorders related to family issues such as severe marital discord, social disadvantage, overcrowding or large family size, paternal criminality, maternal mental disorder, and admission into foster care.

Family planning The process of establishing the preferred number and spacing of one's children, selecting the means by which this plan is best achieved, and effectively using that means.

Federal Emergency Management Agency (FEMA) An agency of the United States Department of Homeland Security. The agency's primary purpose is to coordinate the response to a disaster that has occurred in the United States and that overwhelms the resources of local and state authorities.

Federal role in public health The fundamental purposes of government to provide general welfare.

Fee-for-service In contrast with managed care, a method of paying for medical care in which each visit to a doctor or hospital and each procedure is billed and paid for separately.

Fertility rate Number of live births in a year per 1000 women ages 15 to 44.

Food and Drug Administration (FDA) The federal agency that ensures the safety and nutritional value of the food supply; evaluates all new drugs, food additives, and colorings; and regulates medical devices, vaccines, diagnostic tests, animal drugs, and cosmetics.

Foodborne disease A disease caused by consuming contaminated food or drink.

FoodNet An active surveillance system, meaning that public health officials routinely communicate with more than 650 clinical laboratories serving the surveillance area to identify new cases and conduct periodic audits to ensure that all cases are reported.

Framingham Study A long-term, ongoing cardiovascular cohort study of residents of the city of Framingham, Massachusetts.

G

Gene A unit of hereditary information passed from parents to offspring; the totality of genetic information, contained in DNA (except for some viruses that use RNA), determines the way the offspring develops.

Genetic diseases A disease caused by an abnormality in an individual's genome.

Genetic disorders The group of health conditions that result from genes passed to the embryo from the parents.

Genomics The branch of molecular biology concerned with the structure, function, evolution, and mapping of genomes.

Global warming A gradual increase in the overall temperature of the earth's atmosphere generally attributed to the greenhouse effect caused by increased levels of carbon dioxide, chlorofluorocarbons, and other pollutants.

Greenhouse gas A gas that absorbs radiation of specific wavelengths within the infrared spectrum of radiation emitted by the earth's surface and clouds. The effect is a local trapping of part of the absorbed energy and a tendency to warm the earth's surface. Water vapor, carbon dioxide, nitrous oxide, methane, and ozone are the primary greenhouse gases in the earth's atmosphere.

Gross domestic product (GDP) The market value of the goods and services produced by labor and property located in a country.

H

Hazard analysis critical control points (HACCP) A systematic preventive approach to food safety from biological, chemical, and physical hazards in production processes that can cause the finished product to be unsafe, and designs measurements to reduce these risks to a safe level.

Health As defined by the World Health Organization, a state of physical, mental, and social well-being and not merely the absence of disease and infirmity.

Health Belief Model (HBM) A psychological model that attempts to explain and predict health behaviors.

Health education Instruction that promotes healthy behaviors by informing and educating individuals through the use of materials and structured activities.

Health insurance A type of insurance coverage that pays for medical, surgical, and sometimes dental expenses incurred by the insured.

Health Insurance Portability and Accountability Act (HIPAA) Enacted by the United States Congress and signed by President Bill Clinton in 1996. Title I of HIPAA protects health insurance coverage for workers and their families when they change or lose their jobs. Title II of HIPAA, known as the Administrative Simplification (AS) provisions, requires the establishment of national standards for electronic healthcare transactions and national identifiers for providers, health insurance plans, and employers.

Health maintenance organization (HMO) An organization that manages both the financing and provision of health services to enrolled members.

Health outcomes Results of healthcare interventions.

Health promotion Any planned combination of educational, political, regulatory, and organizational supports for actions and conditions of living conducive to the health of individuals, groups, or communities.

Health savings account A savings account used in conjunction with a high-deductible health insurance policy that allows users to save money tax-free against medical expenses abbreviation HSA.

Health services research The study of the effectiveness, efficiency, and equity of the healthcare system.

Health status indicators Measurements of the state of health of a specified individual, group, or population. Health status may be measured by proxies such as people's subjective assessments of their health; by one or more indicators of mortality and morbidity in the population, such as longevity or maternal and infant mortality; or by the incidence or prevalence of major diseases (communicable, chronic, or nutritional).

Healthcare reform A general rubric used for discussing major health policy creation or changes—for the most part, governmental policy that affects healthcare delivery in a given place.

Healthy People 2020 The fourth generation of an initiative with 10-year targets designed to guide national health promotion and disease prevention efforts to improve the health of all people in the United States.

Herd immunity Protection of individuals who lack immunity to a disease that is provided when a significant majority of the population has been immunized against that disease, either by vaccination or by acquisition of immunity by infection.

Highly active antiretroviral therapy (HAART) Medications used to treat HIV infection.

Hospice A home providing care for the sick, especially the terminally ill.

Human Genome Project An international scientific research project that was set up with the goal of determining the sequence of chemical base pairs which make up human DNA, and of identifying and mapping all of the genes of the human genome from both a physical and functional standpoint.

Human immunodeficiency virus (HIV) The virus that causes acquired immunodeficiency syndrome (AIDS).

Hypertension Abnormally high blood pressure.

I

Immune system The body's natural defense system, which works to eliminate pathogens.

Immunization Stimulating immunity to an infectious disease by exposing an individual to a weakened or inactivated pathogen or a portion of the pathogen.

Incidence A measure of the number of new cases occurring in a population within a given amount of time, usually a year.

Incident Command System (ICS) A standardized approach to the command, control, and coordination of emergency response providing a common hierarchy within which responders from multiple agencies can be effective.

Incubation period The time between infection of an individual by a pathogen and the manifestation of the disease it causes.

Individual factor Risk factors common to many disorders related to individual factors including neurophysiological deficits, difficult temperament, chronic physical illness, and below-average intelligence.

Individual liberty The liberty of an individual to exercise freely those rights generally accepted as being outside of governmental control.

Infant mortality Number of live-born infants who die before their first birthday per 1000 live births.

Infectious disease Disease caused by a microorganism (such as bacteria, protozoans, fungi, or viruses) that enters the body and grows and multiplies there.

Influenza An infectious disease caused by a virus that mutates frequently, causing new strains to spread around the world regularly. Vaccines are effective but must be changed each year.

Injection drug use The use of a needle and syringe to inject illicit drugs (e.g., heroin). This practice places the user at great risk for contracting the human immunodeficiency virus (HIV).

Injury Damage to the body resulting from acute exposure to thermal, mechanical, electrical, or chemical energy or from the absence of such essentials as heat or oxygen. Injury may be intentional, as in the case of suicide, or unintentional, as in the case of accidental drug overdose.

Institutional review board A committee usually comprised of researchers and members of the community that evaluate whether a study's benefits outweight its risks and ensure that the study's subjects are given an opportunity for informed consent.

Insurance exchanges Organizations that facilitate structured and competitive markets for purchasing health coverage.

Intergovernmental Panel on Climate Change (IPCC) The leading international body for the assessment of climate change.

Intentional injury *See* injury.

Intervention A generic term used in public health to describe a program or policy designed to have an impact on a health problem.

Intervention study An epidemiologic study in which the impact of some intervention on one group of subjects is compared with the effect of a placebo or conventional therapy on a control group; for example, a clinical trial.

L

Lead-time bias Occurs when increased survival time after diagnosis is counted as an indicator of success.

Libertarianism A belief system that holds that an individual's rights can only be restricted in order to prevent harm to others.

Life expectancy The number of additional years of life expected at a specified point in time, such as at birth or at age 65.

Local public health agencies Government agencies in the United States on the front lines of public health.

Low birth weight (LBW) Weight at birth of less than 2500 grams. *Very low birth weight* means a weight at birth of less than 1500 grams.

M

Major depressive disorder A combination of symptoms that interfere with a person's ability to work, sleep, study, eat, and enjoy once-pleasurable activities.

Malpractice Improper, illegal, or negligent professional activity or treatment, especially by a medical practitioner, lawyer, or public official.

Mammogram An x-ray of the breast. Mammograms screen for breast cancer.

Managed care A system of administrative controls intended to reduce costs through managing the utilization of health services.

Managed care organization (MCO) An organization that combines the functions of health insurance, delivery of care, and administration.

Maternal death Death of a woman while pregnant or within 42 days of the end of pregnancy from any cause related to or aggravated by the pregnancy or its management, but not from accidental or incidental causes.

Maternal mortality rate The number of registered maternal deaths due to birth- or pregnancy-related complications per 100,000 registered live births.

Medicaid A federally aided, state-operated and state-administered program that provides medical services to eligible low-income populations.

Medicare A national health insurance program for persons over age 65 and certain younger persons who are disabled.

Menthol cigarettes A cigarette flavored with the compound menthol.

Method of transmission The route or method of transfer by which the infectious microorganism moves or is carried from one place to another to.

Minamata Village in southern Japan made famous by the poisoning of its population in the 1950s by mercury released into the bay by a plastics factory. Most severely affected were children born with severe brain damage to mothers who had been exposed while pregnant.

Model State Emergency Health Powers Act A draft of model legislation to increase state powers to respond to bioterrorism or other outbreaks of disease that the Centers for Disease Control and others want the states to pass into law.

Moralism When certain acts or policies are promoted or discouraged based on the person's moral beliefs (e.g., opposition to a condom-distribution public health program because of moral opposition to certain types of sexual activity).

Morbidity The term often used to mean illness or disease.

Morbidity and Mortality Weekly Report (MMWR) A weekly publication issued by the Centers for Disease Control and Prevention (CDC) which is widely distributed in print and electronically via the Internet. MMWR reports on timely public health topics that the CDC deals with, such as outbreaks of infectious diseases and new environmental and behavioral health hazards.

Mortality rate The incidence of deaths per unit of time, most often per year, in a population.

Multidrug resistance (MDR) Antimicrobial resistance shown by a species of microorganism to multiple antimicrobial drugs.

Municipal solid waste Commonly known as trash or garbage in the United States and as refuse or rubbish in Britain, a waste type consisting of everyday items that are discarded by the public.

Mutation The changing of the structure of a gene, resulting in a variant form that may be transmitted to subsequent generations, caused by the alteration of single base units in DNA, or the deletion, insertion, or rearrangement of larger sections of genes or chromosomes.

N

National Center for Health Statistics (NCHS) A principal agency of the U.S. Federal Statistical System which provides statistical information to guide actions and policies to improve the health of the American people.

National Committee for Quality Assurance (NCQA) An independent 501(c)(3) nonprofit organization in the United States that works to improve healthcare quality through the administration of evidence-based standards, measures, programs, and accreditation.

National Comorbidity Survey (NCS) The first large-scale field survey of mental health in the United States.

National Health and Nutrition Examination Survey (NHANES) A survey research program conducted by the National Center for Health Statistics (NCHS) to assess the health and nutritional status of adults and children in the United States, and to track changes over time.

National Highway Traffic Safety Administration (NHTSA) An agency of the Executive Branch of the U.S. government, part of the Department of Transportation. It describes its mission as "Save lives, prevent injuries, reduce vehicle-related crashes."

National Incident Management System (NIMS) A standardized approach to incident management developed by the Department of Homeland Security.

National Institute for Occupational Safety and Health (NIOSH) A U.S. Federal agency responsible for conducting research and making recommendations for the prevention of work-related disease and injury.

National Institutes of Health (NIH) The primary federal agency for biomedical research. The NIH has its own laboratories and also provides funding to biomedical scientists at universities and research centers.

National Survey on Drug Use and Health (NSDUH) An annual nationwide survey on the use of legal and illegal drugs, as well as mental disorders, that has been conducted by the United States federal government since 1971.

Newborn screening A public health program designed to screen infants shortly after birth for a list of conditions that are treatable, but not clinically evident in the newborn period.

Nongovernmental organization (NGO) An organization that is neither a part of a government nor a conventional for-profit business.

Nonpoint-source pollution Water and air pollution from diffuse sources. Nonpoint-source water pollution affects a water body from sources such as polluted runoff from agricultural areas draining into a river, or wind-borne debris blowing out to sea.

Notifiable disease A disease that the law requires to be reported to public health authorities as part of the public health surveillance system.

O

Obesity The condition of being grossly fat or overweight. A person is considered "obese" if their body mass index (BMI) is between 30.0 and 39.9.

Occupational Safety and Health Act A law passed by Congress in 1970 that established the Occupational Safety and Health Administration (OSHA) within the Department of Labor. OSHA was authorized, among other things, to set standards regulating employees' exposure to hazardous substances.

Occupational Safety and Health Administration (OSHA) The federal agency, part of the U.S. Department of Labor, responsible for occupational health and the prevention of occupational injury.

Odds ratio A measure of the strength of an association between an exposure and a disease. The numerator of the odds ratio is the ratio of exposed subjects to nonexposed subjects in the case group; the denominator is the ratio of exposed subjects to nonexposed subjects in the control group.

Office of Emergency Management (OEM) An agency at the local, state or national level that holds responsibility of comprehensively planning for and responding to all manner of disasters, whether man-made or natural.

Opportunistic infections Infections that take advantage of the opportunity offered when a person's immune system has been weakened by the human immunodeficiency virus (HIV). At least 25 medical conditions, including cancers and bacterial, fungal, and viral infections, are associated with HIV infection.

Osteoporosis Reduction of bone mass and a deterioration of the microarchitecture of the bone leading to bone fragility.

Outbreak A sudden increase in the incidence of a disease.

Outcomes research The epidemiologic study of medical care.

Overdiagnosis bias The diagnosis of "disease" that will never cause symptoms or death during a patient's ordinarily expected lifetime.

Overweight Above a weight considered normal or desirable. A person is considered overweight if their body mass index (BMI) is between 25.0 and 29.9.

Ozone layer A layer in the earth's stratosphere at an altitude of about 6.2 miles (10 km) containing a high concentration of ozone, which absorbs most of the ultraviolet radiation reaching the earth from the sun.

P

p value The probability that an observed result or effect could have occurred by chance if there had actually been no real effect.

Pandemic An outbreak of a disease that occurs over a wide geographic area and affects an exceptionally high proportion of the population.

Pap test Microscopic examination of cells collected from the cervix. The Pap test is used to detect changes that may be cancer and can show noncancerous conditions, such as infection or inflammation.

Parasite An organism that lives off another organism (called a host) but does not contribute to the welfare of the host.

Parts per million (ppm) A measure of very low concentrations of pollutants in air, water, or soil (e.g., 1 ppm of an air pollutant is one particle of the pollutant for every million molecules of air). *Parts per billion (ppb)* is similarly used for even smaller concentrations of pollutants.

Passive smoking The involuntary inhaling of second-hand smoke from other people's cigarettes, cigars, or pipes.

Paternalism Restriction of people's individual freedom with the aim of protecting their health and safety.

Pathogen A microorganism that causes illness.

Patient Protection and Affordable Care Act Often called "Obamacare." A law passed in 2010 and fully implemented by 2015 that is designed to provide health insurance to all Americans.

Placebo A supposedly ineffective pill or agent used in a control group to gauge the effect of an actual treatment in another group. Experimenters often must allow for a placebo effect, a response caused by suggestion.

Point-source pollution Water pollution that comes from a single, discrete place, typically a pipe.

Policy development One of the three core functions of public health as specified by *The Future of Public Health*. The process by which a public health agency exercises its responsibility to serve the public interest in the development of comprehensive public health policies by promoting use of scientific knowledge in decision making about public health and by leading in developing public health policy. Agencies must take a strategic approach, developed on the basis of a positive appreciation for the democratic political process.

Political interference with science Manipulating and distorting scientific evidence to fit a political agenda.

Polychlorinated biphenyls (PCBs) A group of chemicals that are common environmental pollutants.

Post-traumatic stress disorder (PTSD) An anxiety disorder that some people get after seeing or living through a dangerous event.

Power The probability that a research study will reveal the presence of an effect if, in fact, an effect exists.

Preferred Provider Organization (PPO) A type of health insurance arrangement that allows plan participants relative freedom to choose the doctors and hospitals they want to visit.

Prematurity Disorders of short gestation and low birth weight.

Prenatal care Pregnancy-related healthcare services provided to a woman between conception and delivery. The American College of Obstetricians and Gynecologists recommends at least 13 prenatal visits in a normal 9-month pregnancy: a visit each month for the first 28 weeks of pregnancy, a visit every 2 weeks until 36 weeks, and then weekly visits until birth.

Prenatal testing Testing for diseases or conditions in a fetus or embryo before it is born.

Preterm (premature) birth Birth occurring before 37 weeks of pregnancy.

Prevalence Proportion of persons in a population who have a particular disease or attribute at a specified point in time or during a specified time period.

Primary care The provision of integrated, accessible healthcare services by clinicians who are accountable for addressing a large majority of personal healthcare needs, developing a sustained partnership with patients, and practicing in the context of family and community.

Primary prevention Activities that are intended to prevent the onset of a disease or injury.

Prion An infectious agent composed entirely of protein that causes rare neurodegenerative diseases such as "mad cow" disease in cattle and Creutzfeldt–Jakob Disease in humans.

Probability A calculation of what may be expected, based on what has happened in the past under similar conditions.

Prohibition A ban on alcohol manufacture, sale, and use passed by a constitutional amendment in 1919. It was repealed 14 years later.

Propogated-source outbreak An infectious-disease outbreak that is spread from one person to another, rather than being spread from a single source to all infected individuals.

Psychosis Any severe mental disorder characterized by deterioration of normal intellectual and social functioning and by partial or complete withdrawal from reality.

Public health As defined by *The Future of Public Health*, organized community efforts to ensure conditions in which people can be healthy. Activities that society undertakes to prevent, identify, and counter threats to the health of the public.

Public health informatics The systematic application of information and computer science and technology to public health practice, research, and learning.

Public Health Information Network (PHIN) A national initiative, developed by the Centers for Disease Control and Prevention (CDC), for advancing fully capable and interoperable information systems in public health organizations.

PulseNet A network run by the Centers for Disease Control and Prevention (CDC), which brings together public health and food regulatory agency laboratories around the United States.

Q

Quality of medical/health care The degree to which health services for individuals increase the likelihood of desired health outcomes and are consistent with current professional standards.

Quarantine Isolation of a patient to prevent him or her from infecting others.

R

Radiation The emission of energy as electromagnetic waves or as moving subatomic particles, especially high-energy particles that cause ionization.

Radon gas A colorless, odorless, radioactive element in the noble gas group. It is produced by the radioactive decay of radium and occurs in minute amounts in soil, rocks, and the air near the ground.

Randomized Division of a sample into two or more comparable groups by some random method that eliminates biased selection.

Random variation The way a coin will successively turn up heads or tails if flipped in just the same way.

Rate The proportion of some disease or condition in a group usually per unit of time, with a numerator and denominator (stated or implied) indicating "so many per so many per year or other unit of time."

Rationing Allocation of goods in the face of scarcity. In medical care, rationing deliberately limits access to some services through tradeoffs between costs and benefits.

Recycling The practice of reusing items that would otherwise be discarded as waste.

Regulatory approach The management of complex systems according to a set of rules and trends.

Relative risk A comparison of two rates (e.g., a comparison of morbidity rates) using a calculation of the ratio of one to the other.

Reportable disease *See* notifiable disease.

Reservoir A place where a pathogen lives and multiplies before invading a noninfected person. Some pathogens infect only humans; some have animal reservoirs and infect humans only occasionally. Contaminated water or food may serve as a reservoir for waterborne or foodborne diseases.

Resource Conservation and Recovery Act (RCRA) The principal federal law in the United States governing the disposal of solid waste and hazardous waste.

Retrovirus A virus that uses RNA as its genetic material instead of the more usual DNA. Retroviruses have long been known to cause cancer in animals, and they were extensively studied for clues to the causes of human cancer, research that proved helpful for understanding the immunodeficiency virus when it was identified.

Risk assessment A quantitative estimate of the degree of hazard to a population presented by some agent or technology or decision. A *risk–benefit assessment* attempts to weigh possible risks against possible benefits.

Risk factor A characteristic that has been demonstrated statistically to increase a person's chance of developing a disease or being injured.

S

Safe Drinking Water Act The principal federal law in the United States intended to ensure safe drinking water for the public.

Sanitary landfill The most common method of municipal waste disposal, replacing open dumps. Requires wastes to be confined in a sealed area.

Schizophrenia A chronic, severe, and disabling brain disorder with symptoms that may include hearing voices that other people do not hear and belief that other people are reading their minds, controlling their thoughts, or plotting to harm them.

Screening Checking for a disease when there are no symptoms.

Second-hand smoke Smoke inhaled involuntarily from tobacco being smoked by others.

Secondary prevention Activities intended to minimize the risk of progression of or complications from a disease or to minimize damage from an injury.

Selection bias When the treatment and control groups of a study are sufficiently different due to the way in which the treatment or control-group subjects were selected, such that inferences about the treatment effect may be incorrect.

Self-efficacy People's sense that they are in control of their lives. High self-efficacy is beneficial to health.

Sensitive/Sensitivity The ability of a test to avoid false negatives; its ability to identify a disease or condition in those who have it.

Sexually transmitted diseases (STDs) Infections caused by bacteria or viruses that are primarily transmitted through sexual activity. Examples of bacterial STDs are syphilis, gonorrhea, and chlamydia. Viral STDs include the human immunodeficiency virus (HIV), genital herpes, and the human papilloma virus.

Shoeleather epidemiology *See* "epidemiologic investigation".

Significance *See* statistical significance.

Sin tax A tax that raises the price of a product that is harmful to oneself or others that is designed to discourage consumption of that product.

Small-area analysis A method of examining how medical practice varies across geographic areas.

Social norms approach An environmental strategy gaining ground in health campaigns. Research in the mid-1980s showed students at a small U.S. college held exaggerated beliefs about the normal frequency and consumption habits of other students with regard to alcohol. These inflated perceptions have been found in many educational institutions, with varying populations and locations. The remedy to the misperception that "everyone is doing it" is to advertise the actual norms on campus. Institutions could reduce high-risk drinking by up to 20 percent over a relatively short period of time by conducting surveys on campus and advertising the results. Although use of the social norms approach is in an early stage, its proponents believe it can be used for a variety of other issues, such as tobacco prevention, seat-belt use, and prevention of high-risk sexual activity.

Social Security A United States federal program of social insurance and benefits developed in 1935. The Social Security program's benefits include retirement income, disability income, Medicare and Medicaid, and death and survivorship benefits.

Social support Emotional and practical help provided by family and friends; social support helps people cope with stress.

Socioeconomic status (SES) A concept that includes income, education, and occupational status; a strong determinant of health.

Special Supplemental Nutrition Program for Women, Infants, and Children (WIC) A federal assistance program of the Food and Nutrition Service (FNS) of the U.S. Department of Agriculture (USDA) for healthcare and nutrition of low-income pregnant women, breastfeeding women, and infants and children under the age of five.

Specificity (Specific) The ability of a test to avoid mistaken identifications—false positives.

State health departments States have the primary constitutional responsibility and authority for the protection of the health, safety, and general welfare of the population, and much of this responsibility falls on the state health departments.

Statistical significance In an experiment or clinical trial, statistical significance means there is only a small statistical probability that the same result could have been found by chance and that the intervention had no real effect.

Statistics As a scientific discipline or method, a way of gathering and analyzing data to extract information, seek causation, and calculate probabilities.

Strategic National Stockpile The United States' national repository of antibiotics, vaccines, chemical antidotes, antitoxins, and other critical medical equipment and supplies.

Stress A psychological and emotional state of tension; "a state that occurs when persons perceive that demands exceed their ability to cope."

Stroke A loss of blood flow to part of the brain caused by a blood vessel bursting or becoming clogged by a blood clot or some other particle.

Substance abuse The problematic consumption or illicit use of alcoholic beverages, tobacco products, and drugs, including misuse of prescription drugs.

Sudden infant death syndrome (SIDS) Sudden, unexplained death of an infant from an unknown cause.

Sugar-sweetened beverage tax A tax or surcharge designed to reduce consumption of drinks with added sugar. Drinks covered under a soda tax often include carbonated soft drinks, sports drinks and energy drinks.

Superfund *See* Comprehensive Environmental Response, Compensation, and Liability Act (CERCLA).

Supplemental Nutrition Assistance Program (SNAP) Formerly known as the Food Stamp Program, SNAP provides food-purchasing assistance for low- and no-income people living in the United States.

Surgeon General The operational head of the U.S. Public Health Service Commissioned Corps (PHSCC) and thus the leading spokesperson on matters of public health in the federal government of the United States.

Surveillance *See* epidemiological surveillance.

Surveillance systems The continuous, systematic collection, analysis and interpretation of health-related data needed for the planning, implementation, and evaluation of public health practice.

Susceptible host A member of a population who is at risk of becoming infected by a disease.

T

Teratogen A substance or agent that causes birth defects.

Tertiary prevention Activities intended to minimize disability caused by a disease or injury. Rehabilitation is one tertiary prevention activity.

"Three E's" of injury prevention Insights first applied to the auto industry designed to prevent injuries. The Three E's of injury are education, enforcement, and engineering.

Toxin Antigenic poison or venom of plant or animal origin, especially one produced by or derived from microorganisms and causing disease when present at low concentration in the body.

Tragedy of the commons The overuse of a shared resource, such as a fish or timber stock, or pollution of a shared resource, such as the air or water, because each individual cares more about his or her own interests than the interests of the population as a whole.

Transtheoretical Model An integrative, biopsychosocial model to conceptualize the process of intentional behavior change.

Treatment group *See* experimental group.

U

Unintended pregnancy A general term that includes pregnancies that a woman states were either mistimed or unwanted at the time of conception (and not at the time of birth).

Unintentional injury *See* injury.

United Network of Organ Sharing (UNOS) An organization that matches available organs with waiting patients. It is a nonprofit organization under contract with the U.S. Department of Health and Human Services and it maintains a computerized network of 58 organ recovery centers in 11 geographic regions of the nation.

United States Census A national survey conducted in United States by the U.S. Census Bureau that provides data on the geographic distribution of the population, its gender, age, and ethnic characteristics, and a wide variety of social and economic characteristics.

Urbanization A population shift from rural to urban areas.

U.S. Department of Health and Human Services (HHS) Also known as the Health Department, is a cabinet-level department of the U.S. federal government with the goal of protecting the health of all Americans and providing essential human services. Its motto is "Improving the health, safety, and well-being of America".

V

Vaccination Treatment with a vaccine to produce immunity against a disease.

Variations in medical practice The variability in the use of specific treatments.

Vector An animal or insect that transmits a pathogen to a human host.

Virus A very small pathogen that is not capable of independent metabolism and can reproduce only inside living cells.

Vital statistics Systematically collected statistics on births, deaths, marriages, divorces, and other life events. More broadly, the statistics of life, health, disease, and death—the statistics that measure progress, or lack of it, against disease.

W

Waist-to-hip ratio (WHR) A health risk indicator given by a person's ratio of the waist circumference to the hip circumference: Waist circumference: measure the circumference of your waist at its smallest point, usually just above the navel.

West Nile virus A single-stranded RNA virus that causes West Nile fever.

X

X-linked disorder Disorders caused by a defective gene on the female sex chromosome, called the X chromosome. These diseases occur predominantly in males. Since females have two X chromosomes, inheritance of the defective gene has minimal impact on them because of the second, normal gene's presence.

Y

Years of potential life lost (YPLL) A measure of the impact of disease or injury in a population, YPLL is years of life lost before a specific age (usually age 75). This approach places additional value on deaths that occur at earlier ages.

Z

Zika virus A virus transmitted by mosquitoes which typically causes asymptomatic or mild infection (fever and rash) in humans. It was originally identified in Africa and later in other tropical regions.

Index

Note: Page numbers followed by *f*, *b*, or *t* indicate material in figures, boxes, or tables, respectively.

$$\frac{3x \cdot y}{3} = \frac{W}{3}$$

$$\frac{x \cdot y}{y} = \frac{W}{34}$$

$$mg \cdot (h) = \frac{E}{mg} \cdot mg$$

$$A = 5B + 11C$$
$$-11C \qquad\qquad -11C$$
$$\frac{A - 11C}{5} = \frac{5B}{5}$$

$$8x - 10y = 4$$
$$+10y \quad +10y$$
$$\frac{8x}{8} = \frac{4 + 10y}{8}$$

$$\frac{m}{9}$$

$$\frac{380}{14} = \frac{418}{x}$$

$$380x = 14(418)$$
$$380x = 5852$$

$$\frac{lb}{mg}$$

$$\frac{162}{216} = \frac{x}{220}$$

$$216x = 162(220)$$
$$216x = 35640$$
$$x = 165$$

$$\frac{mi}{mi}$$

$$\frac{10}{85} = \frac{8}{x}$$

$$10x = 8(85)$$
$$10x = 680$$
$$x = 68$$

$$8750 = 3500 + 250n$$
$$-3500 \quad -3500$$
$$\overline{}$$
$$\frac{5250}{250} = \frac{250n}{250}$$
$$21 = n$$

$$c = 3500 + 250n$$
$$= 3500 + 250(12)$$
$$= 3500 + 3000$$

$$= 107$$
$$T = 4L$$
$$L = ? \quad 22.8$$
$$G = L - 7$$

$$4L + x + L - 7 = 107$$
$$x + 5L - 7 = 107$$
$$x + 5L = 114 \quad {}^{+7}_{+7}$$

$$x = 162 - 6(18)$$
$$x = 162 - 108$$
$$x = 54$$

$$162 = 162 - 6d$$

$$108 = 162 - 6d$$
$$-162 \quad -162$$
$$\overline{}$$
$$\frac{-54}{-6} = \frac{-6d}{-6}$$
$$a = d$$

$$\cancel{\$} \quad \frac{D}{M} \quad \frac{54}{18} = \frac{162}{x}$$

$$162(18) = 54x$$
$$2916 = 54x$$

$$4L + L - 7 = 107$$
$$5L - 7 = 107$$
$$5L = 114$$

$A(t) = 256 - 16t$

$A(t) = 256 - 16t$

$A = 256 - 16(8)$

$A = 256 - 128$

$\quad = 128$

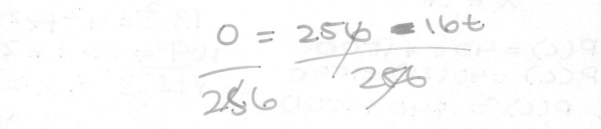
$$0 = 256 - 16t$$
$$\frac{}{256} \quad \frac{}{256}$$

$$0 = \frac{16t}{2}$$
$$\frac{}{0}$$

256 $\xrightarrow{8}$ 128 $\longrightarrow$ 0

$A(W) = 900 - 19W$

$A(W) = 900 - 19(7)$

$577 = 906 - 19W$

$A(W) = 900 - 183$

$-900 \quad -900$

$A(W) = 767$

$$\frac{-323}{19} = \frac{-19W}{-19}$$

$x \le x - 5 + 9$

$W = 17$

$13^2 = 4^2 + x^2$

$P(C) = 40c + 1500$

$169 = 16 + x^2$

$P(C) = 40(21) + 1500$

$\sqrt{153} = x^2$

$P(C) = 840 + 1500$

$P(C) = 2340$

$2780 = 40c + 1500$

28.3693

$-1500 \qquad -1500$

$$\overline{1280 = 40c}$$

$A = \pi r^2$

$C = 32$

$3.14 (3)^2$

$A = \frac{1}{2} bh$

$A = \frac{1}{2} (21) (4)$

$A = \frac{1}{2} (84)$

$C = \pi d$

$3.14 (6)$

$A = 47$

1 plan = 28/month + .14/call

2 plan = 11/month + .19/call

$28 + .14x = 24 + .19x$ 41.$\overset{25}{}$

$2800 + 14x = 2400 + 19x$

$2400 \quad -14x \quad -2400 -14x$

_____

$400 = 5x$ $6(9) - 3 \underset{=}{Z} 21$

           54 -

$\dfrac{27}{\cancel{27}}$ $6000 \times .06 \times 3$

$\left(\dfrac{27}{9} \right.$

3   90 $6v - 3 \underset{=}{Z} -21$

       90     $6(-3)(-3) \underset{=}{Z} -21$

       93     $-18(-3)$

       X

$\dfrac{}{4} = 91$